BIOCHEMICAL ASPECTS OF RENAL FUNCTION

(Proceedings of a symposium held in honour of Professor Sir Hans A. Krebs FRS, held at Merton College, Oxford, England, 16–19 September, 1979)

Guest Editors

Brian Ross and Walter G. Guder

The Organizers and Participants dedicate this volume to

Professor Sir Hans Krebs

in his 80th year
in recognition of his many contributions
to their mutual field of study

PERGAMON PRESS

OXFORD · NEW YORK · TORONTO · PARIS
FRANKFURT · SYDNEY

U.K.	Pergamon Press Ltd, Headington Hill Hall, Oxford OX3 0BW, England
U.S.A.	Pergamon Press Inc., Maxwell House, Fairview Park, Elmsford, New York 10523, U.S.A.
CANADA	Pergamon of Canada, Suite 104, 150 Consumers Road, Willowdale, Ontario M2J 1P9, Canada
AUSTRALIA	Pergamon Press (Aust.) Pty Ltd, P.O. Box 544, Potts Point N.S.W. 2011, Australia
FRANCE	Pergamon Press SARL, 24 rue des Ecoles, 75240 Paris, Cedex 05, France
FEDERAL REPUBLIC OF GERMANY	Pergamon Press GmbH, 6242 Kronberg/Tanus, Hammerweg 6, Postfach 1305, Federal Republic of Germany

ISBN 0 08 025517 5

Published as Volume 12 Number 1/2 of *The International Journal of Biochemistry* and supplied to subscribers as part of their 1980 subscription. Also available to non-subscribers.

Printed in Great Britain by A. Wheaton & Co. Ltd, Exeter

CONTENTS

Contents

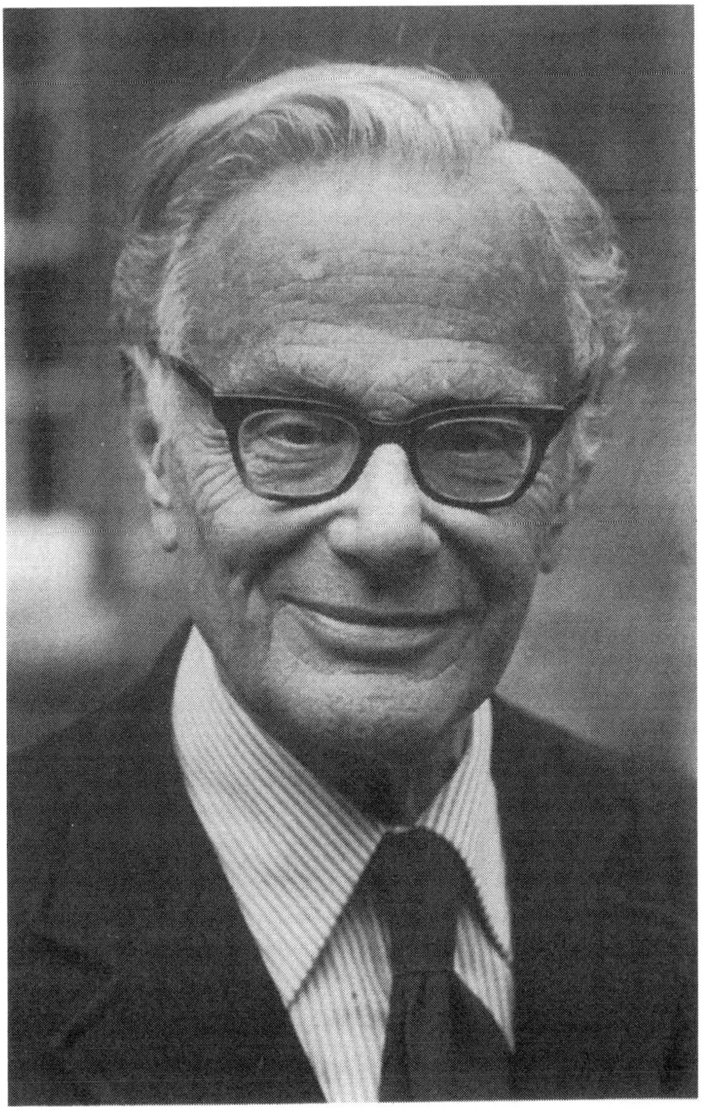

(Photograph by Anton C. Schoolwerth)

Professor Sir Hans A. Krebs FRS
Emeritus Professor of Biochemistry
University of Oxford

Int. J. Biochem. Vol. 12. pp. i to viii
Pergamon Press Ltd 1980. Printed in Great Britain

EXCERPTS FROM AN INTRODUCTORY ADDRESS BY PROFESSOR SIR HANS KREBS FRS

The organizers suggested to the first speakers of each session that before embarking on their own particular subject they should make some general introductory remarks to put the whole session into perspective. After thinking about this suggestion, I came to the conclusion that there was nothing I could say which would do that, but instead I would like to say something else, in response to a challenge which Brian Ross threw out this morning. He said that biochemistry was relevant to this symposium only in connection with renal function. I have some reservations to offer on this comment.

It is true that we are all committed to correlating biochemical events to function. In the case of the kidney—a highly specialized organ—the immediate question arising from any biochemical finding is that of the relation of that finding to urine production. The point I want to make is that it is not always immediately clear what its relevance to function may be and I would like to illustrate this with two examples from my own experience.

In 1935, I had no idea that glutamine synthesis and glutamine degradation in the kidney would be directly connected with urine production—the main function of the kidney. It was when I was systematically studying amino acid metabolism in various tissues that I came across (in a roundabout way which I cannot discuss here) the phenomenon of glutamine synthesis and glutamine degradation in guinea-pig and rabbit kidney. I saw no role for glutamine in the kidney. This did not come to light until 8 years later when van Slyke discovered that glutamine is the main precursor of urinary ammonia. This is one illustration of my point that it is not always possible immediately to relate a biochemical characteristic of the kidney to renal function. If we believe in evolution and accept one of its main principles, namely that non-functional characteristics do not survive, then we must make the assumption, as a working hypothesis, that if we find a chemical process, that process has some relationship to organ functions.

The second example concerns renal gluconeogenesis on which I did a lot of work in the early 1960s. Here again I could find no adequate explanation for the fact that, apart from the liver, the kidney is the only organ which readily synthesizes glucose from lactate, pyruvate and a number of amino acids. The answer to the question of the relationship between renal gluconeogenesis and renal function was provided by Cahill and his associates when they showed in the later 1960s that gluconeogenesis increases under conditions of acidosis. We now look upon renal gluconeogenesis as a salvage reaction for the glutamine carbon which is set free when ammonia has been provided from glutamine. The carbon skeleton that remains is not necessarily needed as a source of energy; it can be salvaged in the form of glucose, a material which can either be stored as glycogen or utilized in other tissues which depend upon carbohydrate as a source of energy.

These are my reservations in accepting the idea that we must pay attention only to those biochemical characteristics which have a bearing on functions. The postulate, of course, is valid but we must bear in mind that we cannot always detect a relationship immediately. This means we must continue to investigate any biochemical characteristic in the expectation that when we have learned more about it, it may be possible to correlate it to function.

FOREWORD AND ACKNOWLEDGEMENTS

This volume represents the collected papers and discussions delivered during the Fifth International Symposium on the Biochemical Aspects of Renal Function, held in Oxford in September, 1979. This Symposium was the successor to four previous meetings which sprang originally from an idea of Dr Max Hohenegger, of Vienna. The earlier meetings, the proceedings of which have also been published, were in Salzburg, Gdansk, Basle and Ulm, and have been highly successful in fostering the study of biochemistry underlying the specialized physiological functions of the kidney.

There is no formal structure to these meetings, which have remained largely European, so that it was somewhat random chance which brought us to Oxford. It was no chance however that the organizers were requested by the participants in the previous meeting to hold this Meeting in honour of Sir Hans Krebs, FRS. So much innovation in biochemistry is owed to this remarkable scientist that it may be forgotten that the earliest work in renal biochemistry was his too. The number of participants in this Symposium who have at some time been associated with Professor Krebs as students or colleagues speaks for his continued contribution to this field. We hope that by holding this Fifth Symposium in Professor Krebs' home city, and with his active participation to demonstrate that the study of biochemistry in relation to renal function remains in the mainstream of science. We also take great pleasure in dedicating this volume to him on the occasion of his eightieth birthday.

This Symposium was made possible by the generous financial support of the National Kidney Research Fund and of a number of other Institutions and Firms in the United Kingdom and from Abroad. They are listed below with sincere thanks for their tangible demonstration of confidence in the outcome of this Meeting. The entire proceedings took place in the confines of Merton College, Oxford and for the ancient comforts of this splendid Institution we are grateful to the Warden, the Domestic Bursar, Colonel Henderson and to Dr George Radda and the other Fellows of the College.

For the speedy preparation of Manuscripts and Discussions for publication in this special volume of the *International Journal of Biochemistry*, we are grateful to Professor Kerkut and the staff of Pergamon Press Ltd (Oxford and Exeter), and to Ms Margaret Smilgin for her expert secretarial help.

B. D. Ross and *W. G. Guder*
(Oxford and Munich)
December 1979

Names of sponsoring organizations

We are grateful for the financial support donated by the following:

Medical Research Council
Physiological Society
Royal College of Pathologists
Oxfordshire Area Health Authority
Nuffield Professor of Surgery, University of Oxford
Lilly Research Centre
Pergamon Press Ltd
Geistlich Sons Ltd
Sardstedt
Braun Melsungen
Vickers Medical
Gambro Ltd
Blackwell Scientific Publications
Boehringer Ingleheim
Merck
Novo Laboratories
Sandoz Products Ltd
Oxford University Chest
Imperial Chemical Industries Ltd
Searle Laboratories
Smith Kline and French (Philadelphia)
British Drugs Houses Ltd
Hoechst UK Ltd
Leo Laboratories Ltd

A SHORT GUIDE TO THIS VOLUME

This Symposium is the record of the papers and discussion during a 3-day meeting. It is invidious for an Editor to select from the 60 papers delivered but by doing so some of the new directions which appear in renal biochemistry are enumerated for the general reader:

1. THE KIDNEY AS A BIOCHEMICALLY HETEROGENEOUS ORGAN

(a) Cells of importance in sodium chloride transport in the thick ascending limb of Henle's loop have been isolated (Eveloff), are responsive to diuretics and have distinctive substrate requirements, which differ from those of the proximal tubule and collecting duct (see also Kurokawa).

(b) Mapping of the phosphorylated products of fructose metabolism along the nephron accords with the distribution of the different primary pathways of metabolism of this sugar. Thus ATP is depleted only in cells of the proximal straight tubule (see paper by Burch) following a fructose load.

(c) In potassium-adaptation, the induction of Na-K-ATPase is limited almost exclusively to cells of the collecting duct (Doucet).

(d) Subcellular localization (mitochondrion vs cytoplasm) of regulatory metabolites (in this case, 2-oxoglutarate) is not uniform (Guder). In kidney as in liver, whole tissue measurements of metabolite changes must, therefore, be treated with some caution.

(e) Heterogeneity of function between long and short-nephrons is established (Giebisch), adding a new complication in localizing biochemical functions in the kidney.

2. METHODOLOGY

A host of new information derives from micromethods (Introduction to Chapter 1) and permits us to think in terms of a "map" of nephron biochemistry. In addition, there are developments in tissue culture (Horster; Mahieu) and in nuclear magnetic resonance (Radda). The perfused rat kidney (Silva; Franke; Schurek; Radda) is extensively used for *in vitro* studies with whole kidney but the problems of heterogeneity have not yet been tackled in this system.

3. MORPHOLOGY

Freeze-fracture and electron microscopy give data which corresponds closely to physiology in defining the "tight-junction" of cells of Henle's loop (Abramow). The greatly improved biochemical definition of function along the nephron is matched by morphometric studies which will permit correlation between rates of transport and membrane surface, substrate concentration and organelle volume and so on for all regions of the rat kidney (Pfaller).

4. ENERGY COST OF SODIUM TRANSPORT

The simple question of how many mols of ATP are hydrolyzed per mol Na-transport has become meaningless (Deetjen; Silva) by virtue of the demonstration of tubular heterogeneity, of passive Na^+ transport and the variability of "basal" oxygen uptake. Even so, a figure of 18 Na/O_2 can be obtained *in vivo* (Kiil) which corresponds to the stoichiometry of Na-K-ATPase.

5. MECHANICS OF SODIUM TRANSPORT

At a molecular level, our understanding of the mechanism of action of the pump enzyme Na-K-ATPase in purified form is almost complete (Jorgensen; Schwartz). The enzyme retains its pump-properties when incorporated into artificial membranes (Anner).

6. FILTRATION AND REABOSRPTION

Disproportionately little time was spent on these topics. The biggest gulfs between physiology and biochemistry remain in those areas, such as glomerular filtration (Baylis) and brush-border function (Kenny), where intracellular events appear to have a rather limited influence. Prostaglandin (Sraer; Mahieu) or cGMP synthesis (Helwig) in isolated glomerulae is documented, but their role uncertain; adenosine may have a regulatory action on GFR but it is unclear how changes within tubular cells can be communicated to glomerular afferent vessels (Osswald). The localization of hydrolases (Le Hir), refined topological studies of membrane-bound enzymes (Kenny; Curthoys) and the extensive application of the method of brush-border membrane vesicles to transport of amino acids (Alleyne; Sacktor; Murer) contribute to a more complete understanding of the mechanisms of tubular transport. Very few workers still believe that the "gamma-glutamyl cycle" is responsible for amino-acid transport in the kidney!

7. METABOLIC REGULATION

The precise site of regulation of ammoniagenesis in acidosis remains unclear; a phosphate transporter (Halperin), malate transport (Brosnan), glutamine uptake (Alleyne), glutamate dehydrogenase (Tannen) and transaminase (Schoolwerth) activity are all of interest. Inter-organ relationships are important in the control of renal metabolism (Krebs; Lemieux; O Donovan). The newest field, that of lipid metabolism (Wirthensohn; Trimble; Hohenegger), still requires some reading between the lines before the conundrum "lipid as the favoured fuel of renal respiration?" has a satisfying answer.

Brian Ross
Walter Guder
Guest Editors

PROCEEDINGS OF PREVIOUS MEETINGS

(Editors and Publishers)

1. M. HOHENEGGER: *Biochemical Aspects of Kidney Function.* Goldmann, Vienna, 1972. ISBN 3 442 50025 7.

2. S. ANGIELSKI and U. C. DUBACH: *Biochemical Aspects of Renal Function.* Hans Huber Verlag, Bern, 1975. ISBN 3 456 80208 0.

3. U. SCHMIDT and U. C. DUBACH: *Renal Metabolism in Relation to Renal Function.* Hans Huber Verlag, Bern, 1976. ISBN 3 456 80304 4.

4. W. G. GUDER and U. SCHMIDT: *Biochemical Nephrology.* Hans Huber Verlag, Bern, 1978. ISBN 3 456 80627 2.

Participants

Professor M. Abramow
Laboratory of Experimental Medicine
Avenue Jean Crocq 1
1020 Bruxelles
Belgium

Professor G. Alleyne
Department of Medicine
University of the West Indies
Kingston 7
Jamaica

Dr N. McFarlane Anderson
Department of Medicine
University of the West Indies
Kingston 7
Jamaica

Professor S. Angielski
Dept of Clinical Chemistry
University Hospital
Gdansk Poland

Madame B. Anner
Ecole de Medicine
Departement de Pharmacologie
20 rue de l'Ecole-de-Medecine
Geneva
Switzerland

Dr G. Baverel
Laboratoire de Physiologie Renale et
Metabolique
Faculte de Medecine Alexis Carrel
Rue Guillaume Paradin
Lyon
France

Dr C. Baylis
Dept of Physiology
University of Manchester
Manchester
England

Dr R. Bogusky
Joslin Diabetics Foundation Inc
1 Joslin Place
Boston Massachusetts
U.S.A.

Dr J. T. Brosnan
Dept of Biochemistry
Memorial University of Newfoundland
Newfoundland
Canada

Dr H. B. Burch
The Edward Mallinckrodt Dept Pharmacology
660 South Euclid Ave
St Louis, Missouri
U.S.A.

Dr A. Booth
Dept of Biochemistry
University of Leeds
9 Hyde Terrace
Leeds
England

Dr N. P. Curthoys
Dept of Biochemistry
School of Medicine
University of Pittsburgh
Pittsburgh, Pennsylvania
U.S.A.

Professor P. Deetjen
Institut fur Physiologie und Balneologie
der Universitat Innsbruck
Fritz-Pregle Strasse 3
Innsbruck
Austria

Dr J. J. H. H. M. de Pont
Dept of Biochemistry
University of Nijmegen
Nijmegen
The Netherlands

Professor D. J. O'Donovan
Dept of Physiology
University College
Galway
Ireland

Dr A. Doucet
Laboratoire de Physiologie Cellulaire
11 Place Marcelin Berthelot
Paris
France

Professor R. Dzurik
Res Lab Exp Ther
3rd Medical Clinic
Bratislava
Czechoslovakia

Professor H. Ebel
Institut fur Klinische Physiologie
Freie Universitat Berlin
Berlin
Federal Republic of Germany

Professor F. H. Epstein
Beth Israel Hospital
330 Brookline Avenue
Boston, Massachusetts
U.S.A.

Dr J. Eveloff
Max Planck Institut fur Biophysik
Heinrich Hoffman Strasse 7
Frankfurt am Main
Federal Republic of Germany

Dr J. Falconer Smith
Dept Clinical Biochemistry
Radcliffe Infirmary
Oxford
England

Dr H. Franke
Phys. Inst. der Christian-Albrechts-University
Olshausenstrasse 40/60 C2
Kiel
Federal Republic of Germany

Dr J. Frolich
Robert Bosch Institute of
Clinical Pharmacology
Auerbachstrasse 112
7000 Stuttgart
Federal Republic of Germany

Dr G. Giebisch
Dept of Physiology
School of Medicine
Yale University
New Haven, Connecticut
U.S.A.

Dr W. G. Guder
Institut Clin Chem
Stadt. Krkh. Munchen-Schwabing
Kolner Platz 1
Munich
Federal Republic of Germany

Dr M. L. Halperin
St Michael's Hospital
Renal-Metabolic Lab
38 Shuter St Annex
Toronto
Canada

Dr J. J. Helwig
Centre de Recherches Chirurgicales Laboratoire Rene Leriche
Hospital Civil
Strasbourg
France

Professor M. Hohenegger
Institut fur allgemeine und expert Pathologie
Wahringerstrasse 13
Vienna
Austria

Dr M. Horster
Physiol Institut der Universitat Munchen
Pettenkoferstrasse 12
Munchen
Federal Republic of Germany

Dr S. Jard
Laboratoire de Physiologie Cellulaire
College de France
11 Place Marcelin Berthelot
Paris
France

Dr P. L. Jorgensen
Institute of Physiology
University of Arhus
Arhus
Denmark

Professor A. L. Katz
Section of Nephrology
University of Chicago
The Division of Biological Sciences and
Pritzker School of Medicine
950 East 59th Street
Chicago, Illinois
U.S.A.

Professor F. Kiil
Institute for Experimental Medical Research
Ulleval Hospital
Oslo
Norway

Professor R. Kinne
Max-Planck-Institut fur Biophysik
Heinrich Hoffman Strasse 7
Frankfurt am Main
Federal Republic of Germany

Dr A. J. Kenny
Dept of Biochemistry
University of Leeds
9 Hyde Terrace
Leeds
England

Dr H. Koepsell
Max-Planck- Institut fur Biophysik
Kennedy-Allee 70
Frankfurt am Main
Federal Republic of Germany

Dr Z. Kovacevic
Dept of Biochemistry
Medical Faculty
2100 Novi Sad
Yugoslavia

Professor H. A. Krebs
Nuffield Dept of Clinical Medicine
Radcliffe Infirmary
Oxford
England

Professor K. Kurokawa
UCLA School of Medicine
VA Wadsworth
Wilshire and Sawtelle Blvds
Los Angeles, California
U.S.A.

Dr J. Ledingham
University of Oxford
Oxford
England

Dr M. Le Hir
Enzyme-Biology Laboratory
Medizinische Universitats-Poliklinik
Kantonsspital Basel
Petersgraben 4
Basel
Switzerland

Professor G. Lemieux
Nephrology-Metabolism Division
Renal Laboratory
Hotel-Dieu Hospital
3840 St-Urbain Street
Montreal, Quebec
Canada

Professor Lowenstein
Boston University Medical Centre
Room 428 Evans Building
80 East Concord Street
Boston, Massachusetts
U.S.A.

Mr M. Lowry
Dept Clinical Biochemistry
Radcliffe Infirmary
Oxford
England

Dr P. Mahieu
Department de Clinique et de Semeiologie
Medicales
Institute de Medicine
Hopital Universitaire de Baviere
Liege
Belgium

Dr C. E. Mogensen
Medical Dept
Arhus Amtssygehus
Arhus
Denmark

Professor F. Morel
Laboratoire de Physiologie Cellulaire
College de France
11 Place Marcelin Berthelot
Paris
France

Dr A. Michell
Dept Physiology
Royal Veterinary College
Hatfield
England

Dr H. Murer
Max-Planck-Institut fur Biophysik
Kennedy-Allee 70
Frankfurt am Main
Federal Republic of Germany

Dr E. A. Newsholme
Dept of Biochemistry
University of Oxford
South Parks Road
Oxford
England

Professor H. Osswald
Abteilung Pharmakologie der Medizinische
Fakultat und der Rhein
Westf. Techn. Hochschule Aachen
Aachen
Federal Republic of Germany

Dr W. Pfaller
Inst. Physiologie u. Balneologie der
Universitat Innsbruck
Fritz-Pregl Strasse
Innsbruck
Austria

Dr R. Price
Dept Biochemistry
Queen Elizabeth College
Campden Hill
London

Dr G. K. Radda
Dept of Biochemistry
University of Oxford
South Parks Road
Oxford
England

Dr G. Robinson
Dept of Biochemistry
University of Oxford
Oxford
England

Dr B. D. Ross
Dept Clinical Biochemistry
Radcliffe Infirmary
Oxford
England

Dr D. Saggerson
Dept of Biochemistry
University of London
Gower Street
London
England

Dr B. Sacktor
Laboratory of Molecular Aging
Gerontology Research Centre
Baltimore City Hospital
Baltimore, Maryland
U.S.A.

Dr A. Schwartz
Dept Pharmacology
University of Cincinnati Medical Centre
Cincinnati, Ohio
U.S.A.

Dr H. J. Schurek
Dept Innere Medizin
Abt Nephrologie
Karl-Wiechert-Alle 9
D 3000 Hannover 61
Federal Republic of Germany

Dr A. C. Schoolwerth
Dept of Medicine/Renal Division
Milton Hershey Medical Center
The Pennsylvania State University
Hershey, Pennsylvania
U.S.A.

Dr S. Silbernagl
Institut fur Physiologie und Balneologie
der Universitat Innsbruck
Fritz-Pregl-Strasse 3
Innsbruck
Austria

Dr P. Silva
Dept of Medicine
Beth Israel Hospital
330 Brookline Avenue
Boston, Massachusetts
U.S.A.

Madame J. Sraer
Hopital Tenon
4 Rue de la Chine
Paris
France

Dr R. Tannen
Dept of Internal Medicine
Division of Nephrology
Medical School, University of Michigan
Ann Arbor, Michigan
U.S.A.

Dr M. E. Trimble
Veterans Administration Hospital
Irving Avenue and University Place
Syracuse, New York
U.S.A.

Dr P. Vinay
Renal Laboratory Hotel-Dieu Hospital
St Urbain
Montreal, Quebec
Canada

Dr M. W. Weiner
Dept of Medicine
Stanford University School of Medicine
Palo Alto, California
U.S.A.

Dr D. H. Williamson
MRC Oxford
Oxford
England

Dr G. Wirthensohn
Institute of Clinical Chemistry
Stadt. Krkh. Schwabing
Kolner Platz 1
Munich
Federal Republic of Germany

Chapter 1

Metabolic studies in kidney; tissue heterogeneity and compartmentation

Int. J. Biochem., Vol. 12, pp. 1 to 2
© Pergamon Press Ltd 1980. Printed in Great Britain

0020-711X/80/0701-0001$02.00/0

INTRODUCTION

Approaches to the problem of Metabolic Heterogeneity in the Kidney

W. G. Guder (Munich) and B. D. Ross (Oxford)

At the outset, we must distinguish "heterogeneite des nephrons" from "heterogeneite du nephron" that is, the differences in function between whole nephrons and between regions along a single nephron. Elegant techniques which take into account the differentiation of the mammalian nephron into its functional parts have enabled renal physiologists to construct a clear map of the intra-renal distribution of reabsorptive and secretory functions. In contrast, most of our biochemical knowledge was, until recently, unrelated to function—the experimental techniques available were either not useful for biochemical studies or were not applied to biochemical questions. Thus, the best known biochemical counterpart of tissue heterogeneity in the kidney, the division between cortical gluconeogenesis and medullary glycolysis, was recognised more than 40 yr ago. The role of gluconeogenesis in renal physiology has only recently been elucidated, while that of medullary glycolysis remains totally obscure.

The picture has changed with the advent of new techniques. The earliest studies necessarily employed rather crude histochemical methods. Specific biochemical techniques were first applied to the kidney by Lowry, and by Dubach, Mattenheimer and Bonting. Today, we are confronted by a large number of techniques which overcome the problems of kidney cell heterogeneity. They range from the direct application of microdissection, with hormone stimulation, enzyme assays or substrate determinations, to *in vivo* isotope dilution methods. In addition, biochemical information can be drawn from morphological or morphometric methods.

Some of the possible applications and limitations of individual techniques are shown below. Detailed methodology is discussed in the articles which follow.

Metabolic heterogeneity in kidney

A. Direct methods	Applications	Limitations
1. *Microdissection*		
(a) Freeze-dried tissue	Enzymes, metabolites	No metabolism, no hormone actions *in vitro*.
(b) Fresh tissue	Enzymes, metabolism, hormone actions	Limited stability, enzyme and metabolite losses
2. *Microperfusion*		
(a) *In situ*	Transport, metabolic inhibition	No metabolic fluxes Limited stability, laborious
(b) *In vitro*	Metabolism, reabsorption, enzymes, metabolites, hormone actions	
3. *Isolated kidney cell preparations*		
(a) Isolated tubules and glomerulae	Metabolism, metabolites, hormone actions	No relation to net transport
(b) Isolated cells	As above, plus ion fluxes	As above
(c) Cell culture	As above	Changes in metabolism during culture
(d) Membrane vesicles	Transport phenomena	No metabolism
4. *Cytosol-mitochondrial localization*		
(a) Digitonin fractionation	Fine analysis of sites of metabolic and hormonal regulation	No relation to transport

continued over

B. Indirect methods	Applications	Limitations
1. *In vivo* studies		
(a) Net balances	Metabolic rates	Only applicable at present for unidirectional pathways
(b) Isotope dilution	As above	Difficulties of interpretation
2. *Isolated perfused kidney*		
(a) Net balances	Metabolism in relation to transport	Limited stability, transport defects
(b) Isotope dilution	As above	As above

With the knowledge derived from microdissection and similar studies, we will be more able to interpret results which are obtained in the whole, functioning kidney. Newer techniques, such as adenyl cyclase mapping, bioluminescence and isotope dilution applied to single tubule structures, cell cultures and isolated cell preparations are likely to lead to a greater understanding of the biochemical processes relating to renal function.

Int. J. Biochem., Vol. 12, pp. 3 to 8
0020-711X/80/0701-0003$02.00/0

METHODS OF LOCALIZING TRANSPORT PROCESSES USING MICROPUNCTURE TECHNIQUES—EVIDENCE FOR NEPHRON HETEROGENEITY

GERHARD GIEBISCH
Department of Physiology, Yale University School of Medicine, 333 Cedar Street, New Haven, CT 06510, U.S.A.

Abstract—1. Available evidence based on free-flow micropuncture of cortical and juxtamedullary nephrons indicates that with respect to the transport of sodium and phosphate ions, these nephron populations show significant differences.

2. From a careful comparison of late distal with collecting tubule delivery of sodium ions during extracellular volume expansion it may be concluded that juxtamedullary nephrons deliver a larger fraction of sodium into the urine. This is abolished by renal papillary necrosis.

3. With respect to phosphate ions, studies in states of either diminished or increased urinary phosphate excretion also show marked differences between cortical and juxtamedullary nephrons.

4. Juxtamedullary nephrons contribute a larger fraction of phosphate during phosphate loading, whereas they conserve phosphate more avidly in the thyroparathyroidectomized state.

5. Potassium ions are extensively reabsorbed along the proximal tubule and Henle's loop of superficial nephrons, and it is potassium secretion along the distal tubule and the collecting ducts that contributes the largest fraction to urinary potassium excretion.

6. Recent evidence has demonstrated potassium recirculation between collecting ducts and the descending limb of Henle's loop, i.e. potassium secretion into juxtamedullary nephrons *prior* to the distal tubule.

7. It is not clear whether such potassium contributes importantly to urinary excretion, but some evidence indicated that juxtamedullary nephrons are not necessary for apparent potassium secretion downstream of the late distal tubule of cortical nephrons.

INTRODUCTION

One of the problems of inferring from experimental manipulations on superficial tubules to the behaviour of the whole kidney is the recognition that superficial (cortical) and deep (juxtamedullary) nephrons may behave differently with respect to the transport of solutes and fluid. Indeed, evidence in favor of such functional heterogeneity has been accumulating in recent years. In principal, two methods are available to study the contribution of individual tubular segments to the formation of ureteral urine. First, it is possible to puncture superficial and juxtamedullary nephrons *in vivo* and infer, from solute and inulin concentration changes at strategic points along the nephron, net transport rates of cortical and juxtamedullary nephrons. Secondly, it has become possible to isolate single nephrons and study their function *in vitro*. Clearly, this is an especially powerful method because it has access to all tubules, including those segments which cannot be punctured *in vivo* from either the cortical surface or from the surface of the exposed renal papilla.

I shall restrict my remarks to the first approach, that of studying problems of nephron heterogeneity *in vivo* by free-flow micropuncture. I shall address the problem of nephron heterogeneity as it affects the excretion of sodium chloride, phosphate and potassium ions.

SODIUM CHLORIDE

The role of medullary, i.e. juxtamedullary nephrons in the maintenance of sodium chloride balance has recently attracted considerable attention. Figure 1 summarizes the experimental approach in these and in similar studies for the study of nephron heterogeneity of sodium, phosphate and potassium transport. Most of those studies have been done in the rat kidney.

Shown are the two principal nephron types in the kidney, a superficial and a juxtamedullary nephron. The loops of Henle of superficial, cortical nephrons extend only to the junction of the inner and outer medulla while those of juxtamedullary nephrons extend to varying levels within the inner medulla (Jamison, 1974). Micropuncture is limited to the strategic points shown. Proximal tubular function can be assessed only in superficial, cortical nephrons, and only some 60–70% of the proximal tubule can be punctured. With respect to cortical nephrons, the next downstream puncture site is the early distal tubule. We have at present no direct information on the function of the loop of Henle of cortical nephrons other than that obtained by comparing late proximal with early distal tubular collections. Specifically, no inferences can be made about transport functions of the descending or ascending limbs of superficial loops. On the other hand, we can study directly the function of superficial distal tubules by early and late distal punctures. Also, by puncturing single collecting ducts at the base of the renal papilla, and by comparing these results with either late distal or final urinary excretion rates, certain functional inferences about nephron inhomogeneity are possible but, as I shall

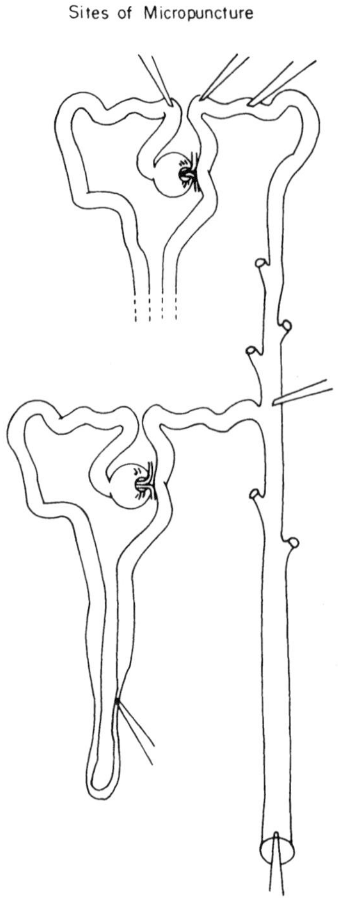

Fig. 1. Cortical and juxtamedullary nephron showing tubular sites available to puncture from either the surface or the exposed papilla. (Modified from Knox, 1977b.)

point out, these have to be done with certain limitations in mind.

With respect to juxtamedullary nephrons, most functional information *in vivo* is based on only one strategic puncture site: the tip area of Henle's loop. Hence, we can only measure delivery to the loop of Henle, mostly to long loops of Henle. At this time, we have no direct measurements that would allow us to measure transport across either the proximal or across the distal tubules of the juxtamedullary nephrons.

Evidence that deep, juxtamedullary nephrons may respond differently than their superficial, cortical counterparts to extracellular volume expansion has been obtained by Stein *et al.* (1976), Osgood *et al.* (1978), Higashimara *et al.* (1978) and by Kokko (1979).

This evidence is based upon micropuncture studies in which extracellular volume expansion was induced by 10% body weight Ringer loading and measurements of the fractional delivery of sodium to the base of the papillary collecting ducts, to the late distal tubule of superficial nephrons, and into the final urine. Relevant results are shown in Fig. 2 for chloride (Higashimara *et al.*, 1978). Very similar results have been obtained for sodium by Stein *et al.* (1976), Osgood *et al.* (1978) and by Reineck *et al.* (1979).

Inspection of Fig. 2 shows that after volume expansion there was a significant increase in the fraction of chloride remaining at the base of the collecting ducts when compared to the fraction remaining at the level of the superficial late distal tubule. Hence, the delivery of chloride (and of sodium) to the base of the papillary collecting duct exceeds that to the late distal tubule of superficial nephrons. It should be noted that such an excess of chloride delivery is absent under non-diuretic conditions. Also, it is apparent that under both experimental conditions, i.e. in the hydropenic as well as volume-expanded state, chloride reabsorption continues along the most terminal segment of the papillary collecting duct despite the very substantial increase in delivery of chloride during volume expansion as contrasted to control hydropenic conditions. These findings are in full agreement with those of Diezi *et al.* (1973) who demonstrated by puncture of single collecting ducts that net sodium chloride reabsorption continues along the most terminal papillary collecting ducts.

Clearly, an alternative explanation to the one commonly given, i.e. greater sodium chloride delivery from juxtamedullary nephrons when compared with sodium chloride delivery from superficial nephrons, would be net sodium addition, i.e. sodium secretion, between the late distal tubule and papillary base, that is along the cortical and medullary collecting tubule. Indeed, Sonnenberg *et al.* (1975) and Bengele *et al.* (1977) have suggested, on the basis of catheterization of single collecting ducts, sodium secretion into collecting ducts under conditions of extreme sodium chloride loading. The precise role of this latter mechanism has to be further explored. The hypothesis of heterogeneity of sodium chloride delivery during volume expansion has recently been greatly strengthened by the observation of Reineck *et al.* (1979) that net addition of sodium between the late distal tubule and the base of the papillary collecting duct was

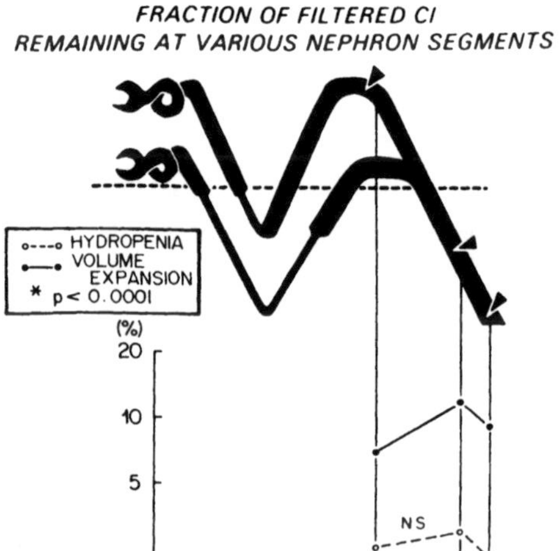

Fig. 2. Fractional excretion rates (ordinate) of chloride in cortical distal tubule and at base (BCD) and tip (TCD) of the papillary collecting duct. Experiments in hydropenia and after 10% body weight isotonic volume expansion. (From Kokko, 1979.)

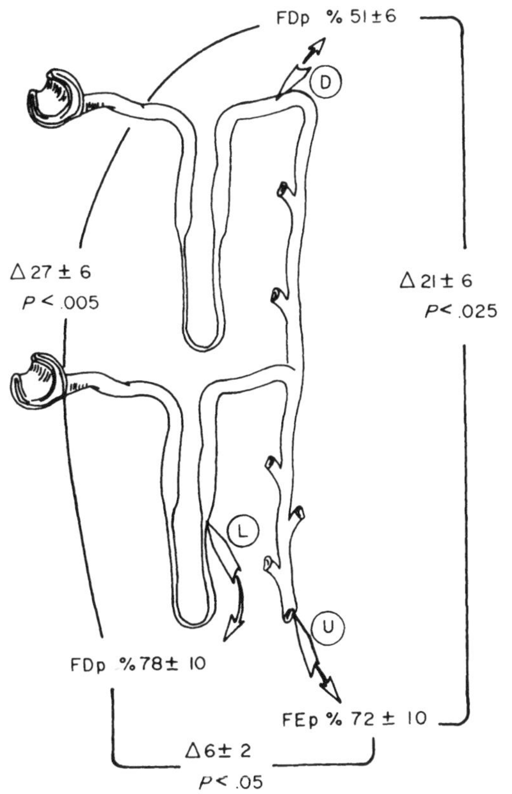

Fig. 3. Fractional phosphate delivery out of distal tubule of cortical nephron and out of loop of Henle of juxtamedullary nephron during phosphate loading. (From Knox *et al.*, 1977a.)

totally abolished by the treatment with bromoethylamine hydrobromide (BEA), an agent which causes selective papillary necrosis in the rat.

The mechanism of proportionately greater sodium delivery of juxtamedullary nephrons after extracellular volume expansion needs further study. What is not clear at present is whether intrinsic transport properties of juxtamedullary and cortical nephrons differ with respect to sodium chloride, or whether extratubular factors (medullary washout etc.) are involved.

PHOSPHATE

The notion that nephron heterogeneity of phosphate reabsorption could be of functional importance, was suggested by studies into the mechanism of apparent phosphate reabsorption and secretion along the collecting duct system. Figure 3 presents data from free-flow micropuncture studies in phosphate-loaded rats of Knox *et al.* (1977a,b). It is apparent that the fractional excretion of phosphate in the final urine (72%) was significantly greater than the fractional delivery from superficial distal tubules (51%). Importantly, the fractional delivery of phosphate to the ascending limb of Henle's loop of justamedullary nephrons was significantly greater than either to the distal tubule of cortical nephrons or to the urine.

Clearly, the difference between late distal phosphate delivery and final urinary phosphate delivery (Δ 21%) could be due either to greater phosphate delivery from deep nephrons in phosphate-loaded rats, a view held by Knox *et al.* (1977a), or, alternatively, by net phosphate secretion in the collecting duct system subsequent to extensive phosphate reabsorption in the ascending limbs of the loop of Henle of juxtamedullary nephrons. Stationary mcirupuncture studies of the ascending limbs of Henle's loop (Lang *et al.*, 1977) and microperfusion studies of the ascending limbs of Henle's loop *in vitro* (Rocha *et al.*, 1977) have shown these tubular segments not to reabsorb phosphate. Although the precise distribution of deep and superficial nephrons with respect to phosphate transport is not known, it seems more likely that greater phosphate delivery from deep nephrons in phosphate-loaded rats contributes to the sharp augmentation of phosphate excretion in the urine.

Nephron heterogeneity of phosphate reabsorption has also been suggested to play a role in animals with low phosphate excretion (Haas *et al.*, 1978). Figure 4 summarizes results from micropuncture studies in chronic thyroparathyroidectomized (TPTX) rats in which the discrepancy in fractional delivery of phosphate between superficial distal tubules and urine is augmented. It is noteworthy that the fractional delivery of phosphate at the point of micropuncture in the ascending limb of juxtamedullary nephrons is significantly lower than from distal tubules of superficial

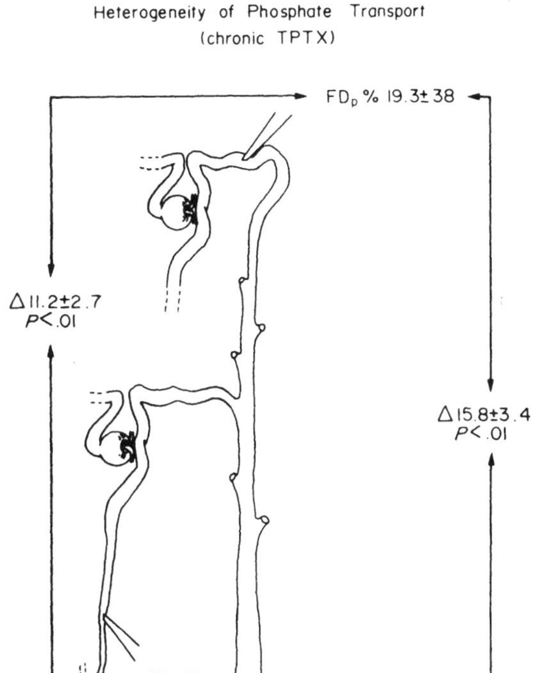

Fig. 4. Fractional phophate delivery out of distal tubule of cortical nephron and out of loop of Henle of juxtamedullary nephron after thyroparathyroidectomy. (From Knox *et al.*, 1978.)

nephrons (8.1 vs 19.3%). Again, in view of the available evidence (i.e. virtual phosphate impermeability of the ascending limb (Lang *et al.*, 1977; Rocha *et al.*, 1977), it is highly unlikely that the difference in fractional excretion rate between deep and superficial nephrons is due to phosphate secretion in the ascending limbs. Although it is likely that some additional, terminal tubule sites are involved in phosphate reabsorption (see the difference (Δ 4.5%) between the phosphate delivery to the tip of Henle's loop and that into the final urine), it is borne out by these experiments that deep nephrons reabsorb phosphate more avidly. Although quantitatively less striking, this is also the case in acute TPTX rats (Haas *et al.*, 1978) and also in animals on a normal phosphate diet. From these data, both in phosphate-loaded as well as phosphate-conserving states, it appears that the range of transport adaptation of deep nephrons exceeds that of superficial nephrons.

POTASSIUM

Studies on single mammalian nephrons have clearly shown that potassium ions are extensively reabsorbed along the proximal tubule and also along the loop of Henle of superficial nephrons. Under almost all circumstances, the extent to which the distal tubular epithelium and the collecting tubules secrete potassium determines the rate of urinary potassium excretion (Malnic *et al.*, 1966; Wright *et al.*, 1978).

Several aspects of tubular potassium transport, relevant to the problem of nephron heterogeneity, have recently been studied. Figure 5 presents a summary of what is presently known about potassium reabsorption and potassium secretion along cortical and juxtamedullary nephrons (Wright *et al.*, 1978).

Although it has been known for some time, Jamison *et al.* (1976) and Battilana *et al.* (1978) have recently carried out a number of studies indicating significant potassium secretion at tubular sites *prior* to the distal tubule. They punctured the loop of Henle of juxtamedullary nephrons and observed fractional amounts of potassium that exceeded those present at the end of the proximal convoluted tubule. This is indicative of secretion along the descending limb of Henle's loop, provided potassium reabsorption along the proximal tubule in these juxtamedullary tubules was similar to that observed in cortical nephrons. Several questions arise in conjunction with this process. Firstly, concerning the origin of this potassium moiety, it was suggested that potassium ions in the collecting duct, where their concentration is high due to both net secretion and fluid abstraction, provide a source for papillary secretion. This thesis is strongly supported by observations that the magnitude of the secretory process in Henle's loop depends on the extent to which potassium ions are secreted into the distal nephron of superficial nephrons. Amiloride and potassium deprivation lower potassium appearance in Henle's loop of juxtamedullary nephrons, whereas potassium loading has the opposite effect.

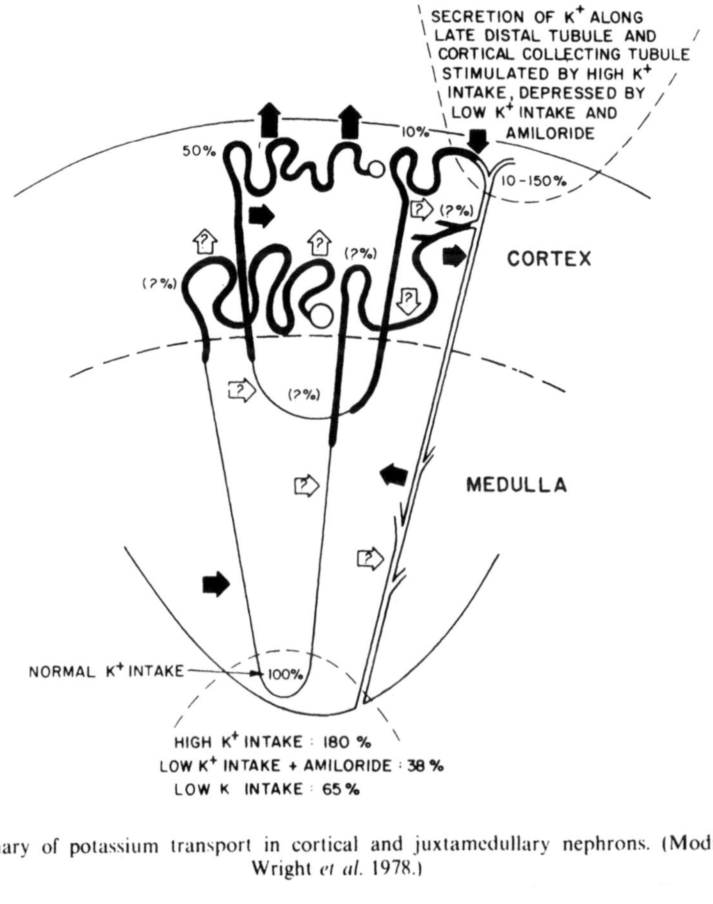

Fig. 5. Summary of potassium transport in cortical and juxtamedullary nephrons. (Modified from Wright *et al.* 1978.)

Secondly, it is of interest to inquire about the fate of the potassium ions secreted into the loop of Henle of juxtamedullary nephrons. This is, essentially, an unresolved problem in view of the fact that distal tubules of juxtamedullary nephrons cannot be punctured. Accordingly, it cannot, at present, be ascertained whether the amount of potassium appearing at the early distal tubule of these deep juxtamedullary nephrons has been reduced to a similar extent, i.e. to some 10% of the filtered load, as that of cortical nephrons. If it has (and if distal tubules of juxtamedullary nephrons were to behave similarly to those of the cortex), the delivery of potassium ions from both cortical and juxtamedullary nephrons into the collecting duct system would be similar.

Although this issue is not fully resolved, some evidence supports this latter view. Reineck *et al.* (1979) have clearly shown net addition of potassium between the late distal tubule of superficial nephrons and the papillary base of collecting ducts. This was interpreted to indicate potassium secretion along cortical collecting ducts. In contrast to sodium, experimentally induced selective papillary necrosis did not affect the increment in delivery between these sites although, as discussed above, it did abolish net addition of sodium between those sites. Hence, it is unlikely that deep juxtamedullary nephrons contribute a disproportionately larger fraction than their cortical counterparts to the potassium fraction at the base of the collecting ducts. These findings indicate that under the experimental conditions of extracellular volume expansion, the observed increment of potassium beyond the superficial distal tubule is due to potassium secretion along the cortical collecting tubule rather than disproportionately larger delivery from juxtamedullary nephrons. This functional behavior is consistent with the strong potassium secretory transport capacity of cortical collecting tubules *in vitro* (Grantham *et al.*, 1970).

REFERENCES

BATTILANA C. A., DOBYAN D. C., LACY F. B., BHATTACHARYA J., JOHNSTON P. A. & JAMISON R. L. (1978) Effect of chronic potassium loading on potassium secretion by the pars recta or descending limb of the juxtamedullary nephron in the rat. *J. clin. Invest.* **62,** 1093–1103.

BENGELE H. H., MCNAMARA E. R. & ALEXANDER E. A. (1977) Volume-expansion natriuresis: nephron function beyond the superficial late distal tubule. *Am. J. Physiol.* **232,** F566–F570.

DIEZI J., MICHOUD P., ACEVES J. & GIEBISCH G. (1973) Micropuncture study of electrolyte transport across papillary collecting duct of the rat. *Am. J. Physiol.* **224,** 623–634.

GRANTHAM J. M., BURG M. B. & ORLOFF J. (1970) The nature of transtubular Na and K transport in the isolated rabbit renal collecting tubules. *J. clin. Invest.* **49,** 1815–1826.

HAAS J. A., BERNDT T. & KNOX F. G. (1978) Nephron heterogeneity of phosphate reabsorption. *Am. J. Physiol.* **234,** F287–290.

HIGASHIMARA E., DUBOSE T. D. & KOKKO J. P. (1978) Direct examination of chloride transport across papillary collect duct of the rat. *Am. J. Physiol.* **235,** F219–F226.

JAMISON R. L. (1974) Countercurrent system. In *Kidney and Urinary Tract Physiology* (Edited by THURAU K.) pp. 199–245. University Press, Baltimore.

JAMISON R. L., LACY F. B., PENNELL J. P. & SANJANA V. B. (1976) Potassium secretion by the descending limb of pars recta of juxtamedullary nephron *in vivo. Kidney Int.* **9,** 323–330.

KNOX F. G., HAAS J. A., BERNDT T., MARCHAND G. R. & YOUNGBERG S. P. (1977a) Phosphate transport in superficial and deep nephrons in phosphate loaded rats. *Am. J. Physiol.* **233,** F150–F153.

KNOX F. G. (1977b) The intrarenal metabolism of phosphate. *Physiologist* **20,** 25–31.

KOKKO J. P. (1979) Mechanism of chloride transport across mammalian collecting duct. *Fedn Proc. Fedn Am. Socs exp. Biol.,* In press.

LANG F., GREGER R., MARCHAND G. R. & KNOX F. G. (1977) Stationary microperfusion study of phosphate reabsorption in proximal and distal nephron segments. *Pflügers Arch. ges. Physiol.* **368,** 45–48.

MALNIC G., KLOSE R. M. & GIEBISCH G. (1966) Micropuncture study of distal tubular potassium and sodium transport in rat nephron. *Am. J. Physiol.* **211,** 529–547.

OSGOOD R. W., REINECK H. J. & STEIN J. H. (1978) Further studies of segmental sodium transport in the rat during expansion of the extracellular fluid volume. *J. clin. Invest.* **62,** 311–320.

REINECK H. J., PARNA R., BARNES J. L. & OSGOOD R. W. (1979) Studies on the role of nephron heterogeneity in renal excretion of sodium and potassium in the rat. *Am. J. Physiol.* In press.

ROCHA A. S., MAGALDI J. B. & KOKKO J. P. (1977) Calcium and phosphate transport in isolated segments of rabbit Henle's loop. *J. clin. Invest.* **59,** 975–983.

STEIN J. H., OSGOOD R. W. & KUNAU R. T. (1976) Direct measurement of papillary collecting duct sodium transport in the rat. *J. clin. Invest.* **58,** 767–773.

SONNENBERG H. (1975) Secretion of salt and water into the medullary collecting duct of Ringer-infused rats. *Am. J. Physiol.* **228,** 565–568.

WRIGHT F. S. & GIEBISCH G. (1978) Renal potassium transport: contributions of individual nephron segments and populations. *Am. J. Physiol.* **235,** F515–F527.

SYMPOSIUM DISCUSSION

Horster: Dr Giebisch, you have demonstrated induction of transport activity and correlated changes in structure. Do you have any information on changes which occur in potassium depletion, or on the reversal after taking animals off the high potassium diet?

Giebisch: After 1 week, the changes of high potassium diet have disappeared. We do not have information on shorter times. The changes in K-depletion are not very striking, and it is difficult to induce net reabsorption of potassium along the superficial, distal tubule of the rat, as can be done by long lasting potassium depletion. There was a 20% reduction in peri-tubular surface area. However, in the cortical collecting tubule, Dr Stensen (in a joint effort) found striking changes in the luminal surface area after prolonged—6 week—potassium depletion. This affected only the dark cells, and involved an increase surface area, rather "bald" with some micro-villi, and in addition, there was an increase in some intracellular particulate material which was absent in the control. In a preliminary study in Amphiuma, a species which only reabsorbs potassium, we find a different change, and that is in the mitochondria which underly the lumen. This coincides with the idea that the potassium pump would be localized in the luminal membrane.

Jorgensen: How far do the changes in luminal surface area extend into the distal tubule?

Giebisch: Wherever you see light-cells, these changes can be observed, so they do extend into the late-distal tubule. Probably the discrepancies in the literature about potassium secretion in later, or earlier parts of the distal tubule arise from this point, as the light cells extend to a variable extent into the distal tubule (late distal tubule in "micro-puncture" nomenclature is the collecting tubule).

Jorgensen: Is this localization the same as that of the response to DOCA shown by Wade *et al.* (*J. Cell Biol.* **81,** 439–445, 1979)

Giebisch: Wade has only studied cortical collecting tubules. We wanted the more physiological stimulus of potassium loading, with 15-fold elevations in aldosterone.

Kiil: The most marked example of nephron heterogeneity that I know of is the old study by Trueta *et al.* (*Studies on the Renal Circulation*, Thomas, Springfield. 1947). He showed that the superficial part of the circulation could be cut off leaving the juxta-medullary circulation. These experiments probably reflect severe sympathetic stimulation. Have you looked at the effects of sympathetic stimulation on nephron heterogeneity?

Giebisch: A very good point, which we have not studied intentionally. But as every micro-puncturist knows sometimes you cannot puncture because the whole cortex is blanched, and the tubules are collapsed. If you give a little dye in this state, it may appear in the final urine. This would be an example of another type of nephron heterogeneity, in response to sympathetic stimulation.

Int. J. Biochem., Vol. 12, pp. 9 to 16
0020-711X/80/0701-0009$02.00/0

TUBULAR REABSORPTION OF L-GLUTAMINE STUDIED BY FREE-FLOW MICROPUNCTURE AND MICROPERFUSION OF RAT KIDNEY*

S. SILBERNAGL
Institut für Physiologie der Universität, A-6010 Innsbruck, Austria

Abstract—1. The free-flow concentration profile of Gln along the proximal convolution was determined by micropuncture. SNGFR was measured by [^{3}H]inulin, glutamine by ultramicro column chromatography. Reabsorption kinetics were determined by microperfusion of the proximal convolution. The equilibrium perfusion fluids contained [^{3}H]inulin and L-[^{14}C]Gln.

2. Gln-reabsorption is saturable. Kinetic constants are: J_{max} = 1.55 ($\pm$0.1 SEM) nmol·m^{-1}·sec^{-1}; K_m = 2.1 ($\pm$0.13 SEM) mmol·l^{-1}.

3. Free-flow concentration profiles predicted from these constants agree with those measured experimentally to a great extent. The endproximal steady state concentration amounts to about 20 μmol·l^{-1} at normal Gln plasma concentrations of 600 μmol·l^{-1}. The endproximal fractional reabsorption amounts to more than 96% up to 6 mmol·l^{-1} Gln plasma concentration.

4. Gln resorption from microperfusate is neither influenced by 2-oxo-glutarate, by mercaptopicolinic acid nor by acute respiratory acidosis.

5. It is concluded that Gln is reabsorbed from the proximal convolution nearly completely at normal as well as at up to 10-fold elevated Gln plasma concentrations. Acute respiratory acidosis and inhibition of cellular gluconeogenesis and mitochondrial Gln uptake does not seem to influence apparent resorption kinetics of Gln.

INTRODUCTION

Although L-glutamine plays an important role in renal ammoniagenesis and has the highest plasma concentration (0.2–0.7 mmol·l^{-1}) of all naturally occurring amino acids, the tubular reabsorption process of this amino acid has not been investigated to a great extent. Early clearance experiments (for reviews see: Lingard *et al.*, 1974; Silbernagl *et al.*, 1975; Young & Freedman, 1971) showed that tubular reabsorption of L-glutamine is quite effective: fractional reabsorption of L-glutamine in mammals ranges normally from 99.3–99.7% of the filtered load suggesting an active transport mechanism for L-glutamine reabsorption. This was confirmed by Lingard *et al.* (1973) and by Oken & Weise (1978) who showed in micropuncture experiments that reabsorption of L-glutamine from the proximal convolution occurs against a steep concentration gradient. Observations of Webber (1962) suggest that L-glutamine shares a reabsorption mechanism with alanine, leucine, phenylalanine and methionine, but not with glutamate. Finally, very recent experiments with tubular brush border vesicles (Macfarlane-Anderson & Alleyne, 1978) showed that the transport step from the tubule lumen into the cell is at least partly dependent from a sodium gradient as has been shown already for other neutral amino acids *in vivo* (Ullrich *et al.*, 1974) and *in vitro* (Ullrich, 1979).

The present study was performed in order to investigate the kinetic parameters of L-glutamine reabsorption and the *in vivo* concentration profile of L-glutamine along the lumen of the proximal convolution. In addition some preliminary experiments were carried out in order to examine a possible influence of intracellular glutamine metabolism and of acute respiratory acidosis on the apparent kinetics of L-glutamine reabsorption.

* This study was supported by grant No. 1740 of the Austrian "Fonds zur Förderung der wissenschaftlichen Forschung".

MATERIALS AND METHODS

Preparation of the experimental animals

Male Wistar rats (Ivanovas, Kißlegg, FRG) weighing 200–350 g were anesthetized with 120 mg/kg body weight (BW) Inactin (Byk-Gulden, Konstanz, FRG). The rats were fed with Altromin standard diet and had free access to food and water prior to the experiment. The animals were infused with Ringer solution at a rate of 0.15 ml·min^{-1} per kg BW during the whole experiment. In the case of the free flow experiments [^{3}H]inulin was added to the infusion fluid (0.1 Ci·l^{-1}) 10 min before the beginning of the sampling period. After a priming infusion of 0.26 ml·min^{-1} per kg BW for a period of 10 min the infusion rate was changed to 0.07 ml·min^{-1} per kg BW for the remainder of the experiment. This procedure resulted in a fairly constant [^{3}H]inulin plasma concentration (*ca.* 4·10^8 dpm·l^{-1} $\pm$ about 10%) throughout the experiment. An uretheral catheter served for sampling the urine. Blood samples were obtained from a catheter in the femoral artery.

Tubular microperfusion

Tubular microperfusion (Deetjen & Silbernagl, 1972; Sonnenberg & Deetjen, 1964) was carried out at a rate of 20 nl·min^{-1}. The equilibrium perfusion fluids of the glutamine experiments contained 200 mCi·l^{-1} [^{3}H]inulin and 40 mCi·l^{-1} L-[^{14}C]glutamine, or 40 mCi·l^{-1} [^{14}C]inulin and 200 mCi·l^{-1} L-[^{3}H]glutamine, respectively. Non-labelled L-glutamine was added to the perfusion fluids in order to adjust the L-glutamine concentration to 1.0, 10 or 50 mmol·l^{-1}, respectively.

The collected perfusion samples were analyzed for their ^{14}C- and ^{3}H-content by a scintillation counter, and some of the microperfusion samples were checked for their specific activity and their radiochemical purity by means of micro column chromatography (see below) combined with scintillation counting. Both values were found to be unchanged compared to the initial perfusion fluid. The perfusion fluid of the 2-oxoglutarate experiments contained 0.31 mmol·l^{-1} (4.6 mCi·l^{-1}), or 2.7 mmol·l^{-1} (40 mCi·l^{-1}) 2-oxo-[5-^{14}C]glutarate. The perfusion distance was measured with the Latex method. Details of the microperfusion technique as used in our laboratory have been published recently (Deetjen & Silbernagl, 1972; Völkl *et al.*, 1979).

Free-flow micropuncture samples

Free flow micropuncture samples were collected with the usual glass capillaries. The sample volume was measured in precalibrated cylindric glass capillaries under the microscope. The free flow micropuncture samples (100–400 nl) and concurrent plasma samples (200 μl) were analyzed for their [^{3}H]inulin content by a scintillation counter as well as for their glutamine content by micro column chromatography sensitive for 0.2 pmol per amino acid (Greger *et al.*, 1978; Silbernagl & Bayliss, 1980). Special care was taken to separate completely the glutamine peak from the neighboured glutamate and asparagine peaks. The distance of the puncture site from the glomerulus was measured by the Latex method (for details see Völkl *et al.*, 1979).

Materials

[^{3}H]inulin (1.7 kCi·mol^{-1}), [hydroxy-^{14}C]methyl inulin (9.9 Ci·mol^{-1}), L-[U-^{14}C]glutamine (228 Ci·mol^{-1}), L-[G-^{3}H]glutamine (20 kCi·mol^{-1}) and 2-oxo-[5-^{14}C]glutarate (14.8 Ci·mol^{-1}) were obtained from the Radiochemical Center, Amersham, England. [^{3}H]inulin (2.37 kCi·mol^{-1}) came from New England Nuclear, Dreieichenhain, FRG and unlabelled L-glutamine from Serva, Heidelberg, FRG. Mercaptopicolinate was a generous gift from Doz. Dr W. Guder, Munich. All other chemical substances were obtained from Merck, Darmstadt, FRG.

Calculations

For the evaluation of the kinetic parameters and for the prediction of the free flow profiles a computer program recently designed in our laboratory was used (Silbernagl, 1975; Völkl *et al.*, 1979). The permeability constant of the tubular wall for glutamine could not be determined directly as has been done recently for other amino acids (Silbernagl & Völkl, 1977) because neither labelled D-glutamine nor a powerful inhibitor of the high-capacity reabsorption system for glutamine is available. A permeability constant of 22.5 $\mu m^2 \cdot sec^{-1}$ was estimated indirectly: this value was obtained when the standard deviation of the mean V_{max} and K_m values was minimal. The permeability constant obtained by these indirect calculations agrees well with the values of other neutral amino acids of a comparable molecular weight (Silbernagl & Völkl, 1977). For the prediction of the free-flow profiles reasonable values of 0.58 nl·sec^{-1} for SNGFR ("1 ×" in Fig. 4F) and of 48 nl·sec^{-1}·m^{-1} ("1 ×" in Fig. 4E) for volume reabsorption were chosen (see also Discussion).

RESULTS

In the first series of experiments sections of single proximal convoluted tubules were microperfused with solutions containing labelled L-glutamine at initial concentrations ranging from 0.1 to 50 mmol·l^{-1}. As can be seen from Fig. 1 at concentrations of 0.1 and 1.0 (corresponding to the physiological plasma concentration which was 0.6 mmol·l^{-1} in our rats) unidirectional L-[^{14}C]glutamine reabsorption is essentially proportional to luminal concentration. Thus, the fractional reabsorption is nearly constant at these initial concentrations and already exceeds 95% at a perfusion distance of 2 mm. At elevated initial concentrations of 10 and 50 mmol·l^{-1} the fractional reabsorption decreases drastically to about 75 or 30%, respectively, at the same perfusion distance of 2 mm. These results clearly indicate that the reabsorption L-glutamine from the proximal convolution is saturable. Taking a small passive diffusion into account (see Calculations) the following kinetic constants of L-glutamine reabsorption were calculated from the single data of Fig. 1.

$$J_{max} = 1.55\,(\pm 0.1,\ \mathrm{SEM})\ \mathrm{nmol \cdot m^{-1} \cdot sec^{-1}}$$
$$K_m = 2.1\,(\pm 0.13,\ \mathrm{SEM})\ \mathrm{mmol \cdot l^{-1}}.$$

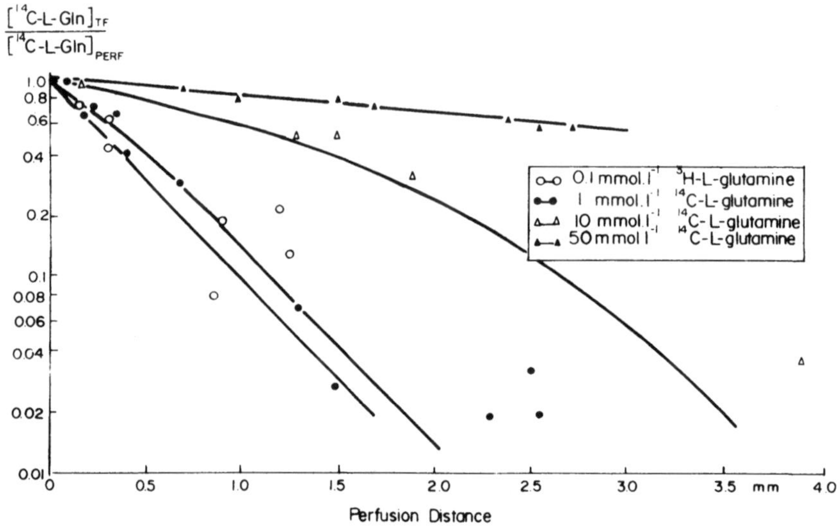

Fig. 1. Unidirectional reabsorption of L-[^{3}H] or L-[^{14}C]glutamine in the proximal convoluted tubule. For calculation of the curves see text.

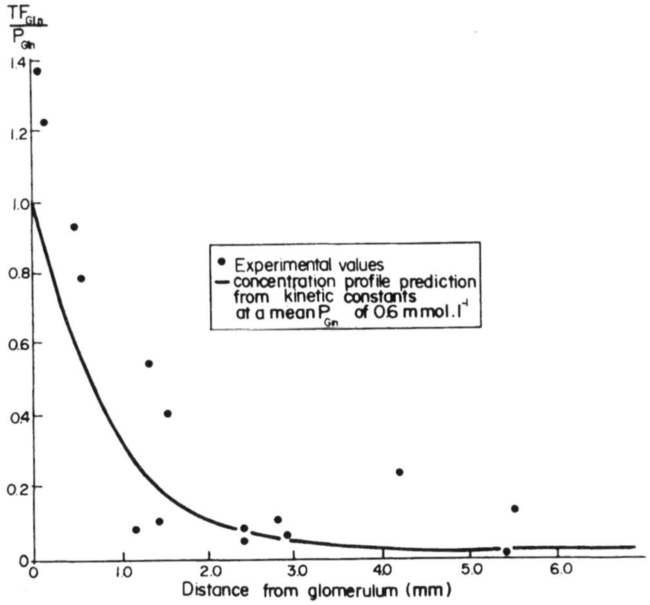

Fig. 2. TF/P glutamine along the proximal convolution. The curve is predicted from the kinetic constants determined from the data of Fig. 1. The dots are obtained by free flow micropuncture.

Using these kinetic constants concentration profiles of L-glutamine along the perfused tubule were calculated by computer (Hewlett-Packard 9100 B). The curves obtained (Fig. 1) are in good agreement with the single experimental data.

In order to predict also the free-flow concentration profile of L-glutamine along the proximal convolution, volume reabsorption, back diffusion ("leak") of L-glutamine into the lumen and the physiological plasma concentration ($0.6\,mmol\cdot l^{-1}$) had to be taken into account additionally (see calculations in Materials and Methods). We now compared the calculated curve (Fig. 2) with experimental free-flow micropuncture data obtained at different distances from the glomerulum (● in Fig. 2). Except at the very beginning of the tubule (see Discussion) the predicted curve is in good agreement with the experimental values.

Furthermore, the results of Fig. 2 indicate that TF/P glutamine decreases to about 0.1 within the first third of the length of the proximal convolution which amounted to 5–6 mm in rats used in these experiments. Along the last third of the proximal convoluted tubule the luminal L-glutamine concentration reaches a constant value of about 3% of the plasma concentration. If the experimental data were converted into percent of filtered load it turns out that about 95% of L-glutamine filtered is reabsorbed within the first third of the proximal convolution.

Some preliminary data show no significant influence of an acute respiratory acidosis (blood pH $\approx$ 7.15) on the reabsorption of L-glutamine ($10\,mmol\cdot l^{-1}$).

Further experiments were performed in order to investigate a possible influence of the intracellular glutamine metabolism on the apparent reabsorption

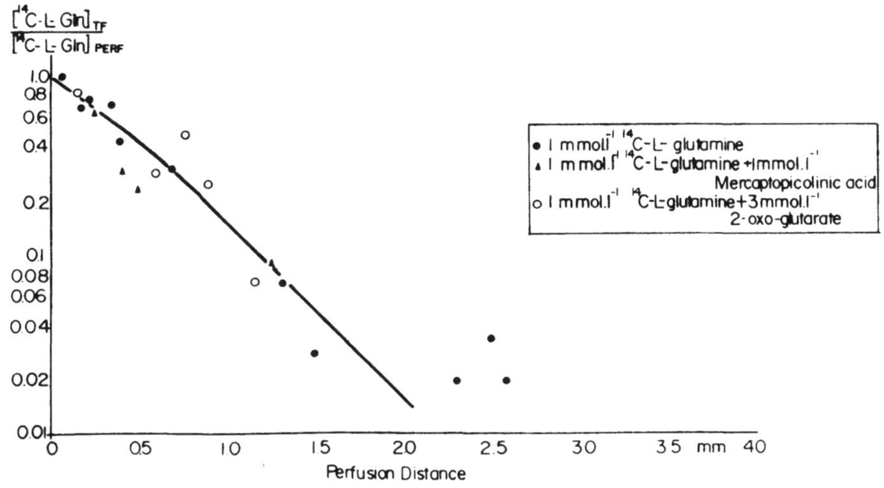

Fig. 3. Unidirectional reabsorption of L-[^{14}C]glutamine from the proximal convolution in presence and absence of mercaptopicolinate or 2-oxo-glutarate both added to the perfusion fluid.

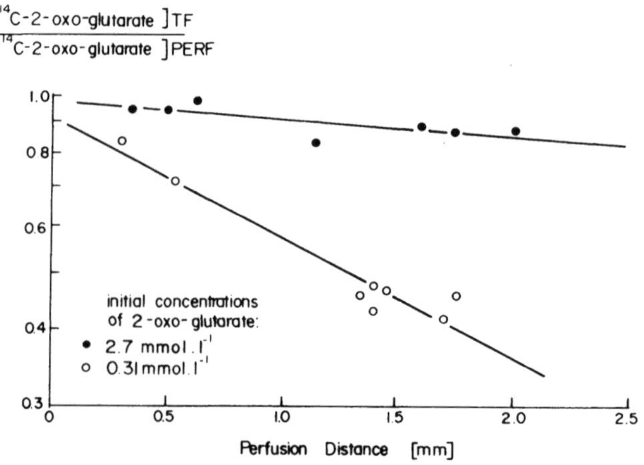

Fig. 4. Unidirectional reabsorption of [2-^{14}C]oxo-glutarate in the proximal convolution.

kinetics of L-glutamine. For this purpose mercapto-picolinate, an inhibitor of renal gluconeogenesis (Ross, 1976), and 2-oxo-glutarate, an inhibitor of glutamine uptake into the mitochondria (Goldstein, 1976), were added to the perfusion fluid. As can be seen from Fig. 3 addition of these inhibitors did not influence L-[^{14}C]glutamine reabsorption. However, these results are only conclusive if a sufficient reabsorption of the inhibitors takes place. That this is the case at least for 2-oxo-glutarate is demonstrated by microperfusion experiments with [2-^{14}C]oxo-glutarate (see Fig. 4). This compound is rapidly removed from the perfused tubule lumen by a saturable transport process (see Fig. 4*).

DISCUSSION

"Little work has been done on the nature of the system(s) transporting glutamine across the plasma membrane of renal cells". This statement by Goldstein (1976) some years ago is still justified today although meanwhile some new insights into these processes have been obtained (Burch *et al.*, 1978; Lingard *et al.*, 1973; Macfarlane-Anderson & Alleyne, 1978; Oken & Weise, 1978). It was the aim of the present study to extend our knowledge on glutamine reabsorption.

The quantitative analysis of the present microperfusion results lead to a maximum rate of tubular L-glutamine reabsorption (J_{max}) of about 1.5 nmol · $sec^{-1} \cdot m^{-1}$ at an affinity constant (K_m) of 2.1 mmol · l^{-1}. If these values are compared with those obtained for other amino acids (see Table 1), the J_{max} value is relatively high and quite similar to the J_{max} values of the reabsorption of cycloleucine, L-histidine and L-methionine. From earlier clearance data of Webber (1962), from microinfusion experiments of Bergeron & Morel (1969) and from microperfusion studies of Chan & Huang (1971) and of our laboratory (Günther & Silbernagl, 1980; Silbernagl, 1976; Silbernagl *et al.*, 1976; Völkl & Silbernagl, 1980) it can be concluded that L-alanine, L-methionine, L-phenylalanine, L-tryptophan and L-histidine share a common reabsorption mechanism with L-glutamine. The latter amino acid seems to have the highest affinity to this "high-capacity-system" for neutral amino acids.

If the luminal concentration is much smaller than the respective K_m value, the effectiveness of the reabsorptive process depends mainly on the ratio J_{max}/K_m at a given luminal concentration. In the units given above this ratio amounts to 0.71 for L-glutamine. Except for L-aspartate (ratio 2.0) this ratio is the highest of all amino acids whose reabsorption kinetics has been hitherto investigated (see Table 1).

Lingard *et al.* (1973) made the first attempt to investigate tubular glutamine reabsorption at the single tubule level. In their split-drop experiments an initial concentration of 7.1 mmol · l^{-1} decreased to about 15% at a contact time of 6 sec. In our continuous microperfusion experiments even a higher initial concentration of 10 mmol · l^{-1} decreased to the same 15% already within about 2.5 sec. This discrepancy may be caused by the different initial pH values of the test solutions pH 5.9 (Lingard *et al.*, 1973) or pH 7.4 (present study), by the presence of acetate in the test fluid (Lingard *et al.*, 1973) or by other principal differences between the two experimental techniques (unstirred layers etc.).

Using the kinetic constants obtained above and reasonable values for SNGFR and volume reabsorption (see calculations in Materials and Methods) a free-flow glutamine concentration profile along the proximal tubule can be predicted. Inserting the normal L-glutamine plasma concentration (0.6 mmol · l^{-1} in our rats) the curve in Fig. 2 is obtained. The TF/P values obtained by free flow micropuncture of the very early part of the tubule are higher than 1 and therefore do not agree very well with the predicted curve in the very beginning of the nephron.

There are several possible explanations for this discrepancy.

(1) Very early proximal micropuncture may cause artificial changes in the glomerular filtration process.
(2) The very early section of the tubule may reasorb glutamine much less rapidly than measured in

* The experiments with 0.31 mmol · l^{-1} were carried out shortly after the symposium. The results were added in proof.

Table 1. Kinetic parameters of amino acid reabsorption determined *in vivo* and *situ* by continuous microperfusion of proximal convoluted tubules of rat kidney (see also Silbernagl, 1979)

Amino acid	K_m (mmol·l^{-1})	J_{max} (nmol·m^{-1}·sec^{-1})	J_{max}/K_m (10^{-3} mm^2·sec^{-1})	Reference
Taurine	0.5	0.06	0.12	Dantzler & Silbernagl (1976)
L-Arginine	1.2	0.5	0.41	Silbernagl & Deetjen (1972)
L-Aspartate	0.1	0.13	1.3	Silbernagl (1979, 1980)
L-Glutamate	0.5	0.26	0.52	As above
Cycloleucine	5.8	2.3	0.4	Silbernagl (1975)
L-Histidine	8.5	1.4	0.16	Günther & Silbernagl (1980)
L-Methionine	6.1	2.5	0.4	Sibernagl *et al.* (1976)
L-Proline, syst. I	11.8	2.5	0.21	Völkl *et al.* (1979)
L-Proline, syst. II	0.03	0.01	0.33	As above
L-Glutamine	2.1	1.5	0.71	Present study

later parts of the proximal tubule. Water reabsorption therefore, here leads to a transient elevation of the tubular glutamine concentration above the plasma level.

(3) For the calculation of the curve a constant volume reabsorption rate per unit of length was inserted. However, it is not commonly accepted that volume reabsorption is really constant; furthermore, volume reabsorption in this early part of the nephron has never been measured. If it is much higher than in later parts of the proximal tubule, the initial concentration increase would be caused by the rapid volume removal.

(4) The curve is calculated for glutamine reabsorption in the absence of any other amino acid. The normal glomerular filtrate, however, contains all other amino acids; the majority of them inhibit glutamine reabsorption which may contribute to the initial delay in glutamine reabsorption.

Except for this discrepancy the prediction from the kinetic parameters fit quite well with the values actually measured. Such an agreement has been already shown for L-proline and L-histidine (Völkl *et al.*, 1979; Günther & Silbernagl, 1980) and lends further force to our supposition that the apparent kinetic constants calculated from microperfusion experiments are also valid for the physiological free flow situation. If this is true, glutamine concentration profiles along the proximal convolution can also be predicted when the transport parameters are varied. The results of such calculations are shown in Fig. 5.

When the plasma concentration is elevated up to about 6 mmol·l^{-1} the TF/P glutamine still reaches the equilibrium value before the end of the proximal convolution (see Fig. 5A). Because the subsequent straight part of the proximal tubule reabsorbs also amino acids (Barfuss & Schafer, 1979; Silbernagl, 1979; Silbernagl, 1980) U/P glutamine will probably not increase before the plasma concentration reaches 10 or 15 mmol·l^{-1}, a conclusion which is in full agreement with the observations of Pilkington *et al.* (1970) in dogs. It should be emphasized that we are dealing here with fractional concentrations. The absolute glutamine excretion will therefore, vary, by the same factor by which the plasma concentration is modified. However, at a fractional excretion of 0.5% it is quantitatively not important whether the absolute glutamine excretion is, for example, elevated two-fold at a doubled plasma concentration. Therefore, the doubled glutamine load will be nearly completely available for the tubule cell. This fact may be of importance for ammoniagenesis in acute acidosis where the glutamine plasma concentration is usually substantially elevated (Relman & Yablon, 1977). It should be noted, that under such conditions not only does the early proximal convolution reabsorb more glutamine but also the more the plasma concentration is elevated the more tubule cells become involved in net glutamine reabsorption. This is a direct consequence of the changed concentration profile as shown in Fig. 5A.

Figure 5B, illustrates that a varied permeability of the tubule wall almost alone influences the end proximal equilibrium TF/P glutamine. Variations by a factor of 3 of the capacity and affinity influences the concentration profile quite impressively (Fig. 5C and D). The same is true for variations by a factor of 2 of SNGFR (Fig. 5F), whereas a modified volume reabsorption rate (factor 2) results in nearly identical concentration profiles (Fig. 5E).

Some preliminary results of this study also show that acute respiratory acidosis does not increase the capacity or affinity of the reabsorption process. From the teleological point of view such an influence would not make sense anyway because, as pointed out above, the increased glutamine load in acute acidosis is completely reabsorbed under these conditions.

2-oxo-Glutarate, a potent inhibitor of mitochondrial glutamine uptake (Goldstein, 1976) does not influence the apparent kinetics of glutamine reabsorption when offered from the luminal side of the cell. It can be concluded from earlier clearance experiments (Balagura & Stone, 1967; Cohen & Wittmann, 1963) and it is demonstrated on the single tubule level by the present results (see Fig. 4) that 2-oxo-glutarate enters the tubule cell quite easily from the luminal cell side. Presuming that the intracellular 2-oxo-glutarate concentration is elevated substantially by the high amount reabsorbed we conclude that luminal reabsorption kinetics do not reflect mitochondrial uptake to a significant extent. Assuming also an efficient reabsorption of 3-mercaptopicolinate, a strong inhibitor of gluconeogenesis (Ross, 1976), it is concluded furthermore that glutamine reabsorption is not influenced by changed rates through this metabolic pathway. However, the influence of intracellular glu-

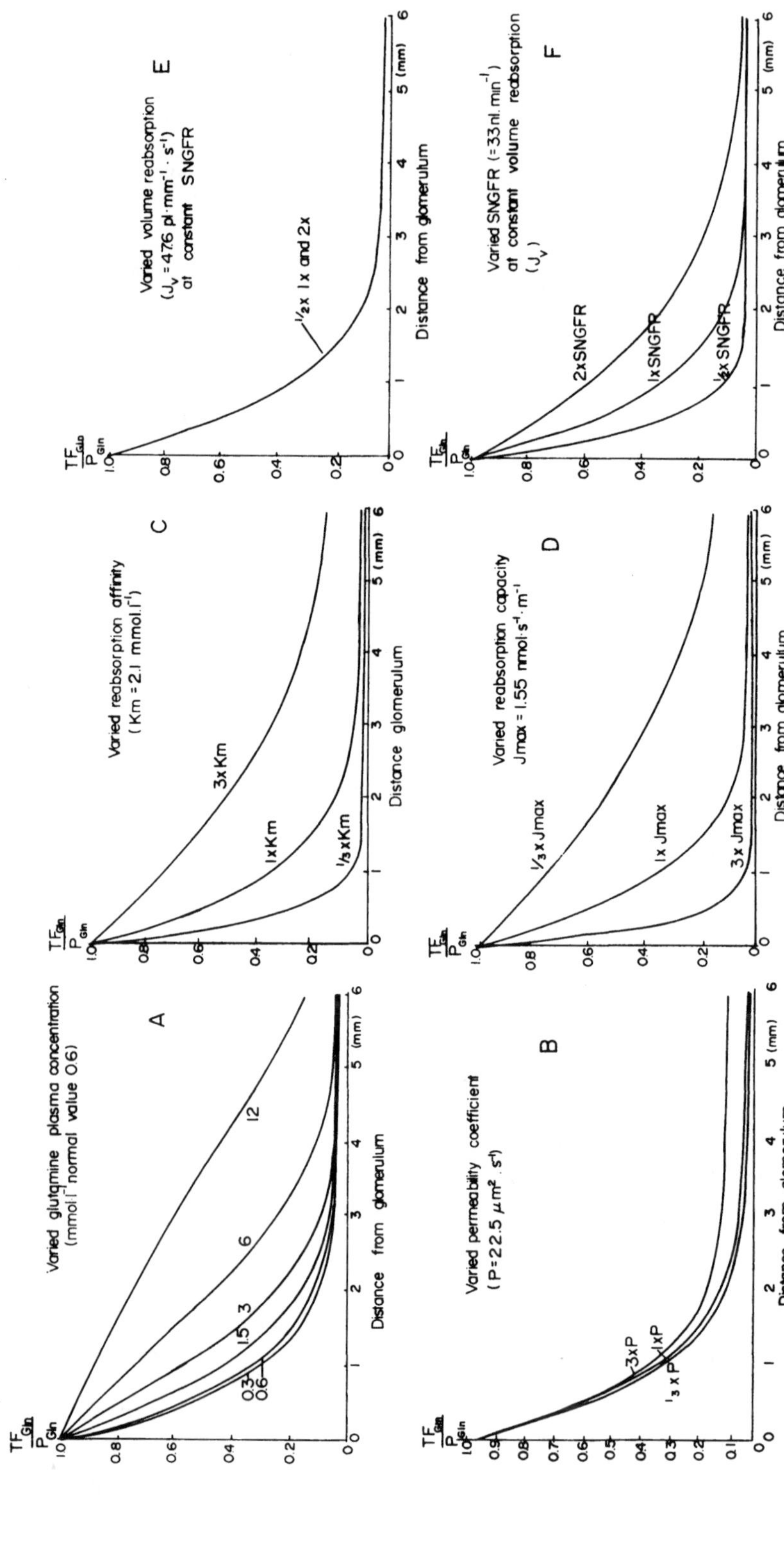

Fig. 5. Predicted concentration profiles of L-glutamine along the proximal convolution when a single parameter is varied.

tamine metabolism on luminal reabsorption of this amino acid has to be investigated in more detail.

Finally, it should be emphasized that glutamine is also taken up into tubule cells from the peritubular blood (Lemieux *et al.*, 1974; Pilkington *et al.*, 1970). Although this uptake contributes significantly to the elevated glutamine supply during increased ammonia-genesis in chronic acidosis, very little is known about the characteristics of this transport step (Lemieux *et al.*, 1974). Further investigations are urgently needed.

REFERENCES

BALAGURA S. & STONE W. J. (1967) Renal tubular secretion of alpha-ketoglutarate in dog. *Am. J. Physiol.* **212,** 1319.

BARFUSS D. W. & SCHAFER J. A. (1979) Active amino acids absorption by proximal convoluted and proximal straight tubules. *Am. J. Physiol.* **236,** F149.

BERGERON M. & MOREL F. (1969) Amino acid transport in rat renal tubules. *Am. J. Physiol.* **216,** 1139.

BURCH H. B., CHAN A. W. K., ALVEY T. R. & LOWRY O. H. (1978) Localization of glutamine accumulation and tubular reabsorption in rat nephron. *Kidney Int.* **14,** 406.

CHAN J. L. & HUANG K. C. (1971) Microperfusion studies on renal tubular transport of tryptophan derivatives in rats. *Am. J. Physiol.* **221,** 575.

COHEN J. J. & WITTMANN E. (1963) Renal utilization and excretion of α-ketoglutarate in dog: effect of alkalosis. *Am. J. Physiol.* **204,** 795.

DANTZLER W. H. & SILBERNAGL S. (1976) Renal tubular reabsorption of taurine, γ-aminobutyric acid (GABA) and β-alanine studied by continuous microperfusion. *Pflügers Arch. ges Physiol.* **367,** 123.

DEETJEN, P. & SILBERNAGL S. (1972) Some new developments in continuous microperfusion technique. *Yale J. Biol. Med.* **45,** 301.

GOLDSTEIN L. (1976) Ammonia production and excretion in the mammalian kidney. In *International Review of Physiology, Kidney and Urinary Tract Physiology II,* Vol. 11 (Edited by THURAU K.) University Park Press, Baltimore.

GOLDSTEIN L. (1976) α-Ketoglutarate regulation of glutamine transport and deamidation by renal mitochondria. *Biochem. biophys. Res. Commun.* **70,** 1136.

GREGER R., LANG F., KNOX F. G. & LECHENE C. (1978) Analysis of tubule fluid In *Methods in Pharmacology,* Vol. 4b (Edited by MARTINEZ-MALDONADO M.) Plenum, New York.

GÜNTHER R. & SILBERNAGL S. (1980) Renal tubular reabsorption of L-histidine. Microperfusion and free-flow micropuncture experiments in rat kidney. In preparation.

LEMIEUX G., VINAY P. & CARTIER P. (1974) Renal hemodynamics and ammonia-genesis. Characteristics of the antiluminal site for glutamine extraction. *J. clin. Invest.* **53,** 884.

LINGARD J., RUMRICH G. & YOUNG J. A. (1973) Reabsorption of L-glutamine and L-histidine from various regions of the rat proximal convolution studied by stationary microperfusion: evidence that the proximal convolution is not homogeneous. *Pflügers Arch. ges Physiol.* **342,** 1.

LINGARD J. M., TURNER B., WILLIAMS D. B. & YOUNG J. A. (1974) Endogenous amino acid clearance by the rat kidney. *Aust. J. exp. Biol. Med. Sci.* **52,** 687.

MCFARLANE-ANDERSON N. & ALLEYNE G. A. O. (1978) Sodium dependent and sodium independent glutamine transport by the rat kidney. *Abstracts of the VIIth International Congress of Nephrology,* p. A-1, Montreal.

OKEN D. E. & WEISE M. (1978) Micropuncture studies of the transport of individual amino acids by the Necturus proximal tubule. *Kidney Int.* **13,** 445.

PILKINGTON L. A., YOUNG T.-K. & PITTS R. F. (1970) Properties of renal luminal and antiluminal transport of plasma glutamine. *Nephron* **7,** 51.

RELMAN A. S. & YABLON S. (1977) The regulation of ammonia production in the rat. In *Current Problems in Clinical Biochemistry,* Vol. 8, p. 198 (Edited by GUDER W. G. & SCHMIDT U.) Huber, Bern.

ROSS B. D. (1976) Effect of inhibition of gluconeogenesis on ammonia production in the perfused rat kidney. *Clin. Sci. Mol. Med.* **50,** 493.

SILBERNAGL S. (1975) Cycloleucine (1-aminocyclopentane carboxylic acid): Tubular reabsorption and inhibitory effect on amino acid transport in the rat kidney (Microperfusion experiments) *Pflügers Arch. ges Physiol.* **353,** 241.

SILBERNAGL S. (1976) Renal tubular reabsorption of amino acids: specificity of the different transport system studied by continuous microperfusion. In *Amino Acid Transport and Uric Acid Transport* (Edited by SILBERNAGL S., LANG F. & GREGER R.) p. 78. Thieme, Stuttgart.

SILBERNAGL S. (1979) Renal transport of amino acids. *Klin Wschr.* **57,** 1009.

SILBERNAGL S. (1980) Tubular transport of acidic amino acids studied by free flow micropuncture and microperfusion in rat kidney. In preparation.

SILBERNAGL S. & BAYLISS E. (1980) Quantitative Columnchromatography of amino acids and oligopeptides in the lower picomol range. In preparation.

SILBERNAGL S. & DEETJEN P. (1972) L-arginine transport in rat proximal tubules. Microperfusion studies on reabsorption kinetics. *Pflügers Arch. ges Physiol.,* **336,** 79.

SILBERNAGL S., FOULKES E. C. & DEETJEN P. (1975) Renal transport of amino acids. In *Reviews of Physiology, Biochemistry and Pharmacology,* Vol. 74, p. 105. Springer, Berlin.

SILBERNAGL S., PFALLER W. & DEETJEN P. (1976) Molecular specificity of tubular amino acid reabsorption. In *Current Problems in Clinical Biochemistry,* Vol. 6, p. 403. (Edited by SCHMIDT U. & DUBACH U. C.) Huber, Bern.

SILBERNAGL S. & VÖLKL H. (1977) Amino acid reabsorption in the proximal tubule of rat kidney: stereospecificity and passive diffusion studied by continuous microperfusion. *Pflügers Arch. ges Physiol.* **367,** 221.

SONNENBERG H. & DEETJEN P. (1964) Methode zur Durchströmung einzelner Nephronabschnitte. *Pflügers Arch. ges. Physiol.* **278,** 669.

ULLRICH K. J. (1979) Sugar, amino acid, and Na^+ cotransport in the proximal tubule. *A. Rev. Physiol.* **41,** 181.

ULLRICH K. J., RUMRICH G. & KLÖSS S. (1974) Sodium dependence of the amino acid transport in the proximal convolution of the rat kidney. *Pflügers Arch. ges Physiol.* **351,** 49.

VÖLKL H., SILBERNAGL S. & DEETJEN P. (1979) Kinetics of L-proline reabsorption studied by continuous microperfusion. *Pflügers Arch. ges Physiol.* **382,** 115.

VÖLKL H. & SILBERNAGL S. (1980) Molecular specificity of tubular reabsorption of L-proline. A microperfusion study in rat kidney. In preparation.

WEBBER W. A. (1962) Interactions of neutral and acidic amino acids in renal tubular transport. *Am. J. Physiol.* **202,** 577.

YOUNG J. A. & FREEDMAN B. S. (1971) Renal tubular transport of amino acid *Clin. Chem.* **17,** 245.

SYMPOSIUM DISCUSSION

Guder: Did you discriminate between cellular and paracellular pathways of transport?

Silbernagl: No we didn't and I don't see a way to do that *in vivo.*

Vinay: Together with Dr Melvin Silverman, we have been interested in glutamine transport in the dog. Using the indicator dilution technique of Chinard, we have looked at luminal and contra-luminal transport of glutamine and found no influence of acidosis on the antiluminal uptake.

Lemieux: Do you think that your TF/P ratio of above 1 in your free-flow study could be due to some uptake of glutamine at the anti-luminal site with some gradient diffusion early in the proximal tubule?

Silbernagl: But then this uptake has to be greater in proportion to the luminal reabsorption than in later parts of the tubule: the profile is determined by the relation between these two.

Silva: Which cation was excreted with oxo-glutarate?

Silbernagl: In these experiments, reabsorption of radioactive oxoglutarate was measured: we did not determine the cation excretion.

Kovacevic: Can you tell us what proportion of glutamine is metabolized compared with that reabsorbed?

Silbernagl: What we are measuring is the disappearance of glutamine from the tubule lumen. We tried to influence intracellular glutamine metabolism by mercaptopicolinate and 2-oxo-glutarate in order to find out whether this manoeuver in turn influences glutamine reabsorption kinetics. We did not find any change but this negative result does not rule out that some glutamine reabsorbed is metabolized within the tubule cells.

Vinay: In the normal dog, around 20% of the glutamine arriving at the antiluminal pole of the proximal tubular cells is extracted. Since this value is greater than the net glutamine extraction, there must be some backflux of glutamine under normal conditions. From calculation of net glutamine extraction and filtration, no more than 60% of the filtered glutamine could be metabolised under normal conditions. In acidosis, the rate of net glutamine extraction exceeds that of glutamine filtration, disclosing a net antiluminal uptake. Our preliminary results indicate that it is not the glutamine uptake which adapts during acidosis in the dog, but efflux of glutamine out of the proximal tubular cells, possibly because of an increased metabolic sink under conditions of chronic metabolic acidosis.

Burch: What is the position along the nephron? In the proximal straight tubule, using different techniques, we have shown (*Kidney Int.* **14,** 406, 1978) that there is a higher concentration of glutamine in this region, and that it can be raised still further when the rat is loaded with glutamine. This is also the site of glutamine synthetase in the rat.

Silbernagl: First to the question of Dr Vinay: in the dog under normal conditions some 10–20% of the arterial plasma glutamine may be extracted by the kidney. Numerically this amount corresponds to 30–60% of the filtered load but it is not known to what extent luminal glutamine uptake participates in this extraction. In the rat Relman & Yablon (In *Biochemical Nephrology* (Edited by GUDER W. G. & SCHMIDT U.) p. 198. Huber, Bern, 1978) did not find any renal glutamine extraction under normal conditions. To the question of Dr Burch: our transport data fit perfectly with what you described. As the load of glutamine increases, the later part of the proximal tubule sees an increasing amount of glutamine. In addition, the microperfusion studies of Barfuss & Schafer (*Am. J. Physiol.* **236,** F 149, 1979) showed in the pars recta, that the passive permeability for amino acids in this zone may be lower, so that the intracellular concentration of the amino acids may be higher there.

Schurek: Did you look at back-flux phenomena in glutamine-free perfusion?

Silbernagl: Yes, it is very small, as expected. Within about 1.5 mm of the perfusion distance the concentration is the same as it is at the end of the proximal tubule.

Franke: I would not expect you to see any effect of inhibiting transport by these metabolic inhibitors, since the concentration of glutamine in the cell is very high.

Guder: I think the conclusion that the inhibition of gluconeogenesis is without effect on glutamine transport is important, since it has been suggested in the past that gluconeogenesis is involved in the reabsorption of anions. It appears to be true only for lactate. (Baumann *et al.* In *Biochemical Aspects of Kidney Function* (Edited by HOHENEGGER M.) pp. 81–93. Goldmann Verlag, Munich, 1972 and Ross & Bullock *Przegl lek.* **34,** 389–400 1977). I want to know if other amino-acids interfere with glutamine transport.

Silbernagl: Phenylalanine, methionine and others inhibit but have affinity constants lower than that of glutamine, so they are not very effective. Basic and acidic aminoacids and proline have no inhibitory effect.

Int. J. Biochem., Vol. 12, pp. 17 to 22
© Pergamon Press Ltd 1980. Printed in Great Britain

0020-711X/80/0701-0017$02.00/0

QUANTITATIVE MORPHOLOGY OF THE RAT KIDNEY

WALTER PFALLER and MICHAEL RITTINGER
Institute of Physiology, University of Innsbruck, Austria

Abstract—1. Light and electron microscopic morphometry was used to determine the volumetric tissue composition within the various zones of the rat kidney.

2. Furthermore, the ultrastructural organization of the nephron along its path from the cortex to the inner medulla was quantified.

3. The subcellular parameters measured were: volume density of nuclei, mitochondria and lysosomes and surface densities of mitochondrial, luminal and baso-lateral plasma membranes.

4. A close correlation between the membrane bound enzymes cytochrome-*c* oxidase and Na-K-ATPase could be demonstrated for mercury induced renal injury.

INTRODUCTION

The application of clearance studies, micropuncture and microperfusion and the use of isolated single nephron segments in nephrologic research has contributed remarkably to our understanding of renal function within the last few years. However, it became also more obvious that the functional heterogeneity due to nephron structure heterogeneity is a limiting factor for quite a few of the applied techniques. This became especially prominent when comparing biochemically determined parameters with physiology.

In general, three methods are available to clarify heterogeneity of the nephron along its path from the glomerulus down to the papillary tip.

1. A detailed quantitative morphologic analysis of all segments forming the nephron.

2. A biochemical analysis of key enzymes driving cell metabolism and their distribution along the nephron segments. This approach includes a mapping of hormonal or "signal" target sites which directly or indirectly may regulate cell metabolism.

3. A functional characterisation in terms of discrete transport mechanisms specific for certain segments. This may be approached using isolated perfused nephrons.

In this presentation we will discuss exclusively the first point, which to our knowledge has not yet been stressed in a quantitative manner. The morphologic heterogeneity of nephrons was recognized as early as histological techniques were available to study kidney tissue. Since than a number of physiological, cytochemical and biochemical parameters have been studied and distinct differences in the reaction patterns have been recognized. In addition some biochemical parameters mainly enzymes involved in intermediary metabolism, the production of high energy phosphates and ion or solute transport are known to be directly related to discrete cellular structures.

Since every biological function must have a clearly defined structural basis any detailed knowledge about nephron cell and renal tissue assembly will potentially contribute to a better understanding of structure-function correlation.

To obtain detailed information on kidney architecture the volumetric and membrane surface composition of nephron cells and the tissue within the various zones were determined by using a stereologic approach. The feasibility by this approach was further tested in $HgCl_2$ induced acute renal failure, where the occurrence of morphologic alterations is well established. These morphologic changes were quantified and correlated with the activity of respiratory chain enzymes, mitochondrial respiration and Na-K-ATPase activity.

MATERIALS AND METHODS

Five male hydropenic Wistar rats (350 ± 20 g body weight) were used in this study. In order to maintain intravital kidney architecture vascular perfusion fixation (Maunsbach, 1967; Pfaller *et al.*, 1974) was carried out using 1% glutaraldehyde buffered by Tyrode solution and rendered isoncotic with dextran. For the deeper zones the fixative buffer systems were adjusted to the increased osmolarity resulting from urine concentration: 750 mOsm$\cdot l^{-1}$ for the inner stripe of outer medulla, 1000 mOsm$\cdot l^{-1}$ for the outer, 1400 mOsm$\cdot l^{-1}$ for the midpart and 1800 mOsm$\cdot l^{-1}$ for the innermost part of the inner medulla. A stereologic analysis was then performed using light and electron microscopy. The following parameters were determined: Fractional volume (volume density; V_V) of nephron epithelium, urinary space, extracellular space, interstitial cells, vascular space, cell nucleus, mitochondria, cytosomes, reabsorptive vacuoles and surface densities (S_V) of the luminal, baso-lateral and mitochondrial outer and inner membranes.

The analysis of volumetric properties is based on the fact that the volumetric composition of a tissue is directly represented by its planimetric composition on sections. By denoting one compartment as i and another as r and measuring their total transectional areas A_i and A_r the ratio of the corresponding volumes will be

$$V_{Vi,r} = V_i/V_r = A_i/A_r$$

V_r may include V_i. Ratios of this type are called volume fractions or volume densities.

A real measurement can be easily performed using point counting (Chalkley, 1943) which leads to the final equation

$$V_{Vi,r} = V_i/V_r = A_i/A_r = P_i/P_r.$$

As a reference various volumes can be utilized. In case of the kidney for example the cytoplasmic volume, the zonal volume or finally the whole sample (organ) volume.

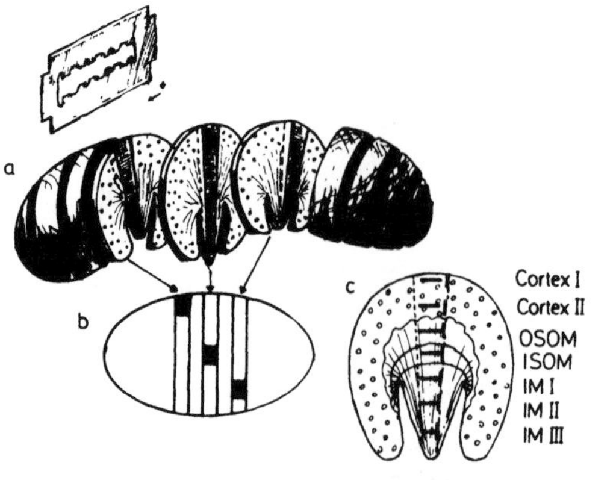

Fig. 1. Schematic presentation of the sampling procedures. (a) and (b) illustrates the random systematic sections of tissue from the kidney's central wedge, (c) shows the location of the sections analysed stereologically.

Surface to volume ratios (surface densities S_V) utilize the relationship $B_{Ai,r} = \frac{\pi}{4} \cdot S_{Vi,r}$ as given by Saltivkov (1958). The phase border length per transectional area B_A is directly proportional to the surface density (S_V). Point counting using a square grid with a spacing d gives the equation

$$S_{Vi,r} = \frac{I_i}{d \cdot P_r}$$

where I_i equals the number of intercepts of test grid lines with the phase border B_i.

The samples used for stereological analysis were obtained from the central wedge of the kidney by random systematic sampling (Fig. 1). Two mutually perpendicular sectional positions were analysed at various locations using a square lattice (for methodological details see Pfaller *et al.*, 1974, 1979; Rittinger, 1979).

The same experimental procedure was used to follow morphologic lesions induced by mercuric chloride at different intervals after administration in order to gain real insight into structure function correlation during acute injury of proximal tubular epithelium. In addition the absolute volume of the kidney was determined by displacement. After processing for light microscopy 15 sections were cut parallel to the kidney's short axis and the zonal volume again determined by point counting. After correcting for the preparative tissue shrinkage absolute volumes and surfaces of tissue and cell structures could be calculated.

RESULTS

The quantitation of tissue compartments is shown in Fig. 2. Always a unit volume of a zone was taken as a reference, so that all values are fractional volumes of the specific zone. This explains the increase in extraepithelial volume in the medulla when compared to the cortex and the reverse behavior for the epithelial volume fraction.

Figure 3a gives the volume density for the mitochondrial volume fraction, Fig. 3b the surface density of mitochondrial outer and inner membrane along the nephron, whereby each column represents a defined sampling position within a zone. The values are referred to a unit volume of cytoplasm. Fig. 3c and d gives an analogous presentation but in contrast to Fig. 3a and b a unit volume of kidney zone is the

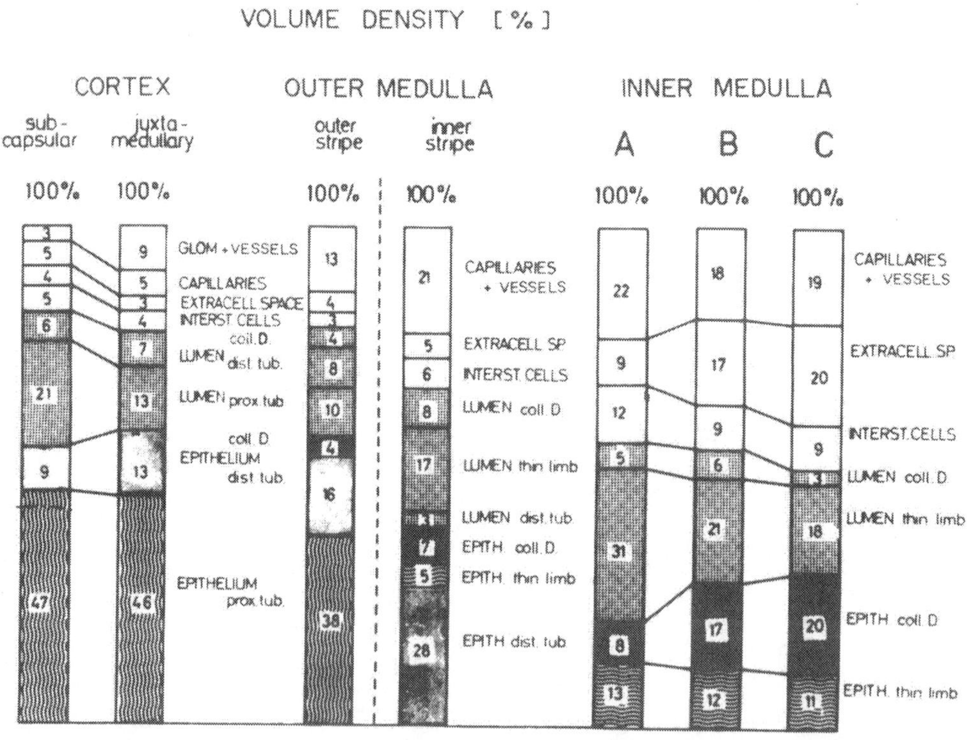

Fig. 2. Quantitation of tissue compartments of normal rat kidney. The relative contributions, by volume, of the epithelium, lumen vessels and interstitial space in the various kidney zones has been determined by stereological analysis. The results are expressed as a percentage of the volume of the given zone.

reference volume. The fairly large variation of baso-lateral and mitochondrial inner membranes is due to the various epithelial types forming the thin limb segment of Henle's loop (Schwartz & Venkatachalam, 1974). For a number of investigations relative values, volume or surface densities (concentrations) may be sufficient, the ultimate aim however are absolute values per standard sized organ. Utilizing the procedure described above, the absolute values of the reference—the zonal tissue and the various components within—can be obtained (Fig. 4).

In cell injury accompanying $HgCl_2$-induced renal failure we can detect changes in respiratory activity of cortical mitochondria and a reduction in proximal tubular sodium and potassium reabsorption 6 and 24 hr after administration of a single dose of $HgCl_2$. If one examines the biochemical mechanisms presumably responsible for this effect we will find an uncoupling of oxidative phosphorylation a reduced respiratory activity represented by the decreased cytochrome-*c* oxidase activity and a decreased activity of the ouabain sensitive Na-K-ATPase (Fig. 5). If we investigate proximal tubular ultrastructure, we find that the corresponding structural sites, the mitochondrial cristae membrane and the basolateral membrane, display a decrease in surface density (Fig. 5). Therefore, one can assume that a reduction in enzyme packing material, a reduction in membrane mass, parallels the proximal tubular injury.

DISCUSSION

The most remarkable result of this investigation was the equidirectional change in mitochondrial volume density, baso-lateral and inner mitochondrial surfaces along those nephron segments known to be involved in ATP dependent solute reabsorption or secretion. This distribution pattern is fairly consistent with that described for marker enzymes of these structural sites. That there is a close correlation between succinate dehydrogenase (SDH), cytochrome-*c* oxidase (CCO) and the mitochondrial cristae membranes in liver and heart muscle was shown by several authors (Plattner, 1973; Reith, 1976). When compar-

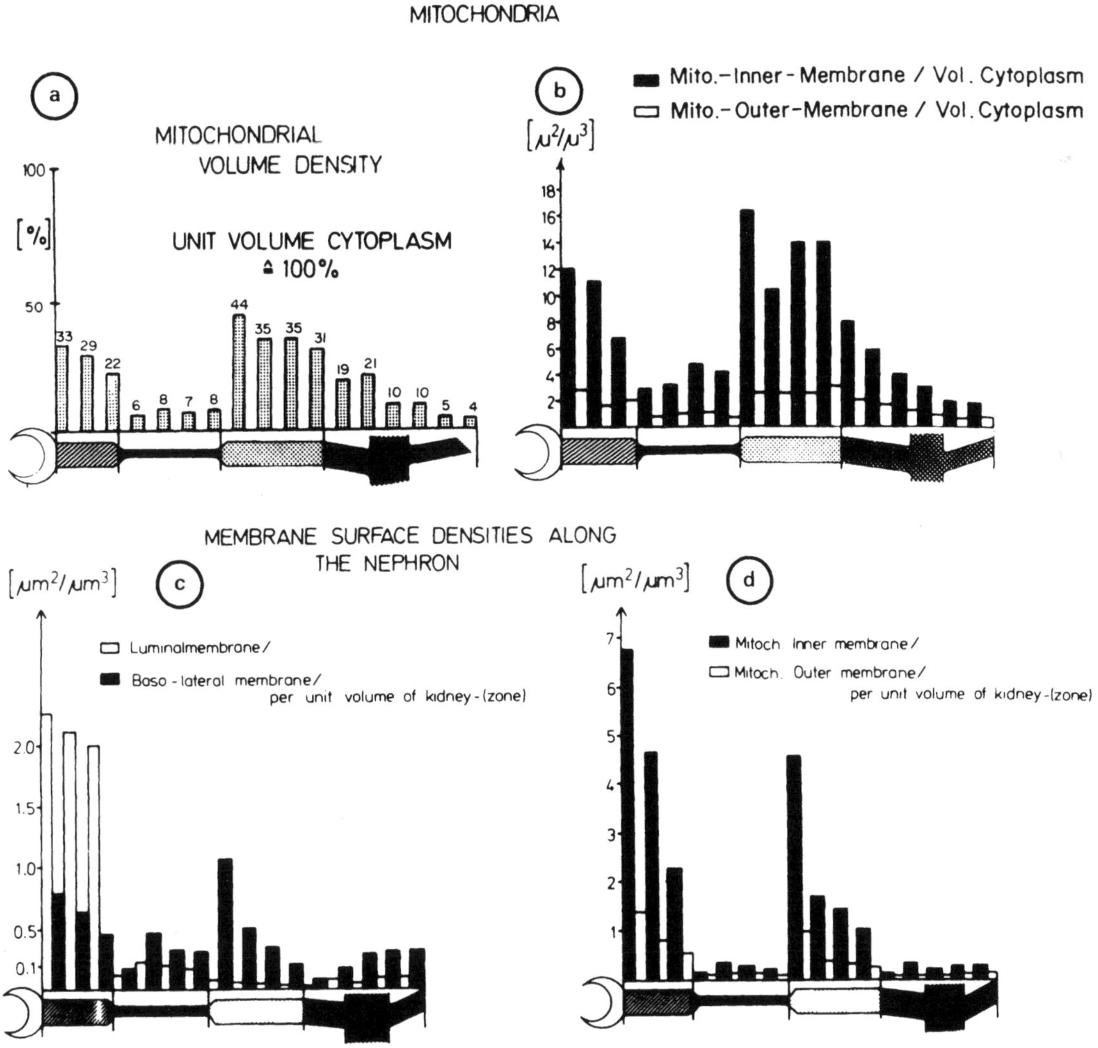

Fig. 3. Graphic representation of volume and surface densities relative to a unit of cytoplasm (3a, b) and to unit of zonal tissue (3c, d). The columns correspond to the section positions shown in Fig. 1.

a — TOTAL KIDNEY VOLUME 1320 μl 100% — ABSOLUTE VOLUMES

	Epithelium P	D	C	TL	Urine space	ECS	Int. cells	Vasc. space
CORTEX 830 μl 63%	386	58	33		195	29	37	91
OUTER STRIPE O.M. 290 μl 22%	110	46	12		63	12	9	38
INNER STRIPE O.M. 160 μl 12%		44	11	8	44	8	9	33
INNER MEDULLA 40 μl 3%			7	5	12	7	4	9
	720 μl or 57,7% of Kidney				314 μl or 23,8%	56 μl or 4,2%	59 μl or 4,5%	171 μl or 13%

b — ABSOLUTE VOLUMES FOR RAT KIDNEY

μl	NUCLEUS P	D	C	TL	MITOCHONDRIA P	D	C	TL	CYTOSOMES P	D	C	TL	VACUOLES P	D	C	TL
KIDNEY 1320 — 100%																
CORTEX 830 — 63%	19	8	4		105	20	6,0		27	0,6	0,2		13	0,5	0,2	
OSOM 290 — 22%	9	5	1,5		27	10	2,0		5,0	0,1	0,09		2,4	0,4	0,06	
ISOM 160 — 12%		4	1,5	1,3		14	1,0	0,5		0,1	0,01	0,04		0,09	0,10	0,04
INNER MED 40 3%			0,9	1,0			0,4	0,3			0,01	0,06			0,06	0,04
	55,2 μl NUCLEI per Kidney or 4,2%				240,2 μl MITOCHONDRIA per Kidney or 18,2%				33,2 μl CYTOSOMES per Kidney or 2,5%				17 μl VACUOLES per Kidney or 1,3%			

c — ABSOLUTE SURFACE [m^2]

	Luminal Prox	Dist	Coll	TL	Baso-lateral Prox	Dist	Coll	TL
CORTEX	1,864	0,021	0,010		0,965	0,291	0,091	
Outer stripe O M	0,600	0,010	0,006		0,190	0,120	0,023	
Inner stripe O M		0,006	0,009	0,021		0,142	0,024	0,038
INNER MEDULLA			0,004	0,008			0,015	0,020
	2,461	0,037	0,029	0,029	1,155	0,553	0,753	0,058
	2,501 m^2				1,919 m^2			

4,420 m^2 nephron cell membranes per kidney

d — MITOCHONDRIAL MEMBRANE ABSOLUTE SURFACE [m^2]

	Inner membrane Prox	Dist	Coll	TL	Outer membrane Prox	Dist	Coll	TL
CORTEX	2,95	0,61	0,18		0,87	0,17	0,05	
Outer stripe OM	0,61	0,30	0,03		0,25	0,11	0,01	
Inner stripe OM		0,57	0,04	0,02		0,15	0,01	0,01
INNER MEDULLA			0,01	0,01			0,005	0,004
	3,56	1,48	0,26	0,03	1,12	0,43	0,075	0,014
	5,33 m^2 Inner membrane surface per kidney				1,639 m^2 Outer membrane surface per kidney			

Fig. 4. Absolute volumes and surface areas of intracellular organelles and zones of the rat kidney. Stereological techniques were applied to kidney of known volume and results expressed in absolute terms for an ideal kidney, volume = 1320 μl. The various kidney zones (O.F.O.M. the outer stripe of outer medulla) and specific structures within each zone have been given separately. a = macroscopic structure; b = organelles; c = surface area of cell membrane; d = surface area of mitochondrial membrane. (P = proximal convoluted tubule; D = distal convoluted tubule; coll = collecting duct; TL = thin limb of Henle's loop.)

ing the mitochondrial inner membrane density pattern along the nephron with the distribution pattern of SDH (Schmidt & Guder, 1976) a close correlation is found.

A similar parallel is present for the mitochondrial volume density and the matrix enzyme malate dehydrogenase (MDH). Distribution of Na-K-ATPase activity as determined on microdissected segments (Schmidt & Dubach, 1971) correlates well with baso–lateral membrane density. The validity of this interpretation seems to be proven further by the fact that during potassium adaptation Na-K-ATPase activity (Doucet & Katz, 1980) increases simultaneously with the baso–lateral surface in the cortical collecting segment (Giebisch, 1980).

The mercuric chloride induced acute renal failure, associated with proximal tubular cell injury, may further illustrate structure–function correlation. This renal insult is characterised by a decreased proximal NaCl and volume reabsorption, a reduction in mitochondrial respiratory control (Pfaller *et al.*, 1979), an inhibition of CCO and a decreased Na-K-ATPase activity already 6 hr after administration (Fig. 4) of a single dose of $HgCl_2$ ($4\ mg \cdot kg^{-1}$ body weight). At this interval a stereologic analysis shows reduced cristae, and baso–lateral membrane surface density in both the proximal convoluted and straight segment (Fig. 4), whereas no changes are present in the distal tubule and the collecting duct.

The data provided by this investigation may be

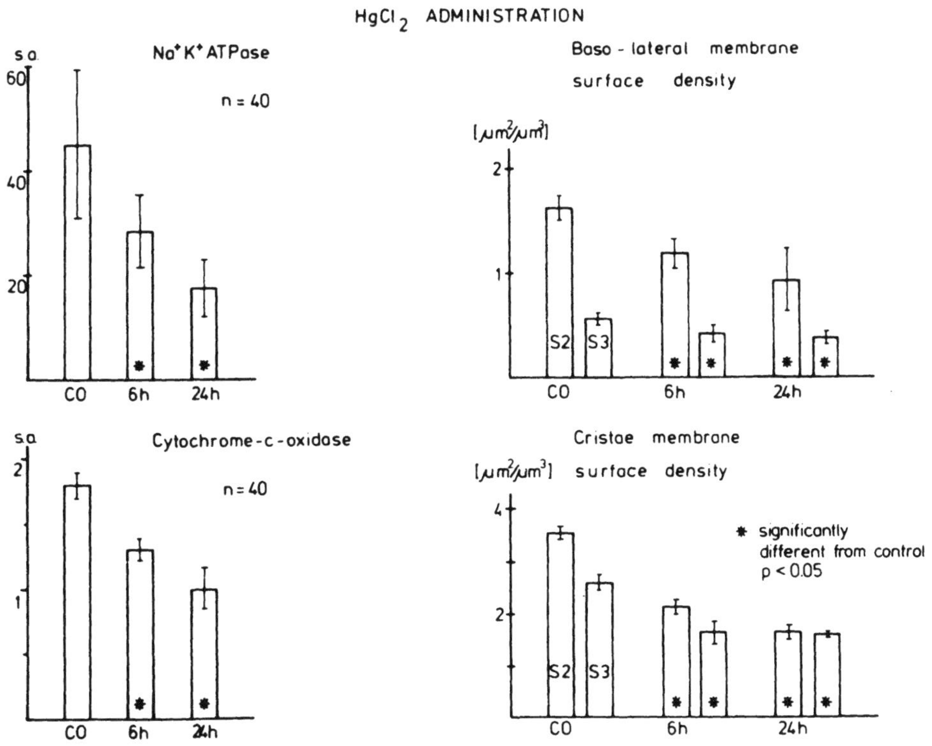

Fig. 5. Biochemical and morphological changes in proximal nephrons following a single dose ($4\ mg \cdot kg^{-1}$) of $HgCl_2$. S_2...proximal convoluted tubule; S_3...proximal straight tubule.

valuable tools for the biochemist in order to control the recovery of organelles after isolation or subfractionation or to refer metabolite concentrations to their real intracellular spaces. In addition changes in activity of membrane bound enzymes may be related to certain structural lesions. The physiologist is supplied with information about solute spaces hardly accessible to *in vivo* measurements. Of course one could argue that this largely depends on fixation, dehydration and embedding. If however, the preparational procedure is adjusted to physiologic conditions the kidney's intravital architecture is well maintained. This is best illustrated by the estimate of renal vascular space, which is 169.5 μl determined *in vivo* using ^{51}Cr-labelled erythrocytes and ^{125}I-labelled immunoglobulin M (Rassmusen, 1973), and 171 μl following our stereologic analysis. Furthermore, values are provided about the absolute surface of membraneous barriers across which active and passive transport takes place.

Last, but not least, it should be mentioned that the stereologic baseline values presented include certain quantitative information which so far cannot be correlated to function. However these data parameters might provide a basis and an aid for future studies on structure–function correlation in the kidney.

REFERENCES

CHALKLEY H. W. (1943) Methods for the quantitative morphologic analysis of tissue. *J. natn. Cancer Inst.* **4**, 47–53.

DOUCET A. & KATZ A. I. (1980) Na-K-ATPase along the mammalian nephron. *Int. J. Biochem.* **12**, 47–51 (This volume).

GIEBISCH G. (1980) Methods of localizing transport processes using micropuncture techniques—evidence for nephron heterogeneity. *Int. J. Biochem.* **12**, 3–8 (This volume).

MAUNSBACH A. B. (1967) The influence of different fixatives and fixation methods on the ultrastructure of rat kidney proximal tubule cells. II. Effects of varying osmolarity, ionic strength, buffer system and fixative concentration of glutaraldehyde solutions. *J. Ultrastruct. Res.* **15**, 283–309.

PFALLER W., FISCHER W. M., STRIEDER N., WURNIG H. & DEETJEN P. (1974) Morphological changes of cortical nephron cells in potassium adapted rats. *Lab. Invest.* **31**, 678–685.

PFALLER W., RITTINGER M. & FISCHER W. M. (1979) A concept for stereologic investigation of rat kidney. *Microsc. Acta* **82**, 137–146.

PFALLER W., TRIFILLIS A., SMITH M. A., KHANG M. W. & TRUMP B. F. (1980) Pathogenesis of $HgCl_2$-induced acute renal failure: A combined morphometric and biochemical analysis. *Kidney Int.* In press.

PLATTNER H. (1973) Quantitative correlation of structure and function on biomembranes. *Prog. Histochem. Cytochem.* **5**, 1–43.

REITH A., BARNARD T. & ROHR H. P. (1976) Stereology of cellular reaction patterns. *Crit. Rev. Toxicol.* **4**, 219–269.

RASMUSSEN S. N. (1973) Intrarenal red cell and plasma volumes in the non diuretic rat. *Pflugers Arch. ges. Physiol.* **324**, 61–66.

RITTINGER M. (1980) Qunatitative Morphologie der Rattenniere. PhD thesis, University of Innsbruck, Austria.

SALTIKOV S. A. (1958) Stereometric metallography. 2nd edn, p. 446. Metallurgizdat, Moscow.

SCHMIDT W. & DUBACH V. C. (1971) Quantitative Histochemie am Nephron, Oxydoreductasen und Na-K-stimmulierte ATPase. *Prog. Histochem. Cytochem.* **2**, 185–298.

SCHMIDT V. & GUDER W. (1976) Sites of enzyme activity along the nephron. *Kidney Int.* **9**, 233–242.
SCHWARTZ M. M. & VENKATACHALAM M. A. (1974) Structural differences in thin limbs of Henle: Physiological implications. *Kidney Int.* **6**, 193–202.

SYMPOSIUM DISCUSSION

Kinne: I think your study raises the problem of associating the surface area and quantitative assays. Can you tell me whether the Na-K-ATPase activity per unit basolateral membrane area is constant along the length of the nephron? Because I think it is very interesting to see that for example, Dr Giebisch, Dr Wayne and others find an increase in contraluminal membranes, together with the increase in the Na-K-ATPase activity, perhaps suggesting that there can only be a limited number of ATPases per unit membrane area.

Pfaller: Yes, we did once do a serial study on potassium adaptation, limiting our study to the distal convolution, and possibly (although it is difficult to identify) on the very early part of the cortical collecting duct. We could not find a change in the basolateral membrane, but we did find a tremendous increase in the inner mitochondrial membrane (about 200%)

Weiner: Could your method be used for the measurement of vascular diameters under various conditions of perfusion, and perhaps as a way of measuring blood flow in the various zones of the kidney?

Pfaller: Answering the first part of your question, I would say yes. There are a number of studies dealing with vascular morphometry, performed for example by the Aarhus group (Osterby, Gundersen). They determined the thickness of basement membranes, lengths of capillaries in the glomerulae, and surface densities of the capillaries. Of course, you can also determine diameters of capillaries and other vessels by morphometry. These values may help to interpret blood flow problems.

Giebisch: Have you looked at any of the parameters along the corticomedullary axis of the cortex? In other words, compared to the superficial nephrons, the juxtamedullary nephrons filter about twice as much, at least in the rat.

Pfaller: Yes, there is a difference along the cortico–medullary axis, which is difficult to interpret. In the deeper cortex, where most of the S_2 segments originate from juxtamedullary glomeruli, we find a lower fractional volume of the tubular lumen than in the same segments which are clearly derived from superficial glomeruli. Whether there are also differences in the subcellular organisation, cannot be answered in this study because of the sampling procedure we had to use.

Kovacevic: Did you observe mitochondrial volume changes under any conditions?

Pfaller: No. We have studied potassium adaptation, and $HgCl_2$ poisoning of the tubule. In the latter case, interestingly, we found no change in the mitochondrial volume fraction, despite considerable cell injury.

Int. J. Biochem., Vol. 12, pp. 23 to 27
© Pergamon Press Ltd 1980. Printed in Great Britain

0020-711X/80/0701-0023$02.00/0

ON THE "TIGHTNESS" OF THE RABBIT DESCENDING LIMB OF THE LOOP OF HENLE—PHYSIOLOGICAL AND MORPHOLOGICAL EVIDENCE*

M. ABRAMOW[1] and L. ORCI[2]
[1]Laboratory of Experimental Medicine, University of Brussels, Belgium and
[2]Institute of Histology and Embryology, University of Geneva, Switzerland

Abstract—1. In order to collect direct information on the nature of the countercurrent multiplier we isolated descending limbs of the loop of Henle in the rabbit inner medulla and perfused them *in vitro*.

2. The transepithelial electrical resistance was high with a mean exceeding 700 $\Omega\,cm^2$ a value typical of tight epithelia.

3. The sodium permeability, calculated from the lumen to bath fluxes of ^{22}Na was very low: $1.7 \times 10^{-6}\,cm \cdot sec^{-1}$.

4. Batches of dissected descending limbs were processed for freeze-fracture electron microscopy. The tight junctions in this segment were characteristic of tight epithelia.

5. Thus functional and morphological evidence indicates that this region of the nephron does not permit free passage of NaCl. These features should facilitate the operation of the countercurrent multiplier according to passive models.

INTRODUCTION

The mechanisms by which the countercurrent multiplier operates in the inner medulla remains a matter of debate. Passive models such as those of Kokko & Rector (1972) and Stephenson (1972) remove the necessity for a pumping mechanism located in the thin ascending limb of the loop of Henle. However, for these models to work, several requirements must be met, particularly regarding the permeability characteristics of the descending limb.

In the model of Kokko & Rector (1972) the wall of the descending limb must be water-permeable. In addition, the reflection coefficient of urea in the interstitium must be high enough so that water can be osmotically extracted from the loop. As a result, the sodium chloride concentration in the loop progressively rises to levels higher than in the interstitium and then the salt diffuses out of the sodium chloride permeable thin ascending limb. Thus dilution in the ascending part of the long loops in the inner medulla can proceed passively.

According to the passive models, the build up of an inside to outside gradient of sodium chloride in the loop requires the epithelium of the descending limb to have a low permeability to sodium.

Several micropuncture studies however (de Rouffignac & Morel, 1969; Jamison *et al.*, 1973) suggest that, during osmotic equilibration along the descending limb, there is a significant entry of urea or even sodium in the lumen. Entry of solutes appears to vary among species and state of hydration. This phenomenon would seriously impair the functioning of the passive models.

The only evidence in favour of the model actually comes from Kokko's laboratory, where isolated perfused descending limbs from rabbits were shown to osmotically equilibrate with their hypertonic environment, essentially by water abstraction (Kokko, 1970, 1972).

Because of the discrepancies we felt it necessary to investigate whether, in the same species, namely the rabbit, the findings could be substantiated by other lines of evidence particularly with respect to the permeability to sodium in the inner medulla.

From the known heterogeneity of the nephron population and from the model it is apparent that the most critical portion of the descending limb to be investigated is that located in the inner medulla. Kokko presumably sampled from the region closest to and including the outer medulla since he had to cannulate short segments still attached to a piece of their pars recta.

We reasoned that, if the inner medullary part of the descending limb has a low permeability to solutes, one should expect it to be tight in terms of resistance to the passage of electrical currents and if the transepithelial leak of solutes is partly through the paracellular shunt pathway, the limiting junctions between adjacent cells should appear tight according to morphological criteria.

PHYSIOLOGICAL EXPERIMENTS

The arrangement for perfusion of isolated tubules has been described previously. We found it particularly important to have an adequate electrical seal at both ends of the tubule using Sylgard 184 (Burg *et al.*, 1966; Abramow, 1974; Burg & Green, 1973).

D.C. signals were injected through the perfusion pipette, the resulting voltage deflection recorded at both ends of the tubule, and transverse resistance calculated using cable analysis.

* This work was supported by the Belgian Fund for Scientific Medical Research (grant No. 3.4540.79) and by the Swiss National Science Foundation (grant No. 3.120.77).

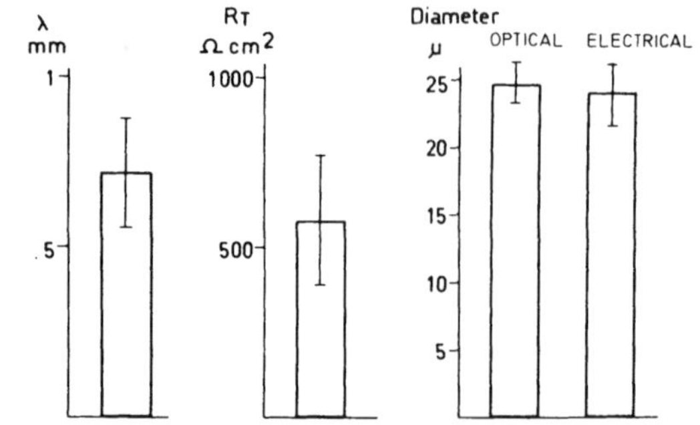

Fig. 1. Electrical resistance of isolated descending limbs of rabbit Henle's loop. λ is the space constant. R_T is the transepithelial electrical resistance. The optical diameter is that measured in the perfusion chamber. The "electrical" diameter was calculated from the cable analysis and the resistivity of the core.

Figure 1 summarizes some results. They reveal that these tubules display a large transverse electrical resistance R_T. The space constant, λ is also shown. The good correspondance between the luminal diameter as measured at the microscope and that calculated from the electrical resistance of the core is an index of the adequacy of the sealing and of the cable analysis.

Comparison of our results in the descending limb with the data obtained by others in other segments of the nephron such as the proximal convoluted tubule, the thick ascending limb of the loop of Henle, the distal tubule *in vivo* and the cortical collecting tubule makes it clear that the descending limb belongs to the category of the tight epithelia.

The evidence that the descending limb must be poorly permeable to Na received a direct confirmation from the measurement of ^{22}Na fluxes. The permeability to sodium calculated from the lumen to bath fluxes is extremely low, a mean of 1.7×10^{-6} cm·sec^{-1} which is lower by about one order of magnitude than that obtained by Kokko.

We made a plot of permeabilities versus electrical resistances in tubules where these parameters were measured simultaneously. Despite the limited number of experiments (three tubules for Na, and three others for urea) an inverse relationship between resistances and permeabilities is suggested, tubules with the highest resistance having the lowest permeabilities to solutes, a behaviour which is not unexpected.

Because *in vivo* the osmotic pressure of the fluids surrounding the cells is changing along the length of the segments we verified if *in vitro* this factor could modify the intrinsic properties of the cells as evaluated by the electrical conductance of the epithelial barrier. Each tubule was incubated and perfused with solutions of stepwise increasing or decreasing osmolalities and the membrane conductance measured in the steady state at each level of tonicity (300, 500 or 700 mOsm·kg^{-1} H_2O). The conductance does not appear to be dramatically altered by these manipulations. There is some indication of an increase in conductance between 500 and 700 mOsm but there are not enough data and in any case this does not alter the basic conclusion that the epithelium remains rather tight.

MORPHOLOGICAL INVESTIGATION

The technique of freeze–fracture enabled the structural organization of the plasma membrane to be examined in detail with special emphasis on the appearance of tight junctions. The morphological complexity of tight junctions is believed to parallel the functional impermeability of the junction which in turn would modulate transepithelial flow (Claude & Goodenough, 1973). Descending limbs were dissected and pooled for freeze–fracture processing as previously described (Humbert *et al.*, 1977). Figure 2 shows a representative fracture of such material. The epithelial cells were mostly cross-fractured but sufficient area of lateral and luminal plasma membrane were present in most cases to allow tight junctions to be visualized (Fig. 2 and inserts). Tight junctions with 1 to 4 ridges or fibrils were observed, junctions containing 3–4 interconnected ridges being most common. The ridges appeared uninterrupted in their exposed segments, a finding characteristic of tight epithelia. Plasma membrane of epithelial cells were, as in the rat (Humbert *et al.*, 1975), richly particulated with variations from very high to moderately high numbers of particles. The tight junctions with most ridges appeared to occur in the least particulated membranes, while the junctions with fewer ridges were found on membranes richest in particles. A systematic, quantitative, evaluation of these variations is now under way to establish whether they represent local changes in the same segment of the tubule or whether they characterize different (i.e. short and long) types of loops. At any rate, the morphology observed in all specimens studied was compatible with that present in a tight epithelium.

In summary, from both points of view, of electrophysiology and morphology, the thin descending limb of the loop of Henle in the rabbit seems to be able to function as a good osmometer which should facilitate the operation of the counter-current multiplier in the inner medulla.

REFERENCES

Abramow M. (1974) Effects of ethacrynic acid on the isolated collecting tubule. *J. clin. Invest.* **53**, 796–804.

Burg M. B., Grantham, J., Abramow M. & Orloff J. (1966) Preparation and study of fragments of single rabbit nephrons. *Am. J. Physiol.* **210**, 1293–1298.

Burg M. & Green N. (1973) Function of the thick ascending limb of Henle's loop. *Am. J. Physiol.* **224**, 659–668.

Claude P. & Goodenough D. A. (1973) Fracture faces of zonulae occludentes from "tight" and "leaky" epithelia. *J. Cell Biol.* **58**, 390–400.

Humbert F., Pricam C., Perrelet A. & Orci L. (1975) Freeze–fracture differences between plasma membranes of descending and ascending branches of the rat Henle's thin loop. *Lab. Invest.* **33**, 407–411.

Humbert F., Abramow M., Perrelet A. & Orci L. (1977) Feasibility of freeze-fracturing single isolated renal tubules. *Kidney Int.* **12**, 66–71.

Kokko J. P. (1970) Sodium chloride and water transport in the descending limb of Henle. *J. clin. Invest.* **49**, 1838–1846.

Kokko J. P. (1972) Urea transport in the proximal tubule and the descending loop of Henle. *J. clin. Invest.* **51**, 1999–2008.

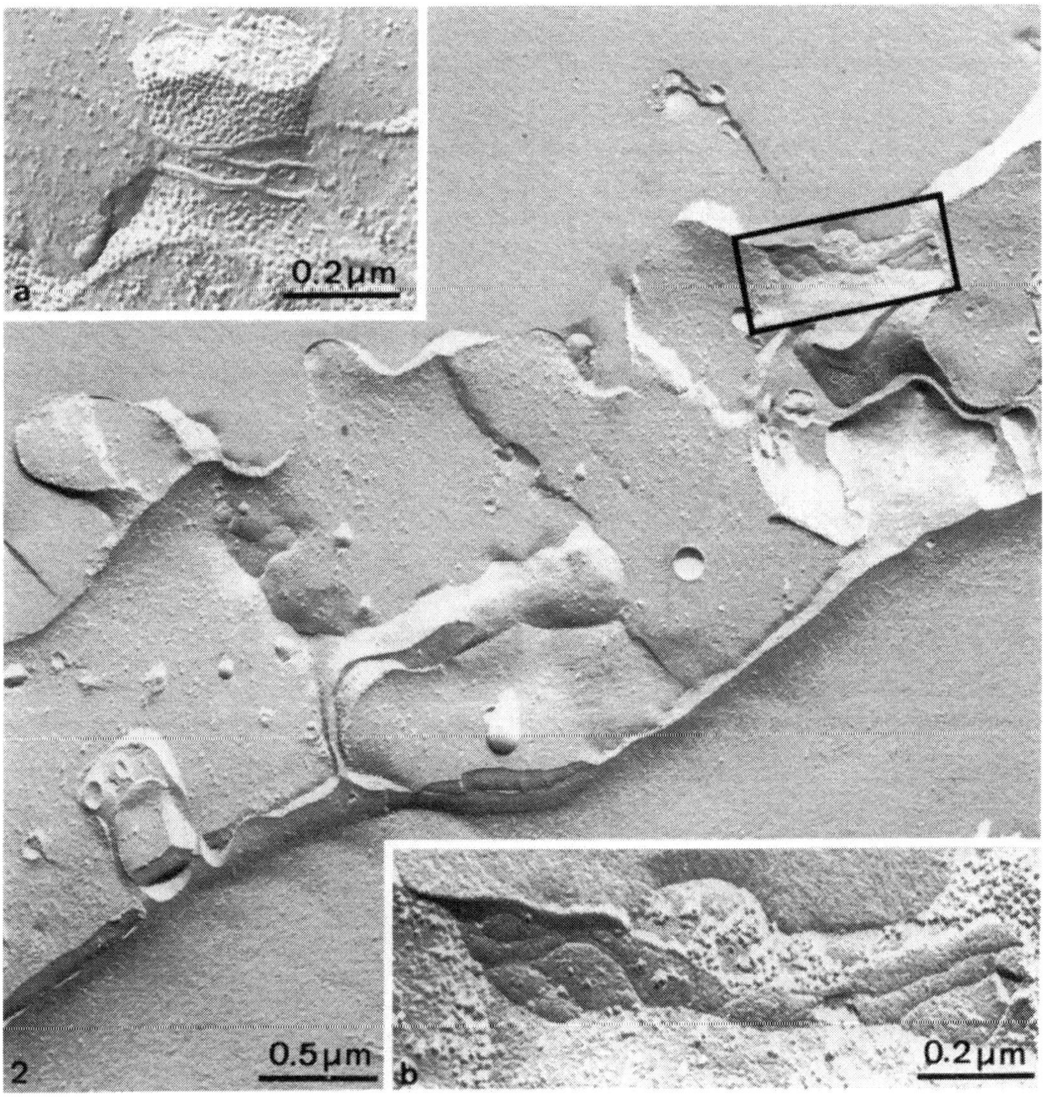

Fig. 2. Typical freeze-fracture image obtained in a pellet of isolated descending thin loops. The luminal surface is upwards, the basal surface is downwards. Although the fracture is mostly across the cell cytoplasm, significant areas of the lateral membrane were exposed near the luminal surface (black rectangle). A magnification of this zone (insert b) reveals the presence of several continuous, interconnected tight junctional strands on the E-fracture face (outer membrane leaflet). Insert (a) shows a three-fibril tight junctions in the P-face (inner membrane leaflet) of another loop. Fibrils are interconnected and continuous in the segment of membrane exposed which shows also the numerous intramembrane particles. Note the thick, "double-stranded" appearance of these junctional fibrils (cf. Humbert *et al.*, 1975; Riddle & Ernst, 1979). Magnifications: Fig 2. ×27,000; insert (a) ×81,000; insert (b) ×81,000.

KOKKO J. P. & RECTOR F. C. JR (1972) Counter-current multiplication system without active transport in inner medulla. *Kidney Int.* **2**, 214–223.

JAMISON R. L., BUERKERT J. & LACY F. (1973) A micropuncture study of Henle's thin loop in Brattleboro rats. *Am. J. Physiol.* **224**, 180–185.

RIDDLE C. V. & ERNST S. A. (1979) Structural simplicity of the zonula occludens in the electrolyte secreting epithelium of the avian salt gland. *J. Membr. Biol.* **45**, 21–35.

ROUFFIGNAC DE C. & MOREL F. (1969) Micropuncture study of water, electrolytes and urea movements along the loop of Henle in Psammomys. *J. clin. Invest.* **48**, 474–486.

STEPHENSON J. L. (1972) Central core model of the renal counterflow system. *Kidney Int.* **2**, 85–94.

SYMPOSIUM DISCUSSION

Kinne: Did your freeze–fracture picture change when you changed the osmolality of your medium? It would be interesting to compare the electrical data with the morphology.

Abramow: We have not done that but we plan to do so. I must remind you of the very low yields of the freeze–fracture samples because of the limited size of tissue which is available.

Weiner: According to the Rector/Kokko model, the thin descending limb should be more permeable to urea than to sodium.

Abramow: No, the descending limb can be neglected in this respect. The model requires only that it should be sufficiently impermeable to both so as to keep the concentration of sodium chloride rising in the lumen.

Giebisch: Do you have similar freeze–fracture data on the thin ascending limb of Henle's loop?

Abramow: No information.

Tannen: Did you measure potassium permeability?

Abramow: Only indirectly, and we concluded that the potassium permeability is much higher than sodium. This was done by comparison. We used an osmotic gradient to see if what happened *in vitro* agreed with what was predicted from the model. Equilibrium was achieved mostly by removal of water, and the ratios of collected over perfused fluid concentration for Na, Cl, osmolality and for the volume marker were identical. The ratio for potassium was much lower, and that fits with the recent observation (BATTILANA *et al.*, *J. clin. Invest.* **62**, 1093, 1978) that, given the appropriate driving force, potassium can penetrate the descending limb even in this situation.

Jorgensen: What is the size of the numerous intramembranous particles in your preparations, and what is their function?

Abramow: Quantitative evaluation in our preparation has not yet been performed. One can only speculate about the function of these particles which have been linked to the preferential pathway for water transfer in this segment in the rat (Humbert *et al.*, *Lab. Invest.* **33**, 407, 1975).

Int. J. Biochem., Vol. 12, pp. 29 to 35

0020-711X/80/0701-0029$02.00/0

HORMONAL STIMULATION AND DIFFERENTIAL GROWTH RESPONSE OF RENAL EPITHELIAL CELLS CULTIVATED *IN VITRO* FROM INDIVIDUAL NEPHRON SEGMENTS

MICHAEL HORSTER
(with the assistance of T. KÖNIG, D. ZAIGLER & R. GLEICH)
Physiologisches Institut der Universität München, Pettenkoferstrasse 12,
D-8000 München 2, Federal Republic of Germany

Abstract—1. Nephron segments (rabbit) were dissected and explanted into primary culture.

2. Outgrowth of epithelial cells and proliferation in monolayer from distal nephron segments was dependent upon cell substratum (plasma or collagen) and upon hormonal supplements of serum-free media.

3. Distal nephron segments from cortex and outer medulla (thick ascending loop of Henle, collecting tubule) have differential requirements for growth-stimulation.

4. Proximal epithelial tissue (embryonic Nephron Anlage) depends on serum or embryo extract for differentiation into convoluted segments.

5. The mammalian nephron can be cultivated *in vitro* to form segmental epithelial monolayers.

INTRODUCTION

The heterogeneity of epithelial functions within the mammalian nephron requires experiments at the level of the single segment. Although substrate and hormone requirements for segmental epithelial work have been studied, e.g. by microperfusion *in vitro* and segmental enzyme analysis during cell differentiation (Horster, 1978b), acute experiments and sample size usually limit the analysis of metabolism and solute transport and their interdependence within the single nephron. A preparation of cell populations derived from defined nephron segments in culture might be a tool for long-term studies on large, defined and homogeneous epithelial cell populations. The present work has sought to establish such a preparation by examining the environmental, nutritional and hormonal conditions necessary for *in vitro* stimulation of cell proliferation from defined mammalian nephron segments.

MATERIALS AND METHODS

Individual nephron segments were obtained by dissection (Horster, 1978a). Renal slices (White New Zealand rabbit) were transferred rapidly into medium (Waymouth 752/1) at 4°C. Microdissection of individual segments from the cortex and the outer medulla and the embryonic Nephron Anlage was carried out without collagenase, using tweezers. Experiments were performed under standard tissue culture conditions (Horster, 1979). Solutions, tools and tissues were sterile or aseptic. Defined segments (1–2 mm in length) were individually placed on the substratum and into a drop (100 μl) of supplemented medium (Fig. 1). The Lucite ring (i.d. 11 mm) facilitated monolayer formation while the outside medium was changed after 2–4 hr, and every 48 hr thereafter. The floor of the culture dish (Petriperm, Heraeus) was a gas-permeable foil which had been covered with a thin layer (about 100 μm) of rabbit plasma (substratum), or with collagen.

Nephron segments dissected from each animal ($n = 92$) were explanted into at least 10 culture dishes. Each dish contained two individual epithelial pieces (about 1–2 mm in length) from each of the six segment types (Fig. 1). The following renal epithelia were systematically tested for culture requirements: embryonic or postembryonic Nephron Anlage; cortical collecting tubule (CTc); cortical thick ascending limb of Henle's loop (TALc); medullary collecting tubule (CTm); medullary thick ascending limb of Henle's loop (TALm); proximal straight tubule (PST).

Cell substrata were decisive for initial outgrowth of cells from the explanted nephron segments. The following substrata were tested: collagen (Ethicon); gelatine 10% (Serva); agar 3% (Gibco); rabbit plasma. Plasma was obtained from cardiac blood by centrifugation (3°C, 2000 rev/min, 10 min). The media and supplements which were tested for their effect on growth response of individual nephron segments are listed in Table 1. Serum-free media (Waymouth 752/1; Ham F12; Leibovitz L15) were supplemented with hormones and the growth response of epithelial segments from the distal nephron to various defined media was recorded. Hormone-supplemented media were also enriched with different serum or extract preparations. These undefined media served to study *in vitro* differentiation of the embryonic Nephron Anlage into convoluted tubules, as well as monolayer growth from the explanted PST.

Cell outgrowth and proliferation as monolayer were recorded (Horster & Gundlach, 1979) on microphotographs, using an inverted-type optical system (Zeiss IM 35) with Differential Interference Contrast Microscopy (Normarski). Cell proliferation in primary nephron culture was measured on coded microphotographs by the number of cells per unit area (Fig. 3b) mutiplied by the number of monolayer area units grown from each of the explanted epithelial segments. Counts were made on day 3 and on day 7 in culture. Control value was an epithelial monolayer of at least 10^5 μm^2, to which the change in area up to day 7 was compared (% of control). Control proliferative rate was measured in Waymouth 752/1, supplemented with Thyroxine (Table 1).

Explanted epithelia were kept at constant temperature (36.5°C) and at controlled O_2 (20 vol%) and CO_2 (3 vol%) of the ambient air. The pH of the medium (5 ml) was maintained at 7.3–7.4 (Hepes buffer).

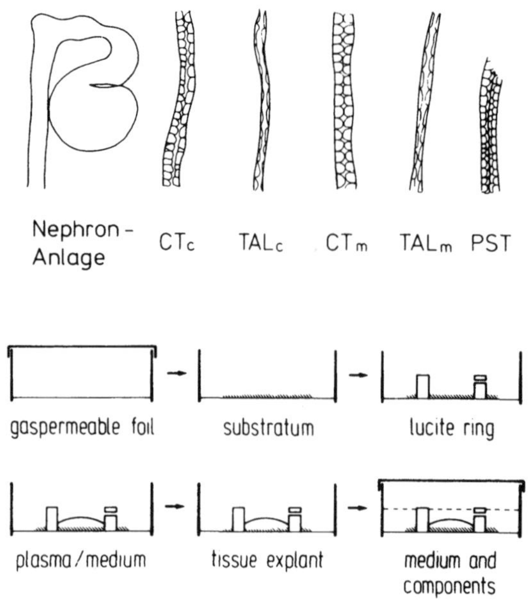

Fig. 1. Procedures for the *in vitro* culture of segmental cell populations from mammalian nephron. Individual epithelial segments were dissected and explanted into primary culture. The gas-permeable foil of the dish, the substratum and the plasma/medium matrix provided favorable environmental conditions for cell proliferation from the Nephron Anlage and from distal nephron segments (modified from Horster, 1979).

RESULTS

The principal findings of this first survey of the growth requirements for nephron cells in primary culture are: (i) mammalian nephron segments can be cultivated *in vitro* to form epithelial monolayers or tubules, (ii) distal nephron epithelia do not require serum for proliferative growth, in contrast to proximal nephron tissue and (iii) epithelia from distal nephron segments depend on hormonal stimulation for proliferation. Some of these hormonal requirements appear to be specific for the different epithelial cell types.

Hormonal stimulation and proliferative response of four different epithelia from renal cortex and outer medulla are depicted in Fig. 2. Striking and differential growth-stimulating effects of hormone-supplemented media on distal cell types were evident. When dexamethasone or thyroxine (see Materials and Methods) were added to the medium, both had growth-stimulating effects on almost all distal nephron segments, except for TALm. In contrast, insulin appears to be less effective for growth-promotion, when compared with thyroxine. The effect was more pronounced in the thick ascending loop segment. However, when dexamethasone was added with insulin, or insulin and thyroxine to the medium, the combination was stimulatory for cell proliferation. This was also true for the corticosteroid when added with thyroxine, except for the cortical collecting tubule. The small effect of insulin, however, could not be enhanced by the addition of thyroxine.

Most interesting was the observation that cortical and medullary segments appear to have differential requirements for cell growth stimulation. Prolactin promotes medullary epithelial growth but does not sustain cortical cell proliferation. Furthermore, progesterone had a stimulatory effect on medullary loop and collecting tubule when compared with the effect of dexamethasone as single supplement. Progesterone also reversed the inhibitory effect of Insulin by inductive action upon medullary loop cells. Lastly, when the epidermal growth factor was added, no additive effect upon cell proliferation was observed, but mitosis of medullary loop cells was stimulated.

Concentrations of hormone supplements were kept constant and close to *in vivo* for most experiments. Some hormone concentrations, however, were altered (Table 1). The proliferative response to dexamethasone was not different at 10^{-8} M when compared with 10^{-10} M. EGF did not alter the proliferative response when added as single component (10^{-8} to 10^{-10} M) or in combination (10^{-8} M) with dexamethasone (Fig. 2). Proximal and distal epithelial growth was inhibited by serum or extract concentrations (Table 1) beyond the *in vivo* range of 3 to 30% (v/v) (Horster, 1979).

Treatment of renal slices with collagenase (Worthington, CLS 2, 1 mg·ml^{-1} medium) during dissection or after monolayer spreading induced cell separation and polylayer aggregates (Horster, 1979).

Epithelial cell polarity, as studied by EM of *in vitro* monolayer culture, was maintained; basal mem-

Table 1. Components used as supplements of synthetic media* for primary *in vitro* culture of epithelial cell populations from explanted mammalian nephron segments (rabbit)

Components and media	Concentration of component	Dishes tested
Dexamethasone	7.4–8.5 × 10^{-10} M	903
(Fortecortin, Merck)	7.4–8.5 × 10^{-8} M	195
Insulin	2.63–3.03 × 10^{-9} M	874
(Hoechst)	6.67 × 10^{-9} M	215
L-Thyroxine (Serva)	5.2–6.0 × 10^{-8} M	425
Prolactin (Ferring)	1.72–1.97 × 10^{-8} M	129
Progesterone	3.2 × 10^{-7} M	289
(Serva)	3.2 × 10^{-6} M	9
Epidermal growth	1.64 × 10^{-10} M	10
factor	1.64 × 10^{-9} M	50
(S. Cohen)	1.64 × 10^{-8} M	30
Fetal calf serum		626
Chick embryo extract		481
Beef embryo extract	0.03–0.3 ml/ml	179
Calf serum, heat inactivated (all Gibco)		339
Waymouth 752/1 (Gibco)		1440
Ham F-12 (Seromed)		76
Leibovitz L-15 (Seromed)		80

The synthetic medium was supplemented with one or more components (Fig. 2) and its effect upon cell proliferation was compared to medium containing L-Thyroxine.
* Antibiotics were not used.

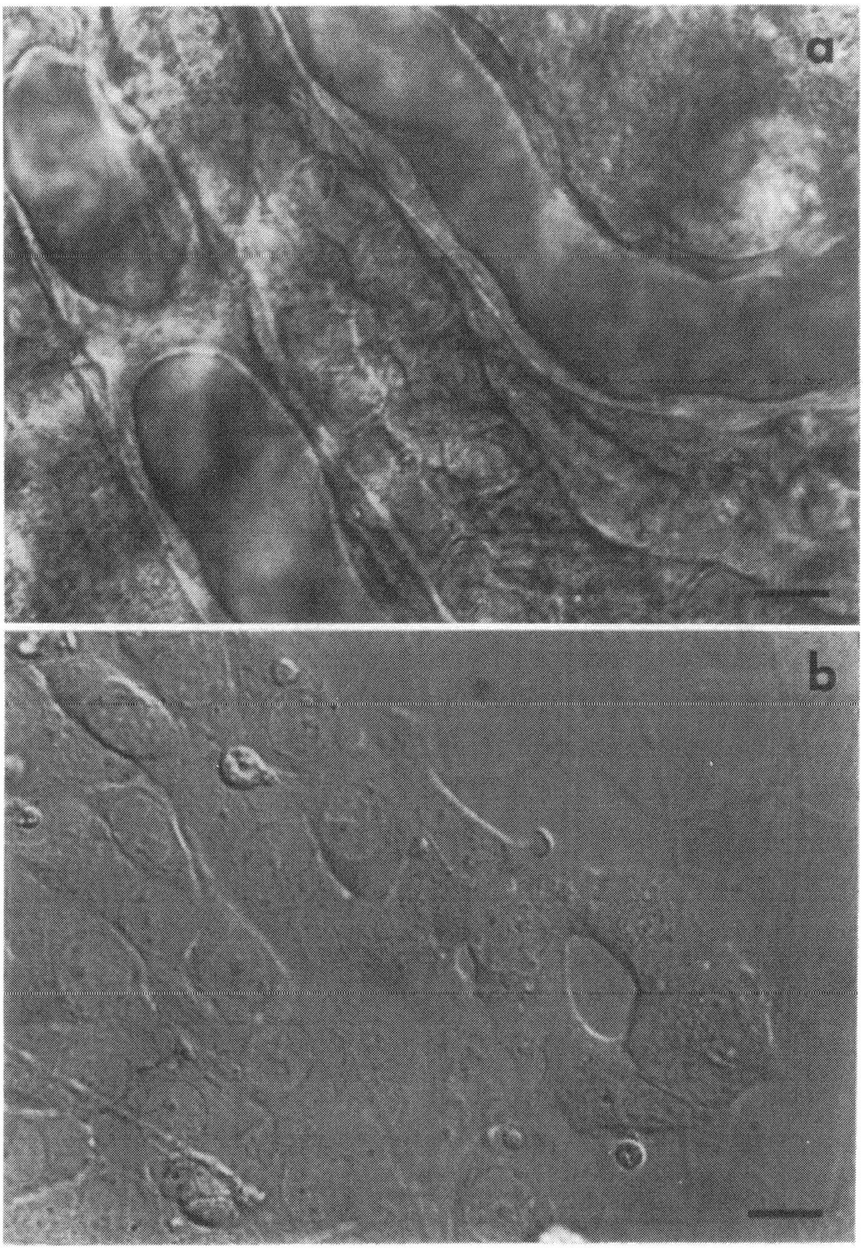

Fig. 3. (a) *De novo* growth of proximal epithelial tissue and formation of tubule lumen (day 11 in culture) in serum-supplemented medium. (b) Proliferative growth of epithelial cell monolayer from medullary thick ascending loop of Henle (day 9 in culture) in serum-free, hormone-supplemented medium on collagen substratum. The bar is 10 μm. Differential Interference Contrast.

branes, cytomembranes, intercellular communications and microvilli were present (Herzog & Horster, unpublished).

DISCUSSION

Environmental, nutritional and hormonal requirements for defined nephron epithelia in primary culture have not been studied, but attempts to cultivate renal tissue *in vitro* date back to the beginning of this century. Champy (1913), in his treatise "Le sort de tissus cultivés en dehors de l'organisme", first demonstrated that a plasma clot sustained peripheral cell proliferation from renal cortex, when explanted at term. This fact had been mentioned earlier (Carrel & Burrows, 1910): "A few tubes, composed of a lumen limited by epithelial-like cells, had passed from the fragment of kidney for a distance into the plasmatic medium". The statement suggests that *in vitro* morphogenesis of convoluted tubules had occurred from tissue explanted into a plasma clot. The present study confirms (Fig. 3a) and extends this finding. Serum or serum constituents are necessary for growth and differentiation of proximal nephron epithelia *in vitro*. The serum factors are more complex than hormones which were studied for growth stimulation. The plasma clot, even when used with medium (Fig. 1), appears to provide a three-dimensional matrix necessary for tubule formation; tubules did not grow on the flat substratum (plasma floor of petridish). *De novo* growth of convoluted tubules and subsequent appearance of lumina (Fig. 3a) were observed only when the chemically defined media had been supplemented with serum. The factors in serum necessary for proximal epithelial growth are unknown. Polypeptides, such as the submaxillary gland derived epidermal growth factor (Fig. 2), may be involved in renal proximal cell proliferation. A fibroblast derived growth factor has been demonstrated to stimulate DNA synthesis in cultured 3T3 fibroblast cells (Bourne & Rozengurt, 1976). Our attempts to stimulate nephron cell proliferation with conditioned media derived from embryonic renal slices were not successful (Horster, 1979). The importance of numerous well-known growth factors (Gospodarowicz *et al.*, 1978) for renal epithelial differentiation, regeneration, and compensatory hypertrophy remains to be demonstrated, using homogeneous segmental cell populations in culture.

Serum also sustains cell proliferation in distal epithelia, when added in final concentrations of 3–30% (v/v) to different media (Horster, 1979). However, various hormones and a defined polypeptide can substitute for serum in distal epithelia (Fig. 2). This role for hormones has been shown in established epithelial cell lines derived, for example, from rat pituitary (Hayashi *et al.*, 1978), and canine total kidney suspension (MDCK) (Taub *et al.*, 1979). The rela-

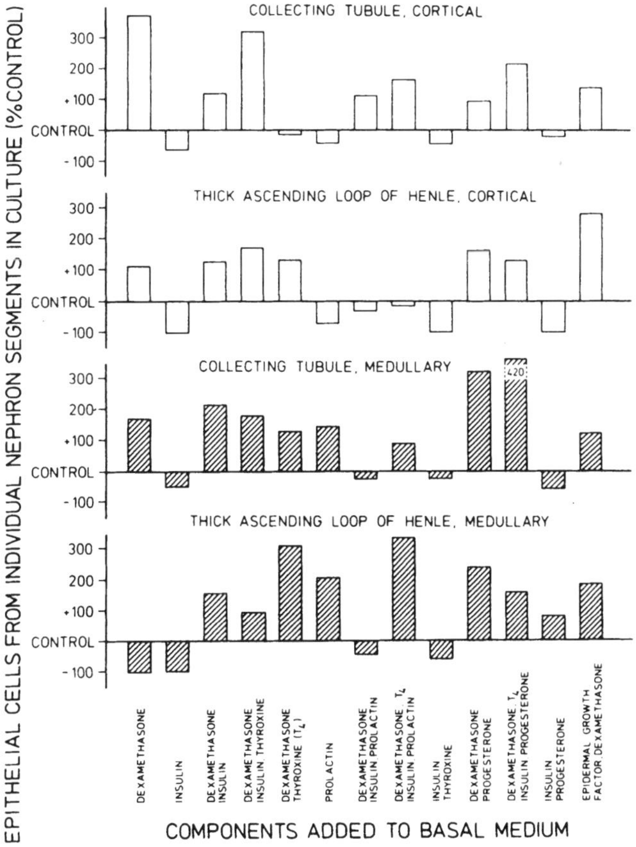

Fig. 2. Hormonal stimulation of *in vitro* cell proliferation from nephron epithelia in serum-free medium. Basal medium was Waymouth 752/1. Control was basal medium supplemented with 3,3′-5,5′-Tetraiodo-L-thyronine. Cell numbers were obtained by planimetry of coherent epithelial monolayers on day 3 and on day 7 in primary culture.

tive mitogenic importance, however, varies among different epithelial organs. Thyroxine, when added (10^{-9} M) to duodenal tissue in culture, accelerates goblet cell proliferation compared with normal *in vivo* differentiation (Black & Moog, 1977). Prostaglandin E_1 appears to be necessary for *in vitro* survival of cells derived from total kidney suspension (Taub *et al.*, 1979), but is not essential for proliferative growth of any of the cell monolayers derived from individual nephron segments (unpublished data). Insulin is an absolute requirement for survival of the pituitary cell line, but is not critical for the MDCK-line or for any of the nephron segmental populations (Fig. 2). However, insulin as well as epidermal growth factor potentiate the effect of vasopressin on DNA synthesis in 3T3 cells (Rozengurt *et al.*, 1979). Similar specific studies for prolactin or progesterone are not available. Their striking differential stimulatory effect on nephron segments (Fig. 2) suggests that the chemical events involved in the initiation and maintenance of cell proliferation might not be identical for cortex and medulla. These events are not yet understood. The first direct evidence, however, that growth-promoting serum initiates membrane permeability changes for Na^+, Ca^{2+} and K^+ (Moolenaar *et al.*, 1979) supports the assumption (Rozengurt, 1979) that extracellular factors (serum constituents) indeed participate in growth control.

Nephron differentiation *in vivo* is a sequence of physical, chemical and structural changes (Horster, 1978b). The *in vitro* culture of segmental epithelial cells and their selective growth stimulation by extracellular factors will be utilized to study the interdependence of these phenomena.

SUMMARY

Individual nephron segments were cultured *in vitro*. Cell proliferation in epithelial monolayers was dependent upon the type of substratum (plasma or collagen). Serum-free, hormone-supplemented media initiated and sustained proliferative growth of cells from thick ascending loop and collecting tubule segments. The growth response of cortical and medullary segments was different, as was the segmental response to specific hormones at *in vivo* concentrations. Combined hormone supplements appeared to have synergistic action upon proliferation. Proximal epithelial tissue differentiated into tubules when serum-supplemented media and a semi-solid matrix were provided. Segmental cell populations derived *in vitro* from the mammalian nephron can be studied for about 2 weeks in primary culture.

Acknowledgements—Work in the author's laboratory is supported by the Deutsche Forschungsgemeinschaft. The expert assistance of T. König, D. Zaigler and R. Gleich in culture maintenance and growth evaluation is gratefully acknowledged. Part of this work was reported in abstract form (*Pflügers Arch. ges. Physiol.* **379**: R58, 1979; **382**: R16, 1979; *Int. J. Biochem.*, **10**(9) 1979).

REFERENCES

BLACK B. L. & MOOG F. (1977) Goblet cells in embryonic intestine: accelerated differentiation in culture. *Science* **197**, 368–370.

BOURNE H. R. & ROZENGURT E. (1976) An 18,000 molecular weight polypeptide induces early events and stimulates DNA synthesis in cultured cells. *Proc. natn. Acad. Sci. U.S.A.* **73**, 4555–4559.

CARREL A. & BURROWS M. T. (1910) Cultivations of adult tissues and organs outside of the body. *J. Am. Med. Ass.* **55**, 1379–1381.

CHAMPY CH. (1913) Le sort des tissus cultivés en dehors de l'organisme. *Rev. gen. Sci.* **24**, 790–801.

GOSPODAROWICZ D., GREENBURG G., BIALECKI H. & ZETTER B. R. (1978) Factors involved in the modulation of cell proliferation *in vivo* and *in vitro*: The role of fibroblast and epidermal growth factors in the proliferative response of mammalian cells. *In vitro* **14**, 85–118.

HAYASHI I., LARNER J. & SATO G. (1978) Hormonal growth control of cells in culture. *In vitro* **14**, 23–30.

HORSTER M. (1978a) Loop of Henle functional differentiation. *In vitro* perfusion of the isolated thick ascending segment. *Pflügers Arch. ges. Physiol.* **378**, 15–24.

HORSTER M. (1978b) Principles of nephron differentiation. *Am. J. Physiol.* **235**, F387–F394.

HORSTER M. (1979) Primary culture of mammalian nephron epithelia. Requirements for cell outgrowth and proliferation from defined explanted nephron segments. *Pflügers Arch.* **382**, 209–215.

HORSTER M. & GUNDLACH H. (1979) Application of differential interference contrast with inverted microscopes to the *in vitro* perfused nephron. *J. Microsc.* **117**, 375–379.

MOOLENAAR W. H., DE LAAT S. W. & SAAG P. T. VAN DER (1979) Serum triggers a sequence of rapid ionic conductance changes in quiescent neuroblastoma cells. *Nature* **279**, 721–723.

ROZENGURT E., LEGG A. & PETTICAN P. (1979) Vasopressin stimulation of mouse 3T3 cell growth. *Proc. natn. Acad. Sci. U.S.A.* **76**, 1284–1287.

TAUB M., CHUMAN L., SAIER M. H. JR & SATO G. (1979) Growth of Madin-Darby canine kidney epithelial cell (MDCK) line in hormone-supplemented, serum-free medium. *Proc. natn. Acad. Sci. U.S.A.* **76**, 3338–3342.

SYMPOSIUM DISCUSSION

Katz: How long have you cultured these cells?

Horster: Primary cultures proliferate for about 14 days, similar to other primary cultures. Subcultures are kept for different periods, depending on the aim of the study. In one type, we aim to keep the cells as close to the primary cell as possible and look for differentiation of function and structure. In another type, we aim, by subculture, to develop cells with some characteristics of a specific nephron segment.

Vinay: Can you get segmental development in order to do transport studies?

Horster: I should stress that we are at present unable to get distal cells into tubular form. The way to go will be to grow the distal cells in sheets on a fluid-permeable support, and that is what we are doing. Proximal cells, by contrast, differentiate into tubules.

Sacktor: Do the cells in culture de-differentiate and become omnipotent? There have been reports that cells in culture show both ADH sensitivity and sodium-dependent glucose transport, characteristics which may indicate they are not derived from a single cell type.

Horster: Without doubt, cells develop differently when obtained from different segments. They respond to hormone-additions in the growth medium by different and segment-specific rates of growth, and this, in turn, may lead to changes in the characteristics of the *in vitro* developed cell. We might even obtain a more uni-potent population of cells if we were able to select them on the basis of their growth response to hormones during the primary culture.

Jorgensen: I do not understand the way in which you express the growth response to various media. What is 100%?

Horster: The "zero" control growth-response was that with Waymouth's medium, with added thyroxine, which affected the growth of cells from all segments. Effects of other hormone additions were expressed as percentage values of the control proliferation.

Osswald: Do you see differences in the structure of the cells growing out of monolayers from the ascending limb, or do they develop uniformly?

Horster: It is too early to answer that question. We expect to see differences between loop-segment types in culture.

Giebisch: Do you have any idea for the collecting duct which cell type is preferentially cultured?

Horster: In the collecting duct, as opposed to all other nephron cell types in culture, the cytosol contains water-filled cysts in some but not in all cultured cells. We are about to study their ultrastructure.

Int. J. Biochem., Vol. 12, pp. 37 to 40
© Pergamon Press Ltd 1980. Printed in Great Britain

0020-711X/80/0701-0037S02.00 0

DIVERSITY OF EFFECTS OF FRUCTOSE LOADS ON DIFFERENT PARTS OF THE NEPHRON*

H. B. BURCH, B. COLE, S. CHOI, T. R. ALVEY and C. DENCE
Department of Pharmacology, Washington University School of Medicine, St Louis, MO, U.S.A.

Abstract—1. Analysis of nine parts of the rat nephron from glomerulus to papilla showed a wide variety of metabolic responses to high loads of fructose among the different segments.

2. There were dramatic increases in fructose-1-P and glucose-6-P in the proximal straight tubule, with lesser changes in the proximal convoluted tubule and none elsewhere.

3. Fructokinase was also confined to the proximal tubule with highest activity in the straight segment.

4. Fructose-1-P aldolase was highest in the proximal convoluted tubule. Fructose bisphosphate aldolase peaked in the distal straight tubule.

5. Glycerol-1-P increased strikingly in the proximal tubule but the peak effect was in the convoluted segment.

6. Highest concentrations of ATP were found in the distal convoluted tubule and did not change with loads of fructose whereas, ATP fell 80% in the proximal straight tubule and somewhat less in the convoluted portion.

INTRODUCTION

Fructose injected or infused into rats produces profound changes in kidney ATP and carbohydrate metabolites (Krebs & Lund, 1966; Raivo *et al.*, 1969; Burch *et al.*, 1970; Bowman, 1970; Hems & Gaja, 1972; Morris *et al.*, 1978). The changes resemble those found in hereditary fructose intolerance–disease in patients in whom fructose-1-phosphate aldolase is low or lacking (Froesch, 1978). Similar changes may also occur in cases where fructose and sucrose contribute excessively to the diet or in clinical situations where fructose treatment may be given. This paper describes metabolic changes along the nephron after large loads of fructose. In view of the structural and metabolic heterogeneity of the nephron it seemed likely that the changes would not be uniformly distributed. Defined parts of the nephron from glomerulus to collecting ducts of the papilla were dissected from freeze-dried microtome slices, and analyzed for appropriate enzymes and metabolites. The different segments were found to contain widely different levels of the enzymes concerned in fructose metabolism and to respond very differently to the fructose loads.

MATERIALS AND METHODS

Male Sprague-Dawley rats weighing 250–280 g were used. They were fed Purina laboratory chow and were given by intraperitoneal injection trypan blue (0.1 mg·g^{-1}) 18–20 hr before the experiment. This dye is concentrated in the proximal convoluted tubules and aids in visualization of these structures in the freeze-dried kidney.

Fed animals were injected with 20 or 40 mmol·kg^{-1} fructose as described previously (Burch *et al.*, 1970). After 40 min, kidneys were removed under light ether anesthesia and quick frozen in Freon-12 (CCl_2F_2) chilled in liquid nitrogen. The frozen tissue was stored at −80°C. Blocks of tissue were mounted, cut into microtome slices, and the slices freeze-dried at −40°C. They were stored under vacuum at −20°C. Plasma samples from tail blood were obtained before and after injection. Neutralized perchloric acid extracts were analyzed for fructose and glucose.

Kidney samples

The general technique for isolation and weighing small identified freeze-dried samples of tissue has been developed and described in detail by Lowry & Passonneau (1972) and associates. Its application to kidney microtome slices has also been reported (Chan *et al.*, 1975). Each sample consisted of a nearly central slice of glomerulus (20–40 ng dry wt) or a 75–150 μm length of tubule (12–30 ng for proximal, 5–20 ng for distal tubules) or 10–30 ng patch of thin limb area or papilla below the inner stripe of outer medulla. The samples were weighed ±2% on a quartz fiber balance (Lowry & Passonneau, 1972).

Analytical methods

The analyses for fructose, metabolites and enzymes utilize methods based on specific enzyme reactions which finally result in oxidation or reduction of pyridine nucleotides. Ultimately the fluorescence of NADH or NADPH is measured directly in a volume of 1 ml in a filter fluorometer (Farrand).

For analysis of parts of the nephron, first steps in the procedure were carried out in small aqueous droplets (0.1–5 μl) in oil wells (Lowry & Passonneau, 1972) and the sensitivity amplified by enzymatic cycling. An improved cycling method was used for NAD (Kato *et al.*, 1973).

For most metabolite assays essentially the same procedures described before were used (Lowry & Passonneau, 1972). For fructose-1-phosphate a method different from that previously reported (Burch *et al.*, 1970) was devised. It utilizes 1-P-fructokinase from *B. symbiosus* (Reeves *et al.*, 1966) generously given us by Dr R. E. Reeves. The first reaction is:

$$\text{Fructose-1-P} + \text{ATP} \xrightarrow{\text{1-PFK}} \text{Fructose bisphosphate} + \text{ADP}.$$

Fructose bisphosphate is then measured as described before (Lowry & Passonneau, 1972) with aldolase, triose-P isomerase and glyceraldehyde-P dehydrogenase as the

* Supported by grants from the U.S. Public Health Service 9 R01-AM22112-11 and 1 KO-8AM-00669-01.

auxiliary enzymes in the presence of arsenate and NAD^+. The NADH formed is then amplified by enzymatic cycling and the analysis completed as described (Kato *et al.*, 1973).

For the two aldolase assays, previous procedures (Burch *et al.*, 1963) were modified to increase sensitivity. The fructokinase assay was based on the spectrophotometric method of Günther *et al.* (1967) in which the fructose-1-P produced is converted to fructose bisphosphate as shown above. Sensitivity was increased by enzymatic cycling.

RESULTS AND DISCUSSION

Distribution pattern of enzymes

The kidney contains two enzymes capable of phosphorylating fructose: hexokinase and fructokinase. Normally, hexokinase is probably of little importance for fructose metabolism because of the very high K_m, 6 mM, whereas fructokinase has a much more favorable K_m, 0.1 mM. Consequently, the first metabolite is predominantly fructose-1-P rather than fructose-6-P. This requires, in turn, the assistance of fructose-1-P aldolase instead of the more common fructose bisphosphate aldolase for further metabolism.

As shown by others (Brannan *et al.*, 1975; Schmidt *et al.*, 1975) hexokinase is much higher in distal portions of the nephron than in the proximal segments (Fig. 1).

In sharp contrast to hexokinase, fructokinase is exclusively located in the proximal tubules with highest levels in the straight segments (Fig. 1). The next enzyme on the metabolic pathway, fructose-1-P aldolase, is also essentially confined to the proximal tubule, but in this case the highest level was found in the convoluted portion, $350\ mmol \cdot kg^{-1}\ (dry) \cdot hr^{-1}$, which is 50% above the activity in the straight portion. This pattern of distribution is completely different from that of the fructose bisphosphate aldolase. This enzyme is present in all parts of the nephron,

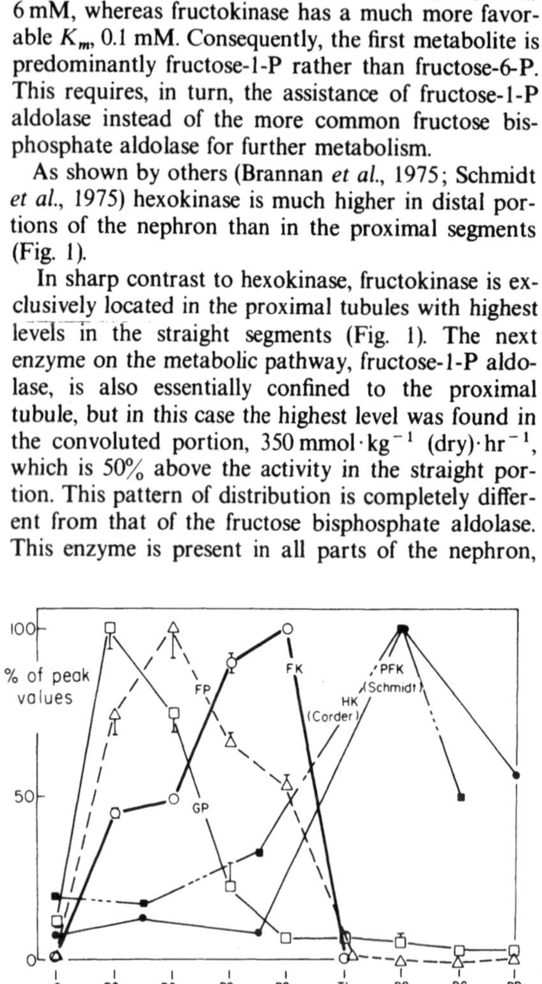

Fig. 1. The distribution along the nephron of fructokinase and related enzymes. Fructokinase was measured in control rats. Each point represents the average ±SEM of 3 animals from which four to six samples of each structure were analyzed. Abbreviations are: fructokinase, FK; hexokinase, HK (14); phosphofructokinase, PFK (17), fructose-bisphosphatase, FP (16), glucose-6-phosphatase, GP (16), glomerulus, G; proximal convoluted tubule, early and late, PC_E, PC_L; proximal straight tubule, early and late, PS_E, PS_L; thin limb area, TL; distal straight tubule, DS; distal convoluted tubule, DC; and papilla area, PP. The points are connected for visualization and separations bear no relation to the length of the tubules.

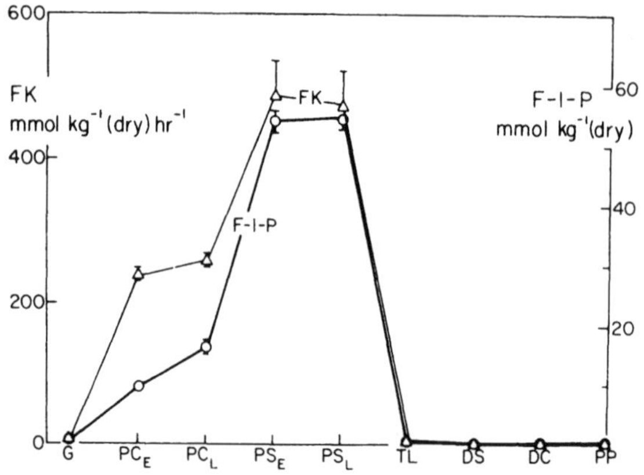

Fig. 2. Comparison of the distribution of fructose-1-P and fructokinase in different parts of the nephron after fructose loads. For fructose-1-phosphate (F-1-P) each point represents the average ±SE of four to eight samples of each structure from a typical rat given $40\ mmol \cdot kg^{-1}$ fructose. For fructokinase the averages ±SE are of 3 control animals. Abbreviations are as in Fig. 1.

with highest levels in the distal portions (data not shown).

Effect of fructose loads on fructose and glucose distribution

A fructose load of $40\ mmol \cdot kg^{-1}$ increased plasma fructose 160-fold (from 0.065 to 10.4 mM) and increased plasma glucose about 2-fold (to 11.7 mM). Fructose distribution in the nephron was not measured in normal kidneys, but must be very low; the concentration is no higher than $0.8\ mmol \cdot kg^{-1}$ dry weight in either whole cortex or whole medulla (Burch *et al.*, 1970). After the fructose load, fructose concentration rose to $100\ mmol \cdot kg^{-1}$ (dry) in the glomerulus and $650\ mmol \cdot kg^{-1}$ in the papilla with intermediate levels in structures between. Glucose also increased in the nephron, but the largest changes were only 3-fold.

Phosphorylated intermediates

Normal fructose-1-P levels in whole kidney cortex are only about $0.4\ mmol \cdot kg^{-1}$. A $40\ mmol \cdot kg^{-1}$ fructose load increased the level of this first fructose metabolite to the extraordinary concentration of $50\ mmol \cdot kg^{-1}$ dry weight in the proximal straight tubule (Fig. 2). There was a remarkable correspondence along the nephron between the levels of fructose-1-P and the activity of fructokinase.

After a fructose load fructose bisphosphate (plus triose phosphate) levels in the proximal tubule were proportional to fructose-1-P but were 40 times lower on an absolute basis (Fig. 3). Elsewhere in the nephron the situation was reversed, with fructose bisphosphate actually higher than fructose-1-P. In the distal straight tubule and thin limb area the bisphosphate was as high as in the proximal straight tubule. Presumably fructose bisphosphate in the proximal tubules arises mainly from fructose-1-P via dihydroxyacetone-P and glyceraldehyde-P. In the other parts of the nephron it is probably formed directly from fructose-6-P, produced either from glucose-6-P or from fructose by hexokinase action. The

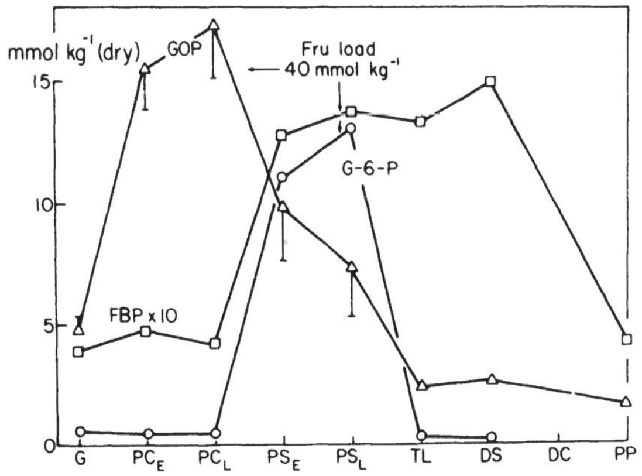

Fig. 3. The distribution of phosphorylated intermediates among different parts of the nephron after fructose loads. Most abbreviations are as in Fig. 1. Glucose-6-P is G6P; glycerol-1-P, GOP; and fructose bisphosphate (plus triose phosphates) FBP. Note FBP levels have been multiplied by 10.

exceedingly high fructose levels would make the latter a likely route in spite of the high fructose K_m.

Glucose-6-P increased almost as dramatically as fructose-1-P as a result of the fructose loads (Fig. 3) and the changes were restricted to the proximal tubule. However, there was one essential difference: The increases in the convoluted portions were minor (3- or 4-fold compared to the 50-fold increases in the straight portions). The much higher level in the straight segments can be reasonably explained by a combination of the 3-fold higher fructose bisphosphate concentration, with nearly as much fructose bisphosphatase and 5- to 15-fold lower glucose-6-P phosphatase activity (Burch *et al.*, 1978).

Another metabolite which accumulated to a remarkable degree in the proximal tubule after fructose loads is glycerol-1-P (Fig. 3). However, in this case the peak occurred in the convoluted segments. We have no explanation for this difference, in the face of the lower level of fructose bisphosphate plus triose phosphates in the convoluted tubules. It cannot be attributed to glycerol-P dehydrogenase which although very active (2.5–3 mol·kg^{-1} (dry)·hr^{-1}) is about the same in both segments. Possibly glycerol-P oxidase, the flavoprotein, is lower in the convoluted portion.

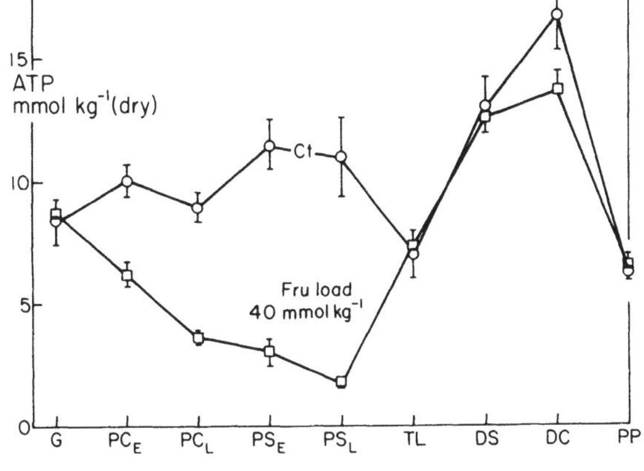

Fig. 4. Distribution of ATP in control and fructose loaded rats. Each point for control animals is the average ±SE of 3 or 4 animals. For a typical fructose loaded animal points are averages ±SE of four to eight samples of each structure.

Distribution pattern of ATP

The highest level of ATP in normal rat nephron is in the distal convoluted tubule where it is twice the level in the proximal convoluted segments (Fig. 4). Lowest levels are in thin limb and papilla areas. After the high fructose loads, ATP fell 58% in proximal convoluted and 80% in proximal straight tubules, with no significant changes elsewhere. The decrease in ATP after giving fructose has been attributed to the depletion of P_i, which is known to occur in both liver and kidney (Raivo *et al.*, 1969; Burch *et al.*, 1970; Morris *et al.*, 1978; Woods *et al.*, 1970) and which in turn is attributed to sequestration of P_i, primarily as fructose-1-P, although in the present case, in the proximal convoluted tubule almost as much phosphate is tied up as glycerol-P. The increases in the metabolites that were measured, and which contain phosphate, total 34 and 56 mmol·kg^{-1} in the convoluted and straight tubules respectively. These far exceed the calculated loss from ATP (5.8 and 8.5 mmol·kg^{-1} respectively).

From the greater changes in ATP in the straight segment, one would predict that this would be the site of the greatest damage from fructose-1-P aldolase deficiency or from giving large fructose loads. Although the proximal tubule is known to be the site of injury, (Yu & Philips, personal communication) which part of the proximal tubule suffers first or most has not been reported.

REFERENCES

Bowman R. H. (1970) Gluconeogenesis in the isolated perfused kidney. *J. biol. Chem.* **245,** 1604–1612.

Brannan T. S., Corder C. N. & Rizk M. (1975) Histochemical measurements of rat kidney hexokinase. *Proc. Soc. exp. Biol. Med.* **148,** 714–719.

Burch H. B., Lowry O. H., Kuhlman A. M., Skerjance J., Diamant E. J., Lowry S. R. & Von Dippe P. (1963) Changes in patterns of enzymes of carbohydrate metabolism in the developing liver. *J. biol. Chem.* **238,** 2267–2273.

Burch H. B., Lowry O. H., Meinhardt L., Max P. Jr & Chyu K. (1970) Effect of fructose, dihydroxyacetone, glycerol and glucose on metabolites and related compounds in liver and kidney. *J. biol. Chem.* **245,** 2092–2102.

Burch H. B., Narins R. G., Chu C., Fagioli S., Choi S., McCarthy W. & Lowry O. H. (1978) Distribution along the rat nephron of three enzymes of gluconeogenesis in acidosis and starvation. *Am. J. Physiol.* **235,** F 246–F253.

Chan A. W. K., Burch H. B., Alvey T. R. & Lowry O. H. (1975) A quantitative histochemical approach to renal transport—I. Aspartate and glutamate. *Am. J. Physiol.* **229,** 1034–1044.

Froesch E. (1978) Essential fructosuria, hereditary fructose intolerance, and fructose-1,6-diphosphatase deficiency. In *Metabolic Basis of Inherited Disease* (Edited by Stanbury J. B., Wyngaarden J. B. & Fredrickson D. S.) pp. 121–136. McGraw-Hill, New York.

GÜNTHER M. A., SILLERO A. & SOLS A. (1967) Fructokinase assay with a specific spectrophotometric method using 1-phosphofructokinase. *Enzym. biol. clin.* **8,** 341–352.

HEMS D. A. & GAJA G. (1972) Carbohydrate metabolism in the isolated perfused rat kidney. *Biochem. J.* **128,** 421–426.

KATO T. S., BERGER S. J., CARTER J. A. & LOWRY O. H. (1973) An enzymatic cycling method for nicotinamide-adenine dinucleotide with malic and alcohol dehydrogenases. *Analyt. Biochem.* **53,** 86–89.

KREBS H. A. & LUND P. (1966) Formation of glucose from hexoses, pentoses, polyols and related substances in kidney cortex. *Biochem. J.* **98,** 210–214.

LOWRY O. H. & PASSONNEAU J. V. (1972) *A Flexible System of Enzymatic Analysis,* pp. 221–260. Academic Press, New York.

MORRIS R. C. JR, NIGON K. & REED E. B. (1978) Evidence that the severity of depletion of inorganic phosphate determines the severity of the disturbance of adenine nucleotide metabolism in the liver and renal cortex of the fructose-loaded rat. *J. clin. Invest.* **61,** 209–220.

RAIVO K. O., KEKOMAKI M. P. & MAENPAA P. K. (1966) Depletion of liver adenine nucleotides induced by D-fructose. Dose dependence and specificity of the fructose effect. *Biochem. Pharmac.* **18,** 2615–2620.

REEVES R. E., WARREN L. G. & HSU D. S. (1966) 1-phosphofructokinase from an anaerobe. *J. biol. Chem.* **241,** 1257–1261.

SCHMID H., SCHOLZ M., MALL A., SCHMIDT U., GUDER W. G. & DUBACH U. C. (1978) Carbohydrate metabolism in rat kidney: heterogeneous distribution of glycolytic and gluconeogenic key enzymes. In *Biochemical Nephrology,* (Edited by GUDER W. G. & SCHMIDT U.) pp. 282–289. Hans Huber, Bern.

SCHMIDT U., MAROSVARY I. & DUBACH U. C. (1975) Renal metabolism of glucose: anatomical sites of hexokinase activity in the rat nephron. *FEBS Lett.* **53,** 26–28.

WOODS H. F., EGGLESTON L. V. & KREBS H. A. (1970) The cause of hepatic accumulation of fructose 1-phosphate on fructose loading. *Biochem. J.* **119,** 501–506.

SYMPOSIUM DISCUSSION

Lemieux: Do you have any idea of the concentration of fructose in the tubular fluid along the nephron when you load animals with fructose?

Burch: We did not measure the difference between fructose of the luminal fluid and the cells. The results on freeze-dried samples represent both. The progressive increase in concentration of fructose along the nephron probably reflects an increase in concentration in the fluid, particularly in more distal structures. To use inulin as a tubular fluid marker would cause difficult analytical problems since it is measured as fructose.

Saggerson: Are these animals hypoglycaemic? How much renal damage in hereditary fructose intolerance could be attributed to hypoglycaemia?

Burch: The animals are moderately hyperglycaemic (11 mM). In hereditary fructose intolerance hypoglycaemia is induced by fructose. The renal damage is more likely to result from the metabolic consequences of the deficiency of fructose-1-P aldolase.

Guder: Your results explain some observations which we have obtained when we studied the interaction of cyclic AMP producing hormones with substrates. When we increased cAMP production in isolated tubule fragments, by adding PTH, we could completely suppress the increase by simultaneous addition of dihydroxyacetone, but we could not do this with fructose (unpublished work in this laboratory). Our conclusion at that time was that there must be some heterogeneity on the proximal tubule between the glycerol-consuming cells which may be PTH-responsive, and the fructose-metabolising cells which are not. If we put your data and Dr Chabardes's data together, we can draw a map between glycerol, fructose metabolism and PTH interaction. Glycerol phosphate production seem to use ATP which might otherwise be used for cAMP formation after PTH.

Brosnan: Can I ask a technical question about this procedure for measuring metabolites? Since you cannot freeze-clamp and still preserve structure, how rapidly can you freeze the inner cells of these kidneys?

Burch: Dropping the kidney into liquid Freon at $-160°C$ it takes a few seconds to freeze (for brain cortex it takes 2–3 sec). We have a more efficient method which uses "pumped out" nitrogen. By preventing the formation of bubbles around the tissue in liquid nitrogen, freezing is accelerated.

Vinay: Have you any measurement of glutamate or aspartate or P_i after fructose?

Burch: No, we have published such figures for glutamate and aspartate after a glutamine load (Burch *et al., Kidney Int.* **14,** 406, 1978). P_i was not measured either, since we know that it falls in parallel with ATP. I did confirm that this was the case in PCA extracts of gross slices of outer cortex and outer stripe of outer medulla.

Angielski: With regard to Dr Guder's comment on your findings, I find if difficult to see even the lowered ATP concentration after fructose being sufficient to compete with the formation of cAMP.

Epstein: The fact that the ATP drops so dramatically in the proximal tubule makes this a wonderful tool for seeing how important the level of ATP is for transport in the tubule. When we did this some time ago, we were disappointed to find no perceptible diuresis. Perhaps, if we had micropunctured the proximal tubule, we might have seen something.

Osswald: Are there haemodynamic changes in kidney following a heavy fructose load?

Burch: I can only report that in the sections after fructose, the vessels along the tubules in the medulla were especially full of blood, but I don't know what this means.

Morel: There is a clear message in this presentation: it is quite possible to measure not only enzymes but also substrates in minute amounts of tissue, with good accuracy, so this will completely change our view of the biochemical approach to kidney function. Biochemical heterogeneity can now be followed at the cellular level.

Burch: This, Dr Morel, is a direct consequence of the many years of work performed by Dr Lowry in developing methods for mapping enzymes and substrates in the brain.

Int. J. Biochem., Vol. 12, pp. 41 to 45
0020-711X/80/0701-0041$02.00/0

DISTRIBUTION OF ACID HYDROLASES IN THE NEPHRON OF NORMAL AND DIABETIC RATS

MICHEL LE HIR and ULRICH C. DUBACH
Medizinische Universitäts-Poliklinik, Enzym-Biologie-Labor, Petersgraben 4, CH 4031 Basel, Switzerland
and
WALTER G. GUDER
Städtisches Krankenhaus München-Schwabing, Klinisch-Chemisches Institut, Kölner Platz 1, 8000 München 40, FRG

Abstract—1. β-D-Galactosidase (β-Gal), N-acetyl-β-D-glucosaminidase (NAG) and acid phosphatase (ac-Pase) have different distribution patterns along the nephron.

2. The main site of reabsorption (heterophagocytosis) for macromolecules coincides with the maximal activity of NAG and, somewhat less distinctly with β-Gal, namely in the first two or three of the five dissected individual parts in the proximal tubule.

3. With the exception for CCD in starved animals, alloxan diabetes and starvation induce activity changes of NAG and β-Gal only in parts where reabsorption of macromolecules occurs (PCT and PSTC2).

4. We conclude that NAG and β-Gal in the last parts of the proximal and in the distal tubule, and ac-Pase in the whole nephron must be mainly involved in cellular turnover (autophagocytosis).

5. Higher activity of NAG and β-Gal in the first parts of the proximal tubule are needed for heterophagocytosis.

6. Our hypothesis: in starvation and alloxan diabetes activity distribution of the glycohydrolases NAG and β-Gal may reflect an impaired reabsorption of proteins in the early proximal tubule.

INTRODUCTION

The lysosomes digest components of the cell (autophagocytosis) as well as extracellular materials (heterophagocytosis. They not only bring about the turnover of organelles and macromolecules, but also participate in the regulation of metabolites. Our understanding of the role of lysosomes in the kidney is complicated by the heterogeneity of the organ. A means of overcoming this obstacle lies in the determination of lysosomal enzymes in microdissected parts of the nephron. In this way, the adaptation of the lysosomal system to various physiological conditions can be studied with respect to known metabolic changes. Because it was observed that lysosomal glycohydrolase activity decreases in diabetes mellitus (Fushimi & Tarui, 1976) and because the metabolic events in this disease are well documented, we studied the distribution of β-D-galactosidase (β-Gal), N-acetyl-β-D-glucosaminidase (NAG) and acid phosphatase (ac-Pase) in 11 parts of the nephron in normal fed, starved and alloxan-diabetic rats.

MATERIALS AND METHODS

Animals

Male Wistar rats, about 200 g body weight, were used. The normal and starved rats (strain B) were killed by decapitation at 10 a.m.

To induce diabetes, alloxan (100 mg·kg^{-1} body weight) was injected in the tail vein (strain A rats). Some animals did not become hyperglycemic (group No Diabetes). The animals, which developed glucosuria were given 4 Units insulin twice daily from the day after alloxan treatment. One group was treated for eight days until sacrificed (group Diabetes + Insulin). In another group insulin was withdrawn after five days. These animals developed hyperglycemia, glucosuria and ketonuria during the following 2 to 3 days.

The kidneys were taken from living animals after blood had been drawn from the aorta under light Nembutal anaesthesia.

Preparation of the tissue

The kidneys were rapidly removed and frozen in liquid N_2. Sections, 16 μm thick, were cut in a cryostat. Each second section was stained with the aqueous P.A.S. method. The other sections were freeze-dried and stored at −40°C. The following parts of the nephron were identified by their position and staining (Fig. 1):

Glomerulus G
Proximal convoluted tubule PCT
Cortical proximal straight tubule PSTC
—PSTC2, localized near the capsule in the medullary rays. It corresponds to the straight part of the segment S2 (nomenclature according to Maunsbach, 1966).
—PSTC3E, early portion of the S3 (Maunsbach, 1966) dissected at the level of the mid-cortex.
—PSTC3L, localized near the cortico-medullary border.
Medullary proximal straight tubule PSTM dissected from the outer stripe.
Distal straight tubule DST:
—DSTI from the inner stripe
—DSTO from the outer stripe
—DSTC from the medullary rays.
Distal convoluted tubule DCT, including the different parts of the distal tubule in the cortical labyrinth (Kaissling *et al.*, 1977)
Cortical collecting ducts CCD.

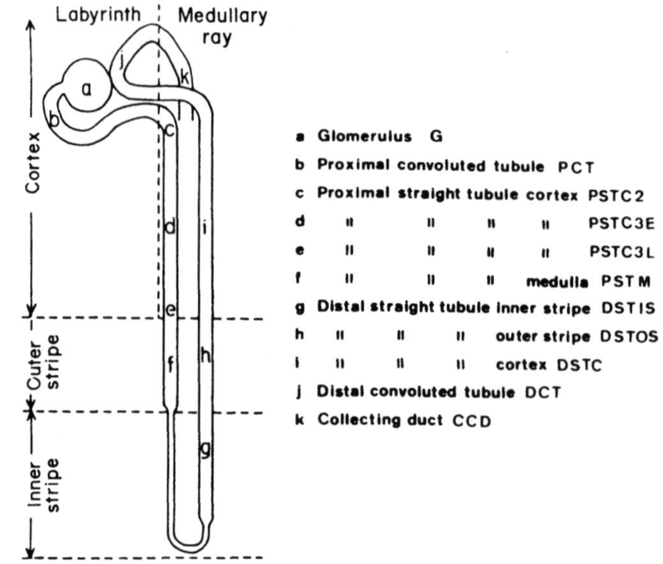

Fig. 1. Diagram of the nephron showing the eleven dissected parts.

The convoluted proximal and distal parts and the glomeruli were dissected out of the superficial half of the cortex including superficial and mid-cortical nephrons. Accordingly, care was taken to choose straight parts from the middle of the medullary rays to be sure that they do not belong to nephrons from deeper seated glomeruli (Kriz *et al.*, 1972). Single dissected pieces were weighed on a quartz-fiber balance.

Enzyme assays

The substrates were derivatives of methylumbelliferon (SERVA, Heidelberg). Previously described procedures for incubation (Robinson, 1970; Hultberg & Oeckermann, 1972; Lake & Ellis, 1976) were adapted with slight modifications for the micromethod.

β-Gal: 0.5 mM methylumbelliferyl-β-D-galactoside in 0.1 M acetate–HCl buffer pH 4.5.

NAG: 0.4 mM methylumbelliferyl-*N*-acetyl-β-D-glucosaminide in 0.1 M phosphate–citrate buffer pH 4.5.

ac-Pase: 0.1 mM methylumbelliferyl-phosphate in 0.1 M citrate–HCl buffer pH 5.

The dissected tissue was transferred to the bottom of a pyrex tube of 3 mm diameter. The tubes were placed in crushed ice and 10 μl of the substrate solution added to each. The blanks contained no tissue. Six tubes received 10 μl of dilutions of methylumbelliferon (100–2000 nM) in

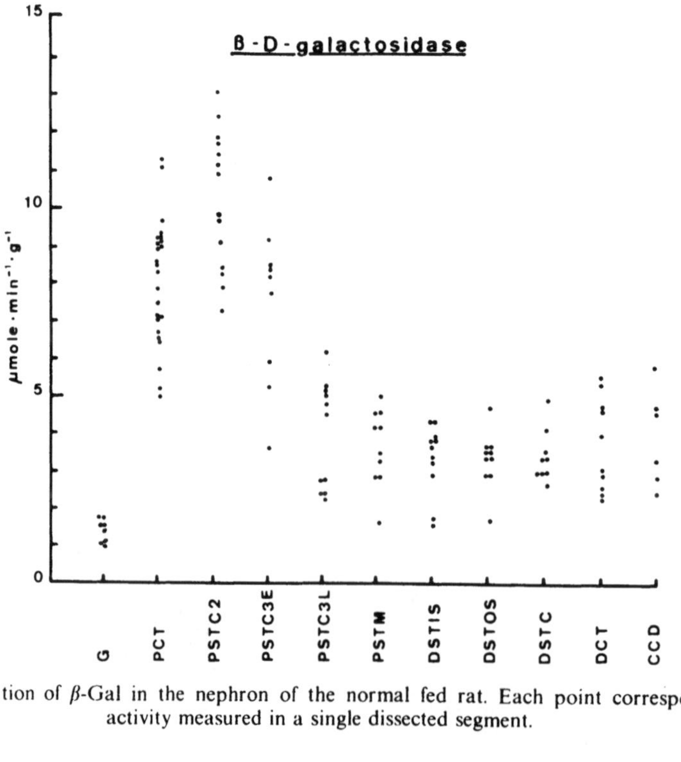

Fig. 2. Distribution of β-Gal in the nephron of the normal fed rat. Each point corresponds to the activity measured in a single dissected segment.

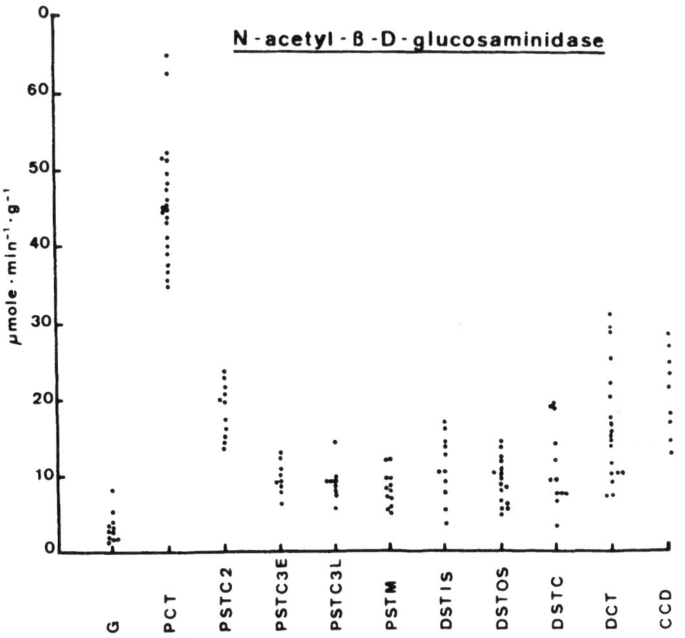

Fig. 3. Distribution of NAG in the nephron of the normal fed rat. Each point corresponds to the activity measured in a single dissected segment.

buffer for the elaboration of a standard curve. The incubation was started at 37°C. After 60 min (NAG) or 120 min (β-Gal and ac-Pase) the reaction was stopped in ice. 200 μl 0.5 M glycine–NaOH buffer pH 10.4 were added to each tube. After mixing, the solution was transferred to fluorimeter cuvettes. Measurements were made at 360 nm (I) and 450 nm (II). The results are expressed in units (μmol methylumbelliferon liberated per min) per g dry tissue.

RESULTS

Normal fed rats

Each enzyme was determined in samples from five animals.

The activity of β-Gal (Fig. 2) is low in glomeruli, and particularly high in the convoluted part and the beginning of the straight part of the proximal tubule. It does not change much along the whole distal tubule where it is similar to that found in the last half of the proximal straight part and the collecting duct. The activity of NAG (Fig. 3) is very low in glomeruli and reaches a maximum in the proximal convoluted tubule. It decreases markedly at the transition to the straight part. Considerable individual differences were found in the straight part of the distal tubule. The activity increases in the distal convolution where large differences are found in the same animal, probably due to the fact that we could not identify the different parts of this segment.

Maximal activity of ac-Pase is found in the straight part of the proximal tubule (Fig. 4). In the distal tubule the activity is lower than in the proximal tubule.

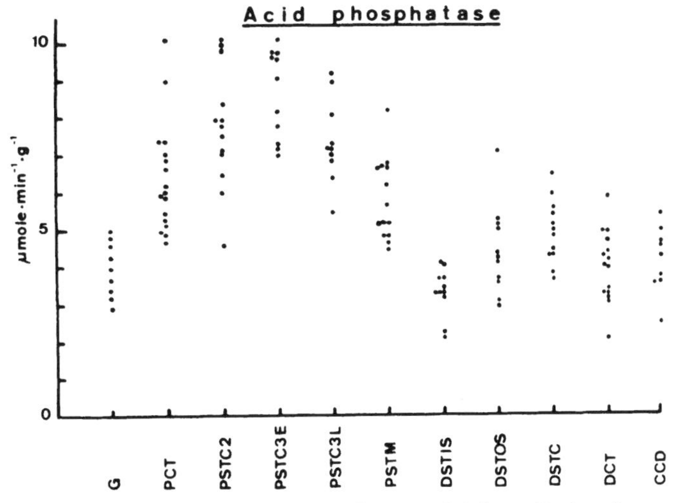

Fig. 4. Distribution of ac-Pase in the nephron of the normal fed rat. Each point corresponds to the activity measured in a single dissected segment.

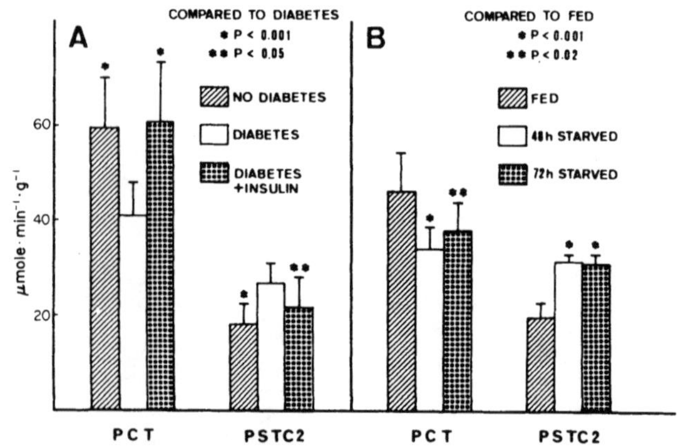

Fig. 5. Activity of NAG in the convoluted part (PCT) and the beginning of the straight part (PST2) of the proximal tubule. A. In alloxan diabetic rats, compared to alloxan treated rats which did not become diabetic and to alloxan diabetic rats treated with insulin up to sacrifice. B. In starved rats, compared with rats fed *ad libitum* up to sacrifice. The animals in the experiments A and B were of two different strains; the activity in controls were somewhat different in A and B, but the distribution was the same.

Starved rats

β-Gal and NAG were assayed in rats starved for 24, 48 and 72 hr (two animals at a time). Animals starved for 24 hr showed the same activities as fed ones. After 48 and 72 hr no significant differences appeared for β-Gal, but the distribution of NAG was clearly modified. The activity decreased about 20% in the proximal convolution, but increased 60% in the first portion of the straight part (Fig. 5A) and 100% in the collecting duct. No changes were induced by starving in other parts.

Diabetic rats

In the absence of hyperglycaemia alloxan treatment (two rats; blood glucose 7.45, 7.59 mM) caused only insignificant changes in the activity of the glycosidases. Their activity pattern is the same as in diabetic animals treated with insulin up to the time of sacrifice (three rats; blood glucose 6.8, 4.2, 2.3 mM). In comparison with these two groups, in diabetic rats deprived of insulin (three rats; blood glucose 32.4, 22, 13.1 mM) the activities of the glycosidases were reduced by 30% ($P < 0.001$) in the proximal convolution. At the beginning of the straight part, NAG—but not β-Gal—was higher than in the control groups (Fig. 5B). No changes were found in any other parts of the nephron.

DISCUSSION

Significant activity of the three hydrolases investigated is present in all segments of rat nephron and may be related to the autophagocytotic function of lysosomes (intracellular turnover).

The particularly high activities of NAG and β-Gal in the two or three first parts of the proximal tubule can be correlated to a high heterophagocytosis at this level (reabsorption). Glycoproteins represent most probably the major substrates for lysosomal NAG and β-Gal in the nephron. The clear peak of NAG in the proximal convolution (Fig. 3) coincides well with the site of maximal reabsorption of proteins (Straus, 1964; Bourdeau *et al.*, 1972). The maximum activity of β-Gal at the beginning of the straight part (PSTC2) is difficult to explain (Fig. 2). The uptake of glycoproteins is strongly affected by the composition of their sugar moieties (Horisberger & Von Lanthen, 1978; Schlesinger *et al.*, 1978; Ullrich *et al.*,1979). Galactose-rich molecules might be reabsorbed in the straight portion, which would explain the very high activity of β-Gal in PSTC2 and PSTC3E. Moreover, while most NAG in the kidney is bound to organelles, a greater part of β-Gal is known to be soluble (Price & Dance, 1967; Chang & Perry, 1979; Pierce *et al.*, 1979) and therefore not related to lysosomal activity. Finally, at least two forms of β-Gal with different substrate affinities exist in the kidney (Price & Dance, 1967), whereas only one form of NAG was found in tubular fragments and glomeruli (Taylor *et al.*, 1971). Therefore the activity of NAG might be a better indicator than β-Gal for the lysosomal system.

Starvation and diabetes mellitus induce similar changes of the activity of NAG in the proximal tubule (Fig. 5). In both cases the lysosomal system could have been directly influenced by insulin deficiency. An increase of fatty acids, ketone bodies and amino acids in plasma is another common feature of starvation and diabetes. A high concentration of acids in the glomerular filtrate could impair the reabsorption of proteins. Prolonged exercise in man may cause proteinuria, which was explained by Viberti *et al.* (1978) as a consequence of increased glomerular permeability. In exercise, too, filtered acids could impair tubular reabsorption of proteins. Severe proteinuria due to altered function of the proximal tubule can be induced by intravenous injection of certain amino acids in man (Mogensen & Sølling, 1977). Possibly, if the quantity of aminoacids reaching the straight part is not excessive, proteins which pass the convolution are taken up here. Activation of the lysosomal system at this level could explain the high activity of NAG we observed.

The recent observation of a decrease of proteinuria in diabetic man during strict control of hyperglycemia by insulin (Viberti *et al.*, 1979) can hardly be explained by a reduction of glomerular filtration alone. We postulate that this observation may be explained in addition by a normalized tubular reabsorption after reduction of blood acids through better control of diabetes mellitus. The normalization of lysosomal enzymes after treatment of alloxan diabetic rats with insulin would support this postulate.

Acknowledgements—We thank Mrs J. Bendy and Mrs H. Vortisch for technical assistance. This research was supported by the Swiss National Foundation No. 3.904.077.

REFERENCES

BOURDEAU J. E., CARONE F. A. & GANOTE C. E. (1972) Serum albumin uptake in isolated perfused renal tubules. Quantitative and electron microscope radioautographic studies in three anatomical segments of the rabbit nephron. *J. cell Biol.* **54,** 382–398.

CHANG A. Y. & PERRY C. S. (1979) Acid glycohydrolase in chinese hamster (*cricetulus griseus*) with spontaneous diabetes—V. Subcellular distribution in the kidney. *Comp. Biochem. Physiol.* **62B,** 557–561.

FUSHIMI H. & TARUI S. (1976) β-Glycosidases and diabetic microangiopathy—I. Decrease of β-glycosidase activities in diabetic rat kidney. *J. Biochem.* **79,** 265–270.

HORISBERGER M & VONLANTHEN M. (1978) Simultaneous localization of an hepatic binding protein specific for galactose and of galactose-containing receptors on rat hepatocytes. *J. Histochem. Cytochem.* **26,** 960–966.

HULTBERG B. & ÖCKERMANN P. A. (1972) Artificial substrates in the assay of acid glucosidases. *Clinica. chim. Acta* **39,** 49–58.

KAISSLING B., PETER S. & KRIZ W. (1977) The transition of the thick ascending limb of Henle's loop into the distal convoluted tubule in the nephron of the rat kidney. *Cell Tissue Res.* **182,** 111–118.

KRIZ W., SCHNERMAN J. & KOEPSELL H. (1972) The position of short and long loops of Henle in the rat kidney. *Z. Anat. Entwickl.-Gesch.* **138,** 301–319.

LAKE B. D. & ELLIS R. B. (1976) What do you think you are quantifying? An appraisal of histochemical methods in the measurement of the activities of lysosomal enzymes. *Histochem. J.* **8,** 357–366.

MAUNSBACH A. B. (1966) Absorption of ferritin by rat kidney proximal tubule cells. Electronmicroscopic observations of the initial uptake phase in cells of microperfused single proximal tubules. *J. Ultrastruct. Res.* **16,** 1–12.

MOGENSEN C. E. & SØLLING K. (1977) Studies on renal tubular protein reabsorption: partial and near complete inhibition by certain amino acids. *Scand. J. clin. Lab. Invest.* **37,** 477–486.

PIERCE R. J., SPIK G. & MONTREUIL J. (1979) Cytosolic location of an endo-*N*-acetyl-β-D-glucosaminidase activity in rat liver and kidney. *Biochem. J.* **180,** 673–676.

PRICE R. G. & DANCE N. (1967) The cellular distribution of some rat-kidney glucosidases. *Biochem. J.* **105,** 877–883.

ROBINSON D. (1970) Fluorimetric detection and assay of kidney and urinary β-glucosidases. In *Proceeding of the 7th Congress on Clinical Chemistry* 1969, Vol. 1, Methods in clinical chemistry, pp. 42–52. Karger, Basel.

SCHLESINGER P. H., DOEBBER T. W., MANDELL B. F., WHITE R., DESCHRYVER C., RODMAN J. S., MILLER M. J. & STAHL P. (1978) Plasma clearance of glycoproteins with terminal mannose and *N*-Acetylglucosamine by liver non-parenchymal cells. Studies with β-glucuronidase, *N*-acetyl-β-D-glucosaminidase, ribonuclease B and agalacto-orosomucoid. *Biochem. J.* **176,** 103–109.

STRAUS W. (1964) Occurrence of phagosomes and phagolysosomes in different segments of the nephron in relation to the reabsorption, transport, digestion, and extrusion of intravenously injected horseradish peroxidase. *J. Cell Biol.* **21,** 295–308.

TAYLOR D. G., PRICE R. G. & ROBINSON D. (1970) The distribution of some hydrolases in glomeruli and tubular fragments from rat kidney by zonal centrifugation. *Biochem. J.* **122,** 641–645.

ULLRICH K., BASNER R., GIESELMANN V. & FIGURA K. VON (1979) Recognition of human urine α-*N*-acetylglucosaminidase by rat hepatocytes. Involvement of receptors specific for galactose, mannose-6-phosphate and mannose. *Biochem. J.* **180,** 413–419.

VIBERTI G. C., JARRETT R. J., MCCARTNEY M. & KEEN H. (1978) Increased glomerular permeability to albumin induced by exercise in diabetic subjects. *Diabetologica* **14,** 293–300.

VIBERTI G. C., PICKUP J. C., JARRETT R. J. & KEEN H. (1979) Effect of control of blood glucose on urinary excretion of albumin and β_2 microglobulin in insulin-dependent diabetes. *New Engl. J. Med.* **300,** 638–641.

SYMPOSIUM DISCUSSION

Helwig: The lysosomal hydrolases are populations of very heterogeneous enzymes. For example, there are at least three isoenzymes of acid phosphatase with different properties. What do you know about the variations and distribution of the isoenzymes in diabetes?

Le Hir: The presence of several isoenzymes of acid phosphatase in the kidney is the reason why we did not measure this enzyme in starvation and diabetes. Changes in the measured activity would be a poor indicator of the physiological adaptation of the lysosomal system. On the contrary, *N*-acetyl-β-D-glucosaminidase exists in a single form in the nephron of the rat (Price & Dance (1967) *Biochem. J.* **105,** 877–883) and, therefore, was the best marker for the lysosomes.

Int. J. Biochem., Vol. 12, pp. 47 to 52
© Pergamon Press Ltd 1980. Printed in Great Britain

0020-711X/80/0701-0047$02.00/0

MICRODETERMINATION OF Na-K-ATPase IN SINGLE TUBULES: ITS APPLICATION FOR THE LOCALIZATION OF PHYSIOLOGIC PROCESSES IN THE NEPHRON

ALAIN DOUCET, FRANÇOIS MOREL and ADRIAN I. KATZ
Laboratoire de Physiologie Cellulaire, Collège de France, Paris, France and
Department of Medicine, The University of Chicago Pritzker School of Medicine, Chicago, U.S.A.

Abstract—1. To define the nephron sites where changes in Na-K-ATPase activity occur during physiologic adaptations we developed a simple micromethod sensitive enough to determine ATPase activity in single segments of the mammalian nephron.

2. In mice chronically loaded with potassium, Na-K-ATPase activity increased by 200% in the cortical and medullary collecting tubule, without being substantially altered in any other segment of the nephron.

3. This observation suggests that the collecting tubule is the major site of renal potassium adaptation in this species.

INTRODUCTION

Several adenosine triphosphatases have been linked to energy-requiring transport systems in the kidney but their physiologic role remains unclear, in part because of the heterogenous composition of the tissue homogenates used for analysis. Determination of enzyme activity in discrete tubule segments and its correlation with transport processes identified in the corresponding region of the nephron with micropuncture and microperfusion techniques could circumvent this difficulty and improve our understanding of the role of ATPases in renal function. To date, the only micromethod available for measurement of ATPase activities in single nephrons is that developed by Schmidt *et al.* (1969, 1978) for the analysis of Na-K-ATPase, the biochemical equivalent of the peritubular Na-K-pump (Glynn, 1973). Although this ingenious method has contributed substantially to our understanding of the role of Na-K-ATPase in the tubular handling of sodium, it is technically demanding and has not yet been introduced in other laboratories. Therefore we sought to develop a simpler micromethod that will allow the measurement of ATPase in large numbers of tubules, yet is sensitive enough to determine the enzyme activity in short nephron segments. Description of this method and its application to the study of another tubular transport function, i.e. potassium adaptation in response to chronic K-loading, are the subject of this report.

Na-K-ATPase ALONG THE MAMMALIAN NEPHRON

The micromethod for ATPase determination, based on the direct measurement of radiolabeled inorganic phosphate released by the hydrolysis of [γ-^{32}P]ATP is outlined in Table 1. Nephron segments 0.2–2 mm long were dissected in the cold from a collagenase treated kidney under stereomicroscopic observation. The various tubule segments were identified on the basis of their appearance, diameter and location within the cortex and outer or inner medulla. Each tubule was photographed at constant magnification in order to confirm its identity and to determine its length, and was then exposed to a hypotonic environment followed by rapid freezing on dry ice to increase its permeability to reactants. Incubation was carried out for 15 min at 37°C without agitation in a 1 μl droplet of assay medium, and the reaction was stopped by addition of cold trichloracetic acid. Unhydrolysed ATP was absorbed on activated charcoal and the labeled inorganic phosphate was separated by filtration through a millipore cellulose filter and the radioactivity determined in a liquid scintillation counter.

To verify that the collagenase used for microdissection did not influence ATPase activity, we compared in preliminary experiments the enzymatic activity of nephron segments dissected from one kidney perfused with collagenase and from its mate, perfused with an identical solution from which collagenase was omitted. Results shown in Table 2 indicate that pretreatment with collagenase did not affect significantly Na-K-ATPase activity in any of the nephron segments studied.

Without maneuvers that increase membrane permeability tubules exhibit a low enzymatic activity, probably due to the limited access of ATP to the catalytic sites. Proximal convoluted tubules from rabbit, rat and mouse kidney were dissected and consecutively exposed to a hypoosmotic environment (distilled water) and rapidly frozen: Na-K-ATPase activity, which was almost undetectable before permeabilization, increased markedly after each step of this procedure. This increment can be correlated with the morphologic changes observed in the tubule.

Figure 1 shows photographs of a rabbit proximal convoluted tubule filmed at constant magnification before and after each stage of the permeabilization procedure. Ruthenium red, a dye with a molecular weight similar to that of ATP, was added to the

Table 1. Micromethod for ATPase determination

$[\gamma\text{-}^{32}P]ATP \rightarrow ADP + {}^{32}P_i$

(1) Microdissection: 4°C; modified Hanks (Ca^{2+} 0.25 mM); freehand
(2) Photography:
(3) Hypoosmotic medium: Distilled water
(4) Freezing: Dry-ice
(5) Incubation: 15 min; 37°C; without agitation
1 μl total ATPase: NaCl 50 mM; KCl 5 mM; $MgCl_2$ 10 mM; EGTA 1 mM; Tris–HCl 100 mM; Na_2-ATP (grade II Sigma) 10 mM; $[\gamma\text{-}^{32}P]$ATP ~10 nCi/μl; pH: 7.4
1 μl Mg-ATPase: As above, −NaCl; −KCl; +ouabain 1 mM. Tris–HCl 150 mM
(6) Reaction stopped: 7 μl; 10% activated charcoal in 5% TCA
(7) Filtration: 0.7 ml; Phosphate buffer 0.1%, pH: 6.0

Table 2. Effect of collagenase treatment of ATPase activity of rabbit nephrons

		Mg-ATPase activity			Na-K-ATPase activity		
	*n**	Without	*P*	With	Without	*P*	With
PCT	6	1004 ± 109†	NS‡	1288 ± 79	2574 ± 238	NS	2926 ± 340
PR	5	903 ± 74	NS	786 ± 85	593 ± 103	NS	485 ± 117
MAL	5	1573 ± 90	NS	2026 ± 234	2545 ± 343	NS	2186 ± 181

* Number of animals.
† $Pmols \cdot mm^{-1} \cdot hr^{-1} \pm SE$.
‡ Not significant.

hypoosmotic medium at the concentration of 10^{-3} M. After 15 min exposure to the hypoosmotic medium at 4°C (middle photograph), cells swelled and the tubular diameter increased. Occasionally, rupture of tubule walls and leakage of cell contents were observed. The freezing–thawing step did not modify further the appearance of the tubule, but it enhanced appreciably the penetration of the dye into cells (right panel).

Concentrations of reactants required for maximal activity of the enzyme were: ATP 10 mM, sodium 70 mM and potassium 5 mM. Na-K-ATPase was completely inhibited by omitting sodium and potassium and addition of 1 mM ouabain to the assay medium. Under these conditions, the enzyme activity was a linear function of the incubation time up to 30 min (or double the time chosen in these experiments), and of the tubule length up to 2 mm.

Figure 2 presents the Na-K-ATPase activity along the rat, mouse and rabbit nephron. The enzyme profile was similar in the three species: Na-K-ATPase activity per mm tubule length was highest in the distal convoluted tubule and thick ascending limb of Henle's loop, intermediate in the proximal convoluted tubule, and lower in the pars recta and collecting tubule. The lower activity measured in the rabbit cortical ascending limb can be correlated with the smaller diameter of this structure compared to its medullary portion, a feature unique to the rabbit nephron. The activity measured in the thin limbs of Henle's loop was very low and close to the sensitivity limit of the method. The highest Na-K-ATPase activities were measured in the rat and the lowest in the rabbit nephrons, with those of the mouse nephron occupying an intermediate position.

SITES OF POTASSIUM ADAPTATION IN THE MOUSE NEPHRON

Animals chronically loaded with potassium survive by increasing potassium excretion by the kidney (Berliner *et al.*, 1950; Silva *et al.*, 1973), as well as by

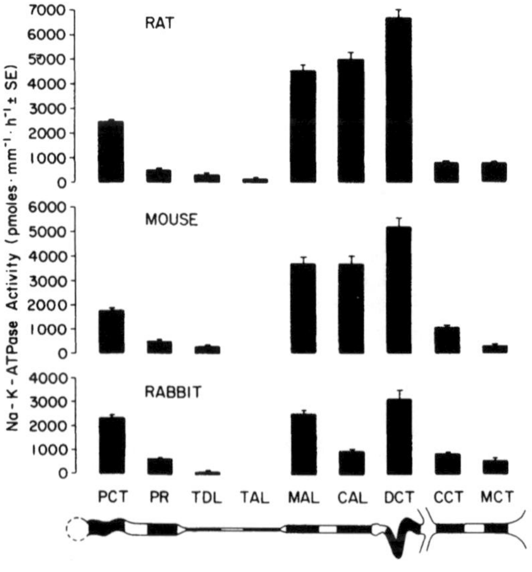

Fig. 2. Na-K-ATPase activity profile in the rat, mouse and rabbit nephron. The enzyme activity profile is similar in the three species. PCT, proximal convoluted tubule; PR, pars recta; TDL, thin descending limb of Henle's loop; TAL, thin ascending limb; MAL, medullary thick ascending limb; CAL, cortical thick ascending limb; DCT, distal convoluted tubule; CCT, cortical collecting tubule; MCT, medullary collecting tubule.

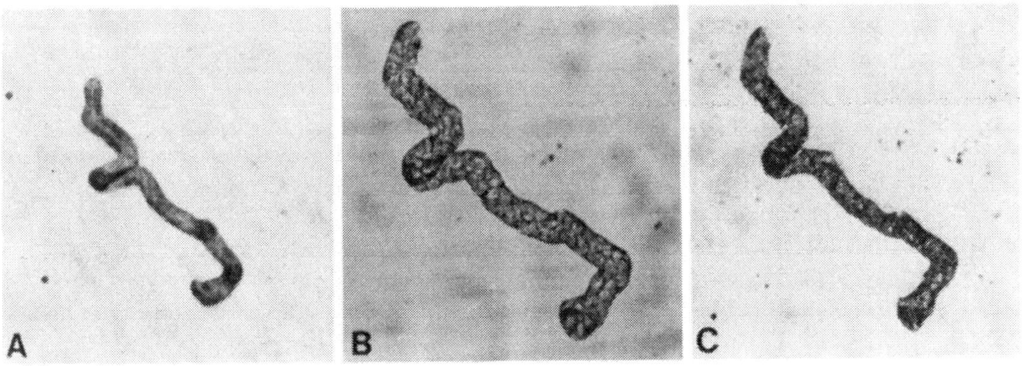

Fig. 1. Rabbit proximal convoluted tubule before treatment (A), after "osmotic shock" (B), and after "osmotic + thermic shock" (C). Ruthenium red 10^{-3} M was added in the hypoosmotic medium. After the "osmotic shock" cells are swollen and the tubule diameter is increased; after the "thermic shock" the dye enters the cells which appear darker.

extrarenal mechanisms (Alexander *et al.*, 1968). During this adaptation net potassium secretion increases in the distal nephron but the site where this increment occurs is disputed. It is generally agreed, however, that the enhanced potassium secretion observed in K-adapted animals is brought about by an increment in intracellular potassium level secondary to the increased activity of the peritubular potassium pump (Schon *et al.*, 1974; Silva *et al.*, 1977; Wright, 1977).

Several lines of evidence indicate that Na-K-ATPase plays an important role in potassium adaptation: first, ouabain, a specific inhibitor of this enzyme, interferes with potassium secretion by the mammalian kidney (Silva *et al.*, 1975), as well as by the isolated rabbit collecting duct (Grantham *et al.*, 1970) and second, the specific activity of Na-K-ATPase measured in kidney homogenates increases during potassium loading (Silva *et al.*, 1973, 1975; Schon *et al.*, 1974; Finkelstein *et al.*, 1975). In an attempt to identify the sites where the enzyme is stimulated, which presumably correspond to the nephron segments where enhanced potassium secretion occurs, we measured the activity profile of Na-K-ATPase along the nephron of K-loaded mice, using the micromethod just described.

Loaded mice fed a potassium-enriched diet (2 mmol KCl/g) for at least 12 days prior to study, ingested 10 times as much potassium as mice fed the standard diet. Urinary potassium excretion paralleled intake, while plasma potassium and GFR were similar in the two groups. Absolute K excretion and its clearance were markedly enhanced in loaded mice, in which fractional potassium clearance averaged 87% compared to 13% in controls.

Figure 3 presents the Na-K-ATPase activity along the nephron of control and K-loaded mice. Enzyme activity increased by 225 and 177%, respectively, in the cortical and medullary portions of the collecting duct of K-loaded mice over the corresponding measurements in control animals. There was no significant effect of potassium loading in any other nephron segment except for the medullary thick ascending limb of Henle's loop in which a slight (25%) increase was observed. The increment in ATPase activity in the collecting tubule and the medullary ascending limb was confined to its Na-K-dependent component, as Mg-dependent ATPase remained unaffected along the entire nephron.

The absence of enzyme activation in the distal convoluted tubule, a segment in which enhancement of potassium secretion during K-loading was previously reported by Wright *et al.* (1971), was unexpected. We searched therefore for a more subtle effect on the distal convoluted tubule enzyme, such as changes in its affinity for K or ouabain, but found no difference between K-loaded and control animals in these measurements as well. A plausible explanation for this discrepancy is that the effect noticed in micropuncture experiments occurred in fact in a later segment, but was attributed to the distal convoluted tubule at a time when the current knowledge of the distal nephron structure was not yet available.

SUMMARY

Na-K-ATPase was measured in all segments of the rabbit, rat and mouse nephron with a simple micromethod based on the direct measurement of radiolabeled phosphate liberated from the hydrolysis of [γ-^{32}P]ATP.

Enzyme activity per mm tubule length was highest in the distal convoluted tubule and the thick ascending limb, intermediate in the proximal convoluted tubule and lower in the pars recta and collecting tubule.

During chronic potassium loading in the mouse Na-K-ATPase activity increases strikingly only in the collecting tubule, suggesting that this nephron segment is the major site of potassium adaptation in this species.

Acknowledgements—This work was supported by grants from C.N.R.S. (to LA 219) and from the National Institutes of Health (AM 13601).

REFERENCES

ALEXANDER E. A. & LEVINSKY N. G. (1968) An extrarenal mechanism of potassium adaptation. *J. clin. Invest.* **47,** 740–748.

BERLINER R. W., KENNEDY T. J. JR & HILTON J. G. (1950) Renal mechanisms for excretion of potassium. *Am. J. Physiol.* **162,** 348–367.

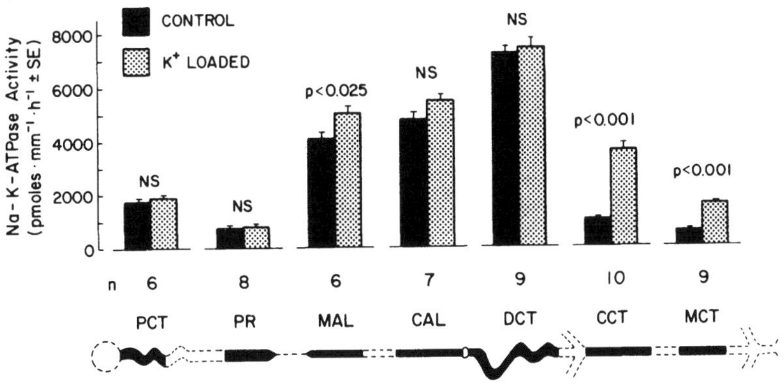

Fig. 3. Na-K-ATPase activity profile along the nephron of control (solid bars) and potassium loaded (hatched bars) mice. Abbreviations are the same as in Fig. 2. *n* represents the number of animals. Enzyme activity increased markedly in the cortical collecting tubule (225%) and medullary collecting tubule (177%) of K-loaded animals.

FINKELSTEIN F. O. & HAYSLETT J. P. (1975) Role of medullary Na-K-ATPase in renal potassium adaptation. *Am. J. Physiol.* **229,** 524–528.

GLYNN I. M. (1973) The nature of the sodium pump. In *Modern Diuretic Therapy in the Treatment of Cardiovascular and Renal Disease.* pp. 179–187. Excerpta Medica, Amsterdam.

GRANTHAM J. J., BURG M. B. & ORLOFF J. (1970) The nature of transtubular Na and K transport in isolated rabbit renal collecting tubules. *J. clin. Invest.* **49,** 1815–1825.

SCHMIDT U. & DUBACH U. C. (1969) Activity of (Na^+–K^+)-stimulated adenosine-triphosphatase in rat nephron. *Pflügers Arch. ges. Physiol.* **306,** 219–226.

SCHMIDT U. & HORSTER M. (1978) Sodium–potassium-activated adenosine triphosphatase: methodology for quantification in microdissected renal tubule segments from freeze-dried and fresh tissue. In *Methods in Pharmacology* (Edited by MARTINEZ-MALDONADO M.) Vol. 4B, pp. 259–296. Plenum Press, New York.

SCHON D. A., SILVA P. & HAYSLETT J. P. (1974) Mechanism of potassium excretion in renal insufficiency. *Am. J. Physiol.* **227,** 1323–1330.

SILVA P., HAYSLETT J. P. & EPSTEIN F. H. (1973). The role of Na-K-activated adenosine triphosphatase in potassium adaptation: Stimulation of enzymatic activity by potassium loading. *J. clin. Invest.* **52,** 2665–2671.

SILVA P., ROSS B. D., CHARNEY A. N., BESARAB A. & EPSTEIN F. H. (1975) Potassium transport by the isolated perfused kidney. *J. clin. Invest.* **56,** 862–869.

SILVA P., BROWN R. S. & EPSTEIN F. H. (1977) Adaptation to potassium. *Kidney Int.* **11,** 466–475.

WRIGHT F. S., STRIEDER N., FOWLER N. B. & GIEBISCH G. (1971) Potassium secretion by distal tubule after potassium adaptation. *Am. J. Physiol.* **221,** 437–448.

WRIGHT F. S. (1977) Sites and mechanisms of potassium transport along the renal tubule. *Kidney Int.* **11,** 415–432.

SYMPOSIUM DISCUSSION

Osswald: Dr Doucet, do you have figures on potassium depletion? In DOCA escape you should see exactly the opposite, with a fall in the ability of the tubules to reabsorb NaCl.

Doucet: We have not studied potassium depletion.

Koepsell: Can you exclude the possibility that the differences in Na-K-ATPase activity which you measure in the different segments of the tubule may be due to different sensitivity of the enzyme to the separation procedure of freezing and hypo-osmotic shock? It is well known that the Na-K-ATPase is sensitive to these procedures in a way which is dependent on the concentrations of ions, and on the lipid composition of the membranes in which the enzyme is found.

Doucet: That is a difficult point to investigate because of the multiplicity of the factors involved. The collagenase treatment does not affect Na-K-ATPase activity (see Table 2). The permeabilisation steps seem to affect the enzyme activity in a similar way in the different structures studied by us (proximal convoluted tubule and medullary ascending limb) in all three species. Finally, we carried out some experiments on sodium and potassium activation of the enzyme from different regions of the nephron and we found that they had the same properties. We did not check structures without the permeabilization procedures, because the activity is undetectable under those circumstances.

Kiil: Sejersted (*Acta physiol. scand.* **99,** 323, 1977) found that within half an hour, during saline loading, an increase of 15–20% in the Na-K-ATPase activity, even in the presence of inhibitors of protein synthesis. This would suggest an effect of an acute increase in sodium load. We find in acute experiments that potassium itself does not have any effect on the enzyme if the plasma concentration is higher than 3–4 mM (Monclair *et al., Scand. J. clin. Lab. invest.*, In press).

Doucet: Sodium excretion probably increases, since the urine volume increases, but we are not dealing with sodium-loading: sodium intake was similar in both groups of animals. Further, we are describing a 300% activation, not 20%.

Kiil: No, I am talking about the thick ascending limb, in which the activity may be very low to start with, so that a rather small increase is required to give a figure of 300%.

Int. J. Biochem., Vol. 12, pp. 53 to 54
© Pergamon Press Ltd 1980. Printed in Great Britain

0020-711X/80/0701-0053$02.00/0

INVITED DISCUSSION

SUBSTRATE OXIDATION BY DEFINED SINGLE NEPHRON SEGMENTS OF RAT KIDNEY

KEITH I. KLEIN, MAW-SONG WANG, SHOZO TORIKAI, WARREN DAVIDSON and KIYOSHI KUROKAWA

Nephrology Sections, Research and Medical Services, VA Wadsworth Medical Center and Harbor General Hospital, and Department of Medicine, UCLA School of Medicine, Los Angeles, CA 90073, U.S.A.

Each defined nephron segment possesses distinct properties of fluid and electrolyte transport. Active solute transport which occurs in some nephron segments is supported by biochemical processes which are accompanied by the metabolism of a variety of substrates to generate high energy compounds such as ATP. It has been generally accepted that metabolism of renal cortex is characterized by aerobic oxidation of substrates and gluconeogenesis while that of renal medulla is characterized by glycolysis. However, little information is available regarding the metabolic characteristics and the specificity of metabolic fuels utilized in each defined nephron segment. Although the distribution of some key enzymes along the nephron segments has been studied by histochemical and microenzyme assays (Schmidt & Guder, 1976), these studies do not necessarily provide information on the metabolic rates and on the substrates preferentially utilized in each nephron segments.

In the present studies, we investigated substrate decarboxylation by the proximal convoluted tubules (PCT) dissected from collagenase-treated rat renal cortex, cortical (CTAL) and medullary (MTAL) thick ascending limb of Henle's loop. These are all sites of active transport probably supported by oxidative metabolism, evidenced by richness in mitochondria in these segments.

Isolated tubules (1–6 segments per incubation) were incubated at 37°C for 60 min in 150 μl KRB buffer containing ^{14}C-labeled substrate at a concentration of 0.05, 0.5 and 1.0 mM, and $^{14}CO_2$ production was determined. In some experiments, a closed system ionization chamber was used to detect $^{14}CO_2$ production (Davidson *et al.*, 1969).

Substrate decarboxylation was linear up to 4 hr in PCT, and for 2 hr for MTAL. Freeze-thawing of tubules resulted in a marked fall in the rates of substrate decarboxylation, and the addition of CN^- (5 mM) completely abolished oxidation of such substrates as succinate and glutamate. PCT demonstrate marked oxidation of succinate, glutamate and 2-oxoglutarate, and a lesser oxidation of glutamine. Little $^{14}CO_2$ was produced from citrate, lactate, and glucose. Significant decarboxylation occurred from glutamate, glutamine and glucose in both MTAL and CTAL. Pentose pathway activity measured by the difference in $^{14}CO_2$ production from [1-^{14}C] and [6-^{14}C]glucose was approx 50% of $^{14}CO_2$ production in both MTAL and CTAL. Palmitate was oxidized in both PCT and MTAL, but not in CTAL. In both MTAL and CTAL, oxidation of malate, citrate, and succinate was undetectable or minimal.

These data demonstrate the clear distinction in the substrate oxidized by these nephron segments all of which are characterized by active transport with oxidative metabolism and rich in mitochondria.

REFERENCES

DAVIDSON W. D., SCHWABE A. D. & THOMPSON J. C. (1969) *Analyt. Biochem.* **26**, 341–349.

SCHMIDT U. & GUDER W. G. (1976) Sites of enzyme activity along the nephron, *Kidney Int.* **9**, 233–242.

SYMPOSIUM DISCUSSION

Baverel: There is a limitation of the interpretation of the data, since low CO_2 production does not exclude metabolism of fatty acid to triglyceride, for example.

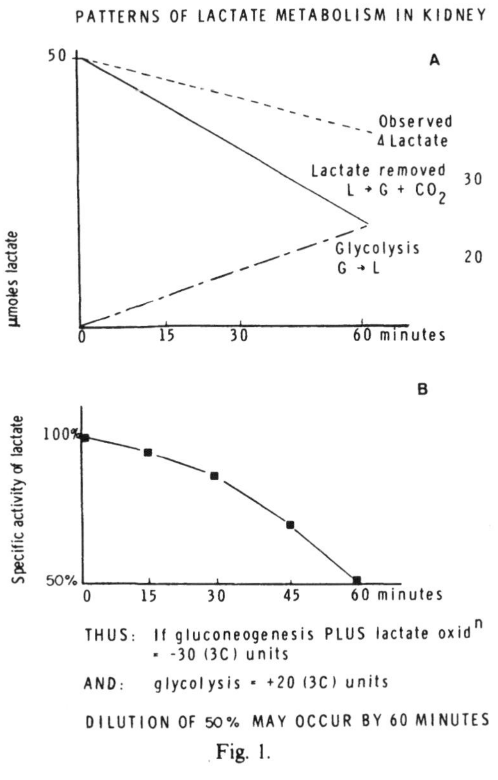

Fig. 1.

Kurokawa: I am well aware of the limitation of interpretation and only wish to show that this can be measured in single segments.

Saggerson: How do you reconcile the lack of palmitate oxidation with the fact that fatty acid can stimulate gluconeogenesis in tubules?

Kurokawa: Palmitate oxidation was actually similar in the proximal convoluted and medullary ascending limb of Henle.

Ross: Many of the new techniques of which we have now learned for the measurement of rates of metabolism in different parts of the nephron can be carried out on isolated segments. There remains the possibility, however, that rates of metabolism may be determined by transport work, so that the data obtained *in vitro* could be misleading. We (Janssens *et al.*, *Biochem. J.* **188,** 1980) are working with a technique of isotope dilution which will permit the measurement of medullary glycolysis in the functioning perfused rat kidney. First, in the kidney of 24 hr fasted rats, there is no loss of specific activity when radioactive lactate is incubated with isolated cortical tubules. This answers, for reasons which we cannot go into here, the question posed by the enzyme localization studies of Schmidt & Guder, and says that, despite the presence of both enzymes in proximal tubule cells, there is no cycling of carbon between PEPCK and pyruvate kinase. This being so, one can take the whole kidney, perfused with glucose and lactate at physiological concentrations, and dilution of lactate specific activity is then a measure solely of medullary glycolysis. The rate of glycolysis which we measure in this way in intact kidney, is very close to the rate of lactate formation from glucose in isolated medullary tissue (Fig. 1) (Bartlett *et al.*, unpublished).

Int. J. Biochem., Vol. 12, pp. 55 to 59
© Pergamon Press Ltd 1980. Printed in Great Britain

0020-711X/80/0701-0055$02.00/0

BIOCHEMICAL AND PHYSIOLOGICAL STUDIES ON CELLS ISOLATED FROM THE MEDULLARY THICK ASCENDING LIMB OF HENLE'S LOOP

J. EVELOFF*†, E. BAYERDÖRFFER‡, W. HAASE and R. KINNE†
Max-Planck-Institut für Biophysik, Heinrich-Hoffmann-Str. 7,
6000 Frankfurt am Main, Federal Republic of Germany

Abstract—1. Viable cells were isolated from the thick ascending limb of Henle's loop (TALH) of rabbit renal medulla.

2. The TALH cells were characterized by high activities of calcitonin-stimulated adenylate cyclase and Na-K-ATPase and low activities of alkaline phosphatase, γ-glutamyl-transpeptidase and ADH-sensitive adenylate cyclase.

3. The oxygen consumption of the TALH cells was inhibitable in a dose dependent manner by furosemide and bumetanide.

4. Ouabain (10^{-4} M) also inhibited oxygen consumption as did replacement of either Na or Cl in the incubation medium.

5. Preliminary experiments with plasma membrane vesicles prepared from the TALH cells indicated the presence of a coupled NaCl transport system.

INTRODUCTION

The thick ascending limb of Henle's loop functions integrally in the countercurrent system for urinary concentration and dilution, the latter being effected by an active transport of sodium chloride out of the tubular lumen in the absence of water movement. In isolated perfused tubules from the thick ascending limb of Henle's loop the active sodium chloride transport has been shown to consist of an active chloride transport and an accompanying passive sodium movement; the biochemical basis for this active chloride is still unclear (Burg & Green, 1973; Rocha & Kokko, 1973).

To date, most of the information on the biochemical parameters of the TALH cells has been derived from studies using kidney slices or intact kidneys. In such preparations, the data obtained reflects the biochemical activity of a variety of different cell types and accordingly information about one specific cell type is almost impossible to obtain.

Thus further investigations on the membrane–molecular mechanism of chloride transport required the isolation of the TALH cells in order to provide homogeneous material for biochemical and physiological studies.

MATERIALS AND METHODS

Rabbits were killed by a blow to the head, the kidney removed and placed in ice-cold Joklik's medium (containing 10% fetal calf serum) (Gibco-Biocult, Karlsruhe, Germany). The kidney was perfused through the renal artery to remove as many red blood cells as possible and the cortex was carefully removed and discarded. Cells from the medullary TALH were prepared as previously described§. In short, tubules were released from the medulla by incubation with 0.2% collagenase–0.25% hyaluronidase in Joklik's buffer for 1 hr at 37°C, gassed with 95% O_2–5% CO_2. The tubules were resuspended in Joklik's buffer containing 0.25% trypsin and incubated 20 min at room temperature with oxygen. The released cells were removed after each incubation by centrifugation, resuspended in Joklik's buffer and kept on ice. The trypsin treatment of the tubules was repeated eight times. The collected medullary cells were separated on a Ficoll® gradient (2.6–30.1%). The cells identified as being of TALH origin were located in the densest fraction of the gradient.

Enzyme activities

Calcitonin stimulated-adenylate cyclase, arginine vasopressin stimulated-adenylate cyclase, Na-K-ATPase, alkaline phosphatase and γ-glutamyltransferase were measured as previously described§. Protein was measured after precipitation with 10% trichloroacetic acid by the method of Lowry *et al.* (1951). Cellular respiration was measured with a Clark Oxygen Electrode (Yellow Springs Instrument Co., Yellow Springs, OH 45387 U.S.A.) at 37°C in a buffer containing in mM: NaCl 137, KCl 5, $MgSO_4$ 0.8, Na_2HPO_4 0.33, NaH_2PO_4 0.44, $MgCl_2$ 1.0, $CaCl_2$ 1.0, Tris–OH, 20.0 pH 7.4, acetate 5, glucose 5.

For the studies on anion and cation dependency Na was replaced isotonically with either $Choline^+$ or Li^+, and Cl^- was replaced isotonically by I^-, SO_4^{2-} or NO_3^-.

After centrifugation of isolated cells through silicone oil (Ar 20:Ar 200,3:1) intracellular sodium and potassium levels were measured in a flame photometer and cellular Cl^- was measured using an Orion chloride electrode (Orion Research Inc., Cambridge, MA 12139, U.S.A.). Intracellular water was measured by drying the cells to a constant weight at 60°C. The contents of intracellular ions and water were corrected for the amount present in adherent extracellular fluid by the use of [^{14}C]inulin as marker.

* Supported by USPHS Grant AM 05841.

† Present address: Albert Einstein College of Medicine, Bronx, NY, U.S.A.

‡ Part of the thesis for an M.D. of E. Bayerdörffer.

§ EVELOFF J., HAASE W. & KINNE R. Isolation of cells from the thick ascending limb of Henle's loop from the rabbit renal medulla. Submitted for publication.

RESULTS

Identification of cells from the medullary TALH

TALH tubules microdissected from the rabbit renal medulla are characterized by high specific activities of calcitonin-stimulated-adenylate cyclase and Na-K-ATPase with low specific activities of the arginine vasopressin (ADH)-stimulated adenylate cyclase and alkaline phosphatase (Charbades *et al.*, 1976; Morel *et al.*, 1976; Schmidt, 1977; Schmidt & Dubach, 1969). These characteristics were also used in developing the isolation procedure. The cells from the TALH showed calcitonin stimulated-adenylate cyclase activity of 700 pmols cAMP$\cdot$mg^{-1} protein × 15 min which corresponds to an enrichment of 5.8 times over the enzyme activity found in the mixed population of medullary cells.

The activity of alkaline phosphatase, an enzyme found mainly in the proximal tubules was only 10% of the activity found in the starting medullary cells (specific activity 32 mU$\cdot$mg^{-1} protein). Similarly, ADH-stimulated adenylate cyclase, an enzyme found predominantly in the collecting ducts, and γ-glutamyl transferase, an enzyme found in high amounts but not specifically in the proximal tubule, had a lower activity in TALH cells (specific activities were 98 pmols cAMP$\cdot$mg^{-1} protein × 15 min for ADH-stimulated adenylate cyclase and 122.8 mU$\cdot$mg^{-1} protein for γ-glutamyl transferase).

In order to further characterize the TALH cells, the effect of furosemide and bumetanide on oxygen consumption was measured (Burg *et al.*, 1973; Imai, 1977). Oxygen consumption was 33.6 μl $O_2\cdot$mg^{-1} protein × hr in the control medium and fell to 25.9 μl$\cdot$mg^{-1} protein × hr (a 23% decrease) upon the addition of 10^{-6} M furosemide to the incubation medium. The oxygen consumption response to furosemide was dose dependent, further additions of furosemide to 10^{-5}, 10^{-4} and 10^{-3} M inhibited oxygen consumption by 40, 48 and 54% of the control. This furosemide effect was less evident in the mixed population of medullary cells. The total medullary cells showed only a 10% inhibition of respiration by 10^{-3} M furosemide. Bumetanide, another TALH diuretic, was an even more potent inhibitor of oxygen consumption than furosemide. Oxygen consumption was inhibited 34, 43 and 51% at 10^{-6}, 10^{-5} and 10^{-4} M bumetanide, respectively.

Amiloride, a distal tubule diuretic assumed not to act in the TALH, had little effect on oxygen consumption in the TALH cells. Oxygen consumption was inhibited 11% by 10^{-4} M amiloride. The dose-dependent furosemide and bumetanide inhibition of respiration and the small effect of amiloride supports further the assumption that these cells are derived from the medullary thick ascending limb of Henle's Loop.

Morphological investigations by transmission electron-microscopy demonstrated that this cell fraction contains at least 90% of medullary thick ascending limb cells as characterized by their large nuclei, dense mitochondria, microvillar surface structure and extensive basal lateral invaginations.

Viability of the TALH cells

Although the isolation period is long, encompassing about six hours and including exposure to proteolytic enzymes, the isolated cells showed a high degree of viability as judged by the following criteria (Baur *et al.*, 1975):

(a) trypan blue was excluded from more than 99% of the cells;

(b) cellular Na and K levels were 9.4 and 139.2 mM, respectively;

(c) respiration was minimally stimulated, 1%, by 1 mM succinate;

(d) 2,4-dinitrophenol (0.05 mM) stimulated respiration by 51%; and

(e) ouabain (10^{-4} M) inhibited oxygen consumption by 51%.

These data indicate, that the cell plasma membrane is intact, (not permeable to trypan blue and succinate as well as not leaky to Na or K), the mitochondria are coupled, the Na-K-ATPase is functional and that overall metabolism and active transport processes are tightly coupled.

Ionic dependence of respiration of TALH cells

Oxygen consumption of the TALH cells was very sensitive to the anion and cation composition of the incubation medium (Fig. 1). The highest oxygen consumption is seen in the presence of both sodium and chloride. When chloride is replaced with iodide, the respiration decreased by 8%, but when sulfate or nitrate replaced chloride as the anion, respiration decreased by 43 and 45% of the control, respectively.

The removal of sodium also decreased oxygen consumption. With LiCl, respiration decreased by 45% and when choline replaced Na, a 47% decrease in respiration was seen. The replacement of both Na and Cl by $LiNO_3$ inhibited respiration to a similar degree, 48%, eliciting no further reduction in oxygen consumption.

The furosemide inhibition of respiration required the simultaneous presence of sodium and chloride, when sodium or chloride (or both) were totally replaced in the incubation medium, no significant inhibition of the respiration by furosemide (10^{-3} M) could be observed (Fig. 1).

Preincubation of the cells with 10^{-4} M ouabain inhibits respiration of the cells to the same extent as the removal of either Na or Cl, (Fig. 1). In the presence of ouabain, neither furosemide nor the removal of Na or Cl had any further significant inhibitory effect (data not shown).

Uptake of ^{22}Na into plasma membrane vesicles prepared from the TALH cells

In preliminary experiments the mechanism of the NaCl entry across the plasma membrane of TALH cells was investigated in a microsomal membrane preparation isolated from TALH cells. In Fig. 2, the uptake of Na into the vesicles in the presence of a chloride or nitrate gradient directed into the vesicles is shown. The uptake of Na was stimulated 2.5-fold in the first 10 sec of uptake in the presence of Cl over that in the presence of nitrate. The addition of 10^{-3} M furosemide to the Cl containing incubation medium inhibited Na uptake (33% in the first 10 sec of incubation). The uptake of D-glucose was measured simultaneously and did not vary when Cl was re-

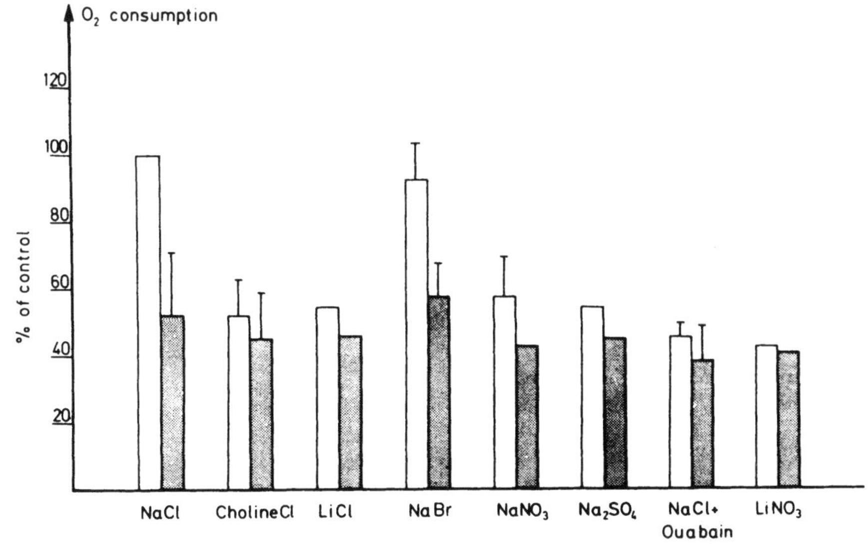

Fig. 1. Oxygen consumption of TALH cells prepared from the rabbit renal medulla. The oxygen consumption was measured at 37°C in a medium containing (in mM): NaCl 137, KCl 5, $MgSO_4$ 0.8, Na_2HPO_4 0.33, NaH_2PO_4 0.44, $MgCl_2$ 1.0, $CaCl_2$ 1.0, Tris–OH 20, pH 7.4, glucose 5, acetate 5. For anion and cation replacement studies, the Cl^- was replaced isotonically with Br^-, NO_3^- or SO_4^{2-}, or the Na^+ was replaced isotonically with choline$^+$ or Li^+. Ouabain inhibition of oxygen consumption was studied in a NaCl medium with 10^{-4} M ouabain. All anion and cation replacement studies were conducted in the absence (□) and presence (■) of 10^{-3} M furosemide. Bars represent means ± SE.

placed by nitrate or in the presence of furosemide, suggesting that the stimulatory effect of Cl and the inhibitory effect of furosemide on Na movement were due to an interaction of these compounds with a sodium transport system in the plasma membranes rather than due to unspecific effects on membrane permeability or size of the vesicles.

DISCUSSION

In the present experiments it has been shown that viable cells from the TALH can be prepared and that their biochemical and physiological parameters are similar to their functions in isolated perfused TALH tubules (Burg & Green 1973; Burg *et al.*, 1973; Imai, 1977; Rocha & Kokko, 1973).

The oxygen consumption studies indicate that in the present preparation 50% of the cellular respiration is related to the movement of sodium and chloride across the cell membrane. This is suggested from the data that the removal of either sodium or chloride decreases respiration by a maximum of 50%. And further, that ouabain (10^{-4} M) and diuretics furosemide and bumetanide maximally inhibit respiration

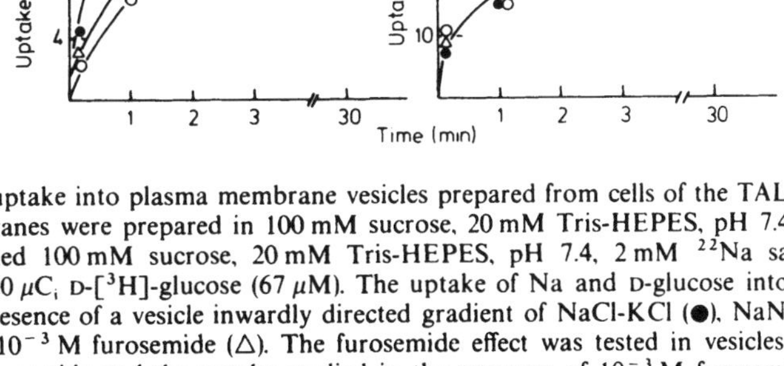

Fig. 2. Sodium uptake into plasma membrane vesicles prepared from cells of the TALH of rabbit renal medulla. Membranes were prepared in 100 mM sucrose, 20 mM Tris-HEPES, pH 7.4. The incubation medium contained 100 mM sucrose, 20 mM Tris-HEPES, pH 7.4, 2 mM ^{22}Na salt (12 μC_i/150 μl) 98 mM K salt, 20 μC_i D-[^{3}H]-glucose (67 μM). The uptake of Na and D-glucose into the vesicles was studied in the presence of a vesicle inwardly directed gradient of NaCl-KCl (●), $NaNO_3$-KNO_3 (○) or NaCl-KCl plus 10^{-3} M furosemide (△). The furosemide effect was tested in vesicles pretreated 2 min with 10^{-4} M furosemide and the uptake studied in the presence of 10^{-3} M furosemide (sodium free). Values are the means of 2 experiments.

by 50%. No additive inhibitory effects could be demonstrated by the combination of any of the above agents, indicating that they all may decrease respiration through inhibition of the active chloride transport system, whether directly, e.g. furosemide, or indirectly, e.g. ouabain. Thus, our data agree well with transport data in isolated perfused TALH tubules where chloride transport was active, sodium dependent and inhibitable by ouabain and furosemide.

In addition, in the isolated cell preparation there was a strong link between the sodium and chloride requirement for respiration. This mutual interdependence was also expressed in the studies with isolated plasma membrane vesicles suggesting that the energy dependent chloride uptake by the cells involves a coupled sodium chloride transport system in the cell membrane. The cellular location of this carrier system is assumed to be in the luminal membranes, but its exact localization remains to be defined. The coupled sodium chloride transport system in the membranes of the TALH cells may be similar to that described in the membranes of the rectal gland of the shark (Eveloff *et al.*, 1978), where chloride accumulation into the cell is driven by the favorable electrochemical gradient for sodium and is involved in the active secretion of chloride by the gland.

SUMMARY

Cells have been isolated from the TALH whose metabolic functions are intact as judged by several viability criteria.

Oxygen consumption of the TALH cells is reduced a maximum of approximately 50% in the presence of the loop diuretics bumetanide and furosemide in a dose dependent manner.

Oxygen consumption of the TALH cells is decreased about 50%, when either Na or Cl is replaced by other ions. Furthermore, when either Na or Cl is lacking in the incubation medium, furosemide has no inhibitory effect.

Oxygen consumption of the TALH cells is decreased approximately 50% by 10^{-4} M ouabain and furosemide has no further inhibitory effect. The oxygen consumption data taken together suggest that approximately 50% of the respiration of the TALH cells is related to the transport of Na and Cl and that these ions may be transported in a coupled manner.

Preliminary experiments with plasma membrane vesicles from the TALH cells show that Na uptake into the vesicles is greater in the presence of Cl than when NO_3 is the accompanying anion. Furthermore, Na uptake into the vesicles in the presence of Cl is inhibited by 10^{-3} M furosemide. The presence of a Na–Cl coupled transport system in the membranes of the TALH cells is suggested.

REFERENCES

Baur H., Kasperek S. & Pfaff S. (1975) Criteria of viability of isolated liver cells. *Hoppe-Seyler's Z. physiol. Chem.* **356,** 827–838.

Burg M. B. & Green N. (1973) Function of the thick ascending limb of Henle's Loop. *Am. J. Physiol.* **224,** 659–668.

Burg M., Stoner L., Cardinal T. & Green N. (1973) Furosemide effect on isolated perfused tubules. *Am. J. Physiol.* **225,** 119–124.

Chabardes D., Imbert-Teboul M., Manetegut M., Clique A. & Morel F. (1976) Distribution of calcitonin-sensitive adenylate cyclase along the rabbit kidney tubule. *Proc. Natn. Acad. Sci. U.S.A.* **73,** 3608–3612.

Eveloff J., Kinne R., Kinne-Saffran E., Murer H., Silva P., Epstein F. H., Stoff J. & Kinter W. B. (1978) Coupled sodium and chloride transport into plasma membrane vesicles prepared from dogfish rectal gland. *Pflügers Arch. ges. Physiol.* **378,** 87–92.

Imai M. (1977) Effect of bumetanide and furosemide on the thick ascending limb of Henle's Loop of rabbits and rats perfused *in vitro. Eur. J. Pharmac.* **41,** 409–416.

Lowry O. H., Rosebrough N. T., Farr A. L. & Randall R. T. (1951) Protein measurements with the folin phenol reagent. *J. biol. Chem.* **193,** 265–275.

Morel F., Chabardes D. & Imbert M. (1976) Functional segmentation of the rabbit distal tubule by microdetermination of hormone-dependent adenylate cyclase activity. *Kidney Int.* **9,** 264–277.

Rocha A. S. & Kokko J. P. (1973) Sodium chloride and water transport in the medullary thick ascending limb of Henle. Evidence for active chloride transport. *J. clin. Invest.* **52,** 612–623.

Schmidt U. (1977) The activities of key enzymes of the γ-glutamyl-cycle in microdissected segments of the rat nephron. *FEBS Lett.* **73,** 220–224.

Schmidt U. & Dubach U. C. (1969) Activity of (Na^+-K^+)-stimulated adenosinetriphosphatase in the rat nephron. *Pflügers Arch. ges. Physiol.* **306,** 219–226.

SYMPOSIUM DISCUSSION

Weiner: Your results are very interesting. We published a report (Cunarro & Weiner, *J. Pharmac. exp. ther.* **206,** 198–206, 1978) on isolated tubules from the rabbit outer medulla, showing that respiration was very sensitive to chloride concentration. The difference from your results was that we found no effect of sodium. Similar to your results, we found furosemide inhibited chloride-dependent respiration, but had no effect on sodium-dependent respiration. My question concerns the mechanism of chloride transport. Does the inhibition of sodium transport or of metabolism affect the intracellular chloride concentration?

Eveloff: We have very preliminary experiments. There are problems measuring intracellular water—our value is about 60 mM Cl. This is decreased by furosemide in a dose-dependent manner, and decreased when sodium is left out. Only the absolute value may be incorrect. Dr Ullrich has reported (*Pflügers Arch. ges. Physiol.* **267,** 207–217, 1958), sodium-dependence of respiration in medullary slices.

Weiner: The fact that the chloride concentration falls suggests that furosemide blocks the entry step.

Eveloff: Yes!

Angielski: Did you use another classical inhibitor of anion transport, since you have now obtained an isolated chloride transport model? Have you tried SITS or DIDS?

Eveloff: No, we have tried other loop diuretics which also inhibit.

Angielski: Can I then ask whether phloretin might be of interest as a specific amino-group agent?

Kinne: This system is different from the one which reacts with DIDS, SITS and phlorrhizin in the erythrocyte, our data suggests that it is a sodium chloride coupled system. In the shark rectal gland, for example, which has such a transport system, it is not inhibited by SITS, DIDS, etc.

Sacktor: Your uptake experiments indicate that the chloride gradient energizes the uptake of sodium. Have you tried the reverse experiment, to see the effect of a sodium gradient on chloride transport?

Eveloff: Those experiments are hard to perform. We tried them in rectal gland membrane vesicles, and in order to get high enough radioactivity, we need a concentration of 30–40 mM Cl. The passive uptake of chloride becomes significant and masks the small active transport component. Theoretically, we should be able to carry out these experiments with radio-active bromide or iodide of high specific activity.

Anner: Is there any potassium counter transport coupled to the sodium-dependent chloride transport?

Eveloff: We do not know. We have done just preliminary experiments.

Guder: Abodeely & Lee (*Am. J. Physiol.* **220,** 1693, 1971) observed dependence of glucose uptake on medium-osmolality in rabbit medullary slices. What was the respiratory substrate in your experiments?

Eveloff: Acetate and glucose. In fact the cells survive better in slightly hypotonic medium (300 mOsm) and have greater oxygen uptake.

Guder: Is there stimulation of oxygen uptake by glucose?

Eveloff: No, but in the presence of glucose and acetate there is a marked stimulation of oxygen uptake by 2,4-dinitrophenol.

Katz: Have you looked at Na-K-ATPases with the anion substitutions?

Eveloff: There is no change with anion substitutions and even with 10^{-3} M furosemide, there was no inhibition of Na-K-ATPase.

Kiil: If you find as great, or greater stimulation with sodium bromide as with chloride, would you then still call it a sodium chloride co-transport system?

Eveloff: Certainly, that is the physiological activity of the thick ascending limb; but other halides could substitute for chloride.

Jorgensen: I have a comment on the significance of your results for the interpretation of the transtubular transport in isolated tubules. Previously it was thought that active chloride transport would continue after removal of sodium. Recently Burg showed that chloride transport is abolished when sodium is removed. This suits your observations very well.

Schurek: I am surprised that when you used succinate there was no stimulation of oxygen uptake. In other studies it has been shown that the kidney responds to addition of succinate with a marked increase in oxygen uptake.

Eveloff: Yes, it is used in liver cell studies as a test of viability. Addition of succinate to intact TALH cells produces no increase in oxygen uptake. We can prove that it is a measure of cellular leakiness in our cells by freezing and thawing to break the cell membrane. We then observe 200% stimulation of respiration by succinate.

Ross: This is an unusual characteristic of a kidney cell as we know them to date, since kidney cells in general are permeable to succinate (Nishiitsutsuji-Uwo *et al.* 1967). The demonstration of succinate impermeability was described by Professor Krebs' group as a special characteristic of the liver cell (Hems, Stubbs & Kreb, *Biochem. J.* **107,** 284–292, 1968). You are, therefore, describing a new property of a kidney cell.

Int. J. Biochem., Vol. 12, pp. 61
© Pergamon Press Ltd 1980. Printed in Great Britain

0020-711X/80/0701-0061$02.00/0

CHARACTERIZATION OF DIFFERENT POPULATIONS OF RABBIT KIDNEY CORTICAL CELLS SEPARATED BY FREE-FLOW ELECTROPHORESIS USING HORMONE-STIMULATED ADENYLATE CYCLASES

A. VANDEWALLE and H.-G. HEIDRICH
Max-Planck-Institut fur Biochemie, D-8033 Martinsried, Federal Republic of Germany

A successful separation of different cell populations from rabbit kidney cortex has been described recently (Heidrich & Dew, 1974). In order to better characterize these different populations of tubular cells we performed adenylate cyclase measurements under basal and stimulated conditions. Morel *et al.* (1978) have demonstrated the existence of a fine functional segmentation of the nephron by measuring different hormone-dependent adenylate cyclase activities on microdissected tubules. These differences should also be detectable in the isolated cell populations thus making it possible to determine from which part of the tubule the cells derive.

The isolated cells were obtained after citrate perfusion and separation using free-flow electrophoresis (Hannig & Heidrich, 1974) (Bender and Hobein, München; 180 mA, 130 V + cm, 5°C). Adenylate cyclase assays were performed on the unseparated cell suspension and on the various fractions obtained after electrophoresis, after a 15 min incubation of the cells in hypo-osmotic medium followed by rapid freezing. The conditions of the test were similar to those described by Morel *et al.* (1978), except that the cells (0.2 to 1.5×10^5) were incubated in a final test volume of 15 μl for 30 min at 30°C. Parathormone (PTH, 10 U/ml), arginine vasopressin (AVP, 10^{-6}M), L-isoproterenol D-bitartrate (ISO, 10^{-6}M) and sodium fluoride (NaF, 5×10^{-3}M) were used for the stimulation experiments. The ratio of stimulated to basal (control) adenylate cyclase activities (s/c) were calculated for each fraction of the separated cells. The table gives the mean (s/c) values of eight experiments for the main fractions of cells isolated by free-flow electrophoresis.

s/c	I	II	III	IV	V
PTH	11.14	21.63	5.98	7.20	3.73
ISO	1.04	1.69	3.72	5.86	2.18
AVP	0.82	1.09	1.46	2.48	2.93
NaF	12.64	23.45	11.03	9.26	6.69

Up to now five cell fractions responding to different hormones were analyzed under the experimental conditions used in this study. Fraction I and II contain the highest number of cells. They present the highest PTH (s/c) ratio which strongly suggests that these fractions contain a pure population of proximal tubule cells. Fraction III responds to both PTH and ISO and is known to contain renin-active cells; thus it is difficult to draw definite conclusions as to the origin of these cells. Fraction IV presents the highest ISO (s/c) ratio ($P < 0.05$ vs fraction I) and also a high AVP (s/c) ratio. This suggests that this population stems from both the distal and the collecting segments. Fraction V shows a similar pattern of stimulation ratios with lower values as in fraction IV. More detailed results can be expected from improvements in the separation particularly in the separation of fractions IV and V.

REFERENCES

HANNIG & HEIDRICH (1974) *Meth. Enzymol.* **31**, 746–761.
HEIDRICH & DEW (1974) *J. Cell Biol.* **74**, 780–788.
MOREL *et al.*, (1978) *Meth. Pharmac.* **4B**, 297–323.

Int. J. Biochem., Vol. 12, pp. 63 to 67
0020-711X/80/0701-0063$02.00/0

THE INTRACELLULAR COMPARTMENTATION OF METABOLITES IN ISOLATED KIDNEY CORTEX TUBULES

WALTER G. GUDER and SUSANNE PÜRSCHEL
Klinisch-chemisches Institut and Institut für Diabetesforschung, Städtisches Krankenhaus München-Schwabing, Kölner Platz 1, D-8000 München 40, Federal Republic of Germany

Abstract—1. A method is described to measure cytosolic and mitochondrial metabolites in isolated kidney tubule suspensions.

2. With the use of digitonin, 95% of cytosolic metabolites are released into the supernatant fraction whereas mitochondrial matrix enzymes are retained in the pellet fraction.

3. In a study of adaptation to acidosis, different α-oxoglutarate gradients between the tubular cell compartments are obtained, when medium pH is changed from 7.0 to 7.8.

INTRODUCTION

Renal metabolite concentrations are thought to be involved in the regulation of renal metabolic fluxes. Thus renal gluconeogenesis and ammoniagenesis have repeatedly been shown to be changed by acute hormonal and metabolic stimuli *in vitro*, which were parallelled by changes in intermediary metabolite levels (Nagata & Rasmussen, 1970; Alleyne & Scullard, 1969; Hems & Brosnan, 1971). The interpretation of results on metabolite levels in the whole kidney or in isolated kidney preparation, however, are complicated by metabolic compartmentation of the kidney. In addition to the heterogeneity of nephron cells, an intracellular compartmentation of metabolites complicates conclusions from whole tissue or cell determinations since the metabolic steps to be regulated are separated in different intracellular compartments. From these difficulties the need for a method to separate cytosolic and mitochondrial metabolites has been recognised in recent papers (Simpson & Hager, 1979; Boyd & Goldstein, 1979). Such methods have been developed for liver (Elbers *et al.*, 1974; Zuurendonk & Tager, 1974; Tischler *et al.*, 1977), adipose tissue (Paetzke-Brunner *et al.*, 1978) and cultured heart cells (Soboll *et al.*, 1979). Due to its rapidity, wide applicability and the extensive experience of collegues from this institute with fractionation studies in liver and adipose cells (Siess *et al.*, 1978; Brocks *et al.*, 1979; Paetzke-Brunner *et al.*, 1978) we adapted the digitonin procedure of Zuurendonk & Tager (1974) for the fractionation of isolated tubule fragments of rats.

MATERIALS AND METHODS

The method of Zuurendonk & Tager (1974) is based on the fact that, due to its higher cholesterol content, the plasma membrane is more sensitive to digitonin treatment than the inner mitochondrial membrane which separates the mitochondrial matrix space from the cytosol. By short-time exposure to low digitonin concentrations at temperatures around 0°C cytosolic metabolites can be separated from the mitochondrial space by rapid centrifugation procedures. During the first experiments with a modified digitonin procedure, it turned out that experience with isolated liver cells could not simply be applied to the tubule suspensions, probably because these form tightly coupled cell groups which are more resistant to digitonin action than isolated cells.

Therefore, additional mechanical disruption of cells by a teflon homogenizer was introduced, as in the fractionation of adipose tissue (Paetzke-Brunner *et al.*, 1978). The detailed procedure is shown in Fig. 1.

After incubation of 10–20 mg tubular protein/1.2 ml Krebs–Henseleit medium in a screw-capped plastic vial for 15 min at 37°C (Guder *et al.*, 1971; Guder, 1979). 0.1 ml of the incubation mixture was deproteinized for total metabolite determination. 10 sec later 0.75 ml was mixed with 3 ml of a precooled solution of digitonin (Merck, Darmstadt, Germany), 1 mg·ml^{-1} in a calcium free Krebs–Henseleit buffer (Krebs & Henseleit, 1932) containing 3 mM EDTA, in a 5 ml glass homogenizer (Braun, Melsungen, Germany). Control vessels, omitting digitonin were performed with each type of experiment.

The mixture was homogenized with a Teflon pestle precooled for 10 sec in liquid nitrogen by two up and down stokes at 1000 rev/min. After 15 sec temperature was controlled with an electric thermometer. Temperature was brought to +2°C by gentle stirring in an ice–salt mixture of −10°C. Care was taken during the whole procedure to prevent freezing of the homogenate. 30 sec after mixing 1 ml samples of the homogenate were layered over 0.5 ml silicon–oil mixture (mixed from AR 20:AR 200, 2:1, Wacker-Chemie, Burghausen, Germany) which was layered before over 0.12 ml 12% $HClO_4$. At 45 sec both samples were spun for 10 sec in an Eppendorf centrifuge at 10,000 ***g*** in a cool chamber at 4°C. To prevent an increase in temperature during the separation the centrifuge was precooled by pouring liquid nitrogen over the rotor shortly before each run. At the same time another 1 ml sample of the homogenate was mixed with 0.1 ml 30% $HClO_4$ as a control for total metabolites and the residue remaining in the homogenizer frozen in liquid nitrogen.

After separation of cells on the centrifuge 0.7 ml of the supernatant fraction was transferred to 0.07 ml 30% $HClO_4$ and the residue stored at 0°C for the determination of supernatant enzymes. The whole procedure was finished after 70 sec. The deproteinized samples were neutralized with KOH and $KHCO_3$ and the neutralized extracts taken for metabolite determinations according to standard procedures (see Siess *et al.*, 1978). Total enzyme activities were measured from the frozen residue after sufficient freezing–thawing cycles (usually three) and compared with the enzyme activities found in the supernatant after separation.

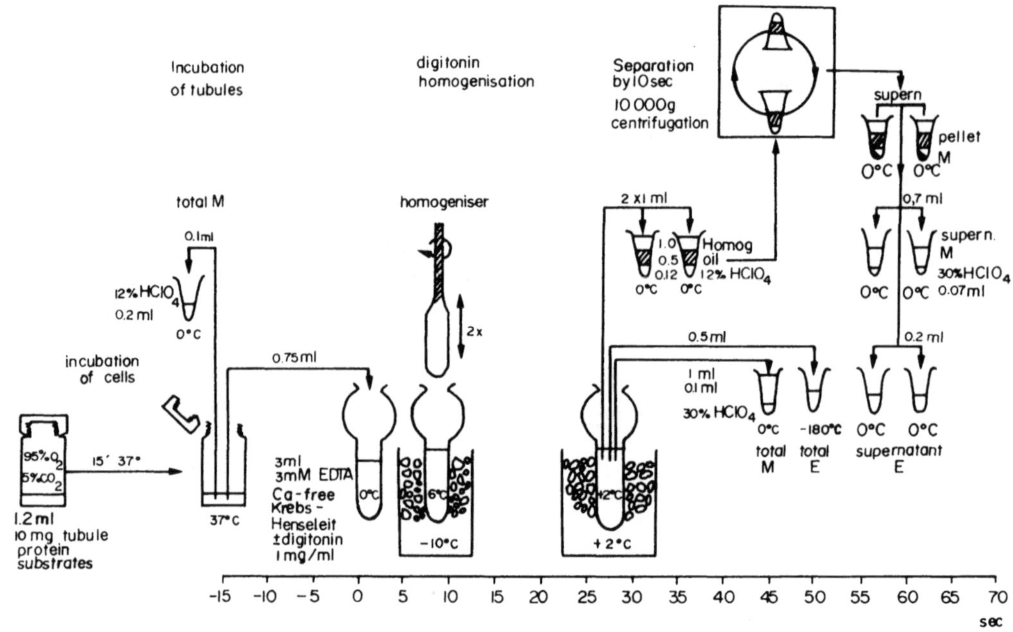

Fig. 1. Procedure for the fractionation of isolated cortical tubule fragments. M = metabolites, E = enzymes.

In some cases sediment enzyme activities were determined by omitting $HClO_4$ in the separation step.

Glutamate dehydrogenase, citrate synthase and lactate dehydrogenase were measured spectrophotometrically with standard procedures using reagents of Boehringer, Mannheim, Germany (Bergmeyer, 1974).

RESULTS

Isolated tubule fragments in suspension proved to be a useful model to study metabolic functions of the proximal tubule. They perform biosynthetic functions at high rates (Guder *et al.*, 1971; Guder & Wirthensohn, 1979), are hormone responsive (Rasmussen & Nagata, 1970; Guder, 1976) and exhibit metabolite levels comparable to the kidney cortex *in situ* (Nagata & Rasmussen, 1970).

When tubules from fed rats were exposed to digitonin, cytosolic metabolites and enzymes are released into the supernatant medium (Fig. 2). At a digitonin concentration of $0.8\ mg \cdot ml^{-1}$ release of α-glycerophosphate was completed after 15 sec. Therefore a lactate dehydrogenase release above 40% was taken as sufficient to assume complete release of cytosolic metabolites into supernatant (Fig. 3). From Figs 2 and 3 it can also be seen that 8–22% of lactate dehydrogenase is already in the supernatant fraction in the absence of digitonin. This is probably the result of autodigestion of tubule cells occurring during incubation (Pfeifer & Guder, 1975).

When mitochondrial matrix enzymes were measured, only 2–3% were recovered in the supernatant in

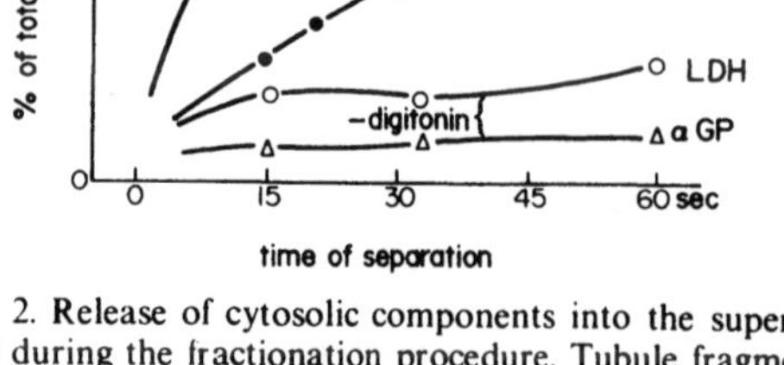

Fig. 2. Release of cytosolic components into the supernatant during the fractionation procedure. Tubule fragments of fed rats were incubated for 15 min with 10 mM glycerol in the presence of 5 mM glutamin and then transferred to the homogenisation procedure in the absence and presence of $1\ mg \cdot ml^{-1}$ digitonin. After the times indicated supernatant fractions were separated by 10 sec centrifugation at 10,000 *g* lactate dehydrogenase (LDH) activity and α-glycerophosphate (α-GP) were measured in the supernatant fractions and are given as % of total activities and levels respectively.

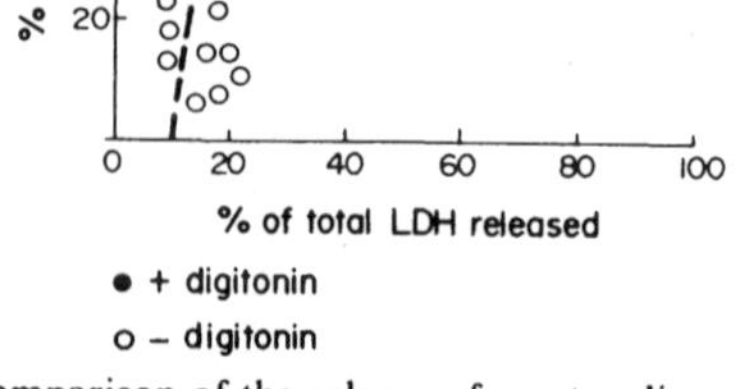

Fig. 3. Comparison of the release of a cytosolic metabolite and a cytosolic enzyme into the supernatant fraction. Experimental details are as described in the legends to Fig. 2 and in Materials and Methods.

Table 1. Distribution of enzymes after fractionation of tubules ($n = 5$)

	Total activity (U/g)	−Digitonin Pellet (%)	−Digitonin Supernatant (%)	+Digitonin Pellet (%)	+Digitonin Supernatant (%)
Lactate dehydrogenase	1057	84	16	45	55
Citrate synthase	116	96	4	91	9
Glutamate dehydrogenase	748	98	2	94	6

the absence of digitonin (Table 1); digitonin increased this percentage to 6–9%. When metabolites were analyzed, only 13% of α-glycerophosphate was found in the supernatant in the absence of digitonin, whereas more than 50% of glutamate and α-oxoglutarate were recovered from this fraction (Table 2). This indicates that α-oxoglutarate and glutamate but not α-glycerophospate are released into the extracellular space.

In the presence of digitonin, however, additional metabolites were released, amounting to over 90% with α-glycerophosphate but only 66% with glutamate and 89% with α-oxoglutarate. If one takes the residual sediment metabolites as mitochondrial and the difference between supernatant levels in the absence and presence of digitonin as cytosolic metabolites, the respective concentration gradients can be estimated. This method has been successfully used to measure the intracellular distributions of glutamate, α-oxoglutarate, phosphoenolpyruvate and glucose. Figure 4 gives an example of the applicability of the method to a regulatory problem, discussed in several recent publications. Goldstein (1976) postulated that cytosolic α-oxoglutarate could be a physiological regulator of renal glutamine metabolism and ammoniagenesis, since whole kidney and kidney cortex α-oxoglutarate levels changed dramatically during acid base changes (Parry & Brosnan, 1978; Boyd & Goldstein, 1976). This postulate was supported by the findings with the fractionation procedure. Changes in tubular α-oxoglutarate during acute acid base changes *in vitro* were found to be due mainly to changes in the supernatant and medium fraction (Fig. 4). Cytosolic α-oxoglutarate represented 60–80% of that of total cells under the different conditions.

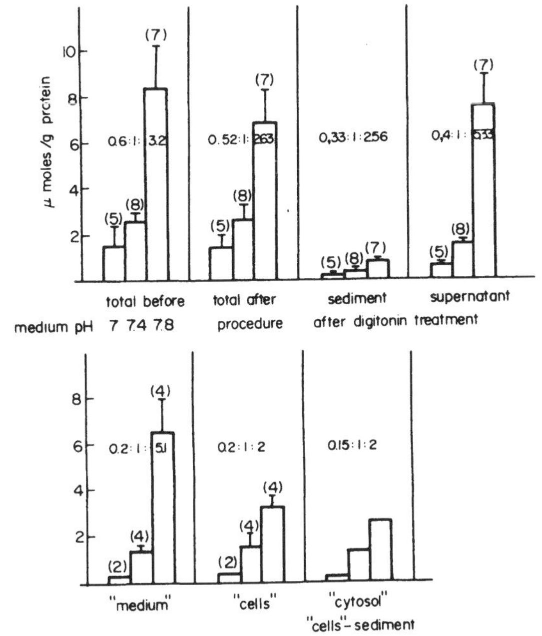

Fig. 4. Effect of pH changes in medium on α-oxoglutarate levels and distribution between mitochondrial, cytosolic and medium spaces. Isolated tubules from fed rats were incubated over 15 min with 5 mM glutamin as described in the methods section. 750 μl samples of these incubations were treated by the homogenisation procedure described in Fig. 1 in the absence and presence of 0.8 mg·ml^{-1} digitonin and the α-oxoglutarate levels measured spectophotometrically in a Perkin–Elmer double-beam spectrophotometer (Siess *et al.*, 1978). "Medium" and "cell" metabolite levels were taken from the experiments in the absence of digitonin. "Cytosol" values were calculated from the supernatant differences between digitonin and digitonin free experiments run from the same tubule experiment. Medium pH was changed by varying bicarbonate concentrations in the incubation medium (Nagata & Rasmussen, 1970). Results are related to total tubule protein and given as means ± SEM with the number of tubule preparations tested in parentheses.

DISCUSSION AND CRITICISM OF THE METHOD

The present paper for the first time describes a method of measuring intracellular compartmentation in kidney cells. Recent evidence from studies with liver indicates that under similar conditions results obtained from the pellet fraction probably represent mitochondrial metabolite profiles, since contamination with cytosolic and medium metabolites is below 10% and can be neglected (Siess *et al.*, 1978).

In fact the metabolite distribution between cytosolic and mitochondrial compartments found with the present method conforms well (Table 2) with the distribution of cytosolic and mitochondrial spaces described for proximal tubules by Pfaller & Rittinger (1980). If changes in cytosolic and mitochondrial spaces during preparation and incubation of tubule fragments can be excluded, these morphometric data may be used to calculate cytosolic and mitochondrial metabolite concentrations. If the data of Pfaller & Rittinger are applied to the present studies, 25% of the cellular volume would be taken by the mitochondrial matrix space, whereas 75% were cytosolic space. Higher amounts (3 times) of metabolites should be recovered from the supernatant fraction, if no mitochondrial cytosolic gradient was to be expected. In fact for α-oxoglutarate a ratio of 2–4 between "cytosolic" and "pellet" α-oxoglutarate was found under different conditions. This would indicate that no steep concentration gradients exist over the mitochondrial membrane under our conditions. Changes in α-oxoglutarate levels by a factor of 10 which occur in the cells when medium pH is changed from 7 to 7.8 are rapidly equilibrated over the mitochondrial, cytosolic and medium compartment.

Table 2. Distribution of metabolites after fractionation of tubules ($n = 5$)

Metabolite	Condition	− Digitonin Pellet (%)	− Digitonin Supernatant (%)	+ Digitonin Pellet (%)	+ Digitonin Supernatant (%)
α-Glycerophosphate	10 mM glycerol 5 mM glutamine	87	13	10	90
α-Oxoglutarate	5 mM glutamine pH 7.8	41	59	34	66
Glutamate	5 mM glutamine pH 7.8	31	69	11	89

In spite of such encouraging results, however, the present method should be used with great caution, unless some of the following possible pitfalls are excluded and better reference values for the respective water spaces are known under the experimental conditions used: the assumption, that the pellet metabolites represent the mitochondrial matrix are valid only if these behave like the matrix enzymes. Unfortunately no metabolite exclusively located in the mitochondria has yet been described, which could serve as a metabolite marker for this space. The comparable results in liver cells, however, between the digitonin and the organic solvent method indicates, that mitochondrial metabolites are well preserved under the present conditions.

In addition to the mitochondrial space, other compartments like nuclei, microsomal vesicles, peroxysomes and brush border membrane vesicles could also sediment with the pellet in the present procedure. This seems of special importance if metabolites are measured which can accumulate in brush border vesicles like amino acids, glucose and phosphate. In order to exclude such artifactual increases in sediment, the metabolite fraction in the pellet should not increase when the metabolite is added to the homogenization medium (Table 3). Total metabolic changes during the separation procedure due to temperature and digitonin can be controlled by the measurement of total metabolites before and after homogenisation. Total metabolites should not be different before and after treatment nor between the control and the digitonin experiment. This control does not however, exclude intracellular redistribution of metabolites during the fractionation procedure. In order to exclude such possibilities, fractionation has been performed in the presence of inhibitors of the respective mitochondrial transport carriers with apparently no change in metabolite distribution (Siess *et al.*, 1978). Likewise temperature effects can be ruled out by using a lower temperature in the presence of DMSO, (Brocks *et al.*, 1979). When considering all these precautions the present method should prove as a useful tool in studying intracellular distribution of metabolites in the kidney.

Table 3. Criteria for good separation experiments

1. More than 85% cytosolic marker metabolites in supernatant.
2. Less than 5% mitochondrial matrix enzymes released by digitonin.
3. Total metabolites before and after separation procedure must be within 20% with the sum of pellet and supernatant fractions.
4. Metabolites added should be recovered by over 90% from the supernatant.
5. Inhibitors of mitochondrial transport added to the digitonin medium should not change metabolite distribution between supernatant and pellet fraction.

SUMMARY

Isolated tubule fragments from fed rats were fractionated into a supernatant and pellet fraction after treatment with 0.8 mg·ml^{-1} digitonin at 2°C. This procedure separated cytosolic and mitochondrial matrix enzymes and metabolites, when several criteria were fulfilled. In the presence of 10 mM glycerol, glycerophosphate was recovered nearly exclusively from the cytosolic fraction. Glutamate and α-oxoglutarate were found to be distributed between mitochondrial, cytosolic and medium fractions. Changes in medium pH resulted in rapid changes in total α-oxoglutarate levels. These changes were found to be more pronounced in the medium and the cytosolic fraction than in the pellet, indicating a rapid equilibration of α-oxoglutarate across the mitochondrial and plasma membranes respectively. These results support the suggestion (Goldstein, 1976), that pH-dependent distribution of α-oxoglutarate over the different cellular compartments can be of regulatory significance in renal metabolism.

Acknowledgements—The present work was supported by the Deutsche Forschungsgemeinschaft (Sonderforschungsbereich 51, München, project D13). Much experienced advice and experimental help came from Elmar Siess, Dietrich Brocks and Ingrid Paetzke, Institut für Diabetesforschung. The authors also wish to thank Professor Dr Otto H. Wieland for continuous support of our work. The help of Mrs E. Rausch and D. Quel during preparation of this manuscript is also gratefully acknowledged.

REFERENCES

Alleyne G. A. O. & Scullard G. H. (1969) Renal metabolic response to acid base changes—I. Enzymatic control of ammoniagenesis in the rat. *J. clin. Invest.* **48,** 364–370.

Bergmeyer H. U. (1974) *Methoden der enzymatischen Analyse*, Verlag Chemie, Weinheim.

Boyd T. A. & Goldstein L. (1979) Kidney metabolite levels and ammonia production in acute acid-base alterations in the rat. *Am. J. Physiol.* **236,** E289–E294.

Brocks D. G., Siess E. A. & Wieland O. H. (1980) The validity of the digitonin method for metabolite compartmentation in isolated hepatocytes. *Biochem. J.* **188,** 207–212.

Elbers R., Heldt H. W., Schmucker P., Soboll S. & Wiese H. (1974) Measurement of the ATP/ADP ratio in mitochondria and in the extramitochondrial compartment by fractionating of freeze-stopped liver tissue in non-aqeous media. *Hoppe Seyler's Z. physiol. Chem.* **355**, 378–393.

GOLDSTEIN L. (1976) α-ketoglutarate regulation of glutamine transport and deamidation by renal mitochondria. *Biochem. biophys. Res. Commun.* **70**, 1136–1141.

GUDER W., WIESNER W., STUKOWSKI B. & WIELAND O. (1971) Metabolism of isolated kidney tubules. Oxygen consumption, gluconeogenesis and the effect of cyclic nucleotides in tubules from starved rats. *Hoppe Seyler's Z. physiol. Chem.* **325**, 1319–1328.

GUDER W. G. (1976) Hormonal regulation of renal gluconeogenesis in isolated tubule fragments in *Renal Metabolism in Relation to Renal Function* (Edited by SCHMIDT U. & DUBACH U. C.) Huber, Bern.

GUDER W. G. (1979) Stimulation of renal gluconeogenesis by angiotensin II. *Biochim. biophys. Acta* **584**, 507–519.

GUDER W. G. & WIRTHENSOHN G. (1979) Metabolism of isolated kidney tubules. Interactions between lactate, glutamine and oleate metabolism. *Eur. J. Biochem.* **99**, 577–584.

HEMS D. A. & BROSNAN J. T. (1971) Effects of metabolic acidosis and starvation on the content of intermediary metabolites in rat kidney. *Biochem. J.* **123**, 391–397.

KREBS H. A. & HENSELEIT H. (1932) Untersuchungen über die Harnstoffbildung im Tierkörper. *Hoppe Seyler's Z. physiol. Chem.* **210**, 33–66.

NAGATA N. & RASMUSSEN H. (1970) Renal gluconeogenesis: effects of Ca^{2+} and H^{+}. *Biochim. biophys. Acta* **215**, 1–16.

PAETZKE-BRUNNER I., SCHÖN H. & WIELAND O. H. (1978) Insulin activates pyruvate dehydrogenase by lowering the mitochondrial acetyl-CoA/CoA ratio as evidenced by digitonin fractionation of isolated fat cells. *FEBS Lett.* **93**, 307–311.

PARRY D. M. & BROSNAN J. T. (1978) Glutamine metabolism in the kidney during induction of, and recovery from, metabolic acidosis in the rat. *Biochem. J.* **174**, 387–396.

PFALLER W. & RITTINGER M. (1980) Quantitive morphology of the rat kidney. *Int. J. Biochem.* **12**, 17–22. (This volume).

PFEIFER U. & GUDER W. G. (1975) Stimulation of cellular autophagy by parathyroid hormone and cyclic AMP in isolated tubular fragments from the rat's kidney cortex. *Virchow's Arch, B. cell. Path.* **19**, 51–67.

RASMUSSEN H. & NAGATA N. (1970) Renal gluconeogenesis: effects of parathyroid hormone and dibutyryl 3',5'-AMP. *Biochim. biophys. Acta* **215**, 17–28.

SIESS E. A., BROCKS D. G. & WIELAND O. H. (1978) Distribution of metabolites between the cytosolic and mitochondrial compartments of hepatocytes isolated from fed rats. *Hoppe Seyler's Z. Physiol. Chem.* **359**, 785–798.

SIMPSON D. P. & HAGER S. R. (1979) pH and bicarbonate effects on mitochondrial anion accumulation. Proposed mechanism for changes in renal metabolite levels in acute acid-base disturbances. *J. clin. Invest.* **63**, 704–712.

SOBOLL S., WERDAN K., BOZSIK M., MÜLLER M., ERDMANN E. & HELDT H. W. (1979) Distribution of metabolites between mitochondria and cytosol of cultured fibroblastoid rat heart cells. *FEBS Lett.* **100**, 125–128.

TISCHLER M. E., HECHT P. & WILLIAMSON J. R. (1977) Determination of mitochondrial/cytosolic metabolite gradients in isolated rat liver cells by cell disruption. *Archs Biochem. Biophys.* **181**, 278–292.

ZUURENDONK P. F. & TAGER J. M. (1974) Rapid separation of particulate components and soluble cytoplasm of isolated rat-liver cells. *Biochim. biophys. Acta* **333**, 393–399.

SYMPOSIUM DISCUSSION

Pfaller: Do you find mono-amino-oxidase in the supernatant fraction, indicating that the space between inner and outer mitochondrial membranes is released?

Guder: That has been done for liver. Adenylate kinase is present in the supernatant.

Radda: Have you looked at ATP? Since the distribution which you may expect to find will depend upon charge, ATP would be an excellent molecule to look at.

Guder: We have indeed tried that but no all of the criteria which I outlined have been fulfilled. For example, we are not sure whether ADP can be phosphorylated during the extraction procedure. We cannot exclude redistribution during extraction. I can tell you that about 75% of ATP is in the cytosol fraction.

Kovacevic: Have you taken account of the possible activation of phospholipase A_2? Because that enzyme may change membrane permeability.

Guder: That is important, particularly for the distribution of phosphorylated intermediates, but we have not measured lysosomal hydrolases.

Ross: Are you suggesting that there is a pH gradient between cytosol and mitochondrion, and that this determined the distribution which you observe for 2-oxoglutarate? If so, how do you explain the effects of the intramitochondrial enzymes (glutamate dehydrogenase and oxo-glutarate dehydrogenase) in setting the concentrations of 2-oxoglutarate when pH is changed outside the cell, and in the cytosol. (See p. 000, this volume.)

GUDER: Our present data do not answer that question.

Chapter 2

Intermediary metabolism and its regulation

Int. J. Biochem., Vol. 12, pp. 69 to 73
© Pergamon Press Ltd 1980. Printed in Great Britain

0020-711X/80/0701-0069$02.00/0

EFFECT OF BICARBONATE ON GLUTAMINE METABOLISM

H. A. Krebs, G. Baverel and P. Lund
Metabolic Research Laboratory, Nuffield Department of Clinical Medicine, Radcliffe Infirmary, Woodstock Road, Oxford OX2 6HE, U.K.

INTRODUCTION

In earlier work by one of us (Krebs, 1935) it was noted that the glutaminases in extracts of rat liver and kidney differ in respect to pH optima and to inhibition by L-glutamate. The kidney enzyme was inhibited by glutamate, the liver enzyme was not. The suggestion was made that kidney glutaminase might be concerned with the synthesis of glutamine *in vivo* because glutamine synthesis occurs in rat kidney, but no satisfactory explanation could be offered at that time for the existence of two enzymes, with different kinetic properties, catalyzing the same reaction.

After this initial work on what now would be called glutaminase isoenzymes Greenstein, Katunuma, Kvamme, Curthoys and Meister have made important contributions to the development of the subject which cannot be discussed in detail here. We emphasize that our study of factors affecting glutaminase activity and the metabolism of glutamine was carried out on freshly prepared hepatocytes or kidney tubules, as opposed to tissue extracts, or purified enzymes, or tissue fragments such as mitochondria. This meant that the enzymic reactions were measured under near-physiological conditions; insofar as the modifiers are concerned the enzymes were present in their natural intracellular environment. The only somewhat unphysiological aspect was the concentration of the added glutamine in the suspension fluid which was 5 mM. *In vivo* it is of the order of 0.5 mM in the blood plasma (but intracellular hepatic glutamine is about 5 mM).

The present work arose from the observation that the metabolic fate of glutamate in liver homogenates is affected by the composition of the incubation medium. In the presence of 10 mM phosphate buffer, 2 mM $MgCl_2$ and 150 mM KCl, the glutamate removed is almost quantitatively converted to aspartate (Krebs & Bellamy, 1960), whereas addition of 25 mM HCO_3^- promoted the formation of additional products, namely glutamine, α-oxoglutarate and citrate. Under these conditions the ammonia appearing as glutamine must have been formed through the glutamate dehydrogenase reaction. As the concentration of HCO_3^- and the rate of metabolism of glutamine and glutamate are linked to the maintenance of the acid–base balance, these experiments were followed up by a study of the effect of the HCO_3^- concentration of glutamine metabolism in hepatocytes, kidney cortex tubules and enterocytes. The methodology is described in detail in Baverel & Lund (1979). The main points to note are (i) the experiments were carried out at constant pH and changes in HCO_3^- concentration were accompanied by the appropriate change in pCO_2, and (ii) L-[1-^{14}C]glutamine was used to allow measurement of flux through α-oxoglutarate dehydrogenase by the determination of $^{14}CO_2$.

ACCELERATION OF GLUTAMINE METABOLISM BY HCO_3^- IN THE LIVER

In hepatocytes HCO_3^- exerts a striking acceleration of glutamine removal and its conversion to glucose and urea. Leucine, which is not metabolized under the test conditions, has an additional accelerating effect (Table 1). The effect of leucine is concentration-dependent over the range tested (0.1–2.5 mM). As the increased glutamine removal is associated with increased glutamate formation, the primary effects of leucine and HCO_3^- are on the glutaminase reaction. Such glutamine as is oxidized is almost quantitatively converted to glucose as indicated by the finding that flux through α-oxoglutarate dehydrogenase (measured as $^{14}CO_2$ production from [1-^{14}C]glutamine) divided by 2 gives the amount of glucose formed, after correction for endogeneous glucose formation (Table 1). These results are consistent with a route for glutamine metabolism via aspartate aminotransferase and not via glutamate dehydrogenase, i.e.

$$\begin{aligned}
2\ \text{L-[1-}^{14}\text{C]glutamine} &\rightarrow 2\ \text{L-[1-}^{14}\text{C]glutamate} + 2\,NH_3\\
2\ \text{L-[1-}^{14}\text{C]glutamate} + 2\ \text{oxaloacetate} &\rightarrow 2\ \alpha\text{-[1-}^{14}\text{C]oxoglutarate} + 2\ \text{aspartate}\\
2\ \alpha\text{-[1-}^{14}\text{C]oxoglutarate} &\rightarrow 2\ \text{oxaloacetate} + 2\ {}^{14}CO_2\\
2\,NH_3 + 2\ \text{aspartate} &\rightarrow 2\ \text{urea} + 2\ \text{fumarate}\\
2\ \text{fumarate} &\rightarrow \text{glucose}
\end{aligned}$$

$$\text{Sum:}\ 2\ \text{L-[1-}^{14}\text{C]glutamine} \rightarrow 2\ \text{urea} + \text{glucose} + 2\ {}^{14}CO_2$$

Table 1. Effects of $[HCO_3^-]$ and leucine on glutamine metabolism in hepatocytes

Buffer system		Glutamine removed	$^{14}CO_2$	Major products formed Glutamate	Glucose	Urea	NH_3
15 mM HCO_3^-; 3% CO_2 in O_2	5 mM [1-^{14}C]gln	1.0	0.9	1.0	1.0	1.6	1.7
15 mM HCO_3^-; 3% CO_2 in O_2	5 mM + 0.1 mM leu	1.5	1.0	1.0	1.0	1.8	1.8
25 mM HCO_3^-; 5% CO_2 in O_2	5 mM [1-^{14}C]gln	2.6	1.3	1.3	1.1	2.3	1.7
25 mM HCO_3^-; 5% CO_2 in O_2	5 mM + 0.1 mM leu	2.9	1.3	1.5	1.3	2.7	1.8
25 mM HCO_3^-; 5% CO_2 in O_2	5 mM + 1 mM leu	3.9	2.0	2.0	1.7	3.7	1.7
25 mM HCO_3^-; 5% CO_2 in O_2	5 mM + 2.5 mM leu	4.5	2.4	2.5	1.7	3.8	3.2
50 mM HCO_3^-; 10% CO_2 in O_2	5 mM [1-^{14}C]gln	3.6	2.0	1.9	1.6	3.7	1.9
50 mM HCO_3^-; 10% CO_2 in O_2	5 mM + 0.1 mM leu	4.1	2.0	2.1	1.7	4.2	1.9
25 mM HCO_3^-; 5% CO_2 in O_2	No substrate	+0.7		0.2	0.5	0.9	0.2

Each flask contained 39.7 mg dry wt (147 mg wet wt) of hepatocytes from a 48 hr starved rat. Incubation was for 30 min at 37°C. Data are from a typical experiment and are expressed as μmol/flask, uncorrected for 1.5 μmol ammonia/flask present as a contaminant of the added glutamine. The amounts of alanine, α-oxoglutarate, citrate and aspartate were each less than 0.2 μmol/flask. As 2 mols of $^{14}CO_2$ are evolved for the formation of each mol of glucose from [1-^{14}C]glutamine, the glucose values (after correction for endogenous glucose formation) show that there is no complete oxidation of the carbon skeleton of glutamine.

This balance of reactions also represents the reactions in the presence of low concentrations of leucine, but not at 2.5 mM and above, when leucine acts both as an accelerator of glutamate dehydrogenase (see Yielding & Tomkins, 1961) and as an inhibitor of urea synthesis (Rognstad, 1977).

The use of 5 mM glutamine may appear unphysiological as the plasma concentration is about 0.5 mM. However, there is virtually no degradation of glutamine by hepatocytes at added concentrations below 2 mM (Lund & Watford, 1976). Recently Joseph & McGivan (1978a) reported that glucagon promotes metabolism at 2 mM glutamine in hepatocytes. We find that 0.05 mM dibutyryl cyclic AMP also promotes glucose and urea synthesis from 2 mM glutamine, and that the accelerating effects of HCO_3^- and leucine persist in the presence of cyclic-AMP. The mechanism by which glucagon or cyclic-AMP increases glutamine degradation in liver is not yet established, though Joseph & McGivan (1978a) provide evidence that it is at the stage of glutaminase and not on glutamine transport.

EFFECT OF HCO_3^- CONCENTRATION ON GLUTAMINE METABOLISM IN KIDNEY CORTEX TUBULES

In kidney tubules glutamine removal is much more rapid than in hepatocytes and, in contrast to liver, is unaffected by changes in the HCO_3^- concentration, but flux through α-oxoglutarate dehydrogenase and the formation of glucose decreases as $[HCO_3^-]$ increases (Table 2). Glucose accounts for about 50% of glutamine removed at 10.5 mM HCO_3^-, but only 30–40% at the higher HCO_3^- concentrations. Endogenous glucose synthesis was negligible. The reason for the decreased flux through α-oxoglutarate dehydrogenase appears to be an inhibition of glutamate dehydrogenase by HCO_3^- because the decrease in glucose formation is roughly paralleled by an increased

Table 2. Effect of $[HCO_3^-]$ on the fate of glutamine in rat kidney tubules

Buffer system	Incubation (min)	Glutamine removed	Major products formed Glutamate	NH_3	$^{14}CO_2$	Glucose	% Distribution of glutamine-carbon As glu	As glucose	Oxidized
10.5 mM HCO_3^-; 2.1% CO_2 in O_2	30	9.4	1.7	16.2	7.8	2.5	18.1	53.2	29.8
25 mM HCO_3^-; 5% CO_2 in O_2	30	9.3	2.3	15.6	7.0	2.3	24.7	49.5	25.8
47 mM HCO_3^-; 9.4% CO_2 in O_2	30	9.1	2.9	15.3	5.9	1.9	31.9	41.8	23.1
10.5 mM HCO_3^-; 2.1% CO_2 in O_2	60	15.8	2.1	27.5	12.9	3.6	13.3	45.6	36.1
25 mM HCO_3^-; 5% CO_2 in O_2	60	15.6	3.0	27.8	11.6	3.2	19.2	41.0	33.3
47 mM HCO_3^-; 9.4% CO_2 in O_2	60	15.6	3.9	26.3	10.5	2.3	25.0	29.5	37.8

The mean dry wt of tubules in each flask was 20 mg. The initial concentration of [1-^{14}C]glutamine was 5 mM. Values (corrected for zero-time) are μmol per flask (mean of 3 experiments). The amounts of each of the following metabolites were less than 0.1 μmol/flask: aspartate, lactate, pyruvate, α-oxoglutarate, malate, fumarate, citrate. The assumption was made that 2 mols $^{14}CO_2$ are evolved at the stage of α-oxoglutarate dehydrogenase during the formation of each mol of glucose. This value was subtracted from total $^{14}CO_2$ to obtain the amount completely oxidized.

accumulation of glutamate. In kidney tubules, in contrast to hepatocytes, the synthesis of glucose from glutamine (or glutamate) is via glutamate dehydrogenase because the pathway via aspartate aminotransferase cannot yield glucose without a stoichiometric accumulation of aspartate:

$$2\ \text{L-}[1\text{-}^{14}\text{C}]\text{glutamine} \rightarrow 2\ \text{L-}[1\text{-}^{14}\text{C}]\text{glutamate} + 2\ NH_3$$
$$2\ \text{L-}[1\text{-}^{14}\text{C}]\text{glutamate} \rightarrow 2\ \alpha\text{-}[1\text{-}^{14}\text{C}]\text{oxoglutarate} + 2\ NH_3$$
$$2\ \alpha\text{-}[1\text{-}^{14}\text{C}]\text{oxoglutarate} \rightarrow 2\ \text{oxaloacetate} + 2\ ^{14}CO_2$$
$$2\ \text{oxaloacetate} \rightarrow \text{glucose}$$

$$\text{Sum}: 2\ \text{L-}[1\text{-}^{14}\text{C}]\text{glutamine} \rightarrow \text{glucose} + 2\ ^{14}CO_2 + 4\ NH_3$$

There was no accumulation of aspartate. The alternative—i.e. that glucose arises from aspartate via the purine nucleotide cycle—is unlikely in that it would mean an obligatory link between this cycle and the rate of gluconeogenesis from those amino acids that, on degradation, form aspartate. There is no evidence of such a link.

The branched-chain amino acids have a slight inhibitory effect on glutamine removal (about 20% by 5 mM leucine). Neither glucagon nor dibutyryl cyclic AMP increases glutamine removal. The stimulation of gluconeogenesis by dibutyryl cyclic AMP is accompanied by a decrease in accumulation and complete oxidation of glutamate. Ammonium ions, which activate glutaminase in the liver (see Joseph & McGivan, 1978a; Haussinger & Sies, 1979) have no effect in kidney cortex tubules.

EFFECTS OF HCO_3^- CONCENTRATION ON GLUTAMINE METABOLISM IN ENTEROCYTES

In view of the importance of arterial glutamine as a respiratory fuel of the mucosa of the small intestine (Windmueller & Spaeth, 1974), similar experiments were carried out in isolated enterocytes. The effect of increasing $[HCO_3^-]$ from 15 to 50 mM is to increase glutamine removal, as in hepatocytes, but the effects are much smaller in the enterocyte. In other respects the effect of increasing $[HCO_3^-]$ is similar to its effect in kidney tubules in that the amount of glutamine carbon passing through the stage of α-oxoglutarate dehydrogenase decreases with increasing $[HCO_3^-]$. In the case of enterocytes, alanine is a major product. Its yield is not influenced by $[HCO_3^-]$. Neither leucine nor dibutyryl cyclic AMP has an effect on the rate of glutamine removal.

DISCUSSION

Differences between the effects of bicarbonate on liver and kidney glutaminase

The experiments show that at constant pH, bicarbonate affects hepatic and renal glutaminases in a strikingly different manner. Increasing the concentration of bicarbonate substantially raises the rate of removal of glutamine and the formation of glucose and urea in hepatocytes. Activation of glutaminase by HCO_3^- has also been observed in isolated liver mitochondria (Joseph & McGivan, 1978b). In contrast renal glutaminase is not affected by variations in the concentration of bicarbonate. The significance of these differences between liver and kidney may be understood by reference to the functional role of glutamine. The need of the kidney for glutamine as a precursor of urinary ammonia in acidosis (i.e. at low bicarbonate concentration) is met by a decreased glutamine degradation in the intestine (Lund & Watford, 1976; Tizianello *et al.*, 1978), liver and possibly other tissues. This preserves glutamine for ammoniagenesis in the kidney. On the other hand when the acid-base balance does not require adjustment by ammonia excretion, the rate of degradation of glutamine in the liver and other tissues rises.

Differences in the effects of glucagon and cyclic AMP on hepatic and renal glutaminase

It has been known for some time that neither hepatocytes nor the isolated perfused liver metabolizes glutamine at near-physiological concentrations in the suspension fluid or perfusion medium (Lund, 1971; Saheki & Katunuma, 1975; Lund & Watford, 1976) while it is readily metabolized at higher concentration (10 mM). This is in keeping with the high apparent K_m for liver glutaminase reported by Huang & Knox (1976). However, glucagon (Joseph & McGivan, 1978a) and dibutyryl cyclic AMP promote metabolism of low concentrations of glutamine in hepatocytes. Presumably glucagon acts through cyclic AMP to decrease the apparent K_m of hepatic glutaminase. In contrast to this the mitochondrial glutaminase of kidney tubules and the isolated perfused kidney responds to low concentrations of glutamine and is not affected by glucagon or cyclic AMP. This regulation of hepatic glutaminase by glucagon and cyclic AMP does not appear to be as directly connected with acidosis as does the regulation by bicarbonate, but indirectly it is connected because it is one of the factors controlling the extent of degradation of glutamine in the body and its preservation for a variety of metabolic processes.

Other modifiers of hepatic glutaminase

Two further activators of hepatic glutaminase have come to light; leucine and ammonium ions. Leucine has been known for some time to be an activator of hepatic glutamate dehydrogenase (Yielding & Tomkins, 1961). The present experiments demonstrate an activating effect for hepatic glutaminase. Leucine has no effect on the renal degradation of glutamine. The activating effect of ammonium ions was first observed by Charles (1968), and subsequently by Nordmann *et al.* (1972) and Haussinger & Sies (1975) and by Joseph & McGivan (1978a). The effect occurs also in isolated mitochondria. Sies interprets the accelerating effect of ammonium ions as a positive feedback. The main function of tissue glutamine is to serve as a store of nitrogen for the synthesis of cell constituents. When the stores are "full" and when there is a surplus of ammonia in the plasma or portal blood, glutamine reaching the liver must be degraded independent of the state of the acid–base balance. Thus ammonia appears to serve as a signal for hepatic glutamine degradation at physiological glutamine concentrations.

The fate of the carbon skeleton of glutamine in kidney and liver

In the liver the endproducts of glutamine degradation are essentially glucose, ammonia and urea. This implies partial oxidation and the liberation of 2 CO_2 but complete oxidation of glutamine does not occur in hepatocytes. On the other hand, a considerable proportion of glutamine carbon is completely oxidized in kidney tubules. This necessitates the formation of pyruvate from malate or oxaloacetate, reactions involving either oxaloacetate decarboxylase (EC 4.1.1.3), or phosphoenolpyruvate carboxykinase (EC 4.1.1.32) plus pyruvate kinase (EC 2.7.1.40), or the NADP-linked (EC 1.1.1.40) or NAD-linked "malic" enzyme. The latter enzyme has been reported to be present in rat liver and rat kidney (Sauer, 1973). Although all are present in extracts of both liver and kidney the factors that control the activities of these enzymes *in situ* must therefore be different for the two tissues.

Intestinal mucosa

The glutaminase of the epithelium of the small intestine ("enterocytes") is again different from those of liver and kidney. In the enterocytes glutamine is the major fuel of respiration; it is the only amino acid which serves this function (Windmueller & Spaeth, 1974). Leucine and cyclic AMP have no effect on the activity of the intestinal glutaminase. Apart from ammonia, a major nitrogenous endproduct of glutamine degradation in enterocytes is alanine, formed by transamination of glutamate with pyruvate, the formation of which must involve the same enzymes as in kidney. All, including the NAD-linked malic enzyme (Sauer *et al.*, 1979) are present in the mucosa of the small intestine. Bicarbonate has a slightly stimulating effect on glutamine removal but much less so than in liver.

Experiments with subcellular preparations

When the cell structure is disrupted by the standard procedure for preparing homogenates, the balance of metabolic processes in the tissue is radically changed. Homogenates may contain more or less intact mitochondria but the cytosol is diluted by the suspension medium. Hence all cytosolic reactions which depend on a specific solute environment, such as gluconeogenesis and urea synthesis, are liable to be impaired. For instance, on addition of glutamate to a liver homogenate, glutamine is synthesized (see Introduction)—a reaction which does not occur in intact hepatocytes. Isolated mitochondria likewise differ from intact cells in their metabolic behaviour. Thus when glutamine is added to isolated kidney mitochondria, aspartate is a major endproduct, while in kidney tubules glucose and ammonia are the main products. This brings home the importance of experimenting with intact cells when attempting to obtain information about events occurring *in vivo*.

Acknowledgements—The work was supported by the Medical Research Council, the U.S. Public Health Services (grant No. AM-11748) and by a grant to G.B. from the Institut National de la Santé et de la Recherche Médicale (grant No. ATP 62-78-94).

REFERENCES

BAVEREL G. & LUND P. (1979) A role for bicarbonate in the regulation of mammalian glutamine metabolism. *Biochem. J.* **184**, 599–606.

CHARLES R. (1968) Mitochondriale citrulline synthese: een ammoniak fixerend en ATP verbruikend proces. Ph.D. Thesis, University of Amsterdam.

HAUSSINGER D. & SIES H. (1975) Activation of glutaminase by ammonium ions in the perfused rat liver. *10th FEBS Meeting*, Abstract No. 1497.

HAUSSINGER D. & SIES H. (1979) Hepatic glutamine metabolism under the influence of the portal ammonia concentration in the perfused rat liver. *Eur. J. Biochem.* **101**, 179–184.

HUANG Y. Z. & KNOX W. E. (1976) A comparative study of glutaminase isoenzymes in rat tissues. *Enzyme* **21**, 408–426.

JOSEPH S. K. & MCGIVAN J. D. (1978a) The effect of ammonium chloride and glucagon on the metabolism of glutamine in isolated liver cells from starved rats. *Biochim. biophys. Acta* **543**, 16–28.

JOSEPH S. K. & MCGIVAN J. D. (1978b) The effects of ammonium chloride and bicarbonate on the activity of glutaminase in isolated liver mitochondria. *Biochem. J.* **176**, 837–844.

KREBS H. A. (1935) Metabolism of amino acids—IV. The synthesis of glutamine from glutamic acid and ammonia, and the enzymic hydrolysis of glutamine in animal tissues. *Biochem. J.* **29**, 1951–1969.

KREBS H. A. & BELLAMY D. (1960) The interconversion of glutamic acid and aspartic acid in respiring tissues. *Biochem. J.* **75**, 523–529.

LUND P. (1971) Control of glutamine synthesis in rat liver. *Biochem. J.* **124**, 653–660.

LUND P. & WATFORD M. (1976) Glutamine as a precursor of urea. In *The Urea Cycle* (Edited by GRISOLIA S., BAGUENA R. & MAYOR F.) pp. 479–488. Wiley and Sons, New York.

NORDMANN R., PETIT M. A. & NORDMANN J. (1972) Recherches sur le méchanisme de l'accumulation intrahépatique d'acides aminés dicarboxyliques au cours de l'intoxication ammoniacale. *Biochimie* **54**, 1473–1478.

ROGNSTAD R. (1977) Sources of ammonia for urea synthesis in isolated rat liver cells. *Biochim. biophys. Acta* **496**, 249–254.

SAHEKI T. & KATUNUMA N. (1975) Analysis of regulatory factors for urea synthesis by isolated perfused rat liver—I. Urea synthesis with ammonia and glutamine as nitrogen sources. *J. Biochem, Tokyo* **77**, 659–669.

SAUER L. A. (1973) An NAD- and NADP-dependent malic enzyme with regulatory properties in rat liver and adrenal cortex mitochondrial fractions. *Biochem. biophys. Res. Commun.* **50**, 524–531.

SAUER L. A., DAUCHY R. T. & NAGEL W. O. (1979) Identification of an $NAD(P)^+$-dependent "malic" enzyme in small-intestinal-mucosal mitochondria. *Biochem. J.* **184**, 185–188.

TIZIANELLO A., FERRARI G. DE, GARIBOTTO G. & GURRERI G. (1978) Effects of chronic renal insufficiency and metabolic acidosis on glutamine metabolism in man. *Clin. Sci. mol. Med.* **55**, 391–397.

WINDMUELLER H. G. & SPAETH A. E. (1974) Uptake and metabolism of plasma glutamine by the small intestine. *J. biol. Chem.* **249**, 5070–5079.

YIELDING K. L. & TOMKINS G. M. (1961) An effect of L-leucine and other essential amino acids on the structure and activity of glutamic dehydrogenase. *Proc. natn. Acad. Sci. U.S.A.* **47**, 983–990.

SYMPOSIUM DISCUSSION

Bogusky: I want to ask Dr Krebs what is the role of hepatic glutaminase in hypokalaemic alkalosis?

Krebs: It might indeed accelerate hepatic glutamine uptake and reduce the amount available for ammoniagenesis in kidney, but there are many factors involved.

Lund: We do not really know the function of glutamine metabolism by the liver *in vivo*. There are multiple factors which it is now known accelerate hepatic glutamine metabolism: cyclic AMP, leucine, bicarbonate and glucagon. These effects are different and I don't, for example, know how the concentration of glucagon might change in hypokalaemia.

Weiner: Professor Krebs, does bicarbonate have its effect in the intact cell, or is this a property of the isolated glutaminase?

Krebs: I have to pass that question to Dr Baverel, who has done experiments on homogenates.

Baverel: The stimulating effect of bicarbonate on glutaminase has also been demonstrated in isolated liver mitochondria (Joseph & McGivan, *Biochem. J.* **176**, 837–844, 1978).

Int. J. Biochem., Vol. 12, pp. 75 to 83
© Pergamon Press Ltd 1980. Printed in Great Britain

0020-711X/80/0701-0075$02.00/0

METABOLIC CHANGES IN SKELETAL MUSCLE DURING CHRONIC METABOLIC ACIDOSIS

GUY LEMIEUX, MALCOLM WATFORD, PATRICK VINAY and ANDRÉ GOUGOUX
Nephrology-Metabolism Division and Renal Laboratory, Hôtel-Dieu Hospital,
Department of Medicine, University of Montreal, Montreal, Quebec, Canada H2W 1T8

Abstract—1. In an attempt to clarify the importance of skeletal muscle as a source of glutamine during chronic metabolic acidosis, *in vivo* and *in vitro* experiments were performed in normal and NH_4Cl acidotic rats.

2. In the acidotic animals, arterial glutamine, glutamate and alanine were significantly lower than in normal rats. The arterio-venous difference for glutamine across the hindlimb was not statistically different in acidotic and normal animals.

3. No net release or uptake of glutamate was observed in either control or acidotic rats. However the uptake of alanine observed in normal animals was completely abolished in the acidotic rats.

4. The metabolite profile of freeze-clamped hindlimb skeletal muscle from acidotic animals revealed a lower concentration of glutamine, glutamate, alanine, aspartate, alphaketoglutarate, lactate and pyruvate and increased ammonia concentration.

5. Alanine aminotransferase activity of the hindlimb skeletal muscle was unchanged by acidosis.

6. *In vitro* glutamine production by the isolated rat diaphragm was not different in acidotic and control animals.

7. The addition of various substrates (valine, leucine and NH_4Cl) stimulated glutamine production to similar extent in control and acidotic animals.

8. While alanine was produced by the diaphragm of the normal animals, it did not occur in the acidotic rats. Furthermore the addition of substrates did not stimulate alanine production by the diaphragm of the acidotic animals.

9. Addition of methionine sulfoximine (MSO) 5 mM to inhibit diaphragm glutamine synthetase activity resulted in a 55% decrease in glutamine synthesis in both normal and acidotic animals.

10. The production of glutamine or alanine was not affected by acidification of the incubation medium from pH 7.4 to 7.0.

11. Our findings suggest that the capacity for glutamine synthesis by the skeletal muscle is not affected by metabolic acidosis.

12. The fall in glutamate and the rise in ammonia concentrations in the skeletal muscle *in vivo* during metabolic acidosis suggest that glutamate availability is rate-limiting for the production of glutamine. This could explain the marked variations in alanine metabolism.

13. In view of the very small changes observed in glutamine production by the skeletal muscle during acidosis, the role of other tissues such as the liver, the brain and, in the rat, the kidney, should be envisaged.

14. The possibility of a significant decrease in glutamine metabolism by the intestine during acidosis making more glutamine available for renal extraction should also be seriously considered.

INTRODUCTION

The renal adaptation to chronic metabolic acidosis is characterized by increased extraction of circulating glutamine (Pilkington *et al.*, 1970; Lemieux *et al.*, 1974; Cartier *et al.*, 1975), increased ammoniagenesis (Lemieux *et al.*, 1974; Cartier *et al.*, 1975) and gluconeogenesis (Cartier *et al.*, 1975) and, in the rat, increased activity of glutaminase I (Rector & Orloff, 1958; Curthoys & Lowry, 1973) and phosphoenolpyruvate carboxykinase (Alleyne & Scullard, 1969). A decrease in arterial glutamine concentration in chronically acidotic rats has been observed by a number of investigators (Lund & Watford, 1976; Squires *et al.*, 1976; Hanson & Parsons, 1977; Parry & Brosnan, 1978). This decrement is insufficient to account for the marked increase in renal glutamine extraction. It therefore follows that extrarenal tissues respond to acidosis either by increasing production or decreasing utilization of circulating glutamine.

In spite of a low glutamine synthetase activity (Iqbal & Ottaway, 1970; Lund, 1971) it has been realized in recent years that skeletal muscle is the primary source of circulating glutamine (Marliss *et al.*, 1971; Hills *et al.*, 1972; Felig *et al.*, 1973; Ruderman & Berger, 1974). However the question of changes in the release of glutamine by muscle during acidosis has not been extensively studied. A small but insignificant release of glutamine has been demonstrated across the hindlimb of chronically acidotic rats (Lund & Watford, 1976). Other studies with the perfused rat hindlimb have shown a small increase in glutamine release with acid (pH 7.06) perfusate but no difference between control and chronically acidotic rats (Oliver *et al.*, 1977). In man, Tizianello *et al.* (1978) reported an increase of questionable significance in the release of glutamine from forearm muscle in normal subjects following 3–6 days of NH_4Cl acidosis. A recent preliminary report by Finley *et al.* (1979) states that increased glutamine efflux from muscle accounts for approx 25% of the augmented renal extraction of glutamine during NH_4Cl acidosis in man.

The purpose of the present work was to clarify changes that might occur in the release of glutamine by skeletal muscle during metabolic acidosis in the rat. To this end studies were carried out *in vivo* and *in vitro*. From *in vivo* measurements of arteriovenous differences across the hindlimb we were unable to demonstrate any significant change in glutamine release between normal and acidotic animals. Using the freeze-clamp technique for the measurement of muscle metabolites *in vivo* we found that acidosis results in marked changes in the concentration of various metabolites involved in glutamine metabolism in skeletal muscle. During *in vitro* studies with the isolated rat diaphragm, chronic acidosis using normal (pH 7.4) or acid (pH 7.0) media had no significant effect on glutamine release.

MATERIALS AND METHODS

Male Wistar rats weighing between 250–300 g for *in vivo* experiments and between 80–120 g for *in vitro* experiments were maintained on a commercial diet (Purina rat chow). The smaller rats were needed to obtain a viable isolated diaphragm preparation (Goldberg *et al.*, 1976). Metabolic acidosis was induced by replacement of drinking water by 1.5% (w/v) NH_4Cl for 6–7 days.

In vivo studies

Rats were anesthetized with pentobarbital and one of two procedures followed. To obtain arterial and venous blood from the same animal, the abdominal cavity was opened and blood (0.5–1.0 ml) was withdrawn from the common iliac vein into a heparinized syringe through a 25-gauge needle. With the venous needle carefully held in place to avoid hemorrhage, arterial blood (1.0–1.5 ml) was obtained from the aorta by a similar procedure. Blood was rapidly added to 1.0 ml 10% (w/v) perchloric acid. Approximately 0.5 ml arterial blood was retained for the determination of blood pH and plasma total CO_2 concentration.

For the determination of metabolite concentrations in skeletal muscle one hindlimb was exposed by removal of the skin. The skeletal muscle of the thigh was rapidly dissected free and frozen between aluminum clamps precooled in liquid nitrogen (Wollenberger *et al.*, 1960). The frozen tissue was extracted and prepared for analyses as previously reported for kidney tissue (Vinay *et al.*, 1978).

In vitro *studies*

Diaphragms were dissected free of the ribs according to the procedure of Goldberg *et al.* (1976), and placed in bicarbonate buffered saline (Krebs & Henseleit, 1932). Quarter-diaphragms were then cut, blotted dry on filter paper, weighed and transferred to 25 ml Erlenmeyer flasks containing 3.0 ml medium with or without glucose 5 mM. Additional substrates 1.0 mM valine, leucine and NH_4Cl were added alone or in combination to the glucose-free or glucose-containing medium. In some experiments the pH of the incubation medium was modified from 7.40 to 7.00 by replacement of some sodium bicarbonate with sodium chloride. The flasks were gassed with O_2/CO_2 (95:5%), stoppered and incubated for up to 2 hr at 37°C, in a shaking water bath. At the end of incubation the diaphragms were rapidly removed, rinsed in fresh medium, blotted dry and frozen in liquid nitrogen. The frozen tissue was carefully pulverized and extracted with 10% (w/v) perchloric acid. The medium was poured into test tubes and placed in a boiling water bath for 2 min to destroy enzymic activity (Garber *et al.*, 1976). In eight experiments, diaphragms from normal and acidotic animals were incubated for 60 min at pH 7.40 with and without methionine sulfoximine (MSO) 5 to 20 mM to inhibit glutamine synthetase. After deproteinization with perchloric acid 40% (w/v) the tissue was homogenized in the flasks and total glutamine and glutamate were measured. The results were corrected for zero time values (no incubation) obtained from flasks treated in the same fashion.

Analytical methods

Blood pH was determined by a glass electrode using an Instrumentation Laboratory Ultramicro Duo-matic blood gas-analyzing system, Model 123-Sl. Plasma total CO_2 was determined with a Natelson manometric microgasometer. Plasma bicarbonate concentration was calculated from the values of blood pH and plasma total carbon dioxide using a value for alpha of 0.0301 in the Henderson–Hasselbalch equation (Lemieux & Gervais, 1964).

Glutamine, glutamate, ammonia, alphaketoglutarate, aspartate, pyruvate, malate, ATP and ADP were assayed by fluorimetric adaptation of standard spectrophotometric procedures previously reported (Vinay *et al.*, 1978). Alanine was measured fluorimetrically by a modification of the spectrophotometric procedure of Williamson (Williamson, 1974). The alanine dehydrogenase used for this technique was dialysed for 4 hr against distilled water to remove branched-chain amino acid dehydrogenase activity (Lund & Baverel, 1978).

Lactate and AMP were measured spectrophotometrically as previously reported (Vinay *et al.*, 1978). Oxaloacetate concentration and the cytosolic redox potential were calculated from components of the malate and lactate dehydrogenase reactions respectively according to Williamson *et al.* (1967). Mass-action ratios for the alanine aminotransferase (GPT) and aspartate aminotransferase (GOT) systems were calculated according to Krebs & Veech (1969). For the measurement of alanine aminotransferase activity at 37°C (Bergmeyer & Bernt, 1974) hindlimb muscle was homogenized in 20 vol of 0.25 M sucrose containing 5 mM Tris buffer pH 7.40. The homogenates were frozen and thawed 3 times to release mitochondrial activity.

Statistical analysis

Statistical analysis was performed using the Student's *t*-test. For repeated comparisons against one control, the Dunnett's *t*-test was used. In all experiments, a *P* value of less than 0.05 was considered significant.

RESULTS

In vivo *studies*

Blood pH in normal rats ($n = 25$) was 7.40 ± 0.02 and plasma bicarbonate 28.3 ± 1.0 mM. In the acidotic animals ($n = 30$) blood pH was 7.12 ± 0.03 and plasma bicarbonate 15.4 ± 1.1 mM.

A marked decrease in the circulating concentration of glutamine, glutamate and alanine was observed in chronically acidotic rats (Table 1). The small output of glutamine by the hindquarter observed in control rats was increased by 76% during metabolic acidosis. However this increase was not statistically significant because of the wide variations in the actual blood glutamine values. Neither net uptake nor release of glutamate were observed across the hindquarter in control or acidotic rats. The small uptake of alanine observed in control animals was completely suppressed during acidosis (Table 1).

The arterial lactate concentration in 8 normal rats (2.08 ± 0.24 mM) was unchanged in 8 acidotic rats (1.79 ± 0.16 mM) while arterial ammonia concentration increased from 0.06 ± 0.01 mM to 0.10 ± 0.01 mM ($P < 0.05$) during acidosis (5 animals in each group).

The concentrations of glutamine, glutamate, alanine, aspartate, alphaketoglutarate, lactate and pyru-

Table 1. Arteriovenous differences for glutamine, glutamate and alanine across the hindlimb of normal and acidotic rats

	Normal (n = 13)			Acidotic (n = 13)		
	Arterial (A)	Venous (V)	A − V	Arterial (A)	Venous (V)	A − V
Glutamine	0.519 ± 0.019	0.535 ± 0.019	−0.016 ± 0.011	0.387 ± 0.019*	0.417 ± 0.018*	−0.030 ± 0.015
Glutamate	0.182 ± 0.009	0.178 ± 0.008	0.004 ± 0.006	0.129 ± 0.008*	0.130 ± 0.007*	−0.001 ± 0.003
Alanine	0.395 ± 0.015	0.358 ± 0.012	0.037 ± 0.005	0.322 ± 0.019*	0.327 ± 0.016	−0.005 ± 0.012*

* $P < 0.05$ acidotic vs normal rats.
Results are expressed as μmols/ml whole blood and are means ± SEM.

vate were all markedly decreased in skeletal muscle during metabolic acidosis (Table 2). A striking increase in tissue ammonia was observed in the acidotic animals (Table 2). Malate concentration was slightly decreased while ATP and ADP were slightly increased during acidosis. The lactate: pyruvate ratio, cytosolic redox state (LDH) and calculated oxaloacetate concentration were unchanged (Table 2). In both control and acidotic rat skeletal muscle the aspartate aminotransferase (GOT) system was close to the equilibrium constant of 6.61 reported by Krebs & Veech (1969). However, the alanine aminotransferase (GPT) system was not close to the equilibrium constant of 1.52 (Krebs & Veech, 1969) (Table 2). Muscle alanine aminotransferase activity was not significantly different in control and acidotic animals (5.98 ± 0.82 vs 7.28 ± 0.54 μmol pyruvate formed per min per gram wet weight). Due to the low glutamate dehydrogenase activity in muscle (Karl *et al.*, 1976) and the large difference observed in tissue and arterial ammonia concentrations, a meaningful mitochondrial redox value could not be calculated from the glutamate dehydrogenase system.

In vitro *studies*

Figure 1 shows the release of glutamine into the incubation medium and the total content of glutamine in the tissue plus medium during incubation for 120 min of diaphragms from normal and acidotic rats. It can be seen that during the first 30 min, glutamine was released into the media while the tissue content of glutamine decreased. This is interpreted as a wash-out effect. Glutamine release was accompanied by a net production for 60 min. From 60 to 120 min glutamine continued to be released into the medium but net production decreased. The pattern was the same in both normal and acidotic animals and the values were not significantly different. It is of interest that in contrast to our findings with freeze-clamped hindlimb muscle, initial glutamine concentration was not significantly different in the diaphragms of acidotic and control rats. In these experiments, initial release of glutamate was observed but it stopped after 30 min and no net production of glutamate was observed throughout the incubation period. Acidotic diaphragms had a lower glutamate concentration than those from normal animals (2.50 ± 0.48 vs 4.43 ± 0.22 μmol per gram wet weight). Figure 2 shows the changes in alanine during the same experiments. Following an initial wash-out, alanine release and production by diaphragms of normal rats continued in a linear fashion. Initial tissue alanine concentration in acidotic rats was 73% of that of normal animals and alanine production was less than 25% of that observed with diaphragms from normal animals (Fig. 2).

The initial decrease in tissue amino acid concentrations as well as that observed between 60 and 120 min were accompanied by simultaneous decrease in the tissue ATP content in both normal and acidotic

Table 2. Metabolite concentrations in freeze-clamped skeletal muscle (hindlimb) of normal and acidotic rats

Metabolites	Normal n = 6	Acidotic n = 6
Glutamine	5.14 ± 0.31	3.48 ± 0.03*
Glutamate	2.51 ± 0.22	1.27 ± 0.14*
Alanine	2.57 ± 0.12	1.72 ± 0.09*
Aspartate	0.65 ± 0.03	0.41 ± 0.09*
NH_4^+	0.16 ± 0.02	1.50 ± 0.38*
Alphaketoglutarate	0.12 ± 0.02	0.04 ± 0.01*
Malate	0.18 ± 0.02	0.14 ± 0.01
Lactate	2.67 ± 0.21	1.93 ± 0.12*
Pyruvate	0.19 ± 0.02	0.14 ± 0.01*
ATP	6.32 ± 0.17	7.26 ± 0.19*
ADP	0.55 ± 0.03	0.75 ± 0.04*
AMP	0.09 ± 0.01	0.07 ± 0.004
L/P	14.1	13.7
OAA (calculated) nmols	3.2	2.5
$NAD^+/NADH_{LDH}$	641	653
K_{GOT}	9.7	5.2
K_{GPT}	0.65	0.39

* $P < 0.05$ acidotic vs normal.
Results are expressed as μmols/g wet wt (except for oxaloacetate) and are means ± SEM.
L/P: lactate/pyruvate.
OAA: oxaloacetate.

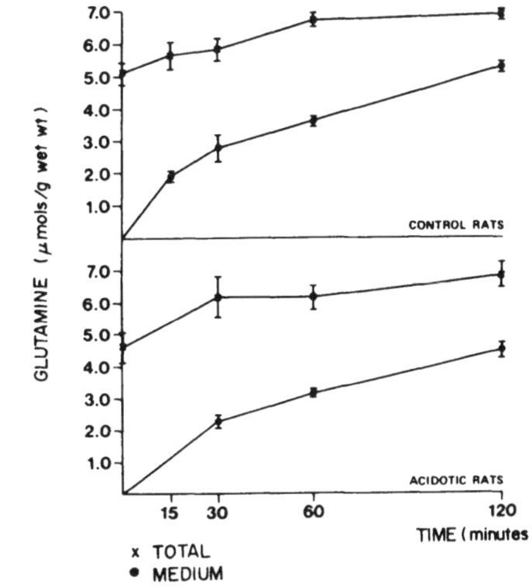

Fig. 1. Time-course of glutamine metabolism by rat diaphragm in control and acidotic animals. The upper line represents the total concentration (tissue + medium) and the lower line that of the medium.

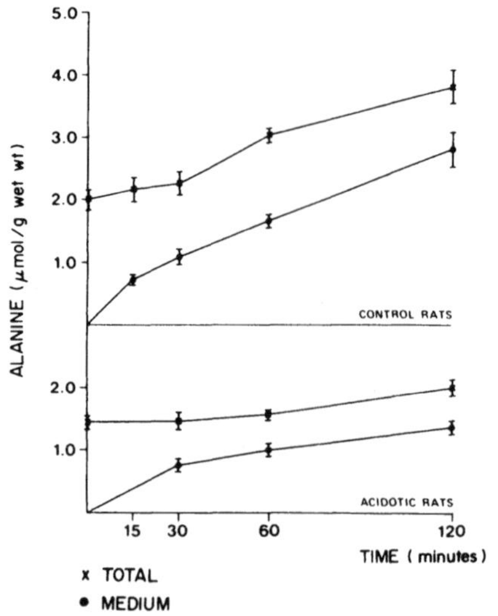

Fig. 2. Time course of alanine metabolism by rat diaphragm in control and acidotic animals. The upper line represents the total concentration (tissue + medium) and the lower line that of the medium.

rats. As the tissue ATP levels were about 75% of the initial values after 60 minutes of incubation and as significant production of glutamine and alanine could be observed at this time, 60-min incubations were used for subsequent experiments. A 15-min pre-incubation period to allow wash-out of metabolites (Goldberg *et al.*, 1976) was not used in this study since it resulted in more pronounced depletion of ATP.

In these experiments, changing the pH of the incubation medium from 7.40 to 7.00 did not modify the release or production of glutamine, glutamate or alanine from diaphragms of either normal and acidotic rats.

Table 3 shows the effect of additional substrates on the metabolism of glutamine, glutamate and alanine in rat diaphragm. Glutamine production was stimulated by ammonium chloride plus valine or leucine in both normal and acidotic rats. However, the diaphragms from acidotic animals did not produce more glutamine than those from normal rats. The total glutamate concentration in tissue plus medium as already mentioned was lower in the acidotic than in the normal animals. The addition of ammonium chloride alone decreased the concentration of glutamate. The latter increased slightly with either valine or leucine both in normal and acidotic rats. The combination of ammonium chloride plus valine or leucine maintained glutamate level near control levels in both normal and acidotic animals. This is interpreted as maintenance of glutamate concentration for increased glutamine production. Alanine released into the medium and total production were unchanged in control animals by the addition of various substrates (Table 3). In acidotic animals, as already noted, alanine production is markedly decreased and could not be restored by the addition of valine, leucine and ammonium chloride alone or in combination.

In all experiments, regardless of the presence or absence of other substrates, the omission of glucose from the incubation medium did not affect the release or production of glutamine, glutamate, and alanine by the diaphragms of normal and acidotic rats. It should be pointed out that tissue ATP levels were maintained throughout the first 60-min period of incubation independent of the presence or absence of glucose. Table 4 shows the results of the experiments using methionine sulfoximine 5 mM to inhibit muscle glutamine synthetase activity in the rat diaphragm. It can be seen that total (tissue plus medium) glutamine fell by 59 and 54% while glutamate rose in the same proportion. Similar results were obtained with MSO concentrations of 10, 15 and 20 mM. The response was the same in normal and acidotic animals (Table 4).

DISCUSSION

The present study confirms that in chronically acidotic rats, arterial glutamine concentration is signifi-

Table 3. Effect of additional substrates on amino acid metabolism in rat diaphragm

Substrate added	Glutamine Medium	Glutamine Total	Glutamate Medium	Glutamate Total	Alanine Medium	Alanine Total
Normal rats ($n = 6$)						
None	3.24 ± 0.19	5.93 ± 0.23	1.33 ± 0.09	3.65 ± 0.25	1.58 ± 0.09	2.99 ± 0.22
Valine	3.79 ± 0.22	6.57 ± 0.42	1.65 ± 0.08	3.96 ± 0.16	1.94 ± 0.14	2.11 ± 0.15
NH_4Cl	3.74 ± 0.19	7.12 ± 0.34	1.16 ± 0.14	2.49 ± 0.20†	1.35 ± 0.05	3.20 ± 0.37
Leucine	3.82 ± 0.25	6.78 ± 0.39	1.80 ± 0.12	4.72 ± 0.28†	1.99 ± 0.24	2.71 ± 0.32
NH_4Cl + valine	4.79 ± 0.19†	8.12 ± 0.41†	1.47 ± 0.24	3.19 ± 0.29	1.85 ± 0.20	2.99 ± 0.16
NH_4Cl + leucine	4.39 ± 0.33†	7.41 ± 0.65†	1.82 ± 0.18	3.60 ± 0.18	2.13 ± 0.16	2.68 ± 0.09
Acidotic rats ($n = 6$)						
None	2.95 ± 0.13	5.06 ± 0.22*	0.79 ± 0.07*	2.66 ± 0.15*	0.91 ± 0.08*	1.53 ± 0.13*
Valine	3.03 ± 0.22*	4.35 ± 0.46*	1.09 ± 0.05*	3.20 ± 0.16	1.30 ± 0.11*†	1.98 ± 0.18*
NH_4Cl	3.21 ± 0.14*	6.11 ± 0.37	0.66 ± 0.11*	1.79 ± 0.18*†	0.68 ± 0.06*	1.08 ± 0.12*
Leucine	3.63 ± 0.39	5.51 ± 0.63	1.36 ± 0.17	3.77 ± 0.21*†	1.29 ± 0.06*†	1.93 ± 0.10
NH_4Cl + valine	4.31 ± 0.41*	7.56 ± 0.72†	0.91 ± 0.16	2.16 ± 0.23*	0.92 ± 0.10*	1.33 ± 0.13*
NH_4Cl + leucine	3.75 ± 0.28	7.12 ± 0.53†	1.33 ± 0.26	2.75 ± 0.15*	1.10 ± 0.08*	1.64 ± 0.12*

* $P < 0.05$—acidotic vs normal rats.
† $P < 0.05$—substrate vs no substrate.
Results are expressed as μmols/g wet wt and are means ± SEM.

Table 4. Effect of methionine sulfoximine (MSO) on the generation of glutamine and glutamate by rat diaphragm

	Normal (n = 4)		Acidotic (n = 4)	
	Glutamine	Glutamate	Glutamine	Glutamate
Medium	2.328 ± 0.225	1.137 ± 0.102	2.031 ± 0.101	1.271 ± 0.207
Medium + MSO 5 mM	0.955 ± 0.130*	2.692 ± 0.313*	0.939 ± 0.118*	2.463 ± 0.180*

* = $P < 0.05$—MSO vs no MSO.
Values are expressed as μmols/g/wet wt after 60 min of incubation and corrected for zero time.
n = number of experiments (8 rats per experiment).

cantly lower than that of normal animals. This is in accord with most other reports (Lund & Watford, 1976; Squires *et al.*, 1976; Hanson & Parsons, 1977; Parry & Brosnan, 1978) although one study has shown an increase in circulating glutamine concentration in acidotic rats (Oliver *et al.*, 1977). Although the arteriovenous difference for glutamine was higher by 76% across the hindquarter of our acidotic rats, this increase was not statistically significant. We are aware of only one other study where the release of glutamine by rat hindlimb in chronic acidosis was studied (Lund & Watford, 1976). The authors of the latter study also failed to demonstrate a significant increase in glutamine release (Lund & Watford, 1976). They attributed this failure to the supplementation of the diet with glucose (Lund & Watford, 1976). It is of interest that increased release of glutamine across the hindquarter of the rat has been reported in animals fed a high-protein diet (Remesy *et al.*, 1978).

The significant decrease in circulating glutamate concentration observed in the present study during chronic acidosis has not been previously reported. Other workers have found either a slight although not significant decrease (Lund & Watford, 1976; Squires *et al.*, 1976) or no change (Hanson & Parsons, 1977). Whereas a slight uptake of glutamate has been reported in starved rats (Ruderman & Berger, 1974; Aikawa *et al.*, 1973), no uptake or release of glutamate by the hindlimb was observed in the present study either in normal or acidotic rats. We also found circulating alanine concentration to be significantly lower in acidotic animals. This is supported by the study of Hanson & Parsons (1977) although Squires *et al.* (1976) reported that alanine concentration remains constant during acidosis. Our finding of an uptake of alanine in normal (fed) rats is in agreement with other reports (Remesy *et al.*, 1978, Macdonald *et al.*, 1976). We are the first, however, to observe that during chronic acidosis the uptake of alanine is completely abolished. Furthermore no net release of alanine was noted.

A detailed profile of metabolites in skeletal muscle has not been previously reported. However most of the values in the normal rat in the present study are in accord with known values from individual reports (Garber *et al.*, 1976; Williamson & Brosnan, 1974). Exceptions are the concentrations of glutamate and alanine which were respectively 2.51 and 2.57 μmols per gram wet weight in the present study versus the reported value of 1.02 and 1.50 by Garber *et al.* (1976).

The marked decrease in the concentration of metabolites observed in skeletal muscle during metabolic acidosis could signify decreased uptake of glutamate and alanine, increased release of metabolites from the cell or increased metabolism to other products. The decrease in glutamate content and the rise in ammonia concentration strongly suggest that glutamate availability is rate-limiting for the synthesis of glutamine and also for alanine after 6–7 days of chronic metabolic acidosis. The large increase in ammonia content of the muscle during acidosis is somewhat unexpected and not easy to explain. It is of interest that in the muscle of our control rats we found a nonequilibrium state for the alanine aminotransferase system thus confirming the observations of Krebs (1975). In the acidotic rat muscle, the alanine aminotransferase system was further removed from equilibrium necessitating the production of alanine which could not be observed either *in vivo* or *in vitro*. This could not be due to lowered alanine aminotransferase activity since it was unchanged in acidotic animals. The absence of alanine production could indicate increased glutamine production from glutamate at the expense of alanine synthesis in the acidotic muscle. The large increment in muscle ammonia observed in the present study could be important in decreasing glutamate availability for alanine synthesis.

Our *in vitro* study with the isolated diaphragm reveals that we used a viable preparation as evidenced by the stable level of ATP during the first 60 min of incubation. The production of glutamine and alanine by the diaphragm in our normal rats was similar to that observed by others (Palaiologos & Felig, 1976; Chang & Goldberg, 1978a,b). Likewise the stimulation of amino acid production by the addition of various substrates (notably branched-chain amino acids and NH_4Cl) was observed although the increments were not as pronounced as those reported by other workers (Palaiologos & Felig, 1976; Chang & Goldberg, 1978b). This is probably due to the omission of pre-incubation procedures and the use of fed animals in the present work. The rate of production of alanine in the normal rats was linear throughout the incubation whereas the rate of glutamine production decreased especially after 60 minutes. This may be related to the energy requirement for glutamine synthesis especially as the decrease in glutamine production was paralleled by a decline in tissue ATP concentration.

Glutamine production by acidotic rat diaphragm was not significantly different from that found in normal rats a finding which is supported by observations in the perfused rat hindlimb (Oliver *et al.*, 1977). However the lowered glutamate levels and the almost complete cessation of alanine production in rat diaphragm during chronic acidosis have not been previously reported. It could be argued that the failure to demonstrate increased glutamine production *in vitro* during acidosis results from low substrate (glutamate) availability. However even when glutamate and NH_4^+ levels are raised by the addition of various substrates, glutamine production is not significantly different between control and acidotic rats. Garber has reported an increase in the production of both alanine and glutamine by epitrochlearis muscle isolated from uremic rats (Garber, 1978a,b). However the maximum rates of release in the presence of additional substrates were not different from control experiments. He concluded that uremia increases the intracellular availability of precursors for alanine and glutamine synthesis presumably by increased proteolysis (Garber, 1978a). Our findings with the diaphragm of the acidotic rat seem to confirm that the capacity for glutamine synthesis is not affected by metabolic acidosis. Despite a report that an acid medium (pH 7.04) causes increased release of glutamine by the perfused rat hindlimb (Oliver *et al.*, 1977), we were unable to demonstrate any such effect in the isolated rat diaphragm in either control or acidotic rats.

The extremely low rates of alanine production observed in diaphragms isolated from acidotic rats add support to the interpretation of our *in vivo* data that during metabolic acidosis glutamine synthesis is favored at the expense of alanine synthesis. The finding that addition of substrates does not significantly affect alanine production in the diaphragm and the fact that alanine aminotransferase activity is unchanged in the hindquarter muscle of acidotic animals are in accord with this concept.

If substrate availability is rate-limiting for glutamine synthesis, then the question of *in vivo* substrates must be considered in the interpretation of the present results. As skeletal muscle uptake of circulating ammonia and glutamate cannot account for glutamine release (Hills *et al.*, 1972; Krebs, 1975), intracellular pathways for substrate provision have been proposed (Krebs, 1975). The catabolism of circulating branched-chain amino acids has been suggested as a possible source of both glutamate and ammonia within the muscle cell (Chang & Goldberg, 1978b; Yamamoto *et al.*, 1974). However, it is unlikely that there is increased utilization of circulating branched-chain amino acids by skeletal muscle during acidosis since their arterial concentration does not change (Squires *et al.*, 1976). Therefore if there is increased production of glutamine by skeletal muscle during acidosis it must arise in part from intracellular proteolysis (Chang & Goldberg, 1978a,b). This raises a problem in using the diaphragm. As diaphragm has an "essential" role, it is possible that other muscles would preferentially undergo proteolysis before the diaphragm although a net loss of protein from diaphragms has been observed in starvation (Snell & Duff, 1977). However, one would expect the biochemical pathways of the diaphragm to be representative of other skeletal muscle (Goldberg *et al.*, 1976; Snell & Duff, 1977). Our studies with methionine sulfoximine indicate that at least half the measured glutamine was generated during incubation. The diaphragm is a special tissue and it is quite possible that the penetration of MSO in this tissue is limited. This would provide a reasonable explanation for the incomplete inhibition of glutamine generation.

Despite our findings of no change in glutamine output by skeletal muscle in chronically acidotic rats both *in vivo* and *in vitro*, these data cannot be taken as conclusive evidence that no augmented release actually takes place. It should be pointed out that in a recent preliminary report Finley *et al.* (1979) suggest that skeletal muscle in man may provide 25% of the extra glutamine required for renal uptake during chronic acidosis. We feel this value is small considering the large mass of muscle in the body and may reflect difficulties similar to ours in assessing the true contribution of skeletal muscle to the generation of circulating glutamine. However, if these findings as well as ours truly reflect the *in vivo* situation, then the question of the provision of the extra glutamine required by the kidney during acidosis remains unanswered. Other possibilities include increased output by the liver, decreased utilization by the intestinal epithelia, contribution from the brain and, in the rat, intrarenal generation of glutamine.

The role of the liver in glutamine metabolism is not clear. It possesses high activity of glutamine synthetase but glutamine synthesis *in vitro* has been shown to occur at very low rates (Lund & Watford, 1976; Lund, 1971). The liver also possesses glutaminase I activity and glutamine at high concentrations is a good precursor for gluconeogenesis and urea synthesis in the perfused rat liver (Ross *et al.*, 1967). However, at more physiological concentrations of glutamine (0.5–1.0 mM) there is no net uptake or release of glutamine by the liver (Lund & Watford, 1976). The available evidence from arterioveneous difference measurements points to the liver as a site of net glutamine synthesis *in vivo* (Lund & Watford, 1976; Remesy *et al.*, 1978; Aikawa *et al.*, 1973; Addae & Lotspeich, 1968) although the quantitative contribution may be small. There are three reports in the literature concerning the effect of chronic acidosis on the synthesis of glutamine by the liver (Oliver *et al.*, 1977, Addae & Lotspeich, 1968; Lueck & Miller, 1970). All three suggest that hepatic glutamine synthesis may be increased during acidosis.

The viscera of the portal bed have been reported to be important in the removal of glutamine from the circulation (Remesy *et al.*, 1978; Ishikawa *et al.*, 1972; Matsutaka *et al.*, 1973). The enterocytes (absorptive columnar epithelial cells of the small intestine) have been shown to be the major site of glutamine metabolism in the portal bed (Windmueller & Spaeth, 1974; Windmueller & Spaeth, 1975). The effect of chronic acidosis on intestinal glutamine metabolism is unclear. Acidosis causes no change in the activity of the phosphate-dependent glutaminase of the small intestine (Macfarlane-Anderson *et al.*, 1976; Pinkus & Windmueller, 1977). Similarly ammonia production from glutamine in intestinal scrapings and slices is unaffected by acidosis (Macfarlane-Anderson *et al.*, 1976). Results from the perfused small intestine of aciacidotic rats have been difficult to interpet since glutamine metabolism is increased when expressed as a factor of intestinal weight but unchanged when expressed as a factor of intestinal length (Hanson & Parsons, 1977). A decrease in utilization of glutamine by the small intestine during acidosis may not be apparent from results expressed as a factor of intestinal weight or length. The peculiar adaptation mechanism of the intestine by increasing or decreasing the total mass' and number of enterocytes very rapidly may be important in this respect. Enterocytes have a life span of 2–3 days (Clarke, 1973). and can disproportionately decrease or increase in number depending on the physiological state of the animals (Alpers & Kinzie, 1973). It is of interest that enterocytes isolated from acidotic rats exhibited similar metabolic characteristics to those from control rats but the yield of cells was less than 50% of that obtained from controls (Watford, unpublished observations). If these changes reflect a true decrease in the population of enterocytes *in vivo* it would mean a considerable decrease in the utilization of glutamine by the small intestine and more glutamine available for renal extraction. Our findings of a decreased arterial alanine concentration in the acidotic rat could indicate reduced alanine production by the small intestine. Alanine and ammonia are the major end products of intestinal glutamine metabolism (Hanson & Parsons, 1977; Ishikawa *et al.*, 1972; Windmueller & Spaeth, 1974; Watford *et al.*, 1979). It should be pointed out that glutamine metabolized by the rat kidney cannot give rise to alanine as this species lacks renal alanine aminotransferase (De Rosa & Swick, 1975). Therefore during acidosis a shift in the site of glutamine metabolism from the small intestine to the kidney could be expected to result in lowered circulating concentrations of alanine.

The brain has been reported as a source of circulating glutamine during acidosis in man (Tizianello *et al.*, 1978). However the importance of this organ in providing glutamine in acidosis remains to be established. The rat kidney, unlike that of man or dog, possesses glutamine synthetase activity (Lemieux *et al.*, 1976). In normal rat this activity is higher in the outer medulla than in the cortex (Lemieux *et al.*, 1976). No increase in activity can be demonstrated during metabolic acidosis (Lemieux *et al.*, 1976). In fact a 40% decrease in the activity of glutamine synthetase in the outer medulla is observed (Lemieux *et al.*, 1976). It is therefore unlikely that the kidney of the rat is an important source of glutamine during acidosis.

Acknowledgement—This study was supported by Program Grant PG-6 from the Medical Research Council of Canada.

REFERENCES

ADDAE S. K. & LOTSPEICH W. D. (1968) Relation between glutamine utilization and production in metabolic acidosis. *Am. J. Physiol.* **215,** 269.

AIKAWA T., MATSUTAKA H., YAMAMOTO H., OKUDA T., ISHIKAWA E., KAWANO T. & MATSUMURA E. (1973) Gluconeogenesis and amino acid metabolism—II. Interorganal relations and roles of glutamine and alanine in the amino acid metabolism of fasted rats. *J. Biochem.* **74,** 1003.

ALLEYNE G. A. O. & SCULLARD G. H. (1969) Renal metabolic response to acid-base changes—I. Enzymatic control of ammoniagenesis in the rat. *J. clin. Invest.* **48,** 364.

ALPERS D. H. & KINZIE J. L. (1973) Regulation of small intestinal protein metabolism. *Gastroenterology* **64,** 471.

BERGMEYER H. U. & BERNT E. (1974) Glutamate-pyruvate transaminase: UV-assay, manual method. In *Methods in Enzymatic Analysis*, (Edited by BERGMEYER H. U.) pp. 752–758. Academic Press, New York.

CARTIER P., BELANGER P. & LEMIEUX G. (1975) Characteristics of *in vitro* ammonia and glucose production by dog kidney cortex. *Am. J. Physiol.* **228,** 934.

CHANG T. W. & GOLDBERG A. L. (1978a) The origin of alanine produced in skeletal muscle. *J. biol. Chem.* **253,** 3677.

CHANG T. W. & GOLDBERG A. L. (1978b) The metabolic fates of amino acids and the formation of glutamine in skeletal muscle. *J. biol. Chem.* **253,** 3685.

CLARKE R. M. (1973) Progress in measuring epithelial turnover in the villus of the small intestine. *Digestion* **8,** 161.

CURTHOYS N. P. & LOWRY O. H. (1973) The distribution of glutaminase isoenzymes in the various structures of the nephron in normal, acidotic and alkalotic rat kidney. *J. biol. Chem.* **248,** 162.

DE ROSA G. & SWICK R. W. (1975) Metabolic implications of the distribution of the alanine aminotransferase isoenzymes. *J. biol. Chem.* **250,** 7961.

FELIG P., WAHREN J., KARL I., CERASI E., LUFT R. & KIPNIS D. M. (1973) Glutamine and glutamate metabolism in normal and diabetic subjects. *Diabetes* **22,** 573.

FINLEY R. J., AOKI T. T., BECKMAN C., CALLAWAY C. W. & CAHILL G. F. JR (1979) Glutamine metabolism during ammonium chloride loading in man. *Clin. Res.* **27,** 484A.

GARBER A. J., KARL I. E. & KIPNIS D. M. (1976) Alanine and glutamine synthesis and release from skeletal muscle—I. Glycolysis and amino acid release. *J. biol. Chem.* **251,** 826.

GARBER A. J. (1978a) Skeletal muscle protein and amino acid metabolism in experimental chronic uremia in the rat. *J. clin. Invest.* **62,** 623.

GARBER A. J. (1978b) The regulation of skeletal muscle alanine and glutamine formation and release in experimental chronic uremia in the rat. *J. clin. Invest.* **62,** 633.

GOLDBERG A. L., MARTE S. B. & KUSHMERICK M. J. (1976) *In vitro* preparations of the diaphragm and other skeletal muscle. *Meth. Enzym.* **39,** 82.

HANSON P. J. & PARSONS D. S. (1977) Metabolism and transport of glutamine and glucose in vascularly perfused small intestine of the rat. *Biochem. J.* **166,** 509.

HILLS A. G., REID E. L. & KERR W. D. (1972) Circulating transport of L-glutamine in fasted mammals: cellular sources of urine ammonia. *Am. J. Physiol.* **223,** 1470.

IQBAL K. & OTTAWAY J. H. (1970) Glutamine synthetase in muscle and kidney. *Biochem. J.* **119,** 145.

ISHIKAWA E., AIKAWA T. & MATSUTAKA H. (1972) The roles of alanine as a major precursor among amino acids for hepatic gluconeogenesis and as a major end product of the degradation of amino acids in rat tissues. *J. Biochem.* **71,** 1097.

KARL I., GARBER A. J. & KIPNIS D. M. (1976) Alanine and glutamine synthesis and release from skeletal muscle—III. Dietary and hormonal regulation. *J. biol. Chem.* **251,** 844.

KREBS H. A. & HENSELEIT K. (1932) Untersuchungen über die Harnstoffbildung im Tierkörper. *Hoppe Seyler's Z. physiol. Chem.* **210,** 33.

KREBS H. A. & VEECH R. L. (1969) Pyridine nucleotide interrelations. In *The Energy Level and Metabolic Control in Mitochondria* (Edited by PAPA S., TAGER J. M., QUAGLIARIELLO E & SLATER E. C.) pp. 329.

KREBS H. A. (1975) The role of chemical equilibria in organ function. In *Advance in Enzyme Regulation.* (Edited by WEBER G. Vol. 13, pp. 449–472. Pergamon Press, Oxford.

LEMIEUX G. & GERVAIS M. (1964) Acute chloride depletion alkalosis: Effect of anions on its maintenance and correction. *Am. J. Physiol.* **207**, 1279.

LEMIEUX G., BAVEREL G., VINAY P. & WADOUX P. (1976) Glutamine synthetase and glutamyltransferase in the kidney of man, dog and rat. *Am. J. Physiol.* **231**, 1068.

LEMIEUX G., VINAY P. & CARTIER P. (1974) Renal hemodynamics and ammoniagenesis. Characteristics of the antiluminal site for glutamine extraction. *J. clin. Invest.* **53**, 884.

LUECK J. D. & MILLER L. L. (1970) The effect of perfusate pH on glutamine metabolism. *J. biol. Chem.* **245**, 5491.

LUND P. (1971) Control of glutamine synthesis in rat liver. *Biochem. J.* **124**, 653.

LUND P. & WATFORD M. (1976) Glutamine as a precursor of urea. In *The Urea Cycle*, (Edited by GRISOLIA S., BAGUENA R. & MAYOR F.) pp. 479–488. Wiley-Interscience, New York.

LUND P. & BAVEREL G. (1978) Interference by branched-chain amino acids in the assay of alanine with alanine dehydrogenase. *Biochem. J.* **174**, 1079.

MACDONALD M., NEUFELDT N., PARK B. N., BERGER M. & RUDERMAN N. (1976) Alanine metabolism and gluconeogenesis in the rat. *Am. J. Physiol.* **231**, 619.

MACFARLANE-ANDERSON N., BENNETT F. I. & ALLEYNE G. A. O. (1976) Ammonia production by the small intestine of the rat. *Biochim. biophys. Acta* **437**, 238.

MARLISS E. B., AOKI T. T., POSEFSKY T., MOST A. S. & CAHILL G. F. JR (1971) Muscle and splanchic glutamine and glutamate metabolism in postabsorptive and starved man. *J. clin. Invest.* **50**, 814.

MATSUTAKA H., AIKAWA T., YAMAMOTO H. & ISHIKAWA E. (1973) Uptake of glutamine and output of alanine and ammonia by non-hepatic splanchnic organs of fasted rats and their metabolic significance. *J. Biochem.* **74**, 1019.

OLIVER J., KOELZ A. M., COSTELLO J. & BOURKE E. (1977) Acid-base induced alterations in glutamine metabolism and ureogenesis in perfused muscle and liver of rat. *Eur. J. clin. Invest.* **7**, 445.

PALAIOLOGOS G. & FELIG P. (1976) Effects of ketone bodies on amino acid metabolism in isolated rat diaphragm. *Biochem. J.* **154**, 709.

PARRY D. M. & BROSNAN J. T. (1978) Glutamine metabolism in the kidney during induction of, and recovery from, metabolic acidosis in the rat. *Biochem. J.* **174**, 387.

PILKINGTON L. A., YOUNG T. K. & PITTS R. F. (1970) Properties of renal luminal and antiluminal transport of plasma glutamine. *Nephron* **7**, 51.

PINKUS L. M. & WINDMUELLER H. G. (1977) Phosphate-dependent glutaminase of small intestine: localization and role in intestinal glutamine metabolism. *Archs Biochem. Biophys.* **182**, 506.

RECTOR F. C. & ORLOFF J. (1959) The effect of the administration of sodium bicarbonate and ammonium chloride on the excretion and production of ammonia. The absence of alterations in the activity of renal ammonia producing enzymes in the dog. *J. clin. Invest.* **38**, 366.

REMESY C., DEMIGRE C. & AUFRERE J. (1978) Inter-organ relationship between glucose, lactate and amino acids in rats fed on high-carbohydrate or high-protein diets. *Biochem. J.* **170**, 321.

ROSS B. D., HEMS R. & KREBS H. A. (1967) The rate of gluconeogenesis from various precursors in the perfused rat liver. *Biochem. J.* **102**, 942.

RUDERMAN N. B. & BERGER M. (1974) The formation of glutamine and alanine in skeletal muscle. *J. biol. Chem.* **249**, 5500.

SNELL K. & DUFF D. A. (1977) The release of alanine by rat diaphragm muscle *in vitro*. *Biochem. J.* **162**, 399.

SQUIRES E. J., HALL D. E. & BROSNAN J. T. (1976) Arteriovenous differences for amino acids and lactate across kidneys of normal and acidotic rats. *Biochem. J.* **160**, 125.

TIZIANELLO A., DE FERRARI G., GARIBOTTO G. & GURRERI G. (1978) Effects of chronic renal insufficiency and metabolic acidosis on glutamine metabolism in man. *Clin. Sci. mol. Med.* **55**, 391.

VINAY P., LEMIEUX G. & GOUGOUX A. (1978) Ammonia detoxification by the rat kidney *in vivo*. *Can. J. Biochem.* **56**, 305.

WATFORD M., LUND P. & KREBS H. A. (1979) Isolation and metabolic characteristics of rat and chicken enterocytes. *Biochem. J.* **178**, 589.

WILLIAMSON D. H., LUND P. & KREBS H. A. (1967) The redox state of free nicotinamide-adenine nucleotide in the cytoplasm and mitochondria of rat liver. *Biochem. J.* **103**, 514.

WILLIAMSON D. H. (1974) L-alanine determination with alanine dehydrogenase. In *Methods in Enzymatic Analysis* (Edited by BERGMEYER H. U.) pp. 1679–1682. Academic Press, New York.

WILLIAMSON D. H. & BROSNAN J. T. (1974) Concentrations of metabolites in animal tissues. In *Methods in Enzymatic Analysis* (Edited by BERGMEYER H. U.) pp. 2266–2302. Academic Press, New York.

WINDMUELLER, H. G. & SPAETH A. E. (1974) Uptake and metabolism of plasma glutamine by the small intestine. *J. biol. Chem.* **249**, 5070.

WINDMUELLER H. G. & SPAETH A. E. (1975) Intestinal metabolism of glutamine and glutamate from lumen as compared to glutamine from blood. *Archs Biochem. Biophys.* **171**, 662.

WOLLENBERGER A., RISTAU O. & SCHOFFA G. (1960) Eine einfache technik der extrem schnellenabkühlung gröberer gewebestücke. *Pflugers Archs. ges. Physiol.* **270**, 399.

YAMAMOTO H., AIKAWA T., MATSUTAKA H., OKUDA T. & ISHIKAWA E. (1974) Interzonal relationships of amino acid metabolism in fed rats. *Am. J. Physiol.* **226**, 1428.

SYMPOSIUM DISCUSSION

Krebs: You seem to take the view that the liver may be a source of glutamine in acidosis. What I said was that the liver prevents the degradation of glutamine in acidosis, so that it becomes available for the kidney. It is a different question, under what conditions the highly active glutamine synthetase of liver may become operative.

Silbernagl: What is the source of plasma glutamine in acute acidosis, in which plasma glutamine levels may be elevated two-fold within the first hour?

Vinay: We agree that there is an impressive rise in plasma glutamine in acute acidosis in dogs, but we have not observed a rise in a–v differences for muscle under these conditions.

Curthoys: What proportion of the extra glutamine required for ammoniagenesis by kidney in acidosis can be accounted for by the increased a–v difference across the hind-limb in your experiments, taking into account the relative masses of muscle and kidney.

Lemieux: I have not calculated that, but Finley *et al.* (*Clin. Res.* **27**, 484A, 1979) from studies of a–v difference across the fore-arm of acidotic man conclude that it accounts for only 25% of the extra glutamine required by kidney. I find this a rather surprising figure, considering the enormous muscle mass.

Weiner: I wonder if the method you used to produce metabolic acidosis with NH_4Cl, the extra ammonia may be converted to glutamine in the liver. If you used a different stimulus, this might be avoided, and a contribution from muscle could be expected.

Lemieux: Data with HCl induced acidosis are precisely the same.

Newsholme: We have data on alanine release form muscle, and observe a heterogeneity of response between different muscles. Amino-acid metabolism in general is greater in Type 2 fibres (white muscle). Diaphragm may fall into the group of muscles with relatively lower rates of aminoacid metabolism. Should you not have looked at another muscle preparation such as epitrochlearis or extensor digitorum longus? There may also be a "hormone" of acidosis as suggested by Alleyne (1977).

Lemieux: I acknowledge your point, but Goldberg's data on the metabolic pathways of diaphragm are convincing. We have had little success with the epitrochlearis preparation of Garber. On the other hand we see a lot of changes in the metabolic profile in muscle in acidosis. A–V differences were also altered. In fed animals there was a slight uptake of alanine *in vivo*. This has been reported by other investigators and is in contrast to the release seen in fasted animals. But in fed-acidotic rats this slight uptake of alanine was completely abolished.

Brosnan: We have, as yet, unpublished results attempting to measure whole body glutamine turnover in rats, using [1-C^{14}]glutamine. To our surprise we see no difference between normal and acidotic rats. This implies that if the kidney is taking up more glutamine, something else is taking up less!

Lund: Lou Welt and I found in 1972 (Lund & Watford in *The Urea Cycle* (Edited by GRISOLIA, BAGHENA & MAYOR) pp. 479–488. Wiley, 1976) that there was no output of glutamine by the hind-limb in chronic acidotic rats, but there was a decreased uptake by the gut; arterio-portal difference was decreased. But this does not answer the question, since a decrease in utilisation still does not provide for an increase in net glutamine production for the kidney.

Alleyne: This is where Dr Curthoys' point is a good one: even a small a–v difference across muscle might explain the amount of glutamine required by the kidney.

Brosnan: It depends more upon blood-flow, and the flow through resting muscle may not even be as great as the blood flow through the kidney!

Alleyne: In reply to Dr Newsholme's question about a hormone of acidosis, we have no data on the effect of serum from acutely acidotic rats on glutamine production by muscle.

GLUTAMINE METABOLISM IN CARBON TETRACHLORIDE-TREATED ACIDOTIC RATS

D. J. O'DONOVAN
Physiology Department, University College, Galway, Ireland

Abstract—1. Rats were given a daily intragastric dose of 1.6 ml $CCl_4 \cdot kg^{-1}$ body weight in liquid paraffin for 7 days.

2. A second group was given 2.5 mEq HCl daily and another group received both substances.

3. Administration of HCl increased the activities of phosphate-independent glutaminase, phosphate-dependent glutaminase and glutamine synthetase in the kidney.

4. CCl_4 increased the activity of glutamine synthetase in the kidney and almost completely abolished the activity of this enzyme in the liver.

5. The adaptive increase in renal phosphate-dependent glutaminase due to acidosis was reduced by CCl_4 treatment.

INTRODUCTION

amine is the primary source of urinary ammonia et al., 1965) and when the demand for urinary onia increases in acidosis the rate of extraction lutamine from the blood by the kidney is nced (Owen & Robinson, 1963). Acidosis does lter the concentration of glutamine in the blood , 1972). It is likely that the increased renal ction of glutamine in acidosis is balanced by an ased extra-renal production in order to maintain lood glutamine level constant.

e liver converts ammonia to glutamine, which is nverted to ammonia in the kidney via the glu-ase enzyme system. Thus, the activity of glu-e synthetase in the liver would appear to be of significance in maintaining the blood level of mine constant in acidosis.

test this hypothesis the liver toxin, carbon tetra-ide, was administered to rats and the activity of glutamine synthetase was monitored. The rats then rendered acidotic by the administration of ochloric acid and the ability of the kidney to bolise glutamine was assayed.

MATERIALS AND METHODS

le Sprague–Dawley rats, weighing approx 200 g were access *ad libitum* to food and water. They were given y intragastric injection of 1.6 ml carbon tetrachloride equal volume of liquid paraffin per kg body weight days. Acidosis was produced by the daily intragastric nistration of 5 ml 0.5 N HCl.

the seventh day the rats were decapitated and exsan-ted. The liver and kidneys were quickly removed, ed and homogenized in a Potter–Elvehjem homogen-For the assay of phosphate-independent glutaminase, phate-dependent glutaminase and protein, 1 g tissue diluted to 10 ml 0.154 M KCl in 0.05 M Tris pH 8.0. the assay of glutamine synthetase, 1 g tissue was d to 10 ml 0.15% deoxycholic acid in 0.32 M sucrose, .5, containing 1 mM EDTA. The phosphate-independent glutaminase and phosphate-dependent glutaminase activities were assayed according to the procedure of Ni Fhaolain & O'Donovan (1971). Glutamine synthetase activity was estimated according to Woolfolk *et al.* (1966) by assaying the γ-glutamylhydroxamate (GHA) liberated. Protein was assayed by the method of Lowry *et al.* (1951).

RESULTS

The intragastric administration of carbon tetrachloride to the rat reduced the activity of liver glutamine synthetase to one-tenth of the control value within 2 days. The activity remained at this low value when the carbon tetrachloride treatment was continued for 15 days (Fig. 1).

A reduction in the rate of glutamine synthesis in the liver should decrease the supply of glutamine available for ammonia production in the kidney. Hence, it was of interest to determine the effect of acidosis on glutamine metabolism during carbon tetrachloride administration. Table 1 shows the effect of administration of hydrochloric acid and carbon tetrachloride, separately and combined, on the rate of glutamine synthesis and degradation. Administration of hydrochloric acid alone increased the rate of synthesis and degradation of glutamine in the kidney, but did not alter the rate of synthesis of glutamine in the liver. This response is similar to that found with other acidifying substances.

In addition to decreasing glutamine synthesis in the liver, carbon tetrachloride increased the activity of glutamine synthetase in the kidney. This indicates that the kidney is compensating for the inability of the liver to produce glutamine. When acidosis was superimposed on carbon tetrachloride treatment kidney glutamine synthetase activity was similar to acidosis alone and liver glutamine synthetase was still not affected by acidosis. Carbon tetrachloride treatment slightly reduced the adaptive increase in kidney phosphate-dependent glutaminase activity.

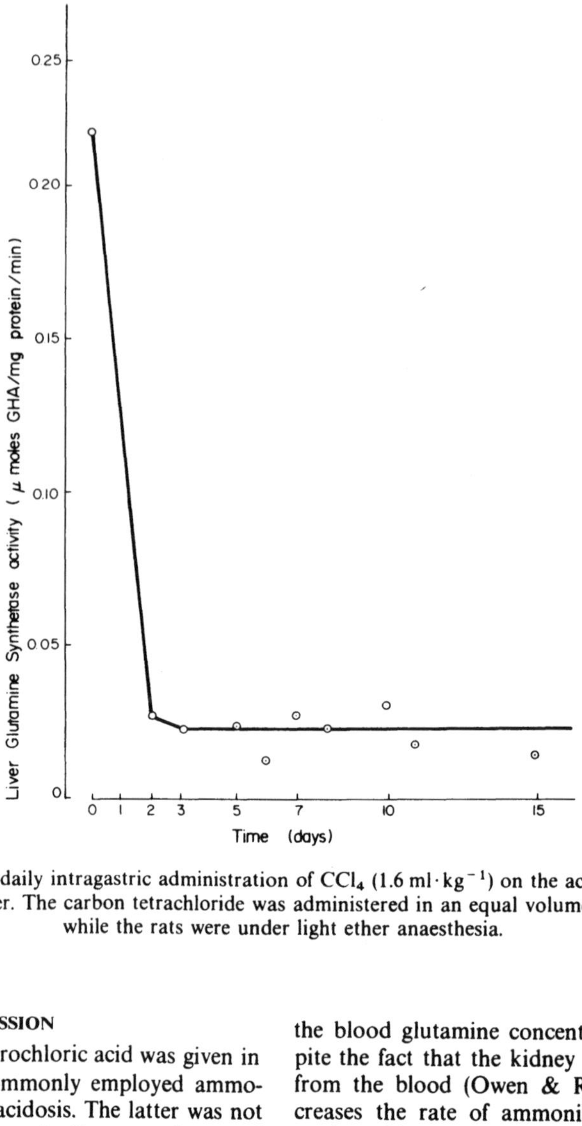

Fig. 1. The effect of daily intragastric administration of CCl_4 (1.6 ml·kg^{-1}) on the activity of glutamine synthetase in rat liver. The carbon tetrachloride was administered in an equal volume of liquid paraffin while the rats were under light ether anaesthesia.

DISCUSSION

In these experiments hydrochloric acid was given in preference to the more commonly employed ammonium chloride to produce acidosis. The latter was not used as it was felt that when the liver was destroyed by carbon tetrachloride it would not be capable of disposing of ammonia. This reservation was supported by the observation that carbon tetrachloride virtually completely destroyed the glutamine synthetic ability of the liver (Table 1). Acidosis does not alter the blood glutamine concentration (Pitts, 1972) despite the fact that the kidney extracts more glutamine from the blood (Owen & Robinson, 1963) and increases the rate of ammonia production from glutamine (O'Donovan & Lotspeich, 1968). The reduction in the phosphate-dependent glutaminase activity of the acidotic kidney by carbon tetrachloride (Table 1) indicates that the adaptation of renal glutaminase in acidosis is partially dependent on the glutamine synthetic ability of the liver.

Table 1. Kidney and liver enzyme activities following daily administration of 2.5 mmol HCl and 1.6 ml·kg^{-1} CCl_4 to the rat for 7 days

	Kidney			Liver
Treatment	P.I.G.*	P.D.G.†	Gln. synthetase	Gln. synthetase
Control	1.98 ± 0.31	7.87 ± 0.63	0.129 ± 0.006	0.218 ± 0.011
HCl	3.29 ± 0.52§	11.07 ± 0.84§	0.214 ± 0.013§	0.186 ± 0.014
CCl_4	1.96 ± 0.27	7.72 ± 0.56	0.183 ± 0.005‡	0.023 ± 0.002§
CCl_4 + HCl	2.02 ± 0.43	9.36 ± 0.47‡	0.227 ± 0.012‡	0.028 ± 0.001§

* P.I.G. = phosphate independent glutaminase.
† P.D.G. = phosphate-dependent glutaminase.
Glutaminase is expressed as μmol NH_3·mg^{-1} protein·hr^{-1}.
Glutamine synthetase is expressed as μmol GHA·mg^{-1} protein·hr^{-1}.
‡ $P < 0.05$ compared to the control value.
§ $P < 0.01$ compared to the control value.

REFERENCES

LOWRY O. H., ROSEBROUGH N. J., FARR L. & RANDALL R. J. (1951) Protein measurement with Folin phenol reagent. *J. biol. Chem.* **193,** 265–275.

NI FHAOLAIN I. & O'DONOVAN D. J. (1971) A relationship between rat kidney mitochondrial swelling and glutaminase activation. *Am. J. Physiol.* **221,** 58–63.

O'DONOVAN D. J. & LOTSPEICH W. D. (1968) Factors affecting the deamidation of glutamine by kidney mitochondria of normal and acidotic rats. *Enzymologia* **35,** 82–92.

OWEN E. E. & ROBINSON R. R. (1963) Amino acid extraction and ammonia metabolism by the human kidney during prolonged administration of ammonium chloride. *J. clin. Invest.* **42,** 263–276.

PITTS R. F. (1972) Control of renal production of ammonia. *Kidney Int.* **1,** 297–305.

PITTS R. F., PILKINGTON L. A. & DE HAAS J. C. M. (1965) ^{15}N tracer studies on the origin of urinary ammonia in the acidotic dog, with notes on the enzymatic synthesis of labeled glutamic acid and glutamine. *J. clin. Invest.* **44,** 731–745.

WOOLFOLK C. A., SHAPIRO B. & STADTMAN E. R. (1966) Regulation of glutamine synthetase. I. Purification and properties of glutamine synthetase from *Escherichia coli. Archs Biochem. Biophys.* **116,** 177–192.

Int. J. Biochem., Vol. 12, pp. 89 to 98
© Pergamon Press Ltd 1980. Printed in Great Britain

0020-711X/80/0701-0089$02.00/0

RESPONSE OF THE RAT AND DOG KIDNEY TO H^+ CONCENTRATION *IN VITRO*—A COMPARATIVE STUDY WITH SLICES AND TUBULES

PATRICK VINAY*, GUY LEMIEUX, ANDRÉ GOUGOUX and CHRISTIANE LEMIEUX
Renal Laboratory, Hôtel-Dieu Hospital and the Department of Medicine,
University of Montreal, Montreal, Quebec, Canada.

Abstract—1. The present study reevaluates the metabolic response of rat and dog renal cortical tissue to changes in H^+ concentration of incubation medium and compares the response of kidney slices to that of isolated tubules.

2. In the rat, acidification (pH 7.1) depresses glutamate accumulation and enhances gluconeogenesis with both slices and tubules, but glutamine extraction and ammonia production increase significantly only with tubules.

3. Alkalinization (pH 7.7) depresses glucose and ammonia production and enhances glutamate accumulation with both slices and tubules but glutamine extraction is also slightly stimulated with tubules only.

4. Thus, in the rat, variations of incubation medium pH modulates (a) glutamate utilization and (b) glutamine transport from the medium to the mitochondria, the second effect being apparent with tubules only. The different response observed with slices and tubules is attributed to a difference of permeability for glutamine between these two preparations.

5. The intracellular metabolite profile of tubules rapidly separated from the incubation medium after 30 min suggests that *in vitro* acidosis increases and alkalosis decreases glutamate utilization and ammonia production probably by affecting the activity of the alpha-ketoglutarate dehydrogenase complex.

6. In the dog, no effect of H^+ concentration on glutamine transport or utilization can be seen. However, H^+ concentration modifies glutamate accumulation and stimulates gluconeogenesis (from glutamate and endogenous substrates).

7. Both effects are in accord with observations in the rat and may involve similar mechanisms.

INTRODUCTION

The metabolic response of renal cortical tissue to changes in hydrogen ion concentration of the incubation medium has been studied in the past as a model to understand the early renal response to metabolic acidosis. Numerous studies have failed to demonstrate any stimulation of renal ammonia production *in vitro* from glutamine by acidification of the incubation medium of rat and dog kidney slices (Cartier *et al.*, 1975; Goodman, 1973; Hems, 1972; Irias & Greenberg, 1972; Pagliara & Goodman, 1970; Preuss *et al.*, 1974; Relman & Narins, 1975; Roobol & Alleyne, 1974). However, a slight but significant increment of glucose production and/or a depression of glutamate accumulation in the flask were generally noted (Cartier *et al.*, 1975; Goodman, 1973; Irias & Greenberg, 1972; Kamm *et al.*, 1967; Nagata & Rasmussen, 1970; Pagliara & Goodman, 1970; Preuss *et al.*, 1974; Roobol & Alleyne, 1974; Simpson & Sherrard, 1968). The present study reevaluates the metabolic response of renal cortical tissue to changes in H^+ concentration. More specifically, it compares the effect of changes of H^+ concentration *in vitro* on glutamine metabolism by slices and by isolated tubules obtained from rat and dog kidney. We demonstrate in the rat that acidification of the incubation medium significantly increases glutamine extraction, ammonia and glucose production with tubules while only glucose production increases with slices. Alkalinization of incubation medium has an opposite effect on glutamine metabolism. The changes in intracellular concentration of metabolic intermediates in tubules following incubation at acid pH are compatible with acute stimulation of the alpha-ketoglutarate dehydrogenase activity. The difference between slices and tubules in the rat is probably related to differences in glutamine permeability. In the dog, no stimulation of glutamine transport or utilization by H^+ concentration can be demonstrated *in vitro*. However, as in the rat, stimulation of gluconeogenesis and depression of glutamate accumulation occur.

* Dr P. Vinay is a Scholar of the Medical Research Council of Canada.

MATERIALS AND METHODS

A. Studies in the rat

Thirty-nine experiments were performed with 88 male or female Wistar rats weighing between 350 and 450 g. All rats were fed with commercial Purina rat chow. Fifty-six rats were in normal acid–base status (arterial pH 7.47 ± 0.01 and plasma HCO_3^- 27 ± 1.2 mM) and 25 rats were made acidotic by drinking 1.5% NH_4Cl for 5 days prior to the experiment (arterial pH 7.28 ± 0.02; HCO_3^- 15.0 ± 1.7 mM).

Experiments with slices

In each of 10 experiments (5 with normal and 5 with acidotic rats), cortical slices were prepared from the kidneys of three rats. Slices were placed in a randomized fashion in incubation flasks (50 ml) ensuring around 200 mg of tissue per flask (3–4 slices/flask). The tissue was incubated in 6 ml Krebs–Henseleit saline containing 2.5 g% of dialysed bovine albumin and adjusted to pH 7.4, 7.1 and 7.7 by varying the bicarbonate concentration. The calcium content of the incubation medium was kept constant at 2.5 mM and sodium at 144 mEq·l^{-1}. Glutamine 1 or 5 mM was the sole substrate added. All flasks were run in duplicate. The flasks were gassed with 5% CO_2–95% O_2 and incubated for 60 min. The incubation was stopped by addition of 0.5 ml 40% perchloric acid. Zero time values with and without substrate were obtained for each experiment. Additional flasks were used to measure the incubation medium pH at the end of incubation.

Experiments with tubules

In each of 12 experiments (7 with normal and 5 with acidotic rats) kidney tubules were prepared as a 60 mg wet wt/ml suspension from the combined kidney cortex slices of two rats according to a modification of the technique of Guder *et al.* (1971). Of this suspension, 0.5 ml was incubated for 30 min in 5.5 ml of Krebs saline containing albumin according to the protocol used for the slices. Amino-oxyacetic acid (AOA) 0.1 mM or L-methionine DL-sulfoximine (MSO) 5 mM were placed in additional flasks containing 1 or 5 mM glutamine in four experiments.

Measurement of glutamine oxidation

In seven additional experiments with tubules obtained from normal rats, the metabolism of [U-^{14}C]glutamine with a specific activity of 0.02 μCi·μmol^{-1} (4.55 × 10^4 dpm·μmol^{-1}) at a final concentration of 1 and 5 mM was studied. $^{14}CO_2$ production and O_2 consumption were simultaneously measured as already described (Vinay *et al.*, 1978). Glutamine oxidation was estimated by drawing a carbon and ammonia balance as already described (Vinay *et al.*, 1979) and from the measurement of $^{14}CO_2$ production, after correction for isotopic dilution (Vinay *et al.*, 1978).

Determination of intracellular metabolites concentration

Ten additional experiments (two normal rats per experiment) were designed to measure the concentration of various metabolites in the tissue. Tubules were incubated for 30 min with 1 or 5 mM glutamine and separated from the incubation medium in special centrifugation tubes and instantly deproteinized according to the technique of Hems (1976). To insure sufficient tissue for the measurements, tubules of four different flasks incubated at the same pH were combined. [^{14}C]inulin was added to these flasks to estimate the amount of incubation medium contaminating the tissue, which represent about 15% of the total tubule volume. Intracellular metabolites concentration was estimated after correction for the amount of metabolites found in extracellular fluid.

B. Studies in the dog

The effect of *in vitro* pH changes was also studied using kidney slices and isolated tubules obtained from 5 normal (arterial pH 7.38 ± 0.02, plasma HCO_3^- 21.9 ± 1.21 mM) and 5 chronically acidotic (pH 7.27 ± 0.03 and HCO_3^- 13.7 ± 1.62 mM) dogs. The methodology involved in preparation and incubation of slices or tubules was similar to that reported for the rat studies.

Analytical measurements

Glutamine, glutamate, glucose, ammonia, alpha-ketoglutarate, lactate, pyruvate, malate, phosphoenolpyruvate, 2-phosphoglyceric acid, 3-phosphoglyceric acid and glucose-6-phosphate were measured enzymatically on the neutralized extract of the incubation fluid or on the isolated tubular tissue by well established methods (Bergmeyer, 1974). Oxaloacetate was calculated from the malate concentration and cytosolic NAD^+:NADH ratio assuming a near-equilibrium situation for the malate/lactate dehydrogenase reactions (Hems & Brosnan, 1971). The pH of the incubation medium as well as arterial blood pH and PCO_2 were measured anaerobically on an Instrumentation Laboratory ultra-micro Duo-matic pH and blood gas-analyzing system, model 213–S1. Results are presented as means ± SEM. Statistical analysis of the data was made with Student's *t*-test for paired or unpaired data whenever applicable.

RESULTS

Effect of H^+ concentration on glutamine metabolism by kidney slices and isolated tubules from normal rats

Table 1 shows that glutamine extraction and ammonia production by cortical slices are unchanged after 60 min of incubation if the tissue is incubated at pH 7.08, 7.45 or 7.73. However, glutamate accumulation in the flask is significantly depressed at acidotic and significantly enhanced at alkalotic pH. Glucose production is stimulated by acidosis and depressed by alkalosis. Similar observations are made if either 1 or 5 mM glutamine is placed in the flasks. At 5 mM, glutamine metabolism proceeds faster than with 1 mM. Furthermore, NH_4 production over glutamine extraction ratio (NH_4:Gln) remains around 2 with 5 mM glutamine while it is significantly higher than 2 with 1 mM glutamine, indicating utilization of endogenous aminoacids by the kidney slices at this concentration of glutamine.

When similar experiments are done with kidney tubules, both glutamine extraction and ammonia production are significantly increased by acidification of the incubation medium (Table 1). In contrast to the observations with slices, acidosis increases glutamate accumulation in the incubation medium. The NH_4:Gln ratio remains around 1.2 with 5 mM and 1.8 with 1 mM suggesting that endogenous utilization of aminoacids is minimal with this preparation.

Alkalinization of the medium also increases glutamine extraction and glutamate accumulation in the flasks and it significantly depresses glucose production at both 1 and 5 mM glutamine levels while ammonia production is little affected. In the four experiments, where additional flasks containing 5 mM MSO to inhibit glutamine synthetase activity or 0.1 mM AOA to inhibit aminotransferases activity were run, the parameters of glutamine metabolism were not different from the results presented in Table 1.

Effect of H^+ concentration on glutamine oxidation by rat kidney tubules

Table 2 shows that complete oxidation of the skeleton carbon of glutamine by kidney tubules is enhanced by acidification of the incubation medium. Using 1 or 5 mM glutamine, and normal incubation pH (7.4), around 20% of the extracted glutamine undergoes complete oxidation. This fraction is not modified by acidification of the medium, suggesting that the increased oxidation follows enhanced extraction of glutamine. No significant effect of alkalinization on glutamine oxidation was observed.

Table 1. Effect of incubation pH on glutamine (1 or 5 mM) metabolism by kidney slices and tubules from normal rats

	Slices $n = 5$			Tubules $n = 7$		
Measured pH	7.08 ± 0.02*	7.45 ± 0.02	7.73 ± 0.02**	7.16 ± 0.03*	7.41 ± 0.04	7.72 ± 0.04**
5 mM Glutamine						
Glutamine extraction	41 ± 2.6	43 ± 4.6	46 ± 7.9	204 ± 25.1*	120 ± 24.2	135 ± 23.1**
Glutamate production	12 ± 2.4* (29.3%)	21 ± 2.6 (48.8%)	36 ± 2.7* (78.3%)	63 ± 8.0* (30.9%)	34 ± 9.1 (28.3%)	41 ± 9.1 (30.4%)
NH_4 production	80 ± 8.4	88 ± 7.2	91 ± 4.7	249 ± 32.2*	151 ± 18.1	160 ± 15.0
Glucose production	15 ± 3.7* (73.2%)	10 ± 2.7 (46.5%)	5 ± 1.2** (21.7%)	22 ± 1.2* (21.6%)	17 ± 1.4 (28.3%)	15 ± 0.9** (22.2%)
NH_4 production/ Gln extraction	1.95	2.05	1.98	1.22	1.26	1.19
1 mM Glutamine						
Glutamine extraction	10 ± 2.8	12 ± 2.2	13 ± 1.8	73 ± 11.0*	34 ± 3.5	49 ± 5.0**
Glutamate production	3 ± 1.0 (30.0%)	4 ± 1.0 (33.3%)	9 ± 2.0** (69.2%)	36 ± 7.8** (49.3%)	15 ± 3.2 (44.1%)	21 ± 4.1** (42.9%)
NH_4 production	30 ± 3.0	34 ± 3.0	37 ± 4.0	131 ± 24.0*	68 ± 9.1	78 ± 9.0
Glucose production	5 ± 0.7* (100.0%)	4 ± 0.7 (66.7%)	3 ± 0.6 (46.2%)	15 ± 0.9 (41.1%)	11 ± 0.9 (64.7%)	10 ± 1.0* (40.8%)
NH_4 production/ Gln extraction	3.00	2.83	2.85	1.79	2.00	1.59

Values are μmols/g wet wt for 60 min (slices) or 30 min (tubules) incubation ± SEM. Glutamate, ammonia and glucose values are corrected for zero-time concentrations in flasks containing 1 or 5 mM glutamine. The fractions of extracted glutamine recovered as glutamate or glucose are indicated as per cent between parentheses. * $P < 0.05$ for comparison of pH 7.4 vs 7.1 and ** for comparison of pH 7.4 vs 7.7, t-test for paired data. n = number of experiments.

Effect of H^+ concentration on glutamine metabolism by kidney slices and isolated tubules from acidotic rats

Slices obtained from acidotic animals extract more glutamine and produce more glucose and ammonia than slices from normal animals ($P < 0.05$) (Table 3). The fraction of the extracted glutamine recovered as glutamate is also smaller in experiments with acidotic animals than with normal ones. Acidification of the incubation medium has no effect on glutamine extraction and ammonia or glucose production (Table 3). Glutamate accumulation again tends to be decreased by this manoeuver. Alkalinization of the incubation medium significantly increases glutamate accumulation while it depresses ammonia and glucose production leaving glutamine extraction more or less intact.

Tubules obtained from acidotic animals extract more glutamine and produce more ammonia and glucose than tubules from normal animals ($P < 0.05$) (Table 3). Again the fraction of the extracted glutamine recovered as glutamate is lower than with normal animals. Acidification of incubation medium decreases glutamine extraction and glutamate production slightly while it has no effect on glucose production (Table 3). On the other hand alkalinization of the incubation medium significantly increases glutamate accumulation and decreases glucose production leaving glutamine extraction and ammonia production unchanged.

Effect of H^+ concentration on the metabolic profile of kidney tubules from normal rats

The various metabolites of the ammoniagenic pathway and of the gluconeogenic chain measured in tubules incubated with 5 mM glutamine at pH 7.1 or 7.7 were compared to the concentrations observed in tubules incubated at pH 7.4 (6 experiments). The data are presented in Table 4 and plotted in Fig. 1 in the manner originaly described by Chance *et al.* (1958). In this figure, the mean concentration of each intermediate in the tissue incubated at pH 7.1 or 7.7 is presented as a percentage of the mean concentration of the same intermediate in the tissue incubated at pH 7.4. Thus increment of concentration will appear above and decrement will appear below the 100% control line. Note that the intracellular concentration of glutamine is around 11 mM after 30 min of incubation i.e. three times greater than the value measured in the incubation medium (Table 4). It is evident from Table 4 and Fig. 1 that acidification of the incubation medium decreases tissue concentration of alpha-ketoglutarate while it increases that of malate and of the calculated oxaloacetate. No significant changes of the intermediates of the gluconeogenic pathway are seen including phosphoenolpyruvate. Incubation in an alkaline medium has the reverse effect on alpha-ketoglutarate concentration but also slightly increases the malate concentration. In addition cellular glutamate rises significantly. No significant changes of lactate or pyruvate could be demonstrated at any pH. In four experiments, the metabolite profile of the tubules was measured after 30 min of incubation with 1 mM glutamine (the intracellular glutamine concentration is then near 4 $\mu mol \cdot g^{-1}$). No significant changes of any of the measured intermediates was observed. The metabolite profile of tubules from acidotic rats was

Table 2. Effect of incubation pH on glutamine (1 and 5 mM) oxidation by isolated kidney tubules from normal rats

		1 mM glutamine	
Measured pH	7.16 ± 0.03*	7.41 ± 0.04	7.72 ± 0.04**
Glutamine extraction	−73 ± 71*	−34 ± 3.5	−49 ± 5.0**
Glutamate production	+36 ± 7.8*	+15 ± 3.2	+21 ± 4.1**
C_3-glucose production	+30 ± 1.8*	+22 ± 1.8	+20 × 2.0**
NH_4 production	+131 ± 24	+78 ± 9.1	+78 ± 9.0
Glutamine to CO_2, from C balance	7.0	0	4.0
Glutamine to CO_2, from NH_4 balance	17.9	9.5	8.5
Glutamine to CO_2, from $^{14}CO_2$ measurement	16.3	10.0	12.8
		5 mM glutamine	
Glutamine extraction	−204 ± 25*	−120 ± 24	−135 ± 23**
Glutamate production	+63 ± 8.0*	+34 ± 9.1	+41 ± 9.1
C_3-glucose production	+44 ± 2.4*	+34 ± 2.8	+30 ± 1.8**
NH_4 production	+249 ± 32*	+151 ± 18	+160 ± 15
Glutamine to CO_2, from C balance	97	52	64
Glutamine to CO_2, from NH_4 balance	49	25	35.5
Glutamine to CO_2, from $^{14}CO_2$ measurement	41.2	20.6	20.4

Values are μmol/g wet wt for 30 min incubation. Mean ± SEM. * $p < 0.05$ for comparison of pH 7.4 vs 7.1. ** For comparison of pH 7.4 vs 7.7; *t*-test for paired data.

not studied in view of the fact that acidification of the incubation medium has little effect on glutamine metabolism in acidotic animals.

Effect of H^+ concentration on glutamine metabolism by kidney slices and isolated tubules from normal and acidotic dogs

Acidification of the incubation medium has no stimulating effect on glutamine (1 and 5 mM) utilization by kidney tubules or kidney slices from normal (Table 5) or acidotic (Table 6) dogs. However, gluconeogenesis from endogenous sources is stimulated by *in vitro* acidosis in both preparations, while glutamate accumulation is depressed. Alkalinization has the reverse effect.

DISCUSSION

Numerous attempts to increase renal ammonia production from glutamine by incubating kidney cortex tissue from normal rats and dogs in acidified incubation medium have failed (Table 7). However, most of these studies have demonstrated that increasing H^+ concentration *in vitro* significantly enhances glucose production and depresses glutamate accumulation in the tissue or in the incubation flasks (Table 7). Most of these studies were performed with slices. Only Nagata & Rasmussen (1970) and Kurokowa & Rasmussen (1973a,b) have incubated rat kidney tubules at different pH. They have also noted a significant acceleration of gluconeogenesis from

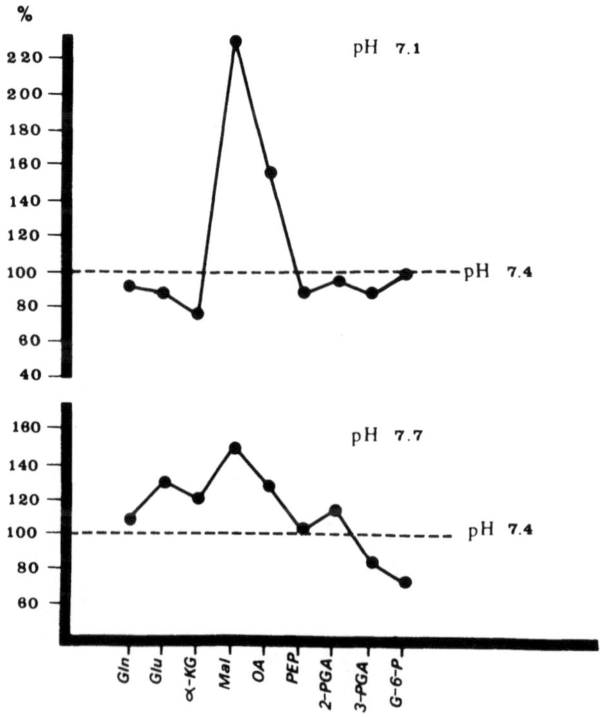

Fig. 1.

Table 3. Effect of incubation pH on glutamine metabolism by kidney slices and tubules from acidotic rats

	Slices $n = 5$			Tubules $n = 7$		
Measured pH	7.12 ± 0.01*	7.38 ± 0.02	7.60 ± 0.02**	7.11 ± 0.03*	7.42 ± 0.04	7.67 ± 0.01**
5 mM Glutamine						
Glutamine extraction	72 ± 3.6	83 ± 6.9	91 ± 6.4	135 ± 3.9*	189 ± 18.5	186 ± 15.8
Glutamate production	17 ± 1.2 (23.6%)	25 ± 3.9 (30.1%)	40 ± 4.2** (44.0%)	47 ± 4.7* (34.8%)	57 ± 4.9 (30.2%)	76 ± 5.4** (40.9%)
NH_4 production	121 ± 16.3*	146 ± 13.3	133 ± 15.2	230 ± 12	237 ± 22	266 ± 10
Glucose production	25 ± 2.8 (69.4%)	27 ± 2.6 (65.1%)	17 ± 2.3** (37.4%)	39 ± 2.6 (57.8%)	35 ± 2.7 (37.0%)	27 ± 1.2** (29.0%)
NH_4 production/ Gln extraction	1.68	1.76	1.46	1.7	1.3	1.4
1 mM Glutamine						
Glutamine extraction	23 ± 0.83	23 ± 0.52	23 ± 0.60	58 ± 4.9	65 ± 5.3	68 ± 4.9
Glutamate production	1.8 ± 0.9* (7.8%)	2.8 ± 0.7 (12.2%)	4.2 ± 1.1** (18.3%)	13 ± 3.9 (22.4%)	16 ± 2.8 (24.6%)	18 ± 3.3 (26.5%)
NH_4 production	49 ± 1.9	48 ± 2.9	50 ± 1.9	117 ± 6.4*	133 ± 9.3	138 ± 9.7
Glucose production	12 ± 0.5 (104.3%)	12 ± 0.6 (104.3%)	10 ± 0.6 (87.0%)	28 ± 21. (96.6%)	26 ± 2.1 (80.0%)	19 ± 2** (55.9%)
NH_4 production/ Gln extraction	2.13	2.09	2.17	2.00	2.00	2.00

Values are μmol/g wet wt for 60 min incubation ± SEM. See Table 1 for description.

various substrates (Kurokawa & Rasmussen, 1973a,b; Nagata & Rasmussen, 1970) including glutamine by acidosis in this preparation, unfortunately, they did not measure ammonia production (Kurokawa & Rasmussen, 1973a,b).

Our experiments performed with kidney slices from normal rats confirm that increment in H^{+} concentration enhances glucose production. However, glutamine extraction is not significantly changed. Therefore, one must postulate that other gluconeogenic precursors than glutamine are used during this process. Glutamate utilization is simultaneously accelerated as less glutamate accumulates in the flasks. The fact that glutamate concentration decreases without stimulating glutamine utilization, even in the presence of 5 mM glutamine, suggests that some permeability barrier prevents this aminoacid gaining access to the mitochondrial deamidation site at sufficient speed to provide enough substrate for the increased glucose synthesis. Increased glutamate utilization without increasing glutamine uptake at the same time will indeed result in a lower intracellular (and presumably intramitochondrial) glutamate as observed in the present study. The fact that endogenous aminoacid utilization is observed when 1 mM glutamine is presented to the slices also indicates a limitation in glutamine permeability in slices.

When glutamine metabolism is studied using kidney tubules, a strikingly different image is seen. First, it is evident that glutamine uptake by tubules after 30 min incubation is far greater with 1 or 5 mM glutamine than that observed in slices after 60 min and that utilization of endogenous aminoacids is undetectable with 1 mM glutamine. This suggests that the permeability for glutamine is greater in the tubule preparation. It is tempting to postulate that the difference of permeability for glutamine observed between slices and tubules is related to the greater surface of contact of the isolated tubules suspension with the incubation medium and to the thickness of tissue inherent to the slice technique.

When tubules are incubated at acid pH glutamine extraction is increased and stimulation of gluconeogenesis from (as well as oxidation of) glutamine occurs. Ammonia production is also significantly accelerated, while glutamate accumulation increases in the flask. This suggests that not only glutamate utilization (for glucose synthesis or oxidation) is significantly increased, but that glutamine gains access to the intramitochondrial deamidation site at a faster rate than glutamate is removed. It is thus reasonable to conclude that increasing the H^{+} concentration *in vitro* modulates the rate of glutamate utilization somewhere between glutamate and phosphoenolpyruvate in slices and tubules and increases glutamine transport inside the cell and/or mitochondria, the second effect being only apparent with tubules. A cellular transport of glutamine is probably involved here since no effect of H^{+} on glutamine transport can be demonstrated with isolated mitochondria (Tannen & Kunin, 1976).

The present experiments stand in contradiction with previous conclusions drawn from experiments with slices in which ammonia production was not only unchanged but actually diminished by acidification of the incubation medium (Relman & Narins,

Table 4. Effect of incubation pH on concentration of metabolic intermediates in isolated rat kidney tubules

Incubation pH	7.1	7.4	7.7
Glutamine	10.6 ± 2.7	11.5 ± 1.6	12.5 ± 1.3
Glutamate	4.3 ± 0.5	4.9 ± 1.0	6.4 ± 0.4**
Alphaketoglutarate	0.22 ± 0.03*	0.29 ± 0.04	0.35 ± 0.04**
Lactate	0.64 ± 0.06	0.63 ± 0.012	0.59 ± 0.09
Pyruvate	0.10 ± 0.03	0.16 ± 0.02	0.13 ± 0.03
Lactate + pyruvate	0.74	0.79	0.72
Malate	0.28 ± 0.05*	0.12 ± 0.02	0.18 ± 0.03**
Oxaloacetate (calculated)	0.011 ± 0.006	0.007 ± 0.004	0.009 ± 0.005
Phosphoenol pyruvate	0.27 ± 0.03	0.31 ± 0.05	0.32 ± 0.07
2-phosphoglycerate	0.25 ± 0.09	0.26 ± 0.011	0.30 ± 0.09
3-phosphoglycerate	0.21 ± 0.05	0.24 ± 0.06	0.20 ± 0.06
Glucose-6-phosphate	0.07 ± 0.009	0.07 ± 0.01	0.05 ± 0.01

The tissue concentration of metabolic intermediates were measured in tubules separated from the incubation medium after 30 min incubation with 5 mM glutamine at pH 7.1, 7.4 or 7.7. Results are expressed as μmols/g wet wt tubules. Values are means ± SEM. * Indicates $P < 0.05$ for comparison 7.1 vs 7.4 and ** for comparison 7.4 vs 7.7.

1975; Roobol & Alleyne, 1974). These results were interpreted as an inhibition of glutaminase I activity (the optimal pH of which is around 8) by the increment in H^+ concentration. Since our data with tubules demonstrating greater rates of deamidation of glutamine at acid pH suggest that such interpretation is unfounded, we propose another explanation for this phenomenon. If a permeability limitation for glutamine exists in slices together with stimulation of the gluconeogenic pathway, then other substrates of endogenous origin will be utilized to support this increased glucose synthesis. Relative competition between glutamine (carrying two nitrogens) and other endogenous substrates (carrying one or no nitrogen) could occur and this would explain a diminution of ammoniagenesis *in vitro* with increased H^+ concentration. Indeed the addition of various gluconeogenic precursors such as lactate (Churchill & Marvin, 1970; Roxe *et al.*, 1974), pyruvate (Irias & Greenberg, 1972), oxaloacetate (Preuss *et al.*, 1974), malate (Irias & Greenberg, 1972), fumarate (Preuss, 1971), succinate (Preuss, 1971), alpha-ketoglutarate (Hems, 1972) will depress glutamine utilization and ammonia production *in vitro*.

With slices, alkalinization of the incubation medium significantly depresses glucose production and enhances accumulation of glutamate in the incubation flasks. Ammonia production does not change significantly as the ammonia produced from glutamate accumulation replaces the ammonia previously formed from glutamate utilization. With kidney tubules alkalinization also depresses significantly glucose production and enhances glutamate accumulation in the flasks. However, glutamine extraction increases in a moderate fashion. Alkalinization of the incubation medium could increase glutaminase I activity secondary to changes of mitochondrial pH or organic acids concentration (O'Donovan & Lotspeich, 1966) as postulated by Preuss (Preuss *et al.*, 1974) and Relman and Narins (1975) and so contribute to the observed accumulation of glutamate. Acute inhibition of the glutamate dehydrogenase enzyme, also critically sensitive to pH *in vitro* (Seyama *et al.*, 1972) is improbable since this would not stimulate glutamine uptake simultaneously. A direct effect of pH on cellular and/or mitochondrial transport or permeability is improbable since it would be surprising that both an increment and a decrement of H^+ concentration would have a similar effect on glutamine transport.

Tubules (or slices) obtained from acidotic rats extract more glutamine and produce more glucose and ammonia than preparations from normal animals. This is usually thought to be the result of an activation of the gluconeogenic pathway at the phosphoenolpyruvate carboxykinase (PEPCK) step (Alleyne, 1970; Alleyne & Scullard, 1969; Kamm *et al.*, 1967). The fact that the fraction of glutamine recovered as glutamate is smaller in experiments with acidotic animals confirms accelerated intramitochondrial utilization of glutamate in this situation. No effect of *in vitro* acidosis on glucose production is noted with tubules or slices from acidotic rats as if gluconeogenesis was already proceeding at maximal rate. Nevertheless glutamate accumulation tends to decrease following acidification and increase following alkalinization, suggesting an additional effect of H^+ somewhere between glutamate and oxaloacetate. Therefore, despite similar glutamine extraction, the metabolism of glutamine is different if the incubation pH is acidotic or alkalotic as already commented upon by Preuss (1974).

In order to pin-point the site of effect of H^+ concentration on the ammoniagenic chain the metabolite profile of kidney tubules were examined after a short incubation at the various pH. With 5 mM glutamine as substrate, a decrement of alpha-ketoglutarate concentration with simultaneous increase in malate concentration creating a cross-over phenomenon between alpha-ketoglutarate and oxaloacetate suggest that alpha-ketoglutarate utilization is increased by acute acidosis. Alkalosis has the opposite effect on the alpha-ketoglutarate concentration which is not accompanied by a depression of malate concentration. The latter observation is consistent with an activation of the glycolytic pathway (Gevers & Dowdle, 1963; Relman, 1972) and of pyruvate carboxylase enzyme by alkalosis (Scrutton & Utter, 1967) preventing a fall in malate or oxaloacetate.

The present findings are only partly in accord with

Table 5. Effect of incubation pH on glutamine metabolism by the kidney cortical tissue of normal dogs

	Slices $n = 5$			Tubules $n = 5$		
Incubation pH	7.11 ± 0.013	7.42 ± 0.022	7.67 ± 0.053**	7.18 ± 0.024	7.45 ± 0.033	7.73 ± 0.049**
5 mM Glutamine						
Glutamine extraction	35.1 ± 3.68	31.5 ± 2.37	33.7 ± 5.21	74.4 ± 17.93	88.9 ± 32.26	92.1 ± 21.17
Glutamate production	14.4 ± 1.04*	18.0 ± 0.72	20.1 ± 1.23**	43.4 ± 4.50	48.8 ± 3.77	48.2 ± 4.25
NH_4 production	38.1 ± 2.58	41.5 ± 3.09	42.6 ± 2.93**	113.8 ± 9.77	115.8 ± 6.66	109.1 ± 6.86
Glucose production	3.14 ± 0.21*	2.63 ± 0.19	2.35 ± 0.14	9.9 ± 1.09*	8.7 ± 1.10	6.9 ± 0.72**
NH_4 production/ Gln extraction	1.09	1.32	0.97	1.52	1.30	1.18
1 mM Glutamine						
Glutamine extraction	10.6 ± 0.62	11.3 ± 0.72	12.2 ± 0.69	23.30 ± 4.51	25.2 ± 5.73	20.91 ± 2.33
Glutamate production	5.05 ± 0.74*	7.83 ± 0.94	10.8 ± 0.71**	24.40 ± 3.13	25.50 ± 3.22	28.61 ± 3.57**
NH_4 production	21.12 ± 1.32	21.24 ± 1.59	19.0 ± 1.07	64.0 ± 6.47	62.5 ± 5.31	62.0 ± 3.30
Glucose production	2.6 ± 0.06*	2.21 ± 0.13	1.8 ± 0.06**	8.2 ± 1.31*	6.3 ± 0.95	4.9 ± 0.79**
NH_4 production/ Gln extraction	1.99	1.88	1.62	2.7	2.48	2.97

Values are μmols/g wet wt for 30 min (tubules) or 60 min (slices) incubation ± SEM. $n = 5$. See Table 1 for description.

Table 6. Effect of incubation pH on glutamine metabolism by kidney cortical tissue of acidotic dogs

	Slices $n = 5$			Tubules $n = 5$		
Incubation pH	7.04 ± 0.04*	7.44 ± 0.01	7.76 ± 0.05**	7.10 ± 0.026*	7.50 ± 0.031	7.80 ± 0.053
5 mM Glutamine						
Glutamine extraction	57.0 ± 13.5	59.4 ± 13.25	64.0 ± 13.27	115.1 ± 19.98	118.0 ± 10.72	135.0 ± 26.67
Glutamate production	12.44 ± 1.08*	16.0 ± 1.83	20.4 ± 2.49	52.2 ± 5.82	55.6 ± 12.9	60.2 ± 14.01
NH_4 production	42.4 ± 3.33	42.5 ± 2.86	45.9 ± 1.41	120.21 ± 4.35**	100.2 ± 7.80	98.0 ± 7.19
Glucose production	4.8 ± 0.40*	3.7 ± 0.33	3.2 ± 0.24**	10.9 ± 1.42*	8.0 ± 1.07	6.3 ± 1.20*
NH_4 production/ Gln extraction	0.74	0.72	0.72	1.05	0.85	0.73
1 mM Glutamine						
Glutamine extraction	14.2 ± 1.19	14.6 ± 1.24	12.3 ± 0.69	36.3 ± 3.14	26.01 ± 5.85	32.3 ± 6.20
Glutamate production	9.8 ± 1.59*	0.1 ± 1.30	10.9 ± 0.66	23.6 ± 2.04*	28.2 ± 2.50	34.9 ± 4.69
NH_4 production	25.0 ± 1.68	22.6 ± 0.99	21.7 ± 0.89	64.6 ± 3.79*	54.5 ± 3.22	45.3 ± 3.48**
Glucose production	3.6 ± 0.33*	2.8 ± 0.19	2.7 ± 0.18	9.1 ± 0.93*	9.1 ± 0.75	5.4 ± 0.89**
NH_4 production/ Gln extraction	1.76	1.55	1.76	1.78	2.10	1.40

Values are μmols/g wet wt for 60 min (slices) or 30 min (tubules) incubation ± SEM. See Table 1 for complete description.

Table 7. Effect of acidification of the incubation medium on glutamine or glutamate metabolism by kidney tissue *in vitro*

Technique	Glutamine concentration	NH_4 production	Glucose production	Flask or tissue glutamate	Author
Rat slices	10 mM	—	↑	—	Kamm *et al.* (1967)
	10 mM	N.C.	—	↓	Goodman (1973)
	10 mM	N.C.	↑	↓	Pagliara *et al.* (1970)
	10 mM	N.C.	—	—	Relman & Narins (1975)
	6 mM	N.C.	↑	N.C.	Irias & Greenberg (1972)
	2 mM	N.C.	↑	↓	Preuss *et al.* (1974)
	2 mM	↓	N.C.	↓	Roobol & Alleyne (1974)
Rat tubules	2 mM	—	↑		Kurokowa & Rasmussen (1973a,b)
Rat perfused kidney	5 mM	N.C.	↑	—	Hems (1972)
	0.5 mM	↑	—	↓	Tannen & Ross (1979)
Dog slices	0.5 mM	—	↑	↓	Simpson & Sherrard (1968)
	1 mM	N.C.	↑	↓	Cartier *et al.* (1975)

N.C. = no change. ↑ = stimulation of glucose. ↓ = depression of ammonia production or tissue glutamate concentration.

previous *in vivo* studies (freeze-clamp) of rat kidney metabolite profile (Hems & Brosnan, 1971; Narins & Relman, 1974) showing lower renal alpha-ketoglutarate and glutamate concentrations in acidotic animal, but with no increment in malate. However, the latter experiments were performed with rats submitted to prolonged acidosis, with secondary stimulation of PEPCK activity (Alleyne & Scullard, 1969), that would prevent the rise in tissue malate concentration. Furthermore, a rapid flux through the ammoniagenic and gluconeogenic pathway, as induced by supra-physiological concentration of glutamine (5 mM), is necessary to show significant changes in malate concentration in our experiments.

It should be noted that the effect of H^+ on alpha-ketoglutarate concentration cannot be due to a primary PEPCK activation by acidosis since malate concentration is not simultaneously depressed. Indeed, no changes in PEPCK activity can be demonstrated before at least 6 hr of metabolic acidosis (Alleyne, 1970; Alleyne & Scullard, 1969) while our observations were made after 30 min. Furthermore, PEPCK activity *in vitro* is stimulated by alkalosis and not by acidosis (Chang *et al.*, 1966; Holten & Nordlie, 1965). A similar fall in alpha-ketoglutarate accumulation induced by increasing H^+ concentration has been reported with isolated rat mitochondria (Relman & Narins, 1975), a preparation lacking PEPCK activity. Acute inhibition of glutamate dehydrogenase by acidification of the medium (Seyama *et al.*, 1972) is also improbable as this would not enhance glutamine uptake or depress glutamate accumulation.

The observed changes in gluconeogenesis and oxidation of glutamine as well as that of alpha-ketoglutarate and malate concentration during acidification could be due to increased alpha-ketoglutarate dehydrogenase activity, increased succinic dehydrogenase activity or increased malate transport across mitochondria. Our studies with AOA and MSO rule out the glutamine synthetase and the aminotransferases reactions as possible sites for the H^+ effect. The fact that increasing H^+ concentration increases glucose production by tubules from substrates before the succinate dehydrogenase step i.e. glutamine, citrate, succinate, alpha-ketoglutarate but not from substrates situated beyond the succinate dehydrogenase reaction i.e. malate, oxaloacetate or lactate (Kurokawa & Rasmussen, 1973a; Nagata & Rasmussen, 1970) is compatible with any of these hypotheses. We have no argument to prove or disprove an effect of H^+ concentration on malate transport or succinate dehydrogenase activity. However, we must imply a direct effect of H^+ on the activity of the alpha-ketoglutarate dehydrogenase complex. As the latter enzyme catalyses the irreversible decarboxylation of alpha-ketoglutarate, this reaction is not expected to be accelerated by removal of its products through succinate dehydrogenase activation or mitochondrial removal of malate. This suggests that alpha-ketoglutarate dehydrogenase itself is modified by H^+ concentration. The reverse effect of alkalosis on alpha-ketoglutarate and glutamate concentration is also compatible with such an action on alpha-ketoglutarate dehydrogenase activity.

It should be noted that H^+ concentration had no detectable effect on glutamine utilization and ammonia production by dog kidney tissue (slices or tubules). However *in vitro* acidosis stimulates gluconeogenesis and depresses glutamate accumulation as in the rat, suggesting that a similar effect (possibly on alpha-ketoglutarate dehydrogenase complex) has occurred but without the accompanying effect on renal glutamine transport.

Acknowledgements—This study was supported by grants from the Medical Research Council of Canada including Program Grant PG 6, and also by a grant from the Jeanne-Mance Foundation. The authors acknowledge Mr Jacques Sénécal, and Misses Pierrette Fournel, Andrée Quennevile, and Syvie Desjardins for their skilled assistance.

REFERENCES

ALLEYNE G. A. O. (1970) Renal metabolic response to acid-base changes. II. The early effects of metabolic acidosis on renal metabolism in the rat. *J. clin. Invest.* **49**, 943–951.

ALLEYNE G. A. O & SCULLARD G. H. (1969) Renal metabolic response to acid-base changes. Enzymatic control of ammoniagenesis in the rat. *J. clin. Invest.* **48**, 364–370.

BERGMEYER H. U. (1974) *Methods of Enzymatic Analysis*. Academic Press, New York.

CARTIER P., BÉLANGER P. & LEMIEUX G. (1975) Characteristics of *in vitro* ammonia and glucose production by dog kidney cortex. *Am. J. Physiol.* **228,** 934–943.

CHANCE B., HOLMES W., HIGGINS J. & CONNELLY C. M. (1958) Localization of interaction sites in multi-component transfer systems: theorems derived from analogues. *Nature* **182,** 1190–1193.

CHANG H., MARUYAMA, MILLER U. J. & LANE M. D. (1966) The enzymatic carboxylation of phosphoenolpyruvate. III. Investigation of the kinetics and mechanism of the mitochondrial phosphoenolpruvate carboxykinase–catalysed reaction. *J. biol. Chem.* **241,** 2421–2429.

CHURCHILL P. C. & MARVIN R. L. (1970) Relation of renal gluconeogenesis to ammonia production in the dog. *Am. J. Physiol.* **218,** 241–245.

GEVERS W. & DOWDLE E. (1963) The effect of pH on glycolysis *in vitro*. *Clin. Sci.* **25,** 343–349.

GOODMAN A. D. (1973) Effect of acid–base changes and dehydration on renal medullary production of ammonia. *J. Lab. clin. Med.* **81,** 905–918.

GUDER W. G., WIESNER W., STUCKOWSKI B. & WIELAND O. H. (1971) Metabolism of isolated kidney tubules: oxygen consumption, gluconeogenesis, and the effect of cyclic nucleotides in tubules from starved rats. *Hoppe Seyler's Z. physiol. Chem.* **352,** 1319–1328.

HEMS D. A. & BROSNAN J. T. (1971) Effects of metabolic acidosis and starvation on the content of intermediary metabolites in rat kidney. *Biochem. J.* **123,** 391–397.

HEMS D. A. (1972) Metabolism of glutamine and glutamic acid by isolated perfused kidneys of normal and acidotic rats. *Biochem. J.* **130,** 671–680.

HEMS R. (1976) Rapid separation of isolated hepatocytes or similar tissue fragments for analysis of cell constituents. In *Use of Isolated Liver Cells and Kidney Tubules in Metabolic Studies* (Edited by TAGER J. M., SOLING H. D. & WILLIAMSON J. R.) pp. 155–157. North Holland, Amsterdam.

HOLTEN D. D. & NORDLIE R. C. (1965) Comparative studies of catalytic properties of guinea pig liver intra and extra-mitochondrial phosphoenolpyruvate carboxylase. *Biochemistry* **4,** 723–730.

IRIAS J. J. & GREENBERG R. E. (1972) Relationship of renal gluconeogenesis to control of ammonia formation. *Am. J. Physiol.* **223,** 750–755.

KAMM D. E., FUISZ R. E., GOODMAN A. D. & CAHILL G. F. (1967) Acid–base alterations and renal gluconeogenesis: effect of pH, bicarbonate concentration and PCO_2. *J. clin. Invest.* **26,** 1172–1177.

KUROKOWA D. & RASMUSSEN H. (1973a) Ionic control of gluconeogenesis. I. The inter-related effects of calcium and hydrogen ions. *Biochim. biophys. Acta* **313,** 17–31.

KUROKOWA D. & RASMUSSEN H. (1973b) Ionic control of renal gluconeogenesis. III. Effects of changes in pH, PCO_2 and bicarbonate concentration. *Biochim. biophys. Acta* **313,** 42–58.

NAGATA N. & RASMUSSEN H. (1970) Renal gluconeogenesis: effects of Ca^{2+} and H^+. *Biochim. biophys. Acta* **215,** 1–16.

NARINS R. G. & RELMAN A. S. (1976) Acute effects of acidosis on ammoniogenic pathways in the kidneys of the intact rat. *Am. J. Physiol.* **227,** 946–949.

O'DONOVAN D. J. & LOTSPEICH W. D. (1966) Activation of kidney mitochondrial glutaminase by organic phosphate and organic acids. *Nature, Lond.* **212,** 930–932.

PAGLIARA A. S. & GOODMAN A. D. (1970) Relation of renal cortical gluconeogenesis, glutamate content and production of ammonia. *J. clin. Invest.* **49,** 1967–1974.

PREUSS H. G. (1970) Ammonia production from glutamine and glutamate in isolated dog renal tubules. *Am. J. Physiol.* **220,** 54–58.

PREUSS H. G., VAVATSI-MANOS O., VERTUNO L. & BAIRD K. (1974) The effects of pH changes on renal ammoniagenesis *in vitro*. *Proc. Soc. exp. Biol. Med.* **146,** 803–808.

RELMAN A. S. (1972) Metabolic consequences of acid–base disorders. *Kidney Int.* **1,** 347–359.

RELMAN A. S. & NARINS R. G. (1975) The control of ammonia production in the rat. *Med. Clin. North. Am.* **59,** 583–593.

ROOBOL A. & ALLEYNE G. A. O. (1974) Controls of renal cortex ammoniagenesis and its relationship to renal cortex gluconeogenesis. *Biochim. biophys. Acta* **362,** 83–91.

ROXE D. M., SCHREINER G. E. & PREUSS H. G. (1974) Regulation of renal gluconeogenesis by physiologic fuels. *Am. J. Physiol.* **225,** 908–914.

SIMPSON D. P. & SHERRARD D. J. (1968) Regulation of glutamine *in vitro* by bicarbonate ion and pH. *J. clin. Invest.* **48,** 1088–1096.

SCRUTTON M. C. & UTTER M. F. (1967) Pyruvate carboxylase: some properties of the activation by certain acyl derivatives of coenzyme A. *J. biol. Chem.* **242,** 1723–1735.

SEYAMA S., SAEKI T. & KATUNUMA K. (1972) Comparison of properties and inducibility of glutamate dehydrogenases in rat kidney and liver. *J. Biochem.* **73,** 39–45.

TANNEN R. L. & KUNIN A. S. (1976) Effect of pH on ammonia production by renal mitochondria. *Am. J. Physiol.* **231,** 1631–1637.

TANNEN R. L. & ROSS B. D. (1979) Ammoniagenesis by isolated perfused rat kidney: the critical role of urinary acidification. *Clin. Sci.* **56,** 353–364.

VINAY P., MAPES J. P. & KREBS M. A. (1978) The fate of glutamine carbon in renal metabolism. *Am. J. Physiol.* **234,** F123–F129.

VINAY P., GOUGOUX A. & LEMIEUX G. (1979) *In vitro* renal ammoniagenesis by rat isolated kidney tubules: a complete carbon and nitrogen balance. *Can. J. Biochem.* **57,** 346–356.

VINAY P., LEMIEUX G., GOUGOUX A. & WATFORD M. (1978) The metabolic fate of glutamine in the renal cells. *Proceedings, VII. International Congress of Nephrology.* KARGER S. Montreal pp. 198–207.

SYMPOSIUM DISCUSSION

Tannen: I should like to agree with what you said, and expand on the observations that Ross and I (1979) made with the isolated perfused rat kidney. Recent studies in my laboratory agree with your findings but do not entirely explain how acute changes in hydrogen ion concentration affect ammonia production. Acute respiratory acidosis increases ammonia production by the isolated perfused kidney comparably with metabolic acidosis in ammonia production. However, it didn't acidify the urine, and ammonia was consequently not trapped in the urine: this result negates the hypothesis that we originally put forward to explain stimulation of ammoniagenesis we observed in the perfused kidney in acute metabolic acidosis. An unexplained finding in perfusion experiments with either in acute metabolic or respiratory acidosis, is that if the urine is allowed to drain into the perfusion medium, we no longer see any increase in ammonia production.

Weiner: How did you lower pH?

Vinay: By modifying the bicarbonate content, keeping CO_2 constant.

Lowry (*Oxford*): The stimulation of ammonia production by acidosis produces a number of responses, each with its own time scale, 24 hr for phosphate dependent glutaminase, 2–3 hr for PEPCK, 15–30 min for the increase in gluconeogenesis and ammonia production. We have identified a much earlier response in the fall in 2-oxoglutarate concentration, which occurs within 5 min in the isolated perfused kidney and even less, 2–3 min, in tubules. This response occurs whether pH is altered by changing HCO_3 or pCO_2, so that we think that this must be a key event in the subsequent series of responses to acidosis (Lowry & Ross, in press).

Kovacevic: You said that in renal tubules, you had increased transport of glutamine. What is your explanation for the differences between tubules and slices?

Vinay: My explanation is that slices are too thick to allow free glutamine entry, so that endogenous substrates are preferentially used. This, in part, could explain why glutamate concentration falls. In tubules, the increased entry of glutamine results in there being no fall, rather a small increase in glutamate concentration. With dog tubules, on the other hand, there is no accumulation of glutamate, presumably because there is no increase in glutamine transport.

Kurokawa: Do you know what happens to succinate levels in the tubules?

Vinay: No.

Guder: We came to a similar conclusion and inferred that 2-oxoglutarate dehydrogenase or succinic dehydrogenase are the regulatory point. We used [1-^{14}C]oxoglutarate and [1,4^{14}C]succinate in experiments in which we acidified the incubating medium. To our surprise, there was a marked increase in glucose formation from both substrates, but no increase in $^{14}CO_2$ production.

Baverel: We did experiments with 1 mM glutamine in dog tubules in which we saw a relatively high rate of oxidation. You have a considerably lower rate of oxidation to CO_2 in your experiments.

Vinay: This may be due to a difference in technique. We have albumin present (presumably with bound fatty acid) while in your experiments you have none. I do not know which experimental system is closer to the *in vivo* state.

Int. J. Biochem., Vol. 12, pp. 99 to 102

0020-711X/80/0701-0099$02.00/0

GLUTAMINE UPTAKE BY CORTICAL SLICES AND LUMINAL BRUSH BORDER VESICLES OF RAT KIDNEY

GEORGE A. O. ALLEYNE, NORMA MCFARLANE ANDERSON and BARBARA SCOTT
Department of Medicine, University of the West Indies, Kingston 7, Jamaica

Abstract—1. Glutamine uptake was measured in cortical slices and brush border vesicles of the rat kidney.
2. Proline inhibited glutamine uptake by kidney slices and this inhibition was markedly less in slices from acidotic rats or in slices incubated in a sodium free buffer.
3. Proline also inhibited glutamine transport less in vesicles from acidotic rats.
4. The effect of metabolic inhibitors sodium maleate and sodium azide disappeared in slices from acidotic rats and in slices incubated in sodium-free buffer.

INTRODUCTION

It has been clearly shown that glutamine is extracted from the arterial blood by the kidney of man and dog and in the latter, this uptake is increased in both acute and chronic metabolic acidosis (Fine *et al.*, 1978; Shalhoub *et al.*, 1963; Pitts 1972). In the rat, while there is debate as to whether there is net uptake of glutamine by the kidney normally, there is no doubt that in acidosis there is considerable uptake of this amino acid in association with enhancement of ammoniagenesis (Yablon & Relman, 1977). In spite of the evidence of increased glutamine uptake and the fact that there must be glutamine reabsorption by the kidney, there are few data on the characteristics of the glutamine transport, in comparison with the numerous studies on the transport of other amino acids by the kidney. Investigators have previously used kidney slices and vesicles from the proximal tubular brush border to study transport of several amino acids (Rosenberg *et al.*, 1961; Sacktor, 1977; Kinne & Schwartz, 1978), but only very recently have some of the characteristics of glutamine transport by brush border vesicles from the rat kidney tubules been established (McFarlane-Anderson & Alleyne, 1979). These studies showed clearly that sodium dependent active transport of glutamine was enhanced in the kidney taken from chronically acidotic rats.

The experiments described here examine the uptake of glutamine by slices and vesicles from control and acidotic rats. We have established that there is a sodium dependent and a sodium independent uptake of glutamine and we propose that the latter persists and is perhaps enhanced by metabolic acidosis.

MATERIALS AND METHODS

Animals were Sprague–Dawley rats. The preparation and incubation of cortical slices and renal brush border vesicles have been described previously (Alleyne, 1970; McFarlane-Anderson & Alleyne, 1979). Chronic metabolic acidosis was induced by giving rats 280 mM NH_4Cl as their sole drinking fluid for 7–10 days while controls received 280 mM NaCl.

When a sodium free buffer was used, 300 mM mannitol was substituted for NaCl and choline bicarbonate for $NaHCO_3$ in the standard Krebs Ringer bicarbonate buffer. All buffers were gassed with an O_2:CO_2 mixture 96:4 and were at pH 7.4.

Glutamine and glutamate were assayed enzymatically (Bergmeyer, 1974) and ammonia by the alkaline phenate method (Kaplan, 1965). Radioactivity was counted in a Beckman LS 150 liquid scintillation counter.

Significance of difference between means was calculated by the Student's *t*-test.

RESULTS

Effect of amino acids on glutamine uptake

The effect of some amino acids on glutamine uptake by cortical slices from normal rats is shown on Table 1. In Krebs–Ringer bicarbonate buffer, alanine, aspartic acid, cysteine and arginine do not alter glutamine uptake which is inhibited 15% by glycine and 50% by proline at the concentrations shown. Glutamine uptake increases curvilinearly with increasing concentration of glutamine and proline (20 mM) competitively inhibits glutamine uptake (Fig. 1). The apparent K_m for glutamine uptake by normal slices is 3.3 mM. The possibility that proline exerts its effects through its metabolism to glutamate was discounted by measuring glutamate levels which are identical in the presence or absence of proline.

When slices are incubated in sodium free buffer, the inhibition by proline and glycine disappears and the only amino acid which depresses glutamine uptake is alanine. Slices from chronically acidotic rats were incubated in glutamine and there is the expected increase in glutamine uptake. However, proline (20 mM) is not as effective in inhibiting glutamine uptake as in slices from control animals (24 vs 50%).

Uptake by vesicles

Proximal tubular brush border vesicles from control animals show that active sodium dependent glutamine uptake is inhibited 67% by proline and in

Table 1. The effect of amino acids (all at 20 mM) on uptake of glutamine (2.0 mM) by renal cortical slices. In sodium free buffer, the standard Krebs–Ringer bicarbonate buffer had NaCl replaced by 300 mM mannitol and $NaHCO_3$ by choline bicarbonate

	Glutamine uptake (μmols/hr/g dry wt) K–R buffer Control	Acidotic	Na$^+$ free buffer Control
Glutamine	252 ± 17	491 ± 37	206 ± 12
+Alanine	240 ± 29		143 ± 13
+Arginine	221 ± 24		186 ± 44
+Aspartic acid	266 ± 26		228 ± 14
+Cysteine	240 ± 33		174 ± 12
+Glycine	189 ± 20		229 ± 28
+Proline	144 ± 17	350 ± 46	224 ± 23

Values are means ± SEM for a minimum of 10 determinations.

vesicles from acidotic animals this is reduced to 20%. There is no effect of proline on sodium independent uptake of glutamine by brush border vesicles from control or acidotic animals.

Effect of metabolic inhibitors

Sodium maleate (2.5 mM) stimulates glutamine uptake by slices from control and acidotic rats in both Krebs–Ringer bicarbonate and sodium-free buffers. In Krebs–Ringer buffer sodium azide (4.0 mM) stimulates glutamine uptake but in sodium free buffer there is no effect of azide on slices from normal animals, while slices from acidotic animals show a depression of glutamine uptake. Both maleate and azide depress ammonia production and glutamate uptake by slices from control and acidotic animals incubated in glutamate (2.0 mM). Maleate is without effect on ammonia production from glycine (2.0 mM).

In vesicles from normal rats, maleate stimulates only the sodium independent uptake of glutamine.

DISCUSSION

Traditionally, uptake of amino acids by slices has been measured by determining the ratios of intracellular to extracellular amino acid after an appropriate period of incubation (Rosenberg *et al.*, 1961). We have found it almost impossible to measure intracellular/extracellular ratios of glutamine in slices. When [^{14}C]glutamine was used, ratios of ^{14}C counts were as high as 4.0 but it was soon established that the majority of the radioactivity was in the form of [^{14}C]glutamate. Deamidation of glutamine in slices is so rapid that it is difficult to establish ratios of glutamine greater than 1. As a first step we chose to obtain data on glutamine uptake rather than ratios. The effect of proline, and to a lesser extent glycine, on glutamine uptake is in keeping with the view that they share a common transport step (Fromter, 1979).

Aminoacid uptake across the luminal membrane and into the renal tubular cell may have two components—one sodium-dependent and the other sodium-independent. The extent to which the sodium-independent step represents active transport or passive diffusion is as yet unclear for glutamine or any other amino acid (Hammerman & Sacktor, 1977). In our studies, proline inhibited the sodium-dependent glutamine uptake but in the sodium free buffer, the effect of proline virtually disappeared. In the acidotic animal sodium-dependent as well as sodium independent glutamine uptake was increased and we found here that proline inhibition of the sodium-dependent uptake was considerably reduced. The similarity of the proline effect in acidosis and in the sodium free buffer might indicate that in chronic acidosis the sodium independent glutamine uptake was enhanced. Another possibility of course is that in chronic acidosis the enhancement of glutamine uptake and metabolism is independent of the presence of sodium:

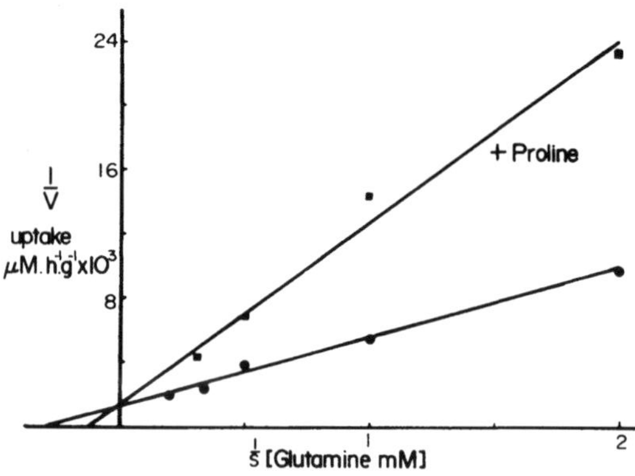

Fig. 1. The effect of proline (20 mM) on the uptake of glutamine by renal cortical slices. Kidney cortex slices were incubated for 1 hr with glutamine alone (●) or with glutamine in the presence of 20 mM proline (■) and the uptake of glutamine measured.

Table 2. The effect of sodium maleate and sodium azide on glutamine uptake by renal cortical slices from normal or chronically acidotic rats incubated in Krebs–Ringer bicarbonate buffer or a sodium free buffer

	Glutamine uptake (μmol/hr/g dry wt). K–R buffer Normal	Acidotic	Na$^+$ free buffer* Normal	Acidotic
Control	285 ± 22	438 ± 50	224 ± 15	328 ± 19
+maleate 2.5 mM	390 ± 29	597 ± 59	346 ± 23	474 ± 30
Control	216 ± 18	370 ± 28	346 ± 19	337 ± 22
+azide 4.0 mM	307 ± 29	391 ± 30	212 ± 19	251 ± 14

* "Na$^+$ free buffer" would contain 2.5 mM Na$^+$ in the case of buffer with sodium maleate and 4.0 mM sodium with sodium azide.

Values are means ± SEM for a minimum of 10 determinations.

passive glutamine diffusion to the sites of metabolic activity is adequate to demonstrate the increased glutamine metabolism. At this stage it is impossible to distinguish between these two possibilities and indeed to state with any certainty that the sodium independent glutamine uptake is anything but passive diffusion of glutamine. To establish this it will be necessary to show that active glutamine transport occurs in the absence of sodium either into slices or into brush border vesicles. We can offer no explanation for the effect of alanine on glutamine uptake in a sodium free buffer.

Previous studies with maleate 2,4, DNP methylene blue, malonate, hydrazine and arsenite have all shown increases in ammonia production from glutamine by the kidney *in vitro* (Strezelecki & Rogulski, 1977) and in a recent study, fluorocitrate *in vivo* was shown to increase glutamine uptake and ammonia production by the kidneys of acidotic as well as alkalotic dogs (Bourke *et al.*, 1979). The mechanism postulated in this last experiment was that there is a decrease in intramitochondrial glutamate levels, deinhibiting glutaminase I and leading to increased deamidation of glutamine. However, in slices, at least with azide and arsenite, glutamate levels increase making this an unlikely mechanism in our studies.

Maleate has been shown to decrease transport of several amino acids into kidney slices (Rosenberg & Segal, 1964), and in addition alters renal metabolism, decreasing ATP levels perhaps by a reduction in the CoA pool through formation of maleyl CoA (Angielski & Rogulski, 1975). In our experiment, incubation of slices with maleate and acetoacetate reverses the maleate effect presumably by protecting the CoA pool and inhibiting the decrease in ATP. Studies in the dog (Gmaj *et al.*, 1973) have shown that maleate causes bicarbonaturia, but it is noticeable from the study of Gougoux *et al.* (1977), also in the dog, that in the first 20 min after maleate, urinary NH_3 actually increased. Maleate may have another effect on renal metabolism through its direct effect on γ-glutamyl transpeptidase enhancing its glutaminase activity or its transport function (Tate & Meister, 1975). The effect of acetoacetate disappears in a sodium-free buffer indicating that in this stituation we are seeing the effect of the maleate ion per se in stimulating glutamine uptake. In the case of azide, the stimulatory effect disappears in sodium-free buffer and in acidotic slices. It is possible that the difference between the effects of maleate and azide on glutamine uptake in the sodium-free buffer and on slices from acidotic rats lies in the dual effects of maleate—one through reduction in ATP and the other through the specific effect of the maleate ion on γ-glutamyl transpeptidase.

SUMMARY

Glutamine uptake by renal cortical slices is competitively inhibited by proline and to a lesser extent by glycine. Alanine, arginine, aspartic acid and cysteine have no effect on glutamine uptake in Krebs–Ringer buffer and with the exception of alanine there is no effect of these amino acids on glutamine uptake in sodium-free buffer. Inhibition by proline disappears in a sodium-free buffer and decreases significantly with slices from acidotic animals. Proximal tubule brush border vesicles show a similar inhibition of glutamine uptake by proline. Metabolic inhibitors maleate and azide, increase glutamine uptake and metabolism. However, whereas the maleate effect persists in a sodium-free buffer, the azide effect disappears. Maleate still retains its effect on slices from acidotic rats while azide does not. These data indicate that proline and glutamine may share a transport step and in acidosis glutamine metabolism may proceed via a mechanism independent of the presence of sodium.

Acknowledgements—This work was supported by grants from the Wellcome Trust and the Medical Research Council of Great Britain. The Wellcome Trust supported Dr McFarlane-Anderson.

REFERENCES

ALLEYNE G. A. O. (1970) Renal metabolic response to acid base changes II. The early effects of metabolic acidosis on renal metabolism in the rat. *J. clin. Invest.* **49**, 943–951.

ANGIELSKI S. & ROGULSKI J. (1975) Metabolic studies in experimental renal dysfunction resulting from maleate administration. In *Biochemical Aspects of Renal Function* (Edited by ANGELSKI S. & DUBACH U. C.) pp. 86–100. Hans Huber, Vienna.

BERGMEYER H. U. (1974) *Methods of Enzymatic Analysis.* Verlag Chemie–Academic Press, New York.

BOURKE E., FRINDT G., SCHREINER G. E. & PREUSS H. G. (1979) Effects of fluorocitrate on renal ammoniagenesis and glutamine metabolism in the intact dog. *Kidney Int.* **15**, 255–264.

FINE A., BENNETT F. I. & ALLEYNE G. A. O. (1978). The effect of acute acid base alterations on glutamine metabolism and renal ammoniagenesis in the dog. *Clin. Sci. mol. Med.* **54**, 503–508.

FROMTER E. (1979) Solute transport across eptihelia: what can we learn from micropuncture studies on kidney tubules. *J. Physiol.* **288**, 1–31.

GOUGOUX A., LEMIEUX G. & LAVOIE N. (1976) Maleate induced bicarbonaturia in the dog: a carbonic anhydrase-independent effect. *Am. J. Physiol.* **231**, 1010–1017.

GMAJ P., HOPPE A., ANGIELSKI S. & ROGULSKI J. (1973) Effects of maleate and arsenite on renal reabsorption of sodium and bicarbonate. *Am. J. Physiol.* **225**, 90–94.

HAMMERMAN M. R. & SACKTOR B. (1977) Transport of amino acids in renal brush border membrane vesicles: uptake of L-proline. *J. biol. Chem.* **252**, 591–596.

KAPLAN A. (1965) Urea nitrogen and urinary ammonia. In *Standard Methods in Clinical Chemistry* (Edited by MEITES S.) Vol. 5, pp. 245–256. Academic Press, New York.

KINNE R. & SCHWARTZ I. L. (1978) Isolated membrane vesicles in the evaluation of the nature, localization and regulation of renal transport processes. *Kidney Int.* **14**, 547–556.

MCFARLANE ANDERSON N & ALLEYNE G. A. O. (1979) Transport of glutamine by rat kidney brush-border membrane vesicles. *Biochem. J.* **182**, 295–300.

PITTS R. F. (1972) Control of renal production of ammonia. *Kidney Int.* **1**, 297–305.

ROSENBERG L. E. & SEGAL S. (1964) Maleic acid induced inhibition of amino acid transport in rat. *Kidney Biochem. J.* **92**, 345–352.

ROSENBERG L. E., BLAIR A. & SEGAL S. (1961) Transport of amino acids by slices of rat kidney cortex. *Biochim. biophys. Acta* **54**, 479–488.

SACKTOR B. (1977) Transport in membrane vesicles isolated

from the mammalian kidney and intestine. *Curr. Top. Bioenerg.* **6,** 39–81.

Shalhoub R., Webber W., Glabman S., Canessa-Fischer M., Klein J., Hass de J. & Pitts R. F. (1963) Extraction of amino acids from and their addition to renal blood plasma. *Am. J. Physiol.* **204,** 181–186.

Strzelecki T. & Rogulski J. (1977) Effect of extracellular pH and inhibitors on the gluconeogenesis and ammonia-genesis relationship in rat kidney cortex slices. *Acta Biochem. polon.* **24,** 253–260.

Tate S. S. & Meister A. (1975) Identity of maleate stimulated glutaminase with γ-glutamyl transpeptidase in rat kidney. *J. biol. Chem.* **250,** 4619–4627.

Yablon S. B. & Relman A. S. (1977) Glutamine as regulator of renal ammonia production in the rat. *Kidney Int.* **12,** 546.

Int. J. Biochem., Vol. 12, pp. 103 to 106

0020-711X/80/0701-0103$02.00/0

INHIBITOR OF RENAL GLUCONEOGENESIS (IGN): ADDITIONAL PHYSIOLOGICAL MODULATOR?

R. DZÚRIK, VIERA SPUSTOVÁ and P. ČERNÁČEK
Research Laboratory of Experimental Therapy, 3rd Medical Clinic 809 46 Bratislava, Czechoslovakia

Abstract—1. A procedure for the partial purification of IGN has been developed: it is insoluble in 80% ethanol but soluble in 6% TCA. It moves in void volume on a column of Sephadex G 25, passes through a membrane with cut-off at 25,000 daltons but not through a membrane with cut-off at 10,000 daltons.

2. IGN inhibits gluconeogenesis both in kidney cortex and liver slices. The inhibition is small during the first 30 min of incubation but it increases during the following periods of time. Liver slices are much less sensitive to the inhibitory action of IGN than kidney cortex slices.

3. IGN exerts its effect even in the absence of either K^+, Ca^{2+} or Mg^{2+} from Krebs–Ringer bicarbonate.

INTRODUCTION

A great number of so-called middle molecular substances accumulate in plasma of patients suffering from renal failure. They accumulate as a consequence of decreased renal excretion or renal breakdown (Bergström *et al.*, 1976). Many of them were found to exert significant metabolic or functional effects (Dzúrik & Simončič, 1968). These effects are usually tested by comparison of diluted control and uraemic sera, which are used as incubation media for various tissues.

Ten years ago, the inhibition of renal gluconeogenesis by uraemic serum was found in two laboratories (Dzúrik, 1979; Heintz & Renner, 1965). Because of shortage of uraemic plasma no further attention was paid to this inhibition. It emerged, after this discovery, that the inhibitor of gluconeogenesis (IGN) was also present in urine of the uraemic and probably also of healthy subjects (Lamberts *et al.*, 1976). The inhibitor was non-dialyzable through Visking tubes and it interfered with gluconeogenesis at the level of *p*-enolpyruvate carboxykinase (Lamberts *et al.*, 1976).

Unfortunately, this crude preparation could not be used in more sophisticated studies. It was found necessary to develop a purification procedure and to define the basic properties of IGN.

MATERIALS AND METHODS

Urine

Urine was obtained from the patients in renal failure with serum creatinine concentrations above 600 $\mu mol \cdot l^{-1}$. Urine was kept freeze dried until used for IGN purification.

Gel filtration

Freeze dried urine was dissolved in 10% of original volume of water, centrifuged and the supernatant was applied to the column.

Sephadex G 25: A column (170 × 7 cm) was packed with Sephadex G 25 fine (Pharmacia, Uppsala) equilibrated and eluted with 0.03 $mol \cdot l^{-1}$ ammonium acetate pH 6.9–7.0. Individual fractions were collected, freeze dried and tested for the inhibitory activity or treated further.

Sephadex G 15: A column (90 × 1.5 cm) packed with Sephadex G 15 (Pharmacia, Uppsala) equilibrated and eluted with 0.02 $mol \cdot l^{-1}$ formic acid was used for the purification of fraction 1.

Ethanol solubility

Fraction 1 was extracted 3 times with precooled 80% ethanol followed by centrifugation. The extracts were discarded, the sediment dried under vacuum after third centrifugation and tested.

TCA solubility

The sediment of 80% ethanol was dissolved in 6% trichloracetic acid (TCA). The insoluble material was removed by centrifugation and the supernatant was extracted three times with diethyl ether to remove TCA. The water phase was freeze dried and tested.

Membrane filtration

Amicon membranes UM 10 with the declared cut off at 10,000 daltons and cone filters CF 25 with cut off at 25,000 daltons were used for membrane filtration.

Measurement of glucose production

Male Wistar rats 180–200 g weight, last fed 24 hr before decapitation in the case of kidney but last fed 48 hr before in the case of liver, were used in the experiments. Kidney cortex slices were prepared "freehand" with razor blade and incubated in Krebs–Ringer bicarbonate buffer containing 5 $mmol \cdot l^{-1}$ alpha-oxoglutarate in atmosphere of 95% O_2 + 5% CO_2 for 1 h if not indicated otherwise. Glucose concentration was determined by the glucose oxidase method (Boehringer commercial kits).

RESULTS

Purification procedure

Gel filtration: IGN moved on a column of Sephadex G 25 eluted with neutral ammonium acetate in void volume (Fig. 1a). This procedure made it easy to separate the inhibitory activity from solutes interfering in the measurement of the inhibitory effect. Fraction 1 obtained on a column of Sephadex G 25 was usually freeze dried and further treated on a column of Sephadex G 15 eluted with formic acid (Fig. 1b). Two to three fractions were usually obtained. The inhibitor moved in fraction 1.1.

Solubility: Ethanol extract of fraction 1 did not contain UV absorbing substances eluted with void volume on the column of Sephadex G 15. On the other hand, the sediment dissolved in water and frac-

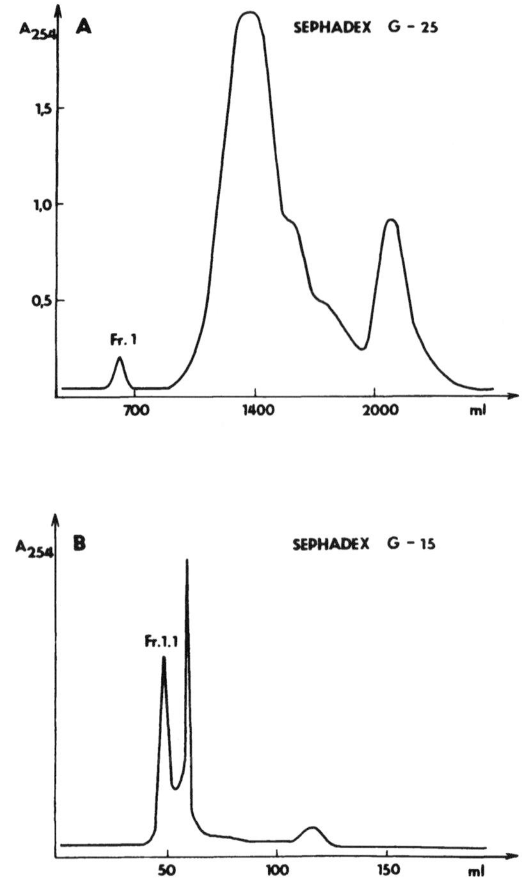

Fig. 1. Fractionation of urine by gel filtration chromatography. A. Fractionation of urine on a column of Sephadex G 25. B. Fractionation of fraction 1 on a column of Sephadex G 15.

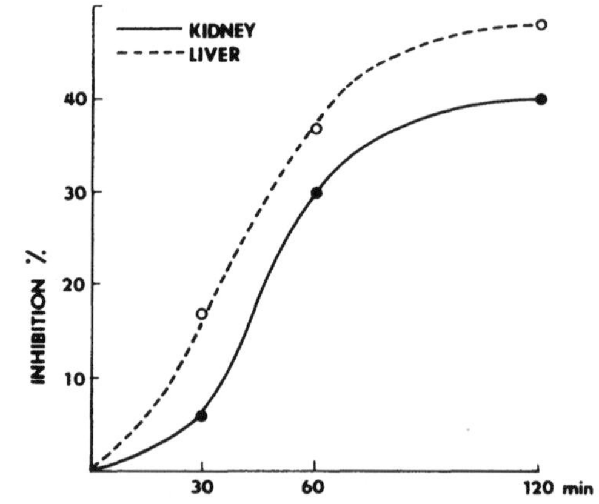

Fig. 2. The relationship between the time of incubation and inhibitory activity.

tionated on a column of Sephadex G 15 contained fraction 1 and the activity of IGN was directly demonstrated (Table 1). The sediment after 80% ethanol elution was further extracted with 6% TCA. The remaining insoluble material was discarded after centrifugation and the supernatant was repeatedly extracted with diethyl ether to remove TCA. Freeze dried water phase contained fraction 1 on a column of Sephadex G 15, and IGN (Table 1).

Membrane filtration: IGN of fraction 1.1 dissolved in 0.1 mol·l^{-1} ammonium acetate did not pass the membrane with a cut off of at 10,000 daltons but it passed the membrane with cut off at 25,000 daltons (Table 1). Thus, its molecular weight was in the range of 10,000–25,000 daltons.

Purification procedure: Freeze dried urine was extracted 3 times with cold 80% ethanol. The ethanol extract was discarded. The sediment was dissolved in

Table 1. Solubility and membrane filtration of IGN

Fraction	Glucose production in kidney cortex slices mg·g wet weight^{-1}·hr^{-1} Control	IGN	*P*	Inhibition %
80% ethanol sediment	12.98 ± 0.84 (6)*	4.53 ± 0.21 (6)	<0.001	65
6% TCA supernatant	13.87 ± 0.99 (6)	6.7 ± 0.48 (6)	<0.001	52
UM-10–0.1 mol·l^{-1} AA				
retained material	8.85 ± 0.19 (6)	5.88 ± 0.24 (6)	<0.001	34
filtrate	7.82 ± 0.17 (6)	8.14 ± 0.33 (6)	NS	
CF 25–0.1 mol·l^{-1} AA filtrate	18.39 ± 1.80 (6)	7.10 ± 0.38 (6)	<0.001	61

* Arithmetic mean ± SEM (number of samples in parentheses).

Table 2. The effect of IGN on glucose production by kidney cortex slices

Substrate	Glucose production mg·g wet weight^{-1}·hr^{-1} Control	IGN	*P*	Inhibition %
α-oxoglutarate (5 mmol·l^{-1})	8.63 ± 0.27 (6)*	6.02 ± 0.57 (6)	<0.01	30
Aspartate (5 mmol·l^{-1})	8.66 ± 0.46 (6)	4.38 ± 0.55 (6)	<0.001	49
Fructose (20 mmol·l^{-1})	17.17 ± 1.61 (6)	8.81 ± 1.07 (6)	<0.002	49

* Arithmetic mean ± SEM (number of samples in parentheses).

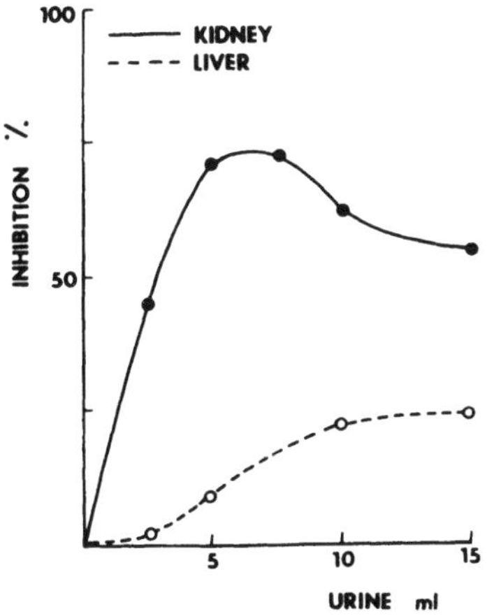

Fig. 3. The relationship between the dose of IGN and inhibitory activity.

6% TCA, centrifuged and the supernatant was extracted 3 times with diethyl ether to remove TCA. Water phase was freeze dried and fractioned on a column of Sephadex G 25. Freeze dried fraction 1 was further fractioned on a column of Sephadex G 15 and fraction 1.1 collected and freeze dried.

The amount of freeze dried substance obtained represented less than 0.01% of the original weight of the freeze dried urine, depending on the osmolality of urine and on its protein content. The increase of the specific activity cannot be presented because it is impossible to measure the inhibitory activity in untreated urine.

Metabolic studies

IGN inhibited glucose production in kidney cortex slices in the presence of various substrates, i.e. alpha-oxoglutarate, aspartate and even fructose (Table 2). IGN inhibited glucose production both in kidney cortex and liver slices (Fig. 2). The inhibition was relatively small at the beginning of incubation but increased later.

There was an apparent difference in the sensitivity of kidney cortex and liver slices to the IGN action, the liver slices being much less sensitive than kidney cortex slices (Fig. 3). It is to be stressed that even at the highest concentrations of IGN used, oxygen consumption of slices did not decrease (Uličná, personal communication).

Kidney cortex slices leached in cold saline for 15 min and incubated in Krebs–Ringer bicarbonate containing no K^+ showed decreased gluconeogenesis, but the effect of IGN was preserved even under these conditions (Fig. 4). Gluconeogenesis also decreased in

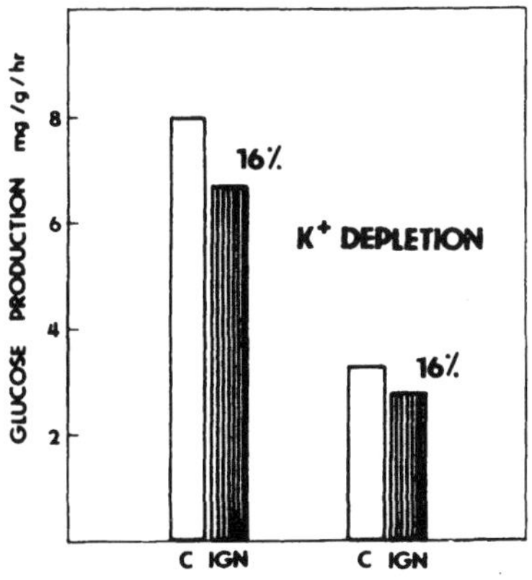

Fig. 4. The effect of K lack on the inhibitory activity of IGN.

absence of Ca^{2+} and Mg^{2+} in Ringer bicarbonate. The relative inhibitory activity of IGN actually increased under these conditions (Table 3).

DISCUSSION

Partial purification and structure of IGN

The described purification procedure has permitted us to isolate sufficient amounts of IGN of satisfactory purity for metabolic studies. Although the active substance is not chemically pure, some of the properties of IGN are suggested.

1. It is a peptide, by virtue of a positive ninhydrin reaction.
2. It is very probably a glycopeptide because of insolubility in 80% ethanol and solubility in 6% TCA.
3. Its molecular weight is between 10,000 and 25,000 daltons.
4. It is not broken down by kidney peptidases *in vitro* because of lasting inhibitory effect.

Metabolic effects of IGN

1. IGN inhibits gluconeogenesis by inhibiting *p*-enolpyruvate carboxykinase (Lamberts *et al*., 1976). However, the inhibition of glucose production in the presence of fructose makes an additional site of action probable.
2. The delay in IGN effect is caused either by a primary action beyond gluconeogenesis or by IGN interference with de novo enzyme synthesis. These possibilities have not been differentiated yet.
3. IGN effect is probably not mediated by K^+, Ca^{2+}, Mg^{2+} or by decreased oxygen consumption. It is impossible to decide on the physiological significance of IGN at the present time, but the studies presented make further investigations justifiable.

Table 3. The effect of Ca and Mg depletion on inhibitory activity of IGN in kidney cortex slices

	Control	IGN	P	Inhibition (%)
Medium with Ca and Mg	9.06 ± 0.79 (5)*	6.57 ± 0.44 (6)	<0.02	27
Medium without Ca and Mg	3.10 ± 0.35 (6)	1.88 ± 0.12 (6)	<0.01	39

* Arithmetic mean ± SEM (number of samples in parentheses).

SUMMARY

Urine from patients in renal failure was used for the study of an inhibitor of gluconeogenesis (IGN). In gel filtration on a column of Sephadex G 25 the active fraction moved in void volume. A procedure for the partial purification of IGN has been developed using an additional gel filtration step (Sephadex G 15) and insolubility of the active substance in 80% ethanol as well as its solubility in 6% TCA. IGN did not pass the membrane with a cut-off at 10,000 daltons, but passed the membrane with a cut-off at 25,000 daltons. This indicates a molecular weight in the range 10,000–25,000 daltons.

IGN inhibits glucose production in kidney cortex slices and liver slices in the presence of alpha-oxoglutarate, aspartate and fructose. The inhibition is small during the first 30 min of incubation but increases during the subsequent period of time. The delay in IGN effect is caused either by its primary action outside of gluconeogenesis or by IGN interference with de novo enzyme synthesis. Liver slices are much less sensitive to the inhibitory action of IGN than kidney cortex slices. In slices acutely depleted of K^+, glucose production was markedly decreased, but action of IGN was unaltered. The same situation was found when Ca^{2+} jnd Mg^{2+} were omitted from the incubation medium.

REFERENCES

Bergström J., Asaba H., Fürst P., Gordon A., Quadracci L. & Zimmerman L. (1976) Middle molecules in uraemia. *Proc. 6th Int. Congr. Nephrol.* Florence 1975 Karger, Basel.

Dzúrik R. & Šimončič E. (1968) Localization of the inhibition of gluconeogenesis in kidney slices by the uremic serum. *Med. Exp.* **18,** 135–138.

Dzúrik R. (1979) *Mittelmoleküle: Gegenwart und Erwartungen.* Vol. 3. Donausymposium Linz. In press.

Heintz R. & Renner D. (1965) Über Hemmwirkungen des Serums von Kranken mit hepatorenalem Syndrom und mit chronischer Urämie auf Sauerstoffverbrauch und Kohlenhydratstoffwechsel von Nieren- und Hirngewebe der Ratte. *Klin. Wschr.* **43,** 1167–1173.

Lamberts B., Brunner H., Ochs H. G. Spellerberg P. & Heintz R. (1976) Effect of urine metabolites from healthy and uremic subjects on gluconeogenesis in slices of rat kidney cortex and liver. *Clin. Nephrol.* **6,** 465–472.

SYMPOSIUM DISCUSSION

Lowenstein: Human uraemic serum may contain insulin or glucagon in varying concentrations. Did you measure these hormones?

Dzúrik: Not in these studies. In these experiments we used tissues from mormal animals, which were incubated in Ringer-bicarbonate with or without the inhibitor. Under these conditions there can be no differences in insulin or glucagon bound to the tissue. We are sure that there was no insulin or glucagon in the preparation of IGN. There is a difference when we use serum from uraemic sources: there is a divergent effect on liver slices and kidney slices, with glucose synthesis being stimulated in liver and inhibited in kidney. This may reflect differences due to glucagon in the serum of uraemic animals.

Guder: Can you exclude the possibility that the factor you describe increased glycolysis?

Dzúrik: IGN does not increase glycolysis either in this tissue or in muscle. We have tested that directly.

Alleyne: Is the concentration of the substance related to the duration of the uraemic process?

Dzúrik: To answer that question, we need to have more material and we have not yet reached that stage of purification.

Int. J. Biochem., Vol. 12, pp. 107 to 111
© Pergamon Press Ltd 1980. Printed in Great Britain

0020-711X/80/0701-0107$02.00/0

REGULATION OF RENAL GLUCONEOGENESIS BY α-ADRENERGIC ACTION

E. David Saggerson, Preminda Kessar and Carol A. Carpenter
Department of Biochemistry, University College London, Gower Street, London WC1E 6BT, U.K.

Abstract—1. Tubule fragments isolated from kidney cortex of fed rats by collagenase treatment were incubated with 5 mM lactate.

2. By use of selective α-adrenergic agonists and blocking agents it was shown that renal gluconeogenesis is stimulated through an α_1-type of adrenoceptor.

3. Catecholamine stimulation of the process is not abolished by omission of extracellular Ca^{2+} and is not accompanied by any change in influx of $^{45}Ca^{2+}$. On the other hand there is an α-adrenergic stimulation of $^{45}Ca^{2+}$ efflux from tubule fragments preloaded with this isotope, suggesting mobilisation of some intracellular calcium store.

4. Ouabain, and removal of extracellular K^+, abolish noradrenaline stimulation of gluconeogenesis suggesting that Na^+ and/or K^+ are involved in transmission of the α-adrenergic stimulus.

INTRODUCTION

Gluconeogenesis in renal cortex can be stimulated by catecholamines (Friedrichs & Schoner, 1973; Klahr *et al.*, 1973; Kurokawa & Massry, 1973; Roobol & Alleyne, 1973; Guder & Rupprecht, 1975; Macdonald & Saggerson, 1977). Studies with selective adrenergic agonists and antagonists have shown that this effect is mediated through an α-type of adrenoceptor (Guder & Rupprecht, 1975; Macdonald & Saggerson, 1977). The intracellular "second messenger" involved in this response is unknown although it is unlikely that cyclic AMP or cyclic GMP are involved (Guder & Rupprecht, 1975; Macdonald & Saggerson, 1977; Guder, 1979). This paper summarises findings from recent studies intended firstly to characterise the type of α-adrenoceptor involved in stimulation of renal gluconeogenesis by noradrenaline and secondly to investigate the possible role of Ca^{2+} and other cations in this process.

MATERIALS AND METHODS

Tubule fragments were prepared by collagenase treatment of kidney cortex pieces from fed rats as described by Macdonald & Saggerson (1977). Glucose formation was measured as described by Macdonald & Saggerson (1977) after incubation of tubule fragments (40–50 μg of DNA per ml) for 1 hr with 5 mM sodium L-lactate in Krebs–Henseleit bicarbonate buffer containing 1.27 mM Ca^{2+}.

RESULTS AND DISCUSSION

Characterization of the α-adrenoceptor

Recently, a considerable body of pharmacological evidence has accumulated consistent with the hypothesis that there may be more than one type of α-adrenoceptor. This distinction was first made between receptors on presynaptic sites and those on postsynaptic sites. Langer (1974) proposed that postsynaptic receptors be referred to as α_1, and the presynaptic α receptors, mediating feedback control by catecholamines of their own secretion from nerve endings as α_2. Subsequently this concept has been generalized to include the possibility that α_2 receptors are also to be found in other than presynaptic sites (Berthelsen & Pettinger, 1977; Kafka *et al.*, 1977; Hoffman *et al.*, 1979; Wood *et al.*, 1979). It is presumed therefore that the distinction between the α_1 and α_2 receptors must be functional rather than anatomical although the reason for this division of α receptors is not understood at present. Ligand binding studies suggest the presence of α_2 receptors in kidney (Jarrott *et al.*, 1979). Furthermore, there is some evidence that inhibition of renin release by catecholamines is mediated through an α_2 receptor (Pettinger *et al.*, 1976). It was therefore of interest to investigate the type of receptor through which noradrenaline stimulates renal gluconeogenesis. This was done with the aid of the selective blocking agents thymoxamine (an α_1 antagonist—Drew, 1976, 1978) and Yohimbine (an α_2 antagonist—Starke *et al.*, 1975; Doxey *et al.*, 1977; Drew, 1978) and by use of the selective agonists methoxamine (α_1—Drew 1977, 1978) and clonidine (α_2—Starke *et al.*, 1974; Drew 1977, 1978).

Figure 1 shows the effects of the selective blocking agents yohimbine and thymoxamine on noradrenaline stimulation of gluconeogenesis. Neither agent had any effect upon the basal rate of glucose formation in the absence of noradrenaline. Only thymoxamine caused any significant shift in the noradrenaline dose curve suggesting that the effect of noradrenaline was through an α_1 type of receptor. Further studies with the selective agonists reinforced this conclusion. Methoxamine was found to stimulate gluconeogenesis in a dose-dependent fashion. The maximum increase due to this agonist was 48 ± 3% (4 experiments) and was seen with 5 μM methoxamine. This may be compared with a 50 ± 3% increase seen with 1 μM noradrenaline in the same experiment. On the other hand clonidine tested over the range 0.1 nM–1 μM had no significant effect on gluconeogenesis (≤6%) whereas in the same experiment 1 μM noradrenaline stimulated glucose formation by 58 ± 7%.

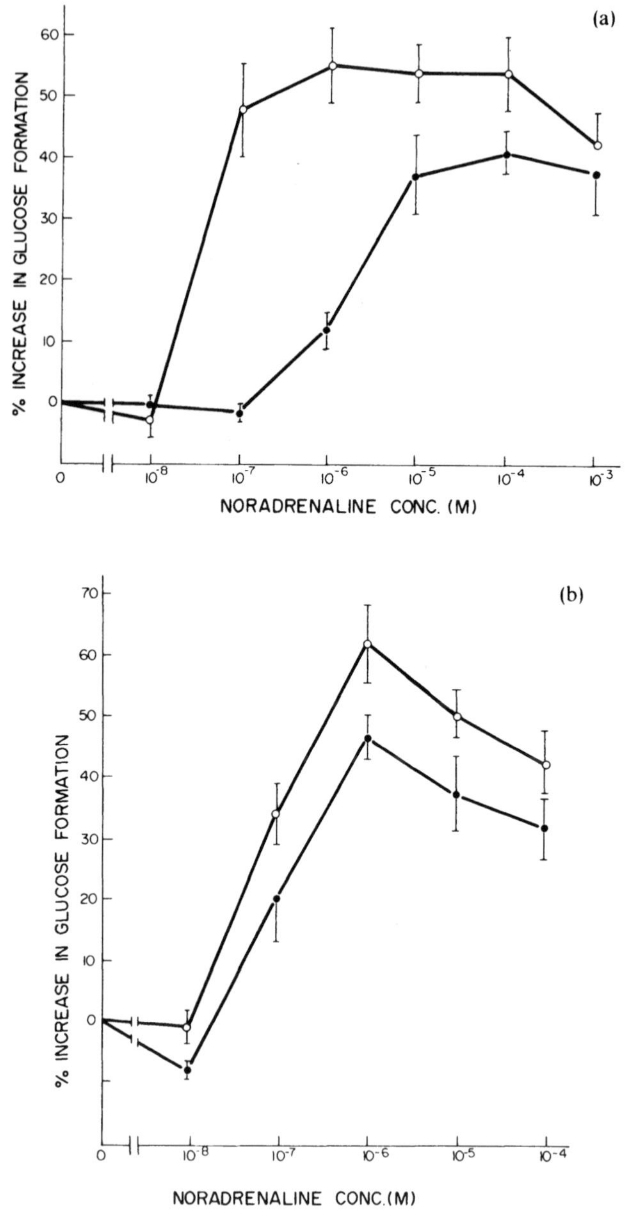

Fig. 1. Effect of selective α-receptor antagonists on noradrenaline stimulation of gluconeogenesis. Tubule fragments were prepared and incubated for 1 hr with 5 mM lactate as described under Experimental Methods. The results are means ± SEM of 4 separate experiments. ○, without α-antagonists; ●, with α-antagonists which were (a) 5 μM thymoxamine and (b) 0.1 μM yohimbine.

A role for Ca^{2+} or other cations in α-adrenergic stimulation of renal gluconeogenesis

The basal rate of renal gluconeogenesis is raised by increasing the concentration of extracellular Ca^{2+} (Krebs *et al.*, 1963; Rutman *et al.*, 1965; Nagata & Rasmussen, 1970) and Ca^{2+} has been assigned the possible role of an intracellular messenger in other systems responding to α-adrenergic stimuli (Keppens *et al.*, 1977; Assimacopoulos-Jeannet *et al.*, 1977; Butcher, 1975). It is therefore reasonable to ask whether Ca^{2+} might play a second messenger role in α-adrenergic stimulation of renal gluconeogenesis. This possibility can be explored by (a) investigating the effect that omission of extracellular Ca^{2+} has on the response of the process to catecholamines (b) investigating the effect of catecholamines on $^{45}Ca^{2+}$ influx into the tissue or on isotope efflux from $^{45}Ca^{2+}$-prelabelled tissue, or (c) investigating the effect of agents found to affect Ca^{2+} movements in other systems.

Macdonald & Saggerson (1977) showed that, although the response was blunted, 1 μM adrenaline was still able to stimulate gluconeogenesis when tubule fragments were incubated without Ca^{2+} in the presence of 0.1 mM EGTA. A possible role for extracellular Ca^{2+} is further discounted by the observation that 1 μM noradrenaline has no effect at all upon

Table 1. Effect of ouabain and extracellular K^+ concentration on noradrenaline stimulation of gluconeogenesis

Experiment number	K^+ concn. (mM)	Ouabain concn. (mM)	Noradrenaline (1 μM)	Glucose formation (μmol/hr per mg DNA)	Increase in glucose formation due to noradrenaline (μmol/hr per mg DNA)
1	6	0	−	3.12 ± 0.21	1.49 ± 0.12 (47 ± 2%)
	6	0	+	4.61 ± 0.31	
	6	0.15	−	2.78 ± 0.20	0.31 ± 0.05 (11 ± 1%)
	6	0.15	+	3.09 ± 0.24	
	6	0.5	−	2.33 ± 0.21	0.14 ± 0.02 (5 ± 1%)
	6	0.5	+	2.46 ± 0.21	
2	6	0	−	2.88 ± 0.16	1.01 ± 0.06 (35 ± 2%)
	6	0	+	3.89 ± 0.20	
	0	0	−	2.71 ± 0.20	0.13 ± 0.06 (4 ± 2%)
	0	0	+	2.84 ± 0.25	

Tubule fragments were prepared and incubated with 5 mM lactate as described under Experimental Methods. The values are means ± SEM of 5 separate experiments in each case. The values in parentheses indicate the percentage increases in glucose formation due to noradrenaline.

$^{45}Ca^{2+}$ entry into incubated tubule fragments (Kessar & Saggerson, unpublished work). On the other hand, when $^{45}Ca^{2+}$-prelabelled tubule fragments are incubated with 5 mM lactate in the presence of 1.27 mM unlabelled extracellular Ca^{2+}, efflux of isotope into the extracellular medium is observed over a period of 70 min (Kessar & Saggerson, unpublished work). This efflux of isotope is significantly increased by 1 μM noradrenaline suggesting that mobilisation of an intracellular Ca^{2+} store may be stimulated. This effect of noradrenaline is abolished by thymoxamine (α_1-blocker) but not by propranolol (β-blocker). The source of the intracellular $^{45}Ca^{2+}$ mobilized by noradrenaline is unknown at present. It is noteworthy though that an α-adrenergic stimulation of intracellular Ca^{2+} mobilization is also seen in rat liver (Assimcopoulos-Jeannet *et al.*, 1977; Blackmore *et al.*, 1978) and this is at least in part, from the mitochondria (Blackmore *et al.*, 1979a).

Experiments with calcium blocking agents have been rather unrewarding in the rat renal tubule system. La^{3+}, Ni^{2+} and ruthenium red have been tested over a range of concentrations and found to have little or no effect upon basal gluconeogenesis at 1.27 mM extracellular Ca^{2+} with 5 mm lactate as substrate. Furthermore, these agents did not interfere with noradrenaline stimulation of gluconeogenesis (Carpenter & Saggerson, unpublished work). D-600 (the methoxy derivative of verapamil) was found to decrease basal gluconeogenesis at concentrations in the range 10–100 μM. This drug also decreased the stimulatory effect of noradrenaline on gluconeogenesis, but this antagonism could be overcome by increasing the concentration of noradrenaline. It is likely that D-600 is acting as an α-receptor blocker in a manner similar to that demonstrated for verapamil by Blackmore *et al.* (1979b) in rat liver.

α-adrenergic action in some systems is associated with changes in K^+ flux (Bülbring & Tomita, 1969; Haylett & Jenkinson, 1972; Perry & Hales, 1970). Furthermore, movement of Ca^{2+} across biological membranes in exchange for Na^+ is now a well documented phenomenon in various tissues (Baker *et al.*, 1969; Blaustein, 1974; Crompton *et al.*, 1978) including the proximal tubule of kidney (Gmaj *et al.*, 1979). The effect of ouabain and of extracellular K^+ removal on noradrenaline stimulation of gluconeogenesis was therefore tested. Table 1 shows that ouabain greatly diminished the noradrenaline effect whilst only causing a small decrease in basal gluconeogenesis. Removal of extracellular K^+ completely abolished the effect of noradrenaline without decreasing basal gluconeogenesis. It is presumed that both ouabain and K^+ removal would lead to a rise in the intracellular Na^+ concentration. It is suggested either that noradrenaline action involves a redistribution of Na^+ and/or K^+, perhaps through regulation of the Na^+/K^+ ATPase activity, or that the movement of some messenger, perhaps Ca^{2+}, is dependent upon "normal" cellular distributions of Na^+ and K^+. Although both ouabain and K^+ removal have previously been shown to diminish β-adrenergic stimulation of rat adipocyte lipolysis (Ho *et al.*, 1967) and to block β-adrenergic effects on contractility and K^+ flux in smooth muscle (Scheid *et al.*, 1979), we are unaware of any previous reports of these treatments affecting α-adrenergic responses.

CONCLUSION

Catecholamines appear to stimulate renal gluconeogenesis through an α_1-type of adrenoceptor. The intracellular messenger(s) involved are unclear at present although it is possible that intracellular Ca^{2+} is mobilised from some store. In addition, Na^+ and/or K^+ movements may also be involved.

REFERENCES

Assimacopoulos-Jeannet F. D., Blackmore P. F. & Exton J. H. (1977) Studies on the α-adrenergic activation of hepatic glucose output. *J. biol. Chem.* **252**, 2662–2669.

BAKER P. F., BLAUSTEIN M. P., HODGKIN A. L. & STEINHARDT R. A. (1969) The influence of calcium on sodium efflux in squid axons. *J. Physiol.*, Lond. **200,** 431–458.

BERTHELSEN S. & PETTINGER W. A. (1977) A functional basis for classification of α-adrenergic receptors. *Life Sci.* **21,** 595–606.

BLACKMORE P. F., BRUMLEY F. T., MARKS J. L. & EXTON J. H. (1978) Studies on α-adrenergic activation of hepatic glucose output. *J. biol. Chem.* **253,** 4851–4858.

BLACKMORE P. F., DEHAYE J. P., STRICKLAND W. G. & EXTON J. H. (1979a) α-adrenergic mobilization of hepatic mitochondrial calcium. *FEBS lett.* **100,** 177–120.

BLACKMORE P. F., EL-REFAI M. F. & EXTON J. H. (1979b) α-adrenergic blockade and inhibition of A23187 mediated Ca^{2+} uptake by the calcium antagonist verapamil in rat liver cells. *Mol. Pharmac.* **15,** 598–606.

BLAUSTEIN M. P. (1974) The interrelationship between sodium and calcium fluxes across cell membranes. *Rev. Physiol. Biochem. Pharmac.* **70,** 33–82.

BÜLBRING E. & TOMITA T. (1969) Suppression of spontaneous spike generation by catecholamines in the smooth muscle of the guinea-pig taenia coli. *Proc. R. Soc. B* **172,** 103–119.

BUTCHER F. R. (1975) The role of calcium and cyclic nucleotides in α-amylase release from slices of rat parotid: studies with the divalent cation ionophore A-23187. *Metab. Clin. Exp.* **24,** 409–418.

CROMPTON M., MOSER R., LÜDI H. & CARAFOLI E. (1978) The interrelationships between the transport of sodium and calcium in mitochondria of various mammalian tissues. *Eur. J. Biochem.* **82,** 25–31.

DOXEY J. C., SMITH C. F. C. & WALKER J. M. (1977) Selectivity of blocking agents for pre- and postsynaptic α-adrenoceptors *Br. J. Pharmac.* **60,** 91–96.

DREW G. M. (1976) Effects of α-adrenoceptor agonists and antagonists on pre- and postsynaptically located α-adrenoceptors. *Eur. J. Pharmac.* **36,** 313–320.

DREW G. M. (1977) Pharmacological characterisation of the presynaptic α-adrenoceptor in the rat vas deferens. *Eur. J. Pharmacol.* **42,** 123–130.

DREW G. M. (1978) Pharmacological characterisation of the presynaptic α-adrenoceptors regulating cholinergic activity in the guinea-pig ileum. *Br. J. Pharmac.* **64,** 293–300.

FRIEDRICKS D. & SCHONER W. (1973) Stimulation of renal gluconeogenesis by inhibition of the sodium pump. *Biochim. biophys. Acta* **304,** 142–160.

GMAJ P., MURER H. & KINNE R. (1979) Calcium ion transport across plasma membranes isolated from rat kidney cortex. *Biochem. J.* **178,** 549–557.

GUDER W. G. (1979) Stimulation of renal gluconeogenesis by angiotensin II. *Biochim. biophys. Acta* **584,** 507–519.

GUDER W. G. & RUPPRECHT A. (1975) Metabolism of isolated kidney tubules. Independent actions of catecholamines on renal cyclic adenosine 3':5'-monophosphate levels and gluconeogenesis. *Eur. J. Biochem.* **52,** 283–290.

HAYLETT D. G. & JENKINSON D. H. (1972) The receptors concerned in the actions of catecholamines on glucose release, membrane potential and ion movements in guinea-pig liver. *J. Physiol.*, Lond. **225,** 751–772.

HO R. J., JEANRENAUD B., POSTERNAK T. & RENOLD A. E. (1967) Insulin-like action of ouabain II. Primary antilipolytic effect through inhibition of adenyl cyclase. *Biochim. biophys. Acta* **144,** 74–82.

HOFFMAN B. B., DE LEAN A., WOOD C. L., SCHOCKEN D. D. & LEFKOWITZ R. J. (1979) Alpha-adrenergic receptor subtypes: Quantitative assessment by ligand binding.

JARROTT, B., LOUIS W. J. & SUMMERS R. J. (1979) The characteristics of [^{3}H]-clonidine binding to an α-adrenoceptor in membranes from guinea-pig kidney. *Br. J. Pharmac.* **65,** 663–670.

KAFKA M. S., TALLMAN J. F. & SMITH C. C. & COSTA J. L. (1977) α-adrenergic receptors on human platelets. *Life Sci.* **21,** 1429–1438.

KAPPENS S., VANDENHEEDE J. R. & DE WULF H. (1977) On the role of calcium as second messenger in liver for the hormonally induced activation of glycogen phosphorylase. *Biochim. biophys. Acta* **496,** 448–457.

KLAHR S., NAWAR T. & SCHOOLWERTH A. C. (1973) Effects of catecholamines on ammoniagenesis and gluconeogenesis by renal cortex *in vitro*. *Biochim. biophys. Acta.* **304,** 161–168.

KREBS H. A., BENNETT D. A. H., GASQUET P. DE, GASCOYNE T. & YOSHIDA T. (1963) Renal gluconeogenesis. The effect of diet on the gluconeogenic capacity of rat-kidney-cortex slices. *Biochem. J.* **86,** 22–27.

KUROKAWA K. & MASSRY S. G. (1973) Evidence for stimulation of renal gluconeogenesis by catecholamines. *J. clin. Invest.* **52,** 961–964.

LANGER S. Z. (1974) Presynaptic regulation of catecholamine release. *Biochem. Pharmac.* **23,** 1793–1800.

MACDONALD D. R. W. & SAGGERSON E. D. (1977) Hormonal control of gluconeogenesis in tubule fragments from renal cortex of fed rats. *Biochem. J.* **168,** 33–42.

NAGATA N. & RASMUSSEN H. (1970) Renal gluconeogenesis: effects of Ca^{2+} and H^{+}. *Biochim. biophys. Acta.* **215,** 1–16.

PETTINGER W. A., KEETON T. K., CAMPBELL W. B. & HARPER D. C. (1976) Evidence for a renal α-adrenergic receptor inhibiting renin release. *Circulation Res.* **38,** 338–346.

PERRY M. C. & HALES C. N. (1970) Factors affecting the permeability of isolated fat-cells from the rat to [^{42}K] potassium and [^{36}Cl] chloride ions. *Biochem. J.* **117,** 615–621.

ROOBOL A. & ALLEYNE G. A. D. (1973) Regulation of renal gluconeogenesis by calcium ions, hormones and adenosine 3':5'-cyclic monophosphate. *Biochem. J.* **134,** 157–165.

RUTMAN J. Z., MELTZER L. E., KITCHELL J. R., RUTMAN R. J. & GEORGE P. (1965) Effect of metal ions on *in vitro* gluconeogenesis in rat kidney cortex slices. *Am. J. Physiol.* **208,** 841–846.

SCHEID C. R., HONEYMAN T. W. & FAY F. S. (1979) Mechanism of β-adrenergic relaxation of smooth muscle. *Nature*, Lond. **277,** 32–36.

STARKE K., MONTEL W., GAYK W. & MERKER R. (1974) Comparison of the effects of clonidine on pre- and postsynaptic adrenoceptors in the rabbit pulmonary artery. *Naunyn-Schmiedeberg's Arch. Pharmac.* **285,** 133–150.

STARKE K., BOROWSKI E. & ENDO T. (1975) Preferential blockade of presynaptic α-adrenoceptors by Yohimbine *Eur. J. Pharmac.* **34,** 385–388.

WOOD C. L., ARNETT C. D., CLARKE W. R., TSAI B. S. & LEFKOWITZ R. L. (1979) Subclassification of alpha-adrenergic receptors by direct binding studies. *Biochem. Pharmac.* **28,** 1277–1282.

SYMPOSIUM DISCUSSION

Vinay: Two questions! First have you looked at the efflux of calcium with verapamil? With Dr Pat Lund in Oxford, we looked at the adenosine effect on glucose formation in tubules from fasted rats (the results are not published) and found no effect. If that is so is there a difference between your findings in fed and fasted rats?

Saggerson: We have not looked at Ca^{2+} efflux with verapamil, and we must obviously try fasted rats. We used lactate, 5 mM, for one hour in these studies.

Alleyne: We looked at an effect of adrenaline in the presence of zero calcium and could see no stimulation of glucose formation.

Saggerson: That is in slices. We found a stimulation even at zero calcium in tubules (Macdonald & Saggerson, 1977. *Biochem. J.* **168,** 33 42).

De Pont: In another tissue viz. the exocrine pancreas, there also exists the problem whether calcium, which plays a role in stimulus–secretion coupling, comes from outside or inside the acinar cell. For a brief initial stimulation of enzyme secretion no extracellular calcium is necessary. However, for continuation of the enzyme secretion calcium from an extracellular source becomes essential. Perhaps the latter process is what you see during your one-hour incubation period; your results might have been different had a much shorter time period been used.

Saggerson: Exton (Blackmore *et al. Mol. Pharmac.* **15,** 598–606, 1979) has looked at fluxes of calcium with D600 (in liver) and does not see anything.

Williamson: In the presence of ouabain, can you get a cAMP stimulation? That would be rather important, wouldn't it?

Saggerson: I haven't looked yet!

Jorgensen: You showed that ouabain prevented the adrenergic stimulation of glucose synthesis. Is this due to the block of Na-K-ATPase or secondary to a loss of potassium from the cell?

Saggerson: I don't know, but as I showed, if you omit K^+ from the medium, you do not affect basal glucose formation, but you completely abolish the noradrenaline stimulation.

Lemieux: Have you looked at the effect of the blockers using other substrates such L-glutamine and glutamate, the metabolism of which was found to be stimulated by isoproterenol? (See Klahr *et al. Biochim. biophys Acta* **304,** 161, 1973).

Saggerson: We have only looked at lactate with the blockers.

Guder: We have done the potassium-dependence experiment. Over the range 0–20 mM, basal glucose formation from lactate or pyruvate is unchanged. If you add noradrenaline, there is no effect up to 2 mM potassium and thereafter the effect increases with increasing potassium.

Tannen: The result with glutamine as substrate is different. With higher potassium concentrations the rate of glucose formation continues to rise.

Guder: We consider that the mechanism of action of ouabain is that blocking ATPase spares ATP, which blocks pyruvate dehydrogenase, liberating substrate for gluconeogenesis. The concentration of ouabain is critical between 0.1 and 1 mM, and, in addition, the source of ouabain appears to be important. We used that from Merck.

Int. J. Biochem., Vol. 12, pp. 113 to 117
© Pergamon Press Ltd 1980. Printed in Great Britain

0020-711X/80/0701-0113S02.00/0

INTRODUCTION

SPECIAL PROPERTIES OF KIDNEY MITOCHONDRIA

MICHAEL W. WEINER
Stanford University Medical Services, Veterans Administration Medical Center, Department of Medicine, 3801 Miranda Avenue (111X), Palo Alto, CA 94304, U.S.A.

The major function of the kidney is filtration of the blood with the subsequent recovery of more than 99% of the filtered water, salt and other solutes by active transport. The reabsorption of the glomerular filtrate requires energy and it is generally accepted that the vast majority of ATP generated within kidney cells is produced by oxidative metabolism in the mitochondria. The very high rate of oxygen consumption by kidney tissue (Cohen & Barac-Nieto, 1973) emphasizes the role of mitochondria.

Before discussing the specific properties of kidney mitochondria, the general properties of mitochondria are briefly listed in Table 1. Although the structural appearance of mitochondria may vary from tissue to tissue, all mitochondria have a double membrane structure. The major function of mitochondria is the production of ATP to be used for a wide variety of biological work functions. Therefore, all mitochondria contain the enzymes of the Krebs cycle, the components of the electron transport chain, the ATP synthetase and the ATP translocase. Finally, mitochondria are capable of transporting a variety of ions: substrate anions are carried into the mitochondria for oxidation by the Krebs cycle, while other substrates are carried out of the mitochondria for gluconeogenesis or other purposes. Therefore, because of mitochondrial substrate transport, there is compartmentation of substrate concentrations within the cell (Klingenberg & Hafen, 1963; Williamson *et al.*, 1970; Greenbaum *et al.* 1971).

Several investigators have previously used different methods to estimate intracellular compartmentation of substrates in liver tissue. The paper by Guder & Pürschel extends this approach to kidney. If this technique is shown to be valid, it will be extremely useful in the investigation of a number of important questions concerning the regulation of renal ammoniagenesis, gluconeogenesis and other processes.

Table 1. General properties of mitochondria

1. Double membrane structure
2. Krebs cycle enzymes
3. Electron transport chain
4. ATP synthesis
5. Ion transport
Substrates
Other ions

Table 2. Special properties of kidney mitochondria

1. Localization near basal-lateral membrane of proximal tubule and thick ascending limb of Henle.
2. Role in ammonium production:
Glutaminase
Glutamine
3. 25-hydroxy cholecalciferol hydroxylase
4. Role in ion transport:
Effects of Na^+
Control of intracellular Ca^{2+}
5. Relatively low respiratory control ratios

Mitochondria also transport inorganic ions such as sodium, potassium, calcium, magnesium and phosphate (Christensen, 1975). The driving force for these transport activities is derived from the membrane potential and pH gradient generated by the electron transport chain (Mitchell, 1966).

Kidney mitochondria have several unique characteristics which are related to specific organ functions (Table 2). In keeping with their major role to produce ATP, kidney mitochondria are localized along the basal lateral membranes of the proximal tubule and thick ascending limb of Henle (Rhodin, 1958). Presumably, the mitochondria are here to produce ATP near its site of utilization by the Na-K-ATPase as it extrudes sodium from the cell (Fig. 1).

It has been known for over 20 yr that renal phosphate dependent glutaminase is an intramitochondrial enzyme, yet only within the last few years has attention been focused on the role of mitochondrial substrate transport in the regulation of renal ammoniagenesis. Several of this session's papers are specifically devoted to the effects of metabolic acidosis on mitochondrial substrate transport.

Although Vitamin D metabolism is not a subject for this symposium, one important and unique property of kidney mitochondria is the production of 1,25-dihydroxycholecalciferol (Gray, *et al.*, 1972).

My own interest in kidney mitochondria has concerned their role in the control of renal transepithelial ion transport. Large quantities of sodium must traverse the renal cell; thus we investigated the effects of sodium on kidney mitochondria. The experiments showed that kidney mitochondria are especially sensi-

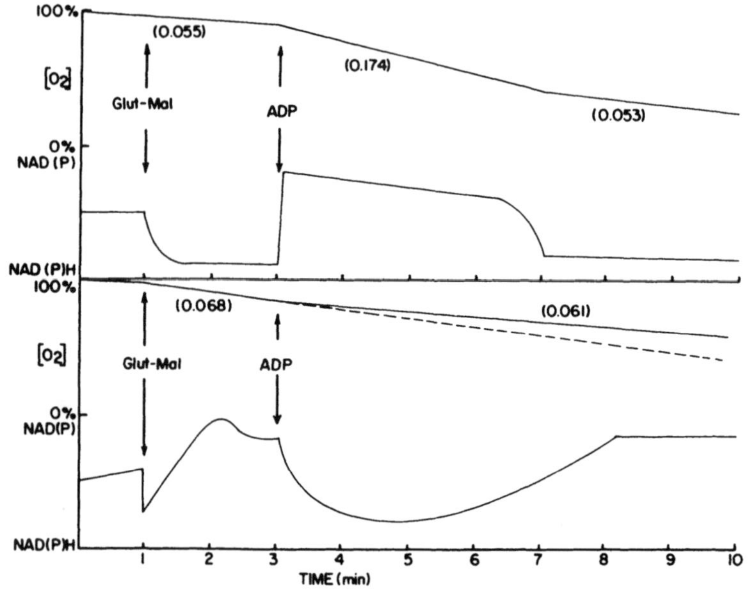

Fig. 2. Effects of ADP on respiration and pyridine nucleotides. Experiments were performed with 1.0 mg of mitochondrial protein, total volume 3.0 ml, 25°C, pH 7.4. Wave length settings of dual wave length spectrophotometer were 340/374. Full scale (set at 5%) equivalent to a Δ[NAD(P)H] of 10.5 nmols. Slit = 3.3 nm. Bracketed numbers refer to respiratory rate (microgram atoms of oxygen $min^{-1} \cdot mg^{-1}$ of protein). Top, incubation medium optimum for oxidative phosphorylation: 0.15 M KCl, 10 mM triethanolamine chloride, 5 mM triethanolamine P_i, 0.25 mM EDTA, 3 mM $MgCl_2$, pH 7.4. Bottom, NaCl–EDTA medium optimum for reverse acceptor control: 0.15 M NaCl, 10 mM triethanolamine chloride, 5 mM triethanolamine P_i, 2.5 mM EDTA, pH 7.4. GlutMal, glutamate–malate (Weiner & Lardy, 1973).

tive to the presence of sodium: when mitochondria from kidney were incubated in sodium-containing solutions, the addition of ADP caused a reduction, rather than an oxidation of NAD(P)H (Weiner & Lardy, 1973) (Fig. 2); this is termed "reverse acceptor control". Liver mitochondria never exhibited this phenomenon. The presence of physiological concentrations of sodium also induces mitochondrial ATPase activity (Weiner, 1975) (Fig. 3). Again, kidney mitochondria are more sensitive to this effect of sodium than are mitochondria obtained from liver (Weiner, 1975). Furthermore, Table 3 shows that kidney mitochondria are uncoupled by the presence of sodium, and that this is reversed by the presence of bovine serum albumin. Liver mitochondria are less sensitive to this effect of sodium.

Recently, the role of kidney mitochondria in the control of intracellular Ca^{2+} concentrations has

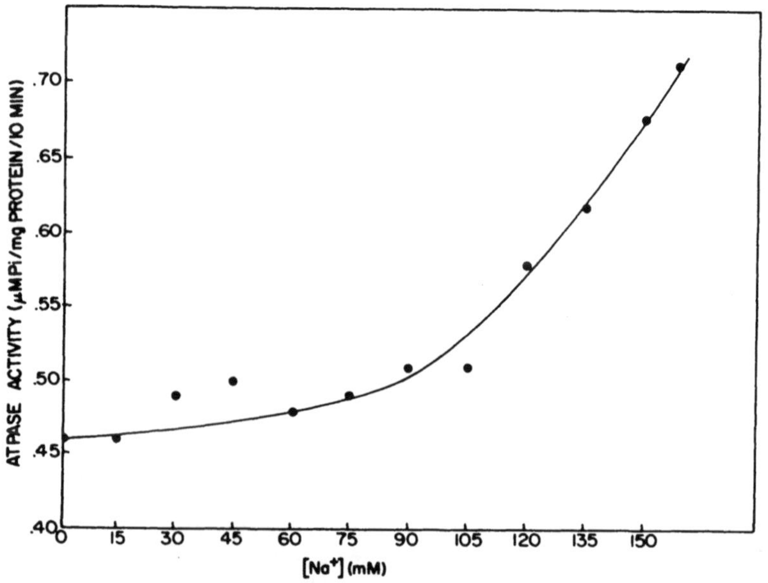

Fig. 3. Effects of sodium concentration on ATPase activity of kidney mitochondria. KCl was added to each tube so that final sodium plus potassium concentration always equaled 150 mM. Incubation media also contained 6 mM ATP, 10 mM triethanolamine Cl, pH 7.4.

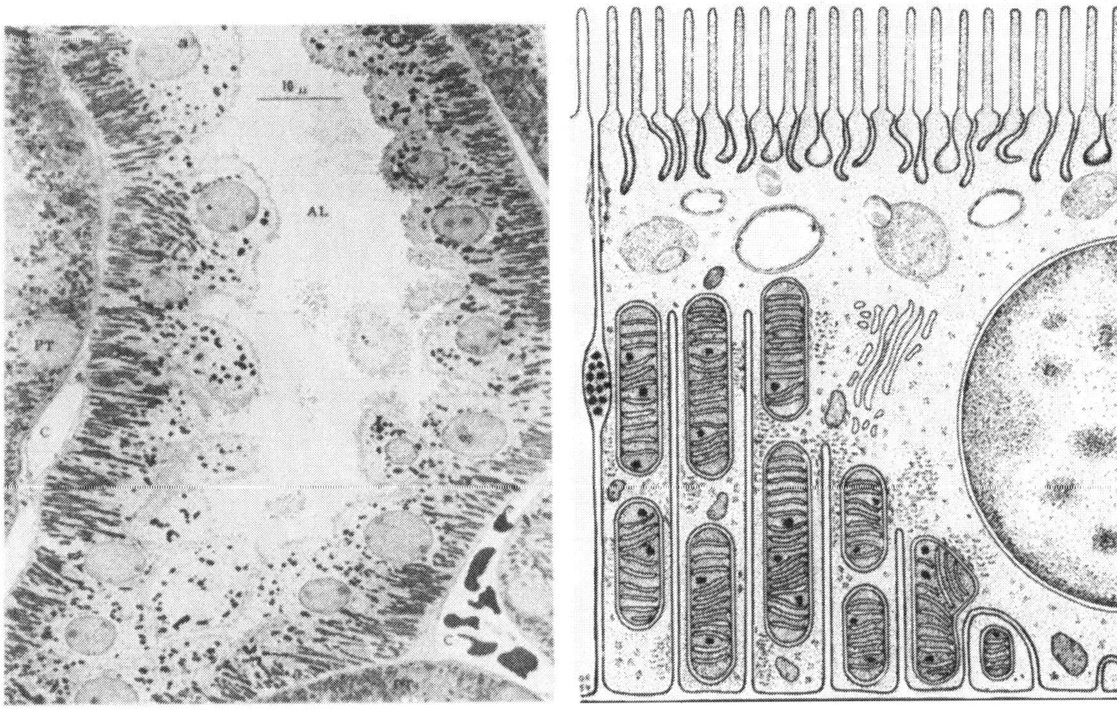

Fig. 1. Left: Low power electron micrograph (× 1250) of a longitudinally sectioned ascending thick limb of Henle's loop. The basal half of the cell is packed with long rod-shaped mitochondria (Rhodin, 1971). Right: Diagramatic representation of a proximal tubular cell with mitochondria lined up within the basal–lateral infoldings (Rhodin, 1958).

Table 3. Oxidative phosphorylation by isolated kidney mitochondria

Incubation medium	State 3*	State 4*	ADP/O†	Respiratory‡ control ratio
KCl (0.15 M)	0.089	0.036	3.5	2.5
NaCl (0.15 M)	0.059	0.053	1.8	2.1
NaCl + BSA	0.082	0.034	3.2	2.4

All media contain: 1.5 mM malate, 1.5 mM glutamate, 5 mM phosphate, 15 mM TeaCl, 3 mM Mg^{2+}, 1 mM EDTA, pH 7.4.

* Respiration = μg atoms O_2. min^{-1}.mg^{-1} mitochondrial protein.

† ADP/O is equivalent to P:O.

‡ Respiratory control ratio = State 3/State 4.

become of increasing interest. Ca^{2+} has been suggested to regulate a wide variety of biological phenomena, including transepithelial sodium transport (Taylor & Windhager, 1979). The vast majority of intracellular Ca^{2+} is thought to be localized within the mitochondria (Carafoli & Crompton, 1978), and Professor Angielski's paper addresses the specific issue of Ca^{2+} efflux from kidney mitochondria. The relationship between Ca^{2+} transport and the other specific functions of kidney mitochondria such as ATP synthesis, vitamin D metabolism, and ammonia production, will surely be topics for future investigation.

Finally, a personal comment concerning investigations of the properties of kidney mitochondria. I believe that the physiological relevance of some of the experiments performed with kidney mitochondria would be greatly enhanced if appropriate controls were performed with mitochondria from other tissues. For example, a large number of papers have shown various effects of changes in acid–base homeostasis on the function of kidney mitochondria. The results of these experiments are usually interpreted within the context of the kidney's role to generate ammonia from glutamine. However, it is possible that the changes in acid–base homeostasis have similar effects on mitochondria obtained from liver or other tissues. Thus, before we associate changes in mitochondrial function with specific physiological functions of the kidney, we must establish that these phenomena are indeed specific for mitochondria obtained from the kidney.

REFERENCES

CARAFOLI E. & CROMPTON M. (1978) The regulation of intracellular calcium in mitochondria. *Ann. N.Y. Acad. Sci.* **307**, 269–284.

CHRISTENSEN H. N. (1975) *Biological Transport*, 2nd edn. Benjamin, New York.

COHEN J. J. & BARAC-NIETO M. (1973) Renal metabolism of substrate, in relation to renal function. In *Renal Physiology*, Section 8: Handbook of Physiology. Chapter 27, pp. 912–916. (Edited by ORLOFF J. & BERLINER R. W.) Am. Physiol. Soc., Washington, D.C.

GRAY R. W. *et al.* (1972) 25-hydroxycholecalciferol-1-hydroxylase. *J. biol. Chem.* **247**, 7528–7532.

GREENBAUM A. L., GUMAA K. A. & MCLEAN P. (1971) The distribution of hepatic metabolites and the control of the pathways of carbohydrate metabolism in animals of different dietary and hormonal status. *Archs Biochem. Biophys.* **143**, 617–663.

KLINGENBERG M. & HÄFEN V. (1963) Hydrogen pathway in mitochondria. Hydrogen transfer from succinate to acetoacetate. *Biochem Z.* **337**, 120–145.

MITCHELL P. (1966) *Chemiosmotic Coupling in Oxidative and Photosynthetic Phosphorylation.* Glynn Research Laboratories. Bodmin, Cornwall, England.

RHODIN J. A. G. (1958) Electron microscopy of the kidney. *Am. J. Med.* **24**, 661–665.

TAYLOR A. & WINDHAGER E. E. (1979) Possible role of cytosolic calcium and Na–Ca exchange in regulation of transepithelial sodium transport. *Am. J. Physiol.* **5**, F505–F512.

WEINER M. W. & LARDY H. A. (1973) Reduction of pyridine nucleotides by adenosinediphosphate in kidney mitochondria: Effects of sodium, magnesium and inhibitors of oxidative phosphorylation. *J. biol. Chem.* **248**, 7682–7687.

WEINER M. W. (1975) ATPase activity of kidney mitochondria stimulated by sodium. *Am. J. Physiol.* **228**, 815–820.

WILLIAMSON D. H., BROSNAN J. T. & KREBS H. A. (1970) Effects of ischaemia on metabolite concentrations in rat liver. *Biochem. J.* **117**, 91–96.

Int. J. Biochem., Vol. 12, pp. 119 to 123
Pergamon Press Ltd 1980. Printed in Great Britain

EFFECT OF UNSATURATED FATTY ACIDS AND MONOVALENT CATIONS ON CALCIUM EFFLUX FROM KIDNEY CORTEX MITOCHONDRIA

S. Angielski, I. Roman, P. Gmaj and C. Nowicka
Department of Clinical Biochemistry, Medical Academy, 80–211 Gdańsk, Poland

Abstract—1. The effect of exogenously added, or endogenously produced, unsaturated fatty acids (UFA) on the uptake and release of Ca^{2+} by rat kidney mitochondria has been studied.

2. Linolenic acid decreases the duration of Ca^{2+} steady state maintenance in mitochondria, and promotes its release.

3. The spontaneous release of Ca^{2+} observed at high temperatures is related to the activation of membrane-bound phospholipases.

4. The effect of endogenously produced, or exogenously added, UFA depends on the cationic composition of the medium, and is strongly inhibited by Na^+ and Li.

5. Evidence is also presented that the releasing effect of UFA is not linked to non-specific alterations in the permeability characteristics of the inner mitochondrial membrane.

INTRODUCTION

Recent evidence has indicated that mitochondria from a variety of tissues possess two separate pathways for transporting Ca^{2+}, one for its uptake, one for its release (Carafoli & Crompton, 1976; Puskin *et al.*, 1976). The uptake pathway has been investigated in a number of laboratories (Washington & Murphy, 1962; Lehninger *et al.*, 1967) and is now generally accepted to be driven electrophoretically by the membrane potential maintained across the inner membrane by respiration or ATP hydrolysis (Mitchell, 1966). Independent pathways of the Ca^{2+} uptake and release have been put forward recently (Harris, 1977; Caroni *et al.*, 1978). In the mitochondria from heart and from other excitable tissues a specific Na^+/Ca^{2+} antiporter was identified which might operate as a Ca^{2+} releasing mechanism (Crompton *et al.*, 1977, 1978). This antiporter is absent from kidney and liver mitochondria, where the efflux pathway still remains to be identified.

No detailed studies of Ca^{2+} release have so far been reported in kidney mitochondria. Clarification of the mechanism responsible for the balance of Ca^{2+} in kidney mitochondria would, on the other hand, be of great significance from a physiological standpoint, given the heavy traffic of Ca^{2+} normally present in kidney tubular cells. In the present paper, the effect of unsaturated fatty acids on kidney mitochondrial Ca^{2+} will be presented. In addition, it will be shown that the effect of unsaturated fatty acids may be regulated by Na^+ and Li.

MATERIALS AND METHODS

Mitochondria were prepared from the kidney cortex and liver of female Wistar rats by a conventional differential centrifugation procedure. The tissue was disrupted in a Teflon–Potter homogenizer. Before homogenization, the medullary portion of the kidneys was excised and discarded.

The homogenization medium consisted of 0.25 M sucrose, 0.01 M Tris–Cl, pH 7.4 and 0.1 mM EGTA. The mitochondrial pellets were washed three times, the last two times without EGTA.

The protein concentration of the mitochondrial preparations was estimated by a biuret procedure.

The standard incubation medium contained in a final volume 1.5 ml:0.12 M KCl or NaCl (see legends to the figures), 0.005 M Hepes–Tris, pM 7.2, 0.5 mM $MgCl_2$, 0.003 M Tris–succinate, 1 μm rotenone (ethanolic solution) and 1 mg mitochondrial protein per ml. The temperature of the reaction medium was thermostatted and the medium was stirred gently by a magnetic flea. Ca^{2+} was added to the medium as the chloride salt in the concentration specified in the legends for the figures. Fatty acids were added as ethanolic solutions, kept at 0°C until used. Other additions were (see legends to figures), fatty acid–free BSA, 0.5% and Na^+-ATP, 0.003 M.

The measurements of O_2 consumption and of Ca^{2+} and H^+ movements were carried out simultaneously in a closed vessel, fitted with a conventional Teflon-coated Clark electrode, connected to a I–31 SU recorder, a combination radiometer pM electrode (PHH 71) and a Ca Specific Phillips electrode. All reagents used were analytical grade.

RESULTS

Effects of temperature on energy-dependent uptake, retention and release of Ca^{2+} by kidney mitochondria

In the energy-linked uptake, the Ca^{2+} distribution between the mitochondria and the suspending medium reaches a steady state, which presumably is maintained by the equilibrium between the Ca^{2+} uptake and release. Figure 1 shows that the steady state of Ca^{2+} distribution and the retention of Ca^{2+} by kidney mitochondria are powerfully influenced by temperature. At 20°C practically all Ca^{2+} added (100 nmol·mg protein^{-1}) was taken up and retained until oxygen had been exhausted, i.e. for at least 8 min. As the temperature was raised, a progressively smaller proportion of the total Ca^{2+} present was taken up and, after a period of steady state maintenance which became shorter the higher the temperature, a spontaneous release of the accumulated Ca^{2+} was clearly seen. Sharp upper deflection points in Fig. 1 correspond to the exhaustion of oxygen in the suspending medium. Apparently, the inside negative membrane potential disappears during anaerobiosis, which results in a rapid and complete release of the

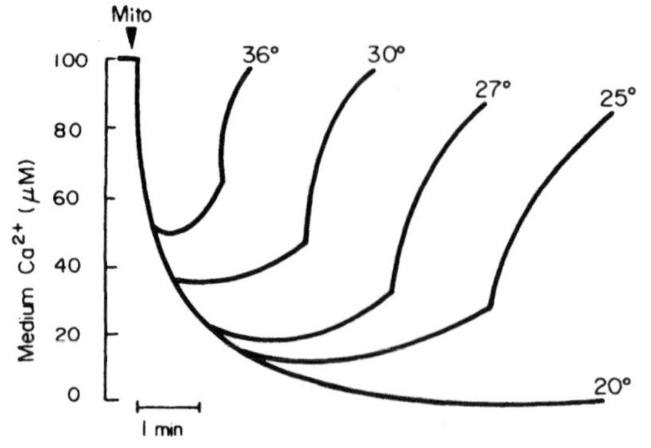

Fig. 1. Temperature dependence of the Ca^{2+} uptake and release by kidney mitochondria. Incubation medium contained: 120 mM KCl, 0.5 mM $MgCl_2$, 5 mM Hepes–Tris pH 7.2, 3 mM Tris–succinate, 1 μM rotenone and 100 μM $CaCl_2$. The Ca^{2+} uptake was started by addition of kidney mitochondria 1 mg/ml.

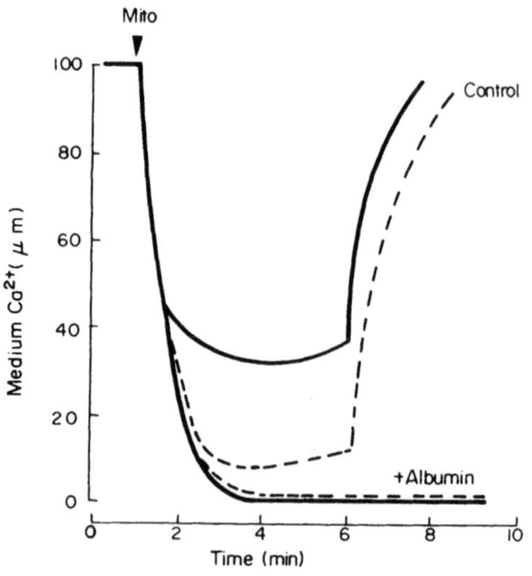

Fig. 2. Effects of Na^+ ions and albumin on the Ca^{2+} uptake and release by kidney mitochondria. Experimental conditions as in Fig. 1. (---) KCl medium, (---) NaCl 120 mM was substituted for KCl in the medium. Albumin concentration 5 mg · ml^{-1}. Incubation temperature 30°C.

accumulated Ca^{2+}. The initial rate of the Ca^{2+} uptake, on the other hand, was much less dependent on temperature than the Ca^{2+} release. This might suggest that the Ca^{2+} uptake and efflux are catalysed by systems with different temperature dependence. The temperature-dependent Ca^{2+} release from liver mitochondria, albeit observable, was much less pronounced than that from kidney mitochondria. This discrepancy will be discussed later on.

Effects of sodium and bovine serum albumin

Figure 2 shows that the usual, spontaneous Ca^{2+} release from kidney mitochondria incubated at 30°C can be abolished if K^+ is substituted for Na^+ as the main cation in the medium. In NaCl medium, the amount of Ca^{2+} taken up was considerably greater, the period of the steady state retention having been prolonged, and the efflux phase much less pronounced. When bovine serum albumin (essentially fatty acid free) was added to the medium, the spontaneous Ca^{2+} release disappeared completely: the mitochondria took up all the Ca^{2+} added and retained it until oxygen had been exhausted. In the presence of bovine serum albumin, Na^+ ions had no effect on both Ca^{2+} uptake and release. These experiments allowed for the following conclusions: (i) the spontaneous temperature-dependent Ca^{2+} release from kidney mitochondria depends on the presence of some factor removable by bovine serum albumin, probably fatty acids and (ii) Na^+ ions inhibit the fatty acid-dependent Ca^{2+} efflux, but have no effect on the Ca^{2+} uptake, having been ineffective in the presence of bovine serum albumin. Therefore, in further experiments the effects of exogenous fatty acids and Na^+ ions on the Ca^{2+} release were investigated in more detail.

Effects of exogenous linolenic acid and sodium ions on Ca^{2+} efflux from kidney and liver mitochondria

In Fig. 3 the effects of exogenous linolenic acid on the Ca^{2+} release from liver and kidney mitochondria are shown. The experiments were performed at 25°C to avoid a large spontaneous Ca^{2+} release. Linolenate, as added after the Ca^{2+} uptake had been completed, evoked an immediate, graded Ca^{2+} release from both liver (panel A) and (panel B) kidney mitochondria. A few minutes after linolenate had been added, a new steady state was established at a much lower Ca^{2+} accumulation level. Upon exhaustion of oxygen from the medium, the residual mitochondrial Ca^{2+} was immediately and completely released. In both liver and kidney mitochondria, the Ca^{2+} efflux induced by linolenate was inhibited by Na^+ ions. Thus, the addition of linolenate at 25°C closely mimicked the spontaneous Ca^{2+} release observed in kidney mitochondria at higher temperatures (compare Figs 2 and 3). In liver, as compared to kidney mitochondria, the concentration of linolenate necessary to evoke Ca^{2+} release was approximately twice as high. A lower sensitivity to exogenous linolenate and a lower spontaneous Ca^{2+} release suggest that the endogenous fatty acid level in liver mitochondria is low. In kidney mitochondria, on the other hand, the effects of endogenous and exogenous fatty acids may sum up producing a higher rate of the Ca^{2+} efflux.

The bottom panels of Fig. 3 show that mitochondrial respiration is activated upon an addition of linolenate. This is the well known uncoupling activity of unsaturated fatty acid. However, the stimulation of respiration is identical in both NaCl and KCl media. Thus, the Ca^{2+} release induced by linolenate cannot be attributed solely to its uncoupling activity and to the collapse of the membrane potential: an inhibition of the Ca^{2+} efflux by Na^+ indicates a specific effect of linolenate on the Ca^{2+} transport. This conclusion had been substantiated by the experiment shown in Fig. 4. The Ca^{2+} efflux from kidney mitochondria, induced by a classical uncoupler CCCP, was not influenced by Na^+ ions. In the latter case, the Ca^{2+} release might indeed result directly from the collapse of the membrane potential.

Effects of linolenate in the presence of ATP and P_i

The effects of linolenate on the Ca^{2+} efflux from kidney and liver mitochondria were further investi-

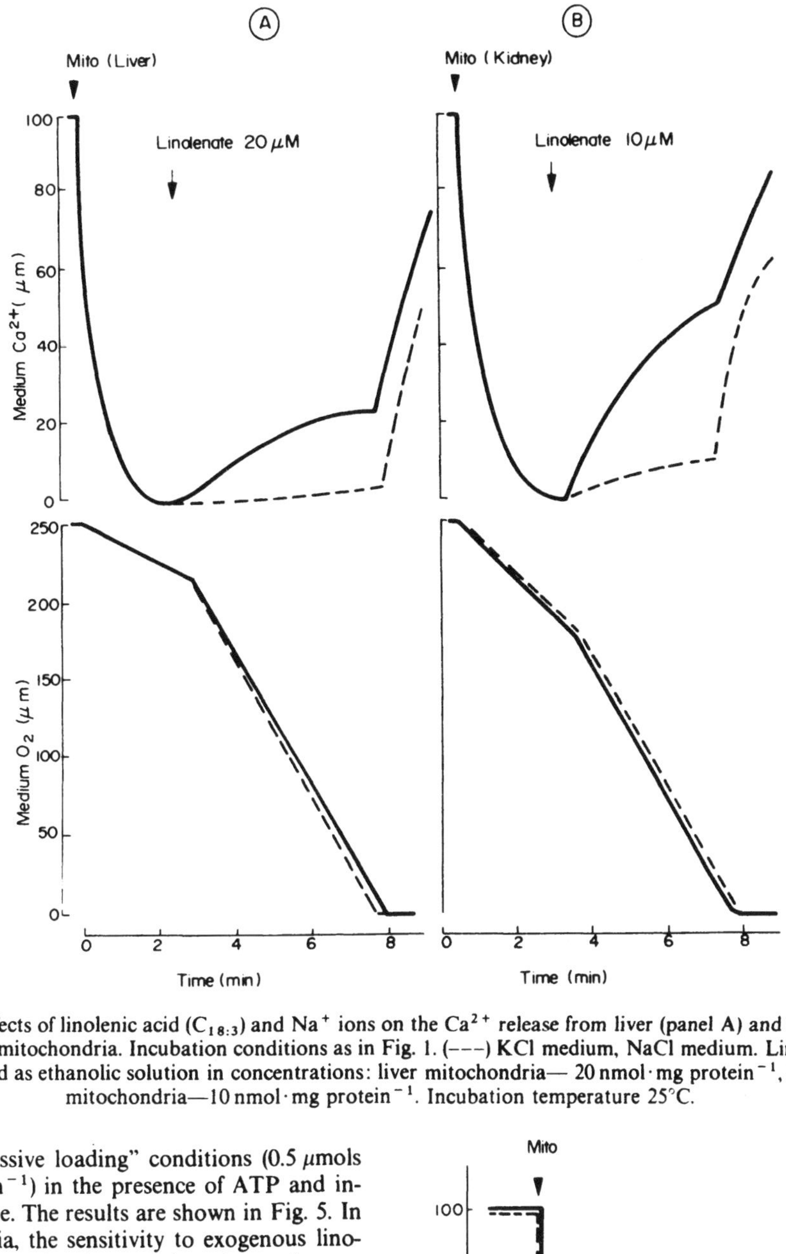

Fig. 3. Effects of linolenic acid ($C_{18:3}$) and Na^+ ions on the Ca^{2+} release from liver (panel A) and kidney (panel B) mitochondria. Incubation conditions as in Fig. 1. (---) KCl medium, NaCl medium. Linolenic acid added as ethanolic solution in concentrations: liver mitochondria— 20 nmol·mg protein^{-1}, kidney mitochondria—10 nmol·mg protein^{-1}. Incubation temperature 25°C.

gated under "massive loading" conditions (0.5 μmols Ca^{2+}·mg protein^{-1}) in the presence of ATP and inorganic phosphate. The results are shown in Fig. 5. In liver mitochondria, the sensitivity to exogenous linolenate was considerably increased under such conditions. 4 nmols linolenate·mg protein^{-1} proved enough to produce an almost complete release of the accumulated Ca^{2+} in KCl medium (as compared to 20 nmols in Fig. 3). This increased sensitivity to linolenate could be related to the increased Ca^{2+} load, rather than to the presence of ATP or P_i, since it was drastically decreased upon lowering of the Ca^{2+} load to 0.1 nmols·mg protein^{-1} (not shown). As in previous experiments, sodium ions strongly inhibited the linolenate-induced Ca^{2+} efflux. In kidney mitochondria, on the contrary, the sensitivity to exogenous linolenate was decreased in the presence of ATP, and higher linolenate concentrations were necessary to induce Ca^{2+} release than those under limited loading conditions. The interpretation of these results are not quite clear yet, but they suggest that the rate of the linolenate-induced Ca^{2+} efflux from liver mitochondria depends on the amount of Ca^{2+} accumulated in the mitochondrial matrix: when it is increased, the

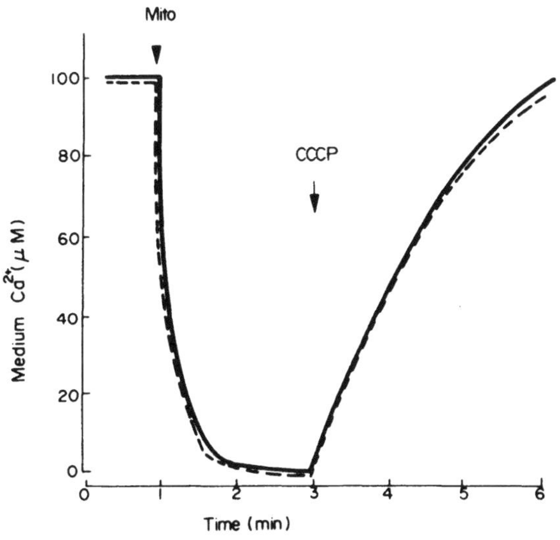

Fig. 4. Effects of Na^+ ions on CCCP-induced Ca^{2+} release from kidney mitochondria. Incubation conditions as in Fig. 1. (---) KCl medium, NaCl medium. CCCP 0.5 nmols·mg protein^{-1} added at arrow. Incubation temperature 25°C.

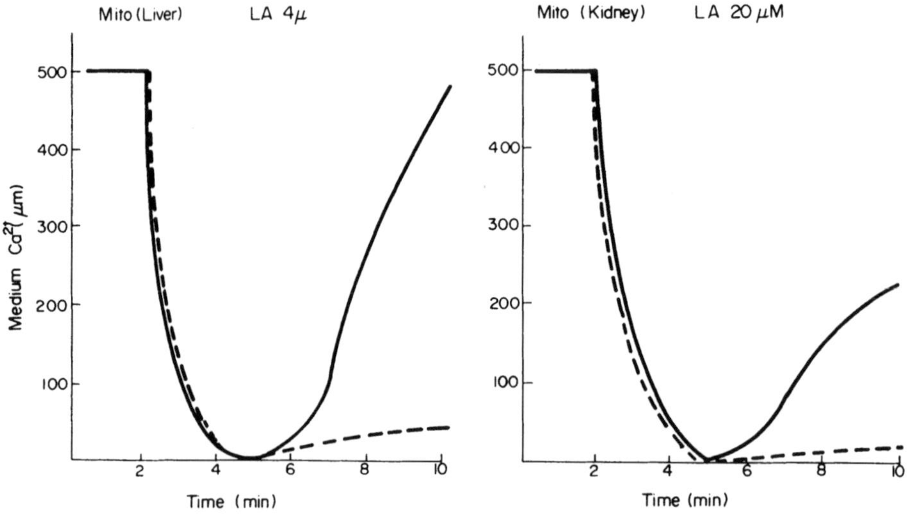

Fig. 5. Effects of linolenic acid on the Ca^{2+} release from liver (panel A) and kidney (panel B) mitochondria under "massive loading" conditions. Incubation medium contained: 120 mM KCl or NaCl, 4 mM $MgCl_2$, 5 mM Hepes–Tris pH 7.2, 3 mM ATP-Na, 4 mM P_i, 3 mM Tris–succinate, 1 mM rotenone and 1 mg·ml^{-1} mitochondrial protein linolenic acid (LA) additions: liver mitochondria—4 nmols·mg protein^{-1}, kidney mitochondria—20 nmols·mg protein^{-1} (——) KCl medium, (---) NaCl medium. Incubation temperature 25°C.

Ca^{2+} efflux rate, at a given level of linolenate, becomes increased too. In kidney mitochondria, the added linolenate may possibly be metabolised in ATP-dependent reactions. This organ specificity requires further investigations.

Effects of monovalent cations

In Fig. 6 the effects of the monovalent cations Li^+, Na^+, K^+ and Cs^+ on the linolenate-induced Ca^{2+} efflux from kidney mitochondria are shown. The fastest Ca^{2+} efflux was observed in CsCl medium, a little slower one in KCl medium. In NaCl and LiCl media the Ca^{2+} efflux was inhibited. The results suggest that the radius, either hydrated or dehydrated, of a monovalent cation may determine its effects on Ca^{2+} transport.

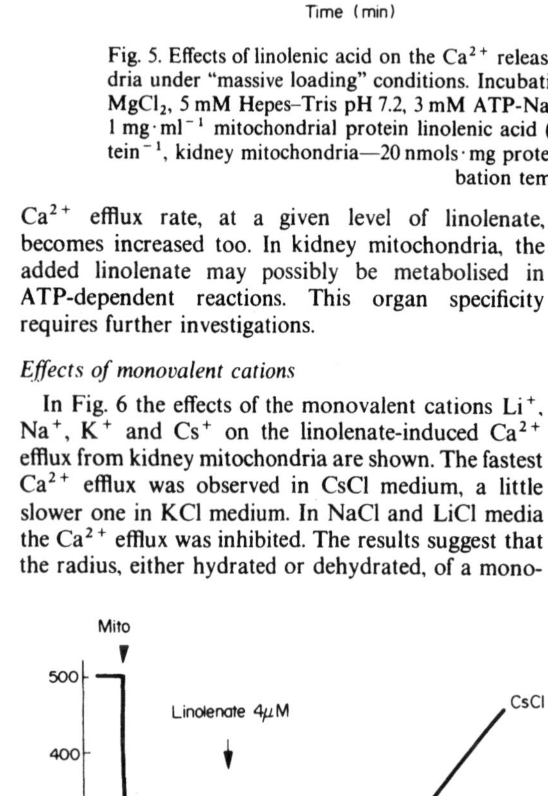

Fig. 6. Effects of monovalent cations on the Ca^{2+} release from kidney mitochondria. Incubation conditions as in Fig. 5 except that KCl was replaced with equal concentrations of CsCl, NaCl or LiCl. Incubation temperature 25°C.

DISCUSSION

The data presented here provide evidence that unsaturated fatty acids can induce the Ca^{2+} efflux from kidney and liver mitochondria by a mechanism at least partly independent of their uncoupling activity. This is indicated by the following observations: (i) the fatty acid-induced Ca^{2+} efflux is inhibited by Na^+ and Li^+ ions (ii) the fatty acid-induced uncoupling, as measured by the stimulation of oxygen uptake, is not influenced by Na^+ and (iii) Ca^{2+} efflux, induced by a classical uncoupler, CCCP, is insensitive to Na^+ (Fig. 4). These results are not easily explained by the fatty acid-induced uncoupling alone. It seems likely that in the presence of small concentrations of fatty acids the uncoupling is not complete, the increased respiration provides enough energy to fully compensate for an increased proton influx, and still the mitochondria maintain a negative potential of sufficient magnitude to drive Ca^{2+} in. Under such conditions, the mitochondria are able to reduce the medium Ca^{2+} concentration to normal low levels, if only the Ca^{2+} efflux has been inhibited by Na^+ ions (Fig. 4). The specific inhibition by Na^+ of the fatty acid-induced Ca^{2+} efflux can be observed only when relatively small concentrations of fatty acids have been used (Roman *et al.*, 1980). When higher concentrations of fatty acids were added, the uncoupling prevailed and the Ca^{2+} efflux could no longer be inhibited by Na^+. The inhibition by Na^+ of the Ca^{2+} efflux can conveniently be explained by a competition between the 2 ions for binding with fatty acids at the inner surface of the membrane, which is readily permeable to Na^+ (Douglas & Cockrell, 1974).

The observation that Na^+ ions inhibit the spontaneous Ca^{2+} efflux from freshly prepared kidney mitochondria (Fig. 2) suggest that the endogenous

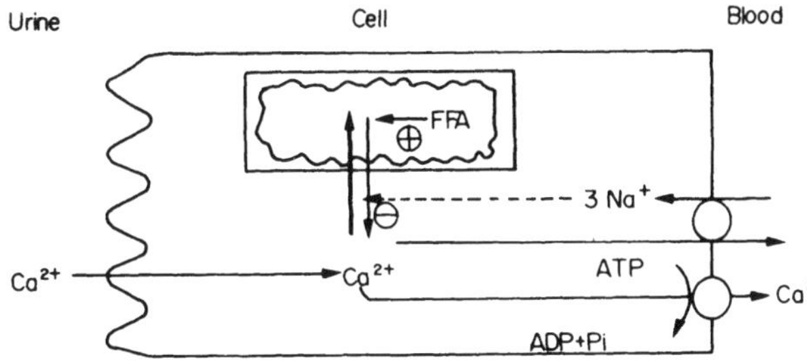

Fig. 7. Regulation of Ca^{2+} transport in kidney cells.

fatty acids may indeed catalyse the Ca^{2+} efflux *in vivo*. It is the membrane phospholipids which are the most likely source of the mitochondrial unsaturated fatty acids. Most phospholipids contain unsaturated fatty acids in position C_2 of glycerol, and the mitochondria show considerable activity of phospholipase A_2 which hydrolyzes phospholipids in the C_2 position (Vignais *et al*., 1971; Scherphof & van Deenen, 1965). The further fates of the split fatty acids, however, and the control of their level in the mitochondrial membranes, are as yet almost completely obscure.

The inhibition by sodium of the Ca^{2+} efflux from kidney mitochondria may have some physiolgical significance. In kidney cells, the extrusion of Ca^{2+} from the cell to the interstitial fluid proceeds via an Na^+/Ca^{2+} exchange mechanism and calcium ATPase (Fig. 7). The Ca^{2+} efflux from the cell is coupled to the Na^+ influx into the cell (Gmaj *et al*., 1979). The inhibition by Na^+ of mitochondrial Ca^{2+} efflux would provide a negative feedback loop between the Ca^{2+} transport in the plasma membrane and in mitochondria. This is just the opposite to the positive feedback observed in the heart (Crompton *et al*., 1977, 1978). Such a mechanism is not unreasonable, however, if we realize that the kidney cells transport large amounts of Ca^{2+} from the tubule lumen to the peritubular fluid. In this situation, the inhibition by sodium of mitochondrial Ca^{2+} efflux may be essential keep the cytosolic Ca^{2+} at low levels in face of varying loads of Ca^{2+} transported across the cell.

REFERENCES

CARAFOLI E. & CROMPTON M. (1976) Calcium ions and mitochondria. *Symp. Soc. exp. Biol.* **30**, 89–115.

CARONI P., SCHWERZMANN K. & CARAFOLI E. (1978) Separate pathways for Ca^{2+} uptake and release in liver mitochondria. *FEBS Lett.* **96**, 339–342.

CROMPTON M., KUNZI M. & CARAFOLI E. (1977) The calcium induced and sodium induced effluxes of calcium from heart mitochondria. *Eur. J. Biochem.* **79**, 549–558.

CROMPTON M., MOSER R. L., LUDI M. & CARAFOLI E. (1978) The interrelations between the transport of sodium and calcium in mitochondria of various mammalian tissues. *Eur. J. Biochem.* **82**, 25–31.

DOUGLAS M. J. & COCKRELL R. S. (1974) Mitochondrial cation–hydrogen ion exchange. *J. biol. Chem.* **249**, 5462–5471.

GMAJ P., MURER H. & KINNE R. (1979) Calcium ion transport across plasma membranes isolated from rat kidney cortex. *Biochem. J.* **178**, 549–557.

HARRIS E. J. (1977) The uptake and release of calcium by heat mitochondria. *Biochem. J.* **168**, 447 456.

LEHNINGER A. L., CARAFOLI E. & ROSSI C. S. (1967) Energy linked ion movements in mitochondrial systems. *Adv. Enzymol.* **29**, 259–320.

MITCHELL P. (1966) *Chemiosmotic Coupling in Oxidative and Photosynthetic Phosphorylation.* Glynn Research Ltd, Bodmin, England.

PUSKIN J. S., GUNTER K. K. & RUSSELL P. R. (1976) Evidence for more than one Ca^{2+} transport mechanism in mitochondria. *Biochemistry* **15**, 3834–3842.

ROMAN J., GMAJ P., NOUSKA C. & ANGIELSKI S. (1980) *Eur. J. Biochem.* Submitted for publication.

SCHERPHOF G. L. & DEENEN L. L. M. VAN (1965) Phospholipase A activity of rat liver mitochondria. *Biochim. biophys. Acta* **98**, 204–206.

VIGNAIS P. M., NACHBAUR J. & COLBEAU A. (1971) In *Membrane-bound Enzymes*. (Edited by PORCELLATI J. & JOSS F. DI) pp. 87–109. Plenum Press, New York.

WASHINGTON F. B. & MURPHY J. V. (1962) Ca^{2+} uptake by rat kidney mitochondria and its dependence on respiration and phosphorylation. *J. biol. Chem.* **237**, 2670–2672.

Int. J. Biochem., Vol. 12, pp. 125 to 129
© Pergamon Press Ltd 1980. Printed in Great Britain

0020-711X/80/0701-0125$02.00/0

CALCIUM-ACTIVATED ADENOSINE TRIPHOSPHATASE ALONG THE RABBIT NEPHRON

ADRIAN I. KATZ and ALAIN DOUCET
Department of Medicine, The University of Chicago Pritzker School of Medicine, Chicago, IL 60637, U.S.A.

Abstract—1. A low-affinity Ca-ATPase was demonstrated along the entire nephron of the rabbit kidney with a micromethod which permits measurement of enzyme activity in discrete tubule segments.

2. This enzyme appears to be present in the plasma membrane as well as in mitochondria, can also be activated by magnesium and is insensitive to sodium and ouabain.

3. Both its activity and distribution profile along the nephron are different from those of Na-K-ATPase.

INTRODUCTION

Several calcium-activated ATPases present in mammalian cells have been linked to active calcium transport by the plasma membrane and by intracellular membrane systems such as mitochondria and sarcoplasmic reticulum (Vincenzi & Hinds, 1976). In the kidney, calcium-activated ATPases have been demonstrated in cortex homogenates (Parkinson & Radde, 1971; Levin *et al.*, 1978) and microsomes or membranes thereof (Moore *et al.*, 1974; Kinne-Saffran & Kinne, 1974; Thompson & Nechay, 1979), as well as in suspensions of cortical tubules (Rorive & Kleinzeller, 1972). Kinne-Saffran & Kinne (1974) have described an ATPase activated by calcium in millimolar concentrations in basal–lateral plasma membranes prepared from rat kidney cortex, and proposed that this enzyme is derived from proximal tubule cells and is involved in active transtubular calcium transport in this segment of the nephron.

Whereas the bulk of filtered calcium is reabsorbed in the proximal tubule accessible to micropuncture, significant net calcium reabsorption also occurs along the pars recta, the thick ascending limb of Henle's loop, the distal convoluted tubule, and the early cortical collecting duct, often by mechanisms that have the characteristics of active transport. To identify the site of origin of calcium-activated ATPase (Ca-ATPase) in the cortex and to determine whether it is also present in the renal medulla, we measured the activity of this enzyme along the rabbit nephron using a micromethod which permits determination of enzyme activity in discrete tubule segments. In addition, we have used several preferential inhibitors of mitochondrial or plasma membrane ATPases to evaluate the relative contribution of the enzyme from these structures to the total Ca-ATPase measured in the intact tubule.

MATERIALS AND METHODS

Kidneys were obtained from male New Zealand rabbits (1.5–2 kg body wt) fed an *ad lib.* diet. Procedures for tubule microdissection, permeabilization and incubation for enzyme microanalysis were identical to those used for the determination of Na-K-ATPase described in detail elsewhere (Doucet *et al.*, 1979). Briefly, tubule segments 0.2–2 mm long from different regions of the nephron were dissected in the cold under stereomicroscopic observation, photographed for subsequent measurement of their length, and incubated individually in 1 μl assay medium for 15 min at 37°C. The reaction was stopped by addition of cold TCA and the enzyme activity was determined from the labeled inorganic phosphate released by the hydrolysis of [γ-^{32}P]ATP and was expressed as a function of tubule length.

Unless otherwise specified, Ca-ATPase was measured in a solution containing Tris–ATP 5 mM, Ouabain 1 mM, and Tris–HCl 50 mM, pH 7.4. In preliminary experiments maximal activity was found in the presence of 5 mM Ca^{2+} while without calcium the enzyme was undetectable, and therefore Ca-ATPase was taken as the difference between the activity measured in the presence of 5 mM Ca^{2+} and in its absence. Seven tubule segments from each region of the nephron were used for enzyme determination in each animal. In addition, five blanks incubated without tubules were used in each assay to measure the nonenzymatic hydrolysis of ATP. Results are expressed as the mean $\pm$SE of the average values measured in each animal.

In separate experiments we prepared mitochondria (10 min × 3; 15,000 ***g***) and microsomes (60 min; 105,000 ***g***) from cortex homogenates of each kidney from three rabbits. The left kidney, which was perfused for microdissection, was homogenized without deoxycholate and the right kidney with 0.2% DOC in a medium containing 0.25 M mannitol and 0.07 M sucrose. Results with and without DOC were comparable and are reported together.

RESULTS

Since microdissection of large numbers of tubules is not possible without the use of collagenase, we verified in preliminary experiments the effect of collagenase on the enzyme activity. Proximal convoluted and straight portions and medullary thick ascending limbs were dissected from one kidney perfused with collagenase (0.1%), and from its mate perfused with an identical solution from which collagenase was omitted. There was no significant difference between the Ca-ATPase measured in these regions of the nephron in the presence or in the absence of collagenase.

The enzyme was independently stimulated by either calcium or magnesium: Maximal activity was observed with 5 mM Ca^{2+} and 1–4 mM Mg^{2+}, and concentrations of either cation in excess of 5 mM were mildly inhibitory (Fig. 1). Neither Ca^{2+} nor Mg^{2+} was required for activation of the enzyme by

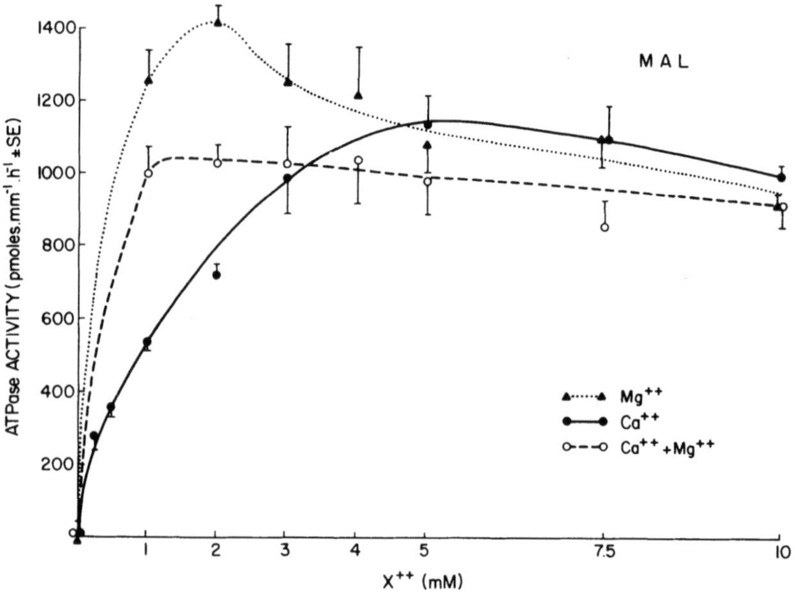

Fig. 1. Effect of Ca^{2+} and Mg^{2+} concentrations on Ca-ATPase from medullary thick ascending limbs (MAL). All MAL were dissected from the same kidney. Maximum stimulation of the enzyme was reached at 5 mM Ca^{2+} and 1–4 mM Mg^{2+} concentrations.

the other cation, and addition of either Ca^{2+} or Mg^{2+} to maximally stimulating concentration of the other cation did not further activate the ATPase. Concentrations of ATP required for maximal activity ranged between 2.5 and 7.5 mM. Sodium (20 and 50 mM) and ouabain (1 mM) had no effect on the enzyme activity.

The Ca-ATPase profile along the nephron is shown in Fig. 2. Total enzyme activity (upper panel) was higher in the distal nephron (except for the cortical

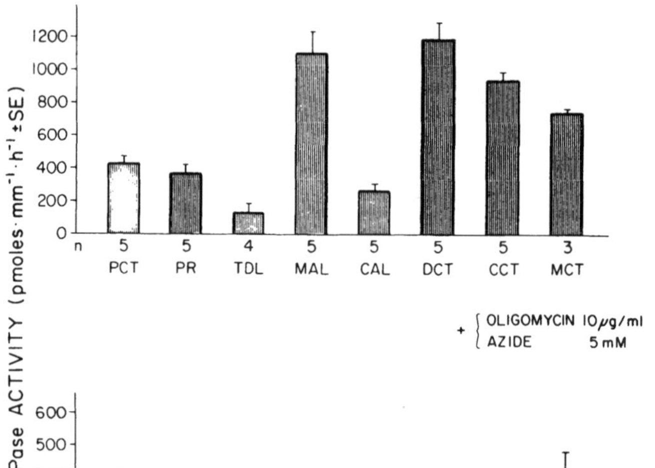

Fig. 2. Distribution of Ca-ATPase activity along the rabbit nephron. Upper panel: Total Ca-ATPase activity. Lower panel: Ca-ATPase measured in the presence of oligomycin (10 μg/ml) and azide (5 mM); under these conditions the enzyme activity contributed by mitochondria is largely inhibited. *n* represents the number of animals. PCT—proximal convoluted tubule; PR—pars recta; TDL—thin descending limb of Henle's loop; MAL—medullary thick ascending limb; CAL—cortical thick ascending limb; DCT—distal convoluted tubule; CCT—cortical collecting tubule; MCT—medullary collecting tubule.

Table 1. Effect of oligomycin and azide on Ca-ATPase from rabbit kidney cortex mitochondria and microsomes. Enzyme activity is expressed as % of control measured without the addition of inhibitors. Incubation medium was as listed for enzyme microdetermination in single tubules

	Ca-ATPase activity (μmols $P_i \cdot$ mg protein^{-1} hr^{-1}) % of control	
Addition to medium	Mitochondria	Microsomes
Oligomycin (10 μg/ml)	18.3 ± 4.1	86.8 ± 6.8
Azide (5 mM)	30.7 ± 3.9	94.0 ± 4.6

ascending limb, which in the rabbit is very thin) than in the proximal nephron. Total Ca-ATPase activity per millimeter tubule length in most nephron segments was substantially lower than that of Na-K-ATPase (averaging between one half and one sixth of the latter), except in the collecting tubule where the activity of the two enzymes was comparable.

Since the enzyme activity was measured in intact tubules, the subcellular component where it originated was not clear. Unlike Na-K-ATPase which has been convincingly located in the basolateral cell membrane, there are several calcium stimulated ATPases in mammalian cells, where besides the cell membrane they are also present in various cell organelles, notably the mitochondria. We therefore used several compounds that inhibit preferentially mitochondrial or membrane ATPase in an attempt to determine the relative contribution of Ca-ATPase from these two structures to the total activity measured in the tubule.

Oligomycin (10 μg$\cdot$ml^{-1}) and azide (5 mM) markedly inhibited mitochondrial Ca-ATPase but had little effect (mitochondrial contamination?) on the microsomal enzyme prepared from rabbit kidney cortex homogenates (Table 1). In single tubules low to moderate (0.2 and 1 μg$\cdot$ml^{-1}) concentrations of oligomycin had no effect on Ca-ATPase, but higher concentrations (5 and 10 μg$\cdot$ml^{-1}) inhibited this enzyme (Fig. 3). Since high concentrations of oligomycin can also inhibit membrane ATPase (Van Groningen & Slater, 1963), we verified their effect on Na-K-ATPase: this enzyme, measured in tubules from the same animals, was not affected by oligomycin at any of the four concentrations tested. Sodium azide, another inhibitor of mitochondrial ATPases, likewise inhibited Ca-ATPase but not the Na-K-ATPase. In contrast, vanadate completely abolished the Na-K-ATPase activity without affecting that of Ca-ATPase, and ruthenium red, reported to inhibit red cell mem-

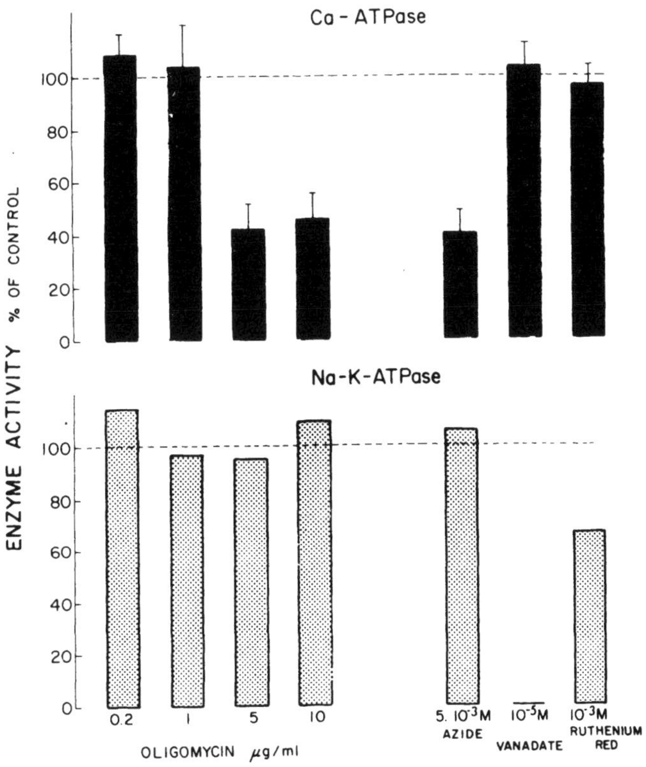

Fig. 3. Effect of ATPase inhibitors on Ca-ATPase and Na-K-ATPase of rabbit nephrons. Enzyme activity in the presence of the inhibitor is expressed as percent of the control activity measured in its absence. Percentage inhibition is the average observed in several segments of the nephron (PCT, MAL, DCT, CCT; abbreviations as in Fig. 2).

brane (Ca + Mg)ATPase (a different enzyme from that discussed here) had a moderate effect only on Na-K-ATPase (Fig. 3).

The inhibitors listed above, with the exception of vanadate, are not entirely specific and therefore it is not possible to draw firm conclusions from the experiments summarized in Fig. 3. Nevertheless, it is obvious that a substantial fraction of the total Ca-ATPase in the rabbit nephron is inhibitable by agents that act preferentially on the mitochondria. To determine the non-mitochondrial Ca-ATPase, we remeasured the activity profile of the enzyme in the presence of both oligomycin ($10\,\mu g \cdot ml^{-1}$) and azide (5 mM). Under these conditions the remaining enzyme activity, which is probably more representative of the plasma membrane Ca-ATPase, showed a different distribution pattern along the nephron: The "membrane" Ca-ATPase activity was highest in the proximal tubule (pars convoluta and pars recta) and in the collecting tubule (cortical and medullary portions) (Fig. 2, lower panel). It should be noted that this activity profile is quite different from that of Na-K-ATPase, another transport ATPase present in the plasma membrane of renal tubular cells.

DISCUSSION

In this paper we describe a renal tubular enzyme that can be activated by millimolar concentrations of either calcium or magnesium, neither of which is required for activation of the enzyme by the other cation. This enzyme is found along the entire nephron and appears to be present both in the plasma membrane and mitochondria (and possibly in other cell organelles); its activity and distribution profile along the nephron are different from those of Na-K-ATPase, the biochemical equivalent of the sodium-potassium pump found in the basal-lateral cell membrane.

A calcium-stimulated ATPase that can also be activated by magnesium has been described in rat kidney cortex homogenates (Parkinson & Radde, 1971), rabbit cortical tubules (Rorive & Kleinzeller, 1972), basal–lateral membranes from rat kidney cortex (Kinne-Saffran & Kinne, 1974) and dog kidney cortex microsomes (Thompson & Nechay, 1979), as well as red cell ghosts (Rosenthal *et al.*, 1970), brain synaptosomal vesicles (Rahamimoff & Abramovitz, 1978), and eel gills (Fenwick, 1979). In all these tissues, the approximate K_m of the enzyme and the calcium concentration required for its maximal activation were in the millimolar range, which is considerably greater than the normal intracellular Ca^{2+} concentration, thought to be no higher than 10^{-5} to 10^{-6} M (Vincenzi & Hinds, 1976). It is surprising therefore that a widespread enzyme, present in numerous organs and different species, should be activated by nonphysiologic concentrations of substrate (calcium), an anomaly which raises the question of the function of this Ca-ATPase in the cell. (While it is possible that calcium may be "compartmentalized" at the inner surface of the plasma membrane where its concentration may be higher than in the rest of the cytoplasm, the ionic activity of the calcium at the inner face of the membrane is unknown and this hypothesis is at present speculative). Kinne-Saffran & Kinne (1974) pointed out, however, that the low affinity of the enzyme for calcium is compensated by its high capacity, so that "at normal intracellular calcium concentrations the enzyme is saturated with the cation only to a very small extent".

An additional difficulty in defining the physiologic role of this Ca-ATPase is raised by the discrepancy between the rates of calcium transport and those of ATP hydrolysis catalyzed by the enzyme. Using the calcium transport rates measured in proximal tubules by Ullrich *et al.* (1976), and in the distal nephron by Rocha *et al.* (1977) and by Shareghi & Stoner (1978), we calculated that the energy requirements for such transport would be provided in ample excess by the rate of ATP hydrolysis measured in the corresponding segment of the nephron.

Moore *et al.* (1974) described by a high affinity Ca-ATPase, which requires magnesium and is activated by calcium in micromolar concentrations, similar to that found in the red cell plasma membrane and considered to be the biochemical expression of the calcium pump (Schatzmann, 1975). It is also of interest that Kinne *et al.* (1977) showed a calcium uptake system in basal–lateral plasma membrane vesicles from rat kidney cortex with an affinity constant in the micromolar range, although the Ca-ATPase of basal lateral membranes reported earlier was activated by calcium in millimolar concentrations. From the considerations discussed above it appears likely that the Ca-ATPase responsible for transmembrane calcium transport in renal tubular cells is a high affinity enzyme. Since such an ATPase appears to be of low capacity there are obvious difficulties in measuring its activity in small tissue samples such as our isolated tubule segments. Nevertheless, preliminary experiments reveal the presence of a high affinity Ca-ATPase in certain segments of the rabbit nephron, with an activity per millimeter tubule length approximately one tenth that of the low affinity Ca-ATPase described in this report.

SUMMARY

Calcium-activated ATPase was determined in the rabbit with a micromethod that permits measurement of enzyme activity in discrete segments of the nephron. The enzyme has a low affinity for calcium (apparent $K_m \simeq 1$ mM; maximal activation $\simeq 5$ mM), can also be activated by magnesium in millimolar concentrations, and is insensitive to sodium and ouabain. Both plasma membranes and mitochondria contribute to the Ca-ATPase activity measured in intact tubule segments.

Ca-ATPase was present in all the segments of the rabbit nephron in which it was determined. The enzyme activity measured in the presence of potent inhibitors of mitochondrial ATPases was highest in the proximal tubule (pars convoluta and pars recta) and in the collecting duct (cortical and medullary portions). Both the absolute activity and the distribution of this enzyme along the nephron were different from those of Na-K-ATPase.

The physiologic role of this Ca-ATPase in transmembrane calcium transport by renal tubular cells remains to be determined.

Acknowledgement—This work was supported by grant AM 13601 from the National Institutes of Health, U.S. Public Health Service.

REFERENCES

DOUCET A., KATZ A. I. & MOREL F. (1979) Determination of Na-K-ATPase activity in single segments of the mammalian nephron. *Am. J. Physiol.* **237,** F105–F113.

FENWICK J. C. (1979) Ca^{2+}-activated adenosinetriphosphatase activity in the gills of freshwater- and seawater-adapted eels (*Anguilla rostrata*). *Comp. Biochem. Physiol.* **62B,** 67–70.

KINNE R., HAASE W., GMAJ P. & MURER H. (1977) ATP-hydrolysis as driving force for transport processes in isolated renal plasma membrane vesicles. In *Current Problems in Clinical Biochemistry,* (Edited by SCHMIDT U. & DUBACH U. C.) Vol. 7, pp. 178–185. Hans Huber, Bern.

KINNE-SAFFRAN E. & KINNE R. (1974) Localization of a calcium-stimulated ATPase in the basal-lateral plasma membranes of the proximal tubule of rat kidney cortex. *J. membr. Biol.* **17,** 263–274.

LEVIN S. R., KASSON B. G. & DRIESSEN J. F. (1978) Adenosine triphosphatases of rat pancreatic islets. Comparison with those of rat kidney. *J. clin. Invest.* **62,** 692–701.

MOORE L., FITZPATRICK D. F., CHEN T. S. & LANDON E. J. (1974) Calcium pump activity of the renal plasma membrane and renal microsomes. *Biochim. biophys. Acta* **345,** 405–418.

PARKINSON D. K. & RADDE I. C. (1971) Properties of a Ca^{2+}- and Mg^{2+}-activated ATP-hydrolyzing enzyme in rat kidney cortex. *Biochim. biophys. Acta* **242,** 238–246.

RAHAMIMOFF H. & ABRAMOVITZ E. (1978) Ca transport and ATPase activity of synaptosomal vesicles from rat brain. *FEBS Lett.* **92,** 163–167.

ROCHA A. S., MAGALDI J. B. & KOKKO J. P. (1977) Calcium and phosphate transport in isolated segments of rabbit Henle's loop. *J. clin. Invest.* **59,** 975–983.

RORIVE G. & KLEINZELLER A. (1972) The effect of ATP and Ca^{2+} on the cell volume in isolated kidney tubules. *Biochim. biophys. Acta* **274,** 226–239.

ROSENTHAL A. S., KREGENOW F. M. & MOSES H. L. (1970) Some characteristics of a Ca^{2+}-dependent ATPase activity associated with a group of erythrocyte membrane proteins which form fibrils. *Biochim. biophys. Acta* **196,** 254–262.

SCHATZMANN H. J. (1975) Active calcium transport and Ca^{2+}-activated ATPase in human red cells. In *Current Topics in Membranes and Transport,* (Edited by BRONNER F. & KLEINZELLER A.) Vol. 6, pp. 125–169. Academic Press, New York.

SHAREGHI G. R. & STONER L. C. (1978) Calcium transport across segments of the rabbit distal nephron *in vitro*. *Am. J. Physiol.* **235,** F367–F375.

THOMPSON J. D. & NECHAY B. R. (1979) Inhibition by metals of a canine renal calcium or magnesium-activated adenosine triphosphatase. *Fedn Proc. Fedn Am. Socs exp. Biol.* **38,** 744. (Abstract)

ULLRICH K. J., RUMRICH G. & KLÖSS S. (1976) Active Ca^{2+} reabsorption in the proximal tubule of the rat kidney. *Pflüger's Arch. ges. Physiol.* **364,** 223–228.

VAN GRONINGEN H. E. M. & SLATER E. C. (1963) The effect of oligomycin on the (Na^+ + K^+)-activated magnesium-ATPase of brain microsomes and erythrocyte membrane. *Biochim. biophys. Acta* **73,** 527–530.

VINCENZI F. F. & HINDS T. R. (1976) Plasma membrane calcium transport and membrane-bound enzymes. In *The Enzymes of Biological Membranes,* (Edited by MARTONOSI A.), Vol. 3, pp. 261–274, Plenum Press, New York.

SYMPOSIUM DISCUSSION

Schwarz: If you pre-incubated your preparation for 10–15 min with sodium or potassium, you will find an effect of vanadate at low concentrations.

Katz: We placed the nephron segments in distilled water at 0°C for 15 min in the process of tubular permeabilization, but did not preincubate them.

Weiner: The use of oligomycin to inhibit mitochondrial ATPase has one drawback, depending on how the tissue has been prepared. Oligomycin sensitivity is only conferred if the F_1 is hooked on to the oligomycin-sensitivity conferring stalk, and if the tissue has been treated in a way that releases the F_1, then the mitochondrial ATPase activity is insensitive to oligomycin.

Katz: The enzyme from mitochondria obtained from kidney homogenates was inhibited 85–90% by oligomycin. In addition, we used azide in combination with oligomycin to ensure more complete inhibition of mitochondrial ATPase in the tubule segments.

Kovacevic: What is the role of mitochondrial Ca-ATPase?

Katz: It pumps calcium from the cytoplasm into the mitochondria. Cytoplasmic Ca^{2+} is probably regulated by the combined activity of membrane and of mitochondrial Ca-ATPase. But the membrane enzyme should have an affinity for calcium in the micromolar range (as the system described by Dr Kinne in the vesicle preparation) whereas the enzyme described today, and by Dr Kinne before, has an affinity for calcium in millimolar concentrations.

Kinne: Indeed, but that precisely reflects the difficulty which we still have with regard to other ATPases: (a) because they are present in many organelles in the cell, and (b) we really have to demonstrate a parallelism between transport and the ATPase activity. This has been done very nicely for Na-K-ATPase, but for Ca-ATPase it has not yet been done, and nor has it been done for the other ATPase that is postulated for kidney, the proton ATPase.

Int. J. Biochem., Vol. 12, pp. 131 to 133
© Pergamon Press Ltd 1980. Printed in Great Britain

0020-711X/80/0701-0131$02.00/0

THE MALATE/2-OXOGLUTARATE TRANSPORTER IN MITOCHONDRIA FROM RAT KIDNEY CORTEX: INCREASED ACTIVITY IN METABOLIC ACIDOSIS

JOHN T. BROSNAN, WAYNE REDMOND, DENIS MORGAN and PATRICK WHALEN
Department of Biochemistry, Memorial University of Newfoundland, St John's, Newfoundland, Canada A1B 3X9

Abstract—1. The malate/2-oxoglutarate antiporter activity of kidney cortex mitochondria from acidotic rats was higher than in mitochondria from control animals as measured by the rate of swelling of these mitochondria in isoosmotic solutions of ammonium 2-oxoglutarate.

2. This finding was confirmed by inhibitor-stop experiments in which [^{14}C]2-oxoglutarate influx into malate-loaded mitochondria was measured at 0°C using phenylsuccinate as an inhibitor.

3. In mitochondria from control rats a transport rate of 13 ± 6 nmol·min^{-1}·mg protein^{-1} and a K_m for external 2-oxoglutarate of 37 ± 6 μM were found.

4. After 7 days of NH_4Cl-induced acidosis there was a significant 70% increase in transporter activity with no change in K_m. The relationship of these changes to glutamine metabolism is discussed.

INTRODUCTION

The increased renal ammonia production that occurs during metabolic acidosis enables the body to excrete strong metabolic acids as ammonium salts (Pitts, 1974). In this connection the regulation of renal glutamine metabolism has been intensively studied since the major portion of urinary ammonia is produced by the renal metabolism of glutamine. The hydrolysis of glutamine by glutaminase is the first enzymatic step in the renal metabolism of glutamine and, since glutaminase is an intramitochondrial enzyme (Kalra & Brosnan, 1974), considerable attention has been paid to the transport processes whereby glutamine enters and its metabolic products exit from renal mitochondria. An increased rate of transport of glutamine into renal mitochondria from acidotic rats has been reported by Goldstein & Boylan (1978). Cheema-Dhadli & Halperin (1978) measured the rate of the malate/phosphate antiporter and found that it was unchanged in metabolic acidosis. In this paper we report on the malate/2-oxoglutarate transporter in mitochondria from rat kidney cortex. Increased activity of this transporter is found in mitochondria from acidotic rats. These findings are discussed in terms of the relationship of this transporter to the pathways of renal glutamine metabolism and their regulation.

MATERIALS AND METHODS

Animals

Male, Sprague–Dawley rats, weighing 250–350 g were used. They were fed *ad libitum* on Purina rat chow. Acidosis was induced by substituting 1.5% (w/v) NH_4Cl for drinking water and recovery was effected by replacing the NH_4Cl solution with tap water. These protocols were described by Parry & Brosnan (1978). Mitochondria were prepared from kidney cortex as previously described (Kalra & Brosnan, 1974) except that, in the case of mitochondria prepared for inhibitor-stop experiments, the homogenization medium also contained 0.5% fat-free bovine serum albumin.

Mitochondrial swelling

Mitochondrial swelling was observed essentially as described by Chappell & Haarhoff (1967). Mitochondria were suspended at room temperature in isotonic solutions (0.1 M) of ammonium malate or of ammonium 2-oxoglutarate, pH 7.2, at a final concentration of 0.25 mg mitochondrial protein per ml. The media also contained 1 mM EGTA (ethylene glycol bis-(β-aminoethyl ether)-N,N^1-tetraacetic acid) and 2.5 μM rotenone. Swelling was measured in a Pye Unicam SP 1800 spectrophotometer as the decrease in apparent absorption at 540 nm that occurred upon addition of 2 mM phosphate or of 2 mM phosphate plus 2 mM malate to the mitochondria suspended in ammonium malate or ammonium 2-oxoglutarate, respectively.

Inhibitor-stop experiments

The malate/2-oxoglutarate transporter was also measured by the inhibitor-stop technique, using 20 mM phenylsuccinate as the inhibitor. Mitochondria were loaded with L-malate as described by Sluse *et al.* (1972). Immediately after loading, mersalyl (0.2 mM) was added so as to prevent malate loss via the dicarboxylate or phosphate transporters (Meijer & Tager, 1969) and after 5 min the suspension was diluted with homogenization medium to which rotenone (10 μM) and antimycin A (2 μg/ml) were added. The mitochondria were washed and resuspended in incubation medium (0.125 M KCl, 0.02 M Tris–HCl, pH 7.4, 10 μM rotenone and antimycin A, 2 μg·ml^{-1}). One aliquot of mitochondria was centrifuged and its malate content measured (Mollering, 1974). The remainder of the mitochondria were employed for the measurement of 2-oxoglutarate transport. Eppendorf centrifuge tubes were prepared containing ice-cold incubation medium and various concentrations (from 5 to 100 μM) [U-^{14}C]2-oxoglutarate (New England Nuclear, Montreal, Canada). Mitochondria were added (0.05 ml containing 0.5–1 mg of mitochondrial protein) with constant stirring and ice-cold sodium phenylsuccinate (final concentration, 20 mM) was added after 5 sec. The mitochondrial suspension was immediately centrifuged for 1 min at 12,000 *g* in the Eppendorf centrifuge. The supernatant was poured off, the pellet dissolved in NCS (Amersham-Searle, Arlington Heights, IL, U.S.A.) and ^{14}C determined by liquid scintillation spectrometry. Experiments were also performed in which phenylsuccinate was added before the mitochondria. These experiments provided zero-time data. All incubations were carried out in triplicate and the means employed for the construction of Lineweaver–Burk plots from which the V_{max} and K_m for 2-oxoglutarate entry were calculated. Preliminary experiments established that the rate of influx was linear over the 5 sec time period employed.

RESULTS AND DISCUSSION

Mitochondrial swelling

Mitochondria from control rats, acidotic rats or from rats recovered from acidosis swelled in ammonium malate at identical rates and to identical extents. Since such swelling occurs as a result of the operation of the dicarboxylate transporter these results imply that the rate of this carrier is unchanged in acidosis. This is in agreement with the inhibitor-stop measurements of Cheema-Dhadli & Halperin (1978). Mitochondria from acidotic rats swelled more rapidly in ammonium 2-oxoglutarate than did mitochondria from normal animals. A two-fold increase in the rate of swelling was evident in mitochondria from 7-day acidotic rats. The rate of swelling returned to control rates after one day of recovery (Data not shown).

Inhibitor-stop experiments

The swelling experiments indicated that an increased activity of the malate/2-oxoglutarate transporter exists in mitochondria from acidotic rats. Inhibitor-stop experiments were carried out so as to obtain more precise information. The concentrations of 2-oxoglutarate, the external substrate, required for half-maximal rates of entry were 38, 54, 53 and 36 μM in mitochondria from control, 1 day acidotic, 7 day acidotic and 1 day recovered rats, respectively (Table 1). There were no significant differences between these values which are similar to the K_m value of 46 μM obtained in rat liver mitochondria by Palmieri *et al.* (1972). The V_{max} of the transporter from control rats was 13.2 nmol$\cdot$min$^{-1}\cdot$mg^{-1} and this was significantly increased to 22 nmol$\cdot$min$^{-1}\cdot$mg^{-1} after 7 days of acidosis. The rate returned to control values after one day of recovery from acidosis. These changes in transporter activity cannot be attributed to alterations in the concentration of the counter anion since there were no differences in the intramitochondrial malate concentration. Thus a significant increase in transporter activity occurred in acidosis. Since there was no change in the K_m for 2-oxoglutarate it seems likely that the increased transporter activity is due to an increase in the number of functioning transporter molecules rather than to a qualitative change in the existing transporter proteins.

Physiological considerations

An *in vivo* activity of 8.8 μmol$\cdot$min$^{-1}\cdot$g^{-1} for control animals and of 14.8 μmol$\cdot$min$^{-1}\cdot$g^{-1} for acidotic animals may be calculated by assuming a Q_{10} of 2 and that 1 g of kidney cortex contains about 60 mg of mitochondrial protein. This is a high rate compared to the rate of most metabolic processes in the kidney but it is likely that it is an overestimate of the actual rate *in vivo* since the transport experiments were carried out at very high concentrations of intramitochondrial malate i.e. about 6 mM.

An increase in an enzyme's activity reflects, in general, an increased flux through the enzyme and it is reasonable to assume that similar considerations apply to an increase in the activity of a transporting process. It is necessary to consider, therefore, the various metabolic pathways in which the malate/2-oxoglutarate transporter plays a role.

The malate/2-oxoglutarate transporter plays an important role in aerobic glycolysis since it is involved in a shuttle mechanism whereby the reducing equivalents of cytoplasmic NADH are ultimately oxidised in mitochondria. There are no reasons to believe that the flux through this pathway may increase during metabolic acidosis.

Gluconeogenesis from lactate also requires the operation of the malate/2-oxoglutarate transporter (Soling *et al.*, 1973). Similar amounts of lactate are removed by the kidneys of normal and acidotic rats (Squires *et al.*, 1976). It is possible, however, that a greater fraction of this lactate is converted to glucose in acidotic rats than in normal animals because of the increased activity of phosphoenolpyruvate carboxykinase (Alleyne & Scullard, 1969). Increased gluconeogenesis from lactate does occur in kidney slices from acidotic rats (Goodman *et al.*, 1966; Parry & Brosnan, 1978).

The most striking alteration in the metabolism of the acidotic kidney is, of course, the increased production of ammonia from glutamine. The metabolic fate of the carbon skeleton of glutamine *in vivo* is uncertain but *in vitro*, at least in the rat, part is converted to glucose and part is oxidized (Vinay *et al.*, 1978). Gluconeogenesis from glutamine does not require the malate/2-oxoglutarate transporter, rather it involves the export of malate from the mitochondrion via the malate/phosphate transporter. Complete oxidation of

Table 1. Kinetic characteristics of the malate/2-oxoglutarate transporter in mitochondria from rat kidneys

State of animals	V_{max} (nmol$\cdot$min$^{-1}\cdot$mg^{-1})	K_m (μM)	Intramitochondrial malate (nmol$\cdot$mg protein^{-1})
Normal (10)	13.2 ± 6.2	38 ± 17	6.5 ± 2.0
Acidotic (10) 1 day	18.7 ± 5.8	54 ± 32	6.6 ± 2.7
Acidotic (8) 7 days	22.0 ± 6.1*	53 ± 24	7.7 ± 1.0
Recovered (6) 1 day	12.3 ± 3.4	36 ± 6	7.2 ± 2.1

* Significantly different from normal, $P < 0.01$.

glutamine to CO_2 may not even involve the export of metabolites from the mitochondrion (Watford *et al.* 1979).

The malate/2-oxoglutarate transporter may play an important role in the regulation of ammoniagenesis by 2-oxoglutarate. Goldstein & Boylan (1978) showed that 2-oxoglutarate, acting on the mitochondrial membrane from the cytoplasmic side, inhibits glutamine entry into mitochondria. It is well appreciated that intramitochondrial 2-oxoglutarate may regulate intramitochondrial glutamate levels, and, hence, glutaminase activity (Krebs & Vinay, 1975). A coordinated regulation by 2-oxoglutarate of glutamine entry and of glutaminase activity would require the malate/2-oxoglutarate transporter so that changes in the concentration of 2-oxoglutarate in one compartment would be rapidly transmitted to the other compartment. The increased malate/2-oxoglutarate transporter activity found in acidosis may be related to this function.

REFERENCES

Alleyne G. A. O. & Scullard G. H. (1969) Renal metabolic response to acid–base changes. I Enzymatic control of ammoniagenesis in the rat. *J. clin. Invest.* **54**, 165–174.

Chappell J. B. & Haarhof K. N. (1967) *Biochemistry of Mitochondria* (Edited by Slater E. C., Kaniuga Z. & Wojtczak L.) pp. 75–91. Academic Press, London.

Cheema-Dhadli S. & Halperin M. L. (1978) Ammoniagenesis in kidney cortex mitochondria of the rat: role of the mitochondrial dicarboxylate anion transporter. *Can. J. Biochem.* **56**, 23–28.

Goodman A. D., Fuisz R. F. & Cahill G. F. Jr (1966) Renal gluconeogenesis in acidosis, alkalosis and potassium deficiency: Its possible role in regulation of renal ammonia production. *J. clin. Invest.* **45**, 612–619.

Goldstein L. & Boylan J. M. (1978) Renal mitochondrial transport and metabolism: studies with a rapid-mixing, rapid-filtration technique. *Am. J. Physiol.* **234**, F514–F521.

Kalra J. & Brosnan J. T. (1974) The subcellular localization of glutaminase isoenzymes in rat kidney cortex. *J. biol. Chem.* **249**, 3255–3260.

Krebs H. A. & Vinay P. (1975) Regulation of renal ammonia production. *Med. Clin. N. Am.* **59**, 595–603.

Meijer A. J. & Tager J. M. (1969) The effect of butylmalonate and mersalyl on anion-exchange reactions in rat-liver mitochondria. *Biochem. biophys. Acta.* **189**, 136–139.

Mollering H. (1974) In *Methods of Enzymatic Analysis* 2nd edn. (Edited by Bergmeyer H.-U.) pp. 1589–1593. Academic Press, London.

Palmieri F., Quagliariello E. & Klingenberg M. (1972) Kinetics and specificity of the oxoglutarate carrier in rat-liver mitochondria. *Eur. J. Biochem.* **29**, 408–416.

Parry D. M. & Brosnan J. T. (1978) Glutamine metabolism in the kidney during induction of, and recovery from, metabolic acidosis in the rat. *Biochem. J.* **174**, 387–396.

Pitts R. F. (1974) *Physiology of the Kidney and Body Fluids*, 3rd edn. pp. 178–241. Year Book Medical Publishers, Chicago.

Sluse F. E., Ranson M. & Liebecq J. (1972) Mechanism of the exchanges catalysed by the oxoglutarate translocator of rat-heart mitochondria. *Eur. J. Biochem.* **25**, 207–217.

Soling H.-D., Kleineke J., Willms B., Janson G. & Kuhn A. (1973) Relationship between intracellular distribution of phosphoenolpyruvate carboxykinase, regulation of gluconeogenesis and energy cost of glucose formation. *Eur. J. Biochem.* **37**, 233–243.

Squires E. J., Hall D. E. & Brosnan J. T. (1976) Arteriovenous differences for amino acids and lactate across kidneys of normal and acidotic rats. *Biochem. J.* **160**, 125–128.

Vinay P., Mapes J. P. & Krebs H. A. (1978) Fate of glutamine carbon in renal metabolism. *Am. J. Physiol.* **234**, F123–F129.

Watford M., Vinay P., Lemieux G. & Gougoux A. (1979) The formation of pyruvate from citric acid-cycle intermediates in kidney cortex. *Biochem. Soc. Trans.* **7**, 753–755.

SYMPOSIUM DISCUSSION

Ross: Since many of the adaptations in ammoniagenesis are now recognised to occur within minutes rather than days, have you done any experiments on the time–course of the adaptation of mitochondrial function which you have just described?

Brosnan: In my opinion, many of these transport adaptations follow flux rather than initiate it, so I should be surprised if they were rapid, but we haven't yet looked.

Halperin: The maximum velocity you observed for the malate/2-oxoglutarate transporter is very rapid. How do you imagine a further increase in the maximum velocity of this transporter can play a role in the regulation of ammoniagenesis?

Brosnan: Calculation (assuming $Q_{10} = 2$ ng and 60 mg mitochondrial protein per gm of kidney), you find a rate of 8 μmols$\cdot$min$^{-1}\cdot$min$^{-1}\cdot$g kidney^{-1}: this is very high, I agree, but we have artificially raised the malate concentration, and this would increase the observed rate, over that which might occur *in vivo*.

Tannen: Have you looked at the effect of changing incubation pH on the transporter?

Brosnan: Not yet.

Int. J. Biochem., Vol. 12, pp. 135 to 137
© Pergamon Press Ltd 1980. Printed in Great Britain

0020-711X/80/0701-0135$02.00/0

REGULATION OF RENAL AMMONIAGENESIS IN THE RABBIT

M. L. HALPERIN and S. CHEEMA-DHADLI
Department of Medicine, University of Toronto, and St. Michael's Hospital, Toronto, Canada

Abstract—1. In order to identify sites of regulation of ammoniagenesis in rabbit renal cortex, the activities of the key steps in this pathway were measured.
2. Results indicate that the flux through the mitochondrial dicarboxylate transporter could limit ammoniagenesis in this species.

INTRODUCTION

Metabolism of a typical North American diet results in the production of about 1 mEq of hydrogen ions per kg body weight. These hydrogen ions are initially removed via the bicarbonate buffer system as alveolar carbon dioxide. Bicarbonate is then regenerated by the kidney as a result of net acid excretion—ammonium being the principal component of this excretion (for review, see Rector, 1976).

Ammonium is synthesized in the renal cortex from glutamine. Although much work has been done in this area, the biochemical mechanisms responsible for regulation of this pathway remain to be fully elucidated (for review, see Tannen, 1978). The most likely sites for this regulation are the mitochondrial glutamine transporter, phosphate dependent glutaminase, glutamate dehydrogenase, phosphoenolpyruvate carboxykinase and the mitochondrial dicarboxylate transporter. In this manuscript, we shall present data concerning the role of the dicarboxylate transporter in ammoniagenesis.

MATERIALS AND METHODS

Male rabbits (2.5–3 kg) were obtained from Reiman's Fur Ranch, St Agatha, Ontario. Bovine serum albumin, free of fatty acid, antimycin A, rotenone and Tris were purchased from Sigma Chemical Co., St Louis, MO L-[U-^{14}C]malic acid and $NaH^{14}CO_3$ were from Amersham/Searle Corp., Don Mills, Ontario. Enzymes and other cofactors were obtained from Boehringer Mannheim Corp., New York, NY. *p*-Iodobenzylmalonic acid was from K & K Laboratories, Inc., Plainview, NY. EGTA was from Eastman Kodak Co. Versilube F-50 silicone fluid was from the General Electric Co., Silicone Products Dept., Waterford, NY.

The preparation of rabbit kidney cortex mitochondria and the loading of mitochondria with L-[U-^{14}C]malate were carried out as described previously (Yu *et al.*, 1976; Cheema-Dhadli & Halperin, 1978; Cheema-Dhadli & Halperin, 1979). The kinetics of the dicarboxylate transporter were determined as previously described (Cheema-Dhadli & Halperin, 1978) by varying the concentration of inorganic phosphate (0.2–5.0 mM) and using *p*-iodobenzylmalonate (5 mM) as the inhibitor stop.

RESULTS

Kinetics of the dicarboxylate anion transporter in renal cortex mitochondria

In mitochondria from either rabbit or rat renal cortex, the K_m for inorganic phosphate for the dicarboxylate transporter was approximately 1 mM whereas the K_m for malate was almost an order of magnitude higher. The V_{max} for this transporter was much lower in the rabbit than in the rat (Table 1).

Observed and calculated velocities in key steps of the ammoniagenesis pathway in the rabbit (Table 2)

The observed maximum velocities of the critical steps of ammoniagenesis exceeded the maximum rate of urinary ammonium excretion by many fold. The maximum *in vivo* rates were obtained by the infusion of inorganic phosphate and glutamine into rabbits with acute metabolic acidosis excreting a urine with a pH less than 6.0 (Cheema-Dhadli & Halperin, 1979). However, the maximum velocities cannot be achieved *in vivo* because the tissue substrate concentrations are usually much lower than required for these rates. We therefore calculated a rate for each of these steps based on the measured K_m for the enzyme and the observed substrate concentrations. To evaluate the glutamine transporter and phosphate dependent glutaminase, we elected to measure glutamine deamination by intact mitochondria because intramitochondrial glutamine was too difficult to measure with accuracy. The glutamine concentration required for half maximal rates was 2.5 mM and the maximum velocity was 30 nmol per min per mg of mitochondrial protein or about 20 μmol. min^{-1} via both kidneys (for details of calculations, see Cheema-Dhadli & Halperin, 1979). The tissue concentrations of glutamate and oxaloacetate were not very different from the K_m of their respective enzymes. However, the tissue content of inorganic phosphate and especially intramitochondrial malate were very much lower than the concentrations required to support the maximum velocity of flux through the dicarboxylate transporter (Cheema-Dhadli & Halperin, 1979).

DISCUSSION

The biochemical pathway of ammoniagenesis has a significant intramitochondrial component. For continued flux in this pathway, the major carbon skeleton of glutamine must exit from the mitochondrion via the dicarboxylate transporter. This statement implies that the malate formed is not metabolized at a significant rate by the intramitochondrial malic enzyme. Flux through the dicarboxylate transporter results in carbon, nitrogen, electrical and pH balance in the various intracellular compartments during active

Table 1. Kinetic parameters for dicarboxylate carrier in rabbit and rat kidney mitochondria

Species	Substrate	K_m (mM)	V_{max} (nmols. mg protein$\cdot^{-1}$ min^{-1} at 0°C)
Rabbit	Inorganic phosphate	1.6 ± 0.2*	
			1.60 ± 0.6
	Malate	14	
Rat	Inorganic phosphate	1.0 ± 0.1	
			10.5 ± 0.02
	Malate	7.0	

* Mean ± SEM.

ammoniagenesis (for review, see Cheema-Dhadli & Halperin, 1978, 1979).

The rabbit has a low rate of ammoniagenesis during acute or chronic metabolic acidosis despite much higher activities of the enzymes of the early steps of this pathway (Cheema-Dhadli & Halperin, 1979; Richterich & Goldstein, 1958). In fact, this rate can be markedly increased when phosphate is infused (Yu *et al.*, 1976; Cheema-Dhadli & Halperin, 1979). Studies with mitochondria suggest that this stimulation can be localized to exit of the basic TCA cycle four-carbon intermediates via the dicarboxylate transporter for the following reasons:

1. It is prevented when this step is inhibited by 2-n-butylmalonate (Yu *et al.*, 1976).
2. It can be reproduced by compounds which lead to the net exit of intramitochondrial metabolites (Yu *et al.*, 1976).
3. Phosphate does not lead to additional stimulation of the ammoniagenesis pathway if intramitochondrial metabolite levels are already lowered (Yu *et al.*, 1976).
4. The rate of renal mitochondrial ammoniagenesis with glutamine as substrate is inversely proportional to the intramitochondrial glutamate level (see Fig. 3 of Cheema-Dhadli & Halperin, 1979).

In order to evaluate what factors might regulate dicarboxylate transporter activity in renal cortex mitochondria, the kinetic properties of this transporter were determined in both the rabbit and the rat. There was no increase in the activity of this transporter during acute or chronic metabolic acidosis in the rabbit or rat (Cheema-Dhadli & Halperin, 1978, 1979). Furthermore, the K_m for its extramitochondrial substrate, inorganic phosphate, was approximately 1 mM in both species and this value did not decrease during metabolic acidosis (Cheema-Dhadli & Halperin, 1978). In addition, the apparent K_m for intramitochondrial malate was very high and again did not change during metabolic acidosis. With respect to the V_{max} of this step, this value was about an order of magnitude lower in the rabbit than the rat and by calculation, could limit the flux in the ammoniagenesis pathway (Cheema-Dhadli & Halperin, 1979). However, these calculations must be interpreted with caution as concentrations of compartmented metabolites were only estimated.

Table 2. Rate of flux in critical steps in ammoniagenesis in the rabbit*

Step	Velocity (μmol. min^{-1}) Observed V_{max}	Derived velocity
Glutamine deamination	20	4
Glutamate dehydrogenase	700	300
PEPCK	200	50
Dicarboxylate transporter	50	1
Ammonia excretion	4	—

* For description, see text.

From the above, we suggest the following hypothesis to account for the low rates of ammoniagenesis in the rabbit. High rates of flux through the dicarboxylate transporter require that the concentration of its substrate, intramitochondrial malate, rise to more than 14 mM. However, this is unlikely to occur without a concomitant rise in intramitochondrial precursors such as glutamate. High glutamate concentrations, by feedback inhibition (Goldstein, 1966), would lead to inhibition of phosphate dependent glutaminase and thus prevent high rates of ammoniagenesis. This sequence of events is not as important in the rat because of the much greater activity of the dicarboxylate transporter, a more than 10-fold higher maximum velocity and lower K_m for intramitochondrial malate.

SUMMARY

The purpose of these investigations was to review factors which may regulate ammoniagenesis in the kidney cortex of the rabbit. Emphasis was placed on the segment of the pathway by which the carbon derived from glutamine must exit from the mitochondrion; the *in vivo* rate of ammoniagenesis could be increased about ten-fold by inorganic phosphate infusion which seemed to act by promoting malate exit from mitochondria. The dicarboxylate transporter, which is essential for ammoniagenesis, has a maximum velocity which was low in the rabbit. The malate concentration required for half maximal rates of transport was 14 nmols per mg mitochondrial protein. There was no effect of chronic metabolic acidosis on dicarboxylate transporter activity. The maximum velocity of phosphate dependent glutaminase, glutamate dehydrogenase and PEPCK were all much greater than the maximal rate of ammoniagenesis observed in the rabbit *in vivo*. Therefore, the low rates of ammoniagenesis and the failure to adapt to acidosis in the rabbit can be explained by the properties of the dicarboxylate transporter.

Acknowledgements—The authors are very grateful to Drs Brian H. Robinson, Marc B. Goldstein and Bobby J. Stinebaugh for helpful advice and discussions, and to Ms Barbara Gardner and Mr Ching-Bun Chen for expert technical assistance. This research was funded by the Medical Research Council of Canada (MT3363).

REFERENCES

CHEEMA-DHADLI S. & HALPERIN M. L. (1978) Ammoniagenesis in kidney cortex mitochondria of the rat: role of the mitochondrial dicarboxylate anion transporter. *Can. J. Biochem.* **56,** 23–28.

CHEEMA-DHADLI S. & HALPERIN M. L. (1979) Role of the mitochondrial anion transporters in the regulation of ammoniagenesis in renal cortex mitochondria of the rabbit and rat. *Eur. J. Biochem.* **99,** 483–489.

GOLDSTEIN L. (1966) Relation of glutamate to ammonia production in the rat kidney. *Am. J. Physiol.* **210,** 661–666.

RECTOR F. C. JR (1976) Renal acidification and ammonia production; chemistry of weak acids and bases; buffer mechanisms. In *The Kidney*, (Edited by BRENNER B. M. & RECTOR F. C. JR) Vol. 1, pp. 318–348. W. B. Saunders, Philadelphia.

RICHTERICH R. W. & GOLDSTEIN L. (1958) Distribution of glutamine metabolizing enzymes and production of urinary ammonia in the mammalian kidney. *Am. J. Physiol.* **195,** 316–320.

TANNEN R. L. (1978) Ammonia metabolism. *Am. J. Physiol.* **235**(4), F265–F277.

YU H. L., GIAMMARCO R., GOLDSTEIN M. B., STINEBAUGH B. J. & HALPERIN M. L. (1976) Stimulation of ammonia production and excretion in the rabbit by inorganic phosphate. *J. clin Invest.* **58,** 557–564.

SYMPOSIUM DISCUSSION

Lemieux: You equate ammonia excretion and ammonia production. Have you actually measured ammonia production directly *in vivo* in the rabbit? What is blood ammonia in the rabbit?

Halperin: First, we measured only ammonia excretion and not ammonia production in these studies. Second, the blood ammonia concentration was similar to that in other species.

Epstein: What is the serum phosphate, and how much do you increase it by your infusion of phosphate?

Halperin: The normal plasma phosphate of rabbits is 1.5–2.0 mM. We did not measure plasma phosphate following the infusion.

Alleyne: Suppose you keep a rabbit on a high phosphate diet, to chronically increase its NH_3 production, do you see any adaptation in the dicarboxylic acid carrier?

Halperin: We have fed rabbits a diet which was supplemented with inorganic phosphate for several weeks. Ammonia excretion was increased somewhat under these conditions but there was no detectable change in the kinetic properties of the renal cortex dicarboxylate carrier activity.

Guder: We know (H. Radda *et al.* pp. , this volume) that you cannot decrease intracellular phosphate *in vitro* by leaving phosphate out of the medium. Have you measured whether you can increase intracellular phosphate by incubating with increased phosphate? How quickly does the response of ammonia production occur?

Halperin: First, we did not measure the renal cortex phosphate content following the infusions. Second, the phosphate induced rise in ammonia excretion was very rapid—the peak response was usually observed 30 min after starting the infusion of phosphate.

Weiner: What is the effect of phosphate in other species?

Halperin: There are only small changes in ammonia excretion when phosphate was infused into rats. However, the dicarboxylate transporter has both different kinetic properties and a much higher maximum velocity in the rat.

O'Donovan: Do you use sodium or potassium phosphate? What effect does phosphate have without acidosis?

Halperin: Sodium phosphate. Even when the rat has an alkaline urine, ammonia excretion was increased.

Kovacevic: Using sodium phosphate, what is the effect of sodium?

Halperin: The control is the experiment with sodium sulphate which I showed in which there was no increase in ammonia production following sodium sulphate administration.

Int. J. Biochem., Vol. 12, pp. 139 to 143
0020-711X/80/0701-0139$02.00/0

VOLUME CHANGES OF RAT KIDNEY MITOCHONDRIA, TRANSPORT OF GLUTAMINE AND ITS INHIBITION BY MERSALYL

Z. Kovačević, K. Bajin and M. Pavlović
Department of Biochemistry, Medical Faculty, 21000 Novi Sad Yugoslavia

Abstract—1. The use of different —SH reagents (mersalyl, NEM, pCMB and DTNB) showed that the glutamine carrier and phosphate-dependent glutaminase (PGD) of rat kidney mitochondria are two different proteins and that activity of the enzyme is not necessary for the transport of glutamine.

2. However, it is interesting that there is a very similar sensitivity of these two proteins to the thiol blocking agents.

3. Further investigation showed that volume changes of the mitochondria have a significant influence on glutamine transport and the mechanism of its inhibition by mersalyl.

4. It is suggested that swelling of the mitochondria leads to unmasking of the functional —SH groups of glutamine carrier resulting in the stimulation of its activity and a higher sensitivity to the inhibition by mersalyl.

INTRODUCTION

In order to elucidate the regulation of ammoniagenesis during the adaptation to metabolic acidosis and the mitochondrial metabolism of glutamine in general, great attention has been paid to the understanding of glutamine transport across the inner mitochondrial membrane. It was suggested that transport of glutamine is the rate-limiting step in ammonia production and that it is increased in acidosis. However, the mechanism and kinetics of glutamine transport are still poorly understood and are the matter of a very controversial discussion (Tannen, 1978). This is for the following reasons: transport was investigated under conditions where glutamine hydrolysis by PDG was not inhibited so that it was impossible to study strictly the initial rate of kinetics of the transport process. One of the main factors showing the existence of glutamine carrier was the decrease of [^{14}C]glutamine-permeable space caused by mersalyl, a thiol blocking agent which affects a lot of different mitochondrial functions. For this reason the question arose as to whether mersalyl specifically inhibits glutamine carrier or the influx of glutamine is blocked due to inhibition of some other processes involved in the transport of the metabolite. It was also assumed that the changes of mitochondrial energy-state might change transport of glutamine due to volume change of the organelles and that this may influence the inhibition by mersalyl.

The present investigation showed that mitochondria undergo a significant volume change in the presence of mersalyl and that the change has an influence on the mechanism of inhibition. It was also found that there is a correlation between the amount of different —SH reagents and the degree of PDG inhibition in intact and lysed mitochondria.

MATERIALS AND METHODS

Rats of Wistar strain of both sexes were used. Kidney mitochondria were located and purified by velocity Ficoll step gradient centrifugation (Kovačević *et al.*, 1979; Curthoys *et al.*, 1978). Purification was essential if phosphate-dependent glutaminase activity was measured. This was done by measuring the formation of [^{14}C]glutamate from [U^{14}C]glutamine.

Reduced glutathione was estimated by 5,5(-dithio-bis-(2-nitrobenzoic acid) (DTNB) (Jocelyn, 1976).

Volume changes of the mitochondria were followed by measuring the spaces for [^{3}H]-H_2O, [^{14}C]sucrose and [^{14}C]glutamine (Chappell, 1968). It is assumed that the inner mitochondrial membrane is not permeable for [^{14}C]sucrose whereas it is freely permeable for tritiated water. Radioactivity was measured by means of a Beckman LS-250 liquid scintillation counter.

RESULTS AND DISCUSSION

Effect of thiol blocking agents on the activity of PDG in intact and lysed mitochondria

Since it is known that PDG is sensitive to —SH reagents investigation was undertaken to determine whether mersalyl primarily inhibits the enzyme activity which then results in the inhibition of the transport of glutamine. It was assumed that this possibility might exist even if PDG and glutamine carrier are two different proteins; activity of the enzyme may be the driving force for the influx of glutamine by maintaining a high concentration gradient of glutamine. It was found that there is a correlation between the amount of mersalyl and some other —SH reagents (pCMB, DTNB and NEM) and the degree of the inhibition of PDG in intact and lysed mitochondria (Fig. 1). It is interesting that *N*-ethylmaleimide (NEM), which is known as a much weaker inhibitor of PDG compared to organic mercurials (Kvamme *et al.*, 1968) is also much less efficient in inhibiting the enzyme in intact mitochondria. In addition the amount of NEM which inhibits PDG activity does not inhibit the influx of [^{14}C]glutamine into the mitochondria (not shown). It should be noted that a higher amount of —SH reagents is needed for the inhibition of PDG in lysed mitochondria. This is because the lysis of the mitochondria leads to the liberation of additional —SH groups which mainly

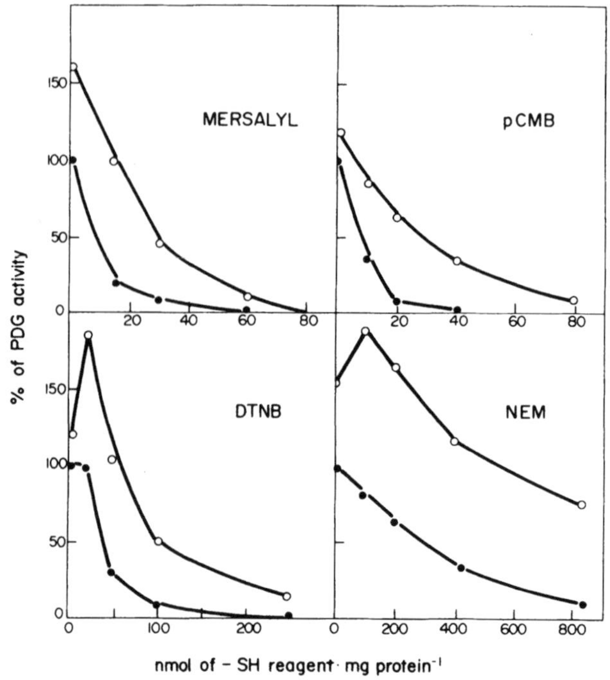

Fig. 1. Inhibition of PDG activity in intact (●) and lysed (○) mitochondria by mersalyl, PCMB, DTNB and NEM. The mitochondria (1 mg protein) were incubated in the medium of the following composition: 100 mM Tris–Cl, 30 mM Tris–phosphate, 8 mM [^{14}C]glutamine; pH 7.5. The final volume was 1.2 ml and temperature 30°C. Concentration of Triton X-100 (if present) was 0.02%.

belong to glutathione (GSH). Further investigations showed that mersalyl in the amount which completely inhibits PDG in intact mitochondria does not decrease the amount of intramitochondrial GSH, indicating that the inhibitor does not penetrate the inner membrane (Table 1). Therefore, if PDG is located on the inner side of the inner membrane (Kovačević, 1976) it could not be inhibited by mersalyl.

Swelling of the mitochondria in a hypotonic medium and inhibition of PDG activity and transport of glutamine by mersalyl

If the inhibitory effect of mersalyl is mainly due to the inhibition of glutamine carrier, a decrease of the osmolarity of the incubation medium should result in a simple, non carrier-mediated diffusion of glutamine and a significant removal of PDG inhibition. It was found that the increase of hypotonicity of the incubation medium does not decrease the percentage of the inhibition of PDG, suggesting that mersalyl primarily inhibits the enzyme (Fig. 2). However, further investigations gave quite surprising results. It was found that the mitochondrial membrane is still impermeable for a simple, non carrier-mediated diffusion of glutamine since mersalyl completely inhibited penetration of [^{14}C]glutamine into the inner space (Fig. 3). Although the matrix space was increased several times the phospholipid bilayer was still a barrier for simple diffusion of the metabolite. It was also observed that energized mitochondria do not swell in the hypotonic medium in the presence of mersalyl whereas deenergized mitochondria undergo marked swelling (Fig. 4). We have found earlier that the glutamine carrier is more sensitive to mersalyl inhibition in de-energized mitochondria, whereas energization removes the inhibition (Kovačević, 1976). Preliminary experiments showed that swollen mitochondria are more sensitive to the mersalyl inhibition. These and other findings suggest that swelling unmasks —SH groups of glutamine carrier so that they become more accessible to the thiol blocking agent.

Table 1. Reaction of mersalyl and NEM with intramitochondrial glutathione and inhibition of PDG activity in intact mitochondria

Conditions	nmol. GSH/mg. protein	% of PDG inhibition
Control	4.5	
+15 nmol. mersalyl/mg. protein	4.5	78
+30 nmol. mersalyl/mg. protein	4.0	100
+60 nmol. mersalyl/mg. protein	3.7	100
+30 nmol NEM/mg. protein	0.4	

The mitochondria (3 mg protein) were incubated in a medium of the following composition: 120 mM Tris–Cl, 10 mM Tris–phosphate, pH 7.4. The final volume was 1.3 ml.

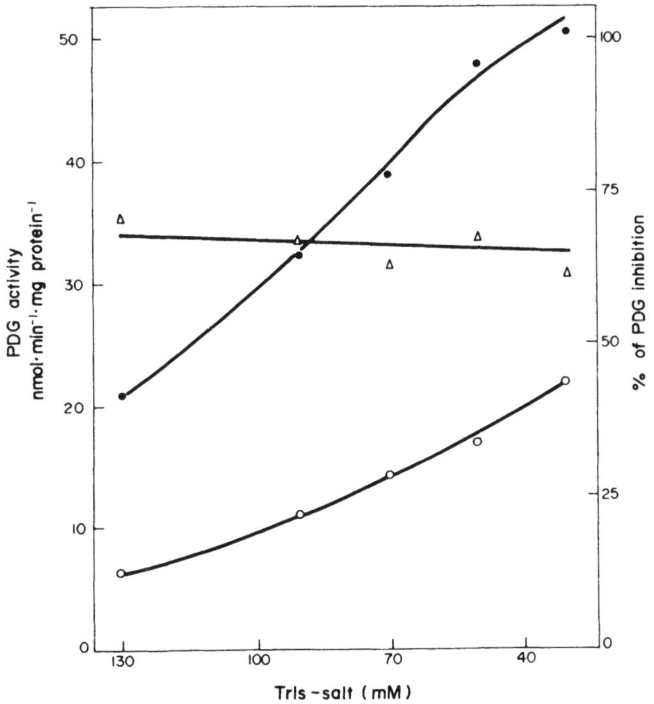

Fig. 2. The effect of decrease of osmolarity on PDG activity (control, ●) and its inhibition by mersalyl (○). △, percentage of the inhibition. Isotonic medium had the following composition: 100 mM Tris–Cl, 30 mM Tris–phosphate; pH 7.5. Osmolarity was decreased by decreasing concentration of Tris–Cl to zero. Concentration of [^{14}C]glutamine was 8 mM. The amount of mersalyl was 12.5 nmol. mg protein.^{1}

Figure 2 shows another phenomenon which still lacks a satisfactory explanation. Swelling of the mitochondria in the hypotonic medium increases activity of PDG 2–3 times although the membrane is not freely permeable for the substrate. Since there is a decrease of the K_m of PDG for glutamine (Kovačević *et al.*, 1979) the swelling probably increases the influx of substrate on a specific carrier by unmasking its functional —SH groups. It was also observed previously that energy-induced swelling stimulates PDG activity (Kovačević *et al.*, 1970). Together with our present finding this suggests that transport of glutamine is the rate-limiting step in the enzyme activity.

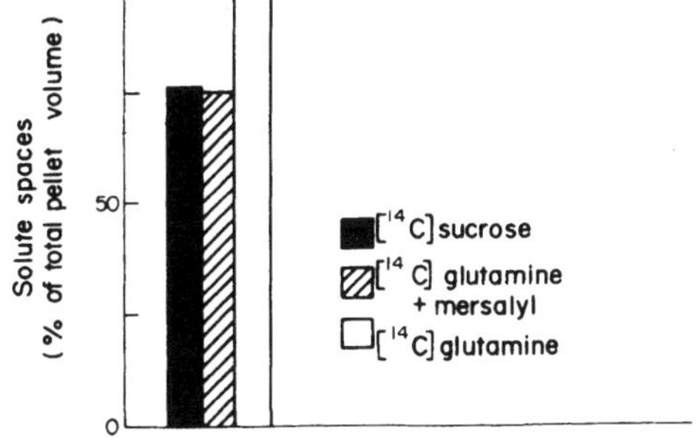

Fig. 3. Inhibition by mersalyl of the influx of [^{14}C]glutamine into the mitochondria suspended in a hypotonic medium. The incubation medium was of the following composition: 30 mM K^{+}-phosphate plus rotenone (1 μg/mg protein^{-1}); pH 7.4. Mersalyl (30 nmol/mg protein^{-1}) was added after the mitochondria.

Does glutamine uptake by kidney mitochondria represent transport or a binding process

For the understanding of the mechanism of glutamine influx into the mitochondria it is important to know whether the uptake of glutamine represents transport or a binding process (Azzone *et al.*, 1973). This is especially relevant if one wants to know whether glutamine appears in the matrix space or not. Even if the mitochondria accumulate glutamine this still does not prove that the metabolite appears in the

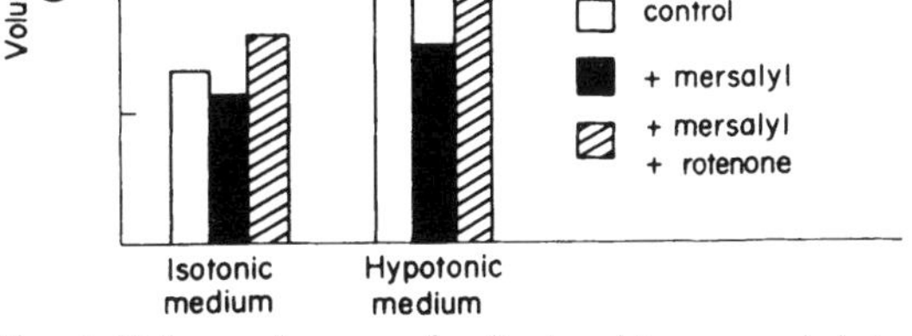

Fig. 4. Volume changes of mitochondria suspended in an isotonic or a hypotonic solution and effect of mersalyl. Composition of the media: Isotonic—100 mM KCl, 30 mM K^{+}-phosphate; pH 7.4. Hypotonic—30 mM K^{+}-phosphate; pH 7.4. The volume changes were determined by measuring [^{14}C] sucrose spaces.

Table 2. Swelling of the mitochondria and uptake of ^{14}C label from [^{14}C]glutamine as a function of osmotic pressure of the incubation medium

mM K ± salt	Inner space (μl)	nmol. Glu. NH_2 + Glu·mg^{-1} protein
130	3.5	8.1
60	12.0	24.0
30	13.1	25.8

The isotonic medium was of the following composition: 100 mM KCl, 30 mM K^+-phosphate, 8 mM [^{14}C]glutamine; pH 7.4. Osmolarity was decreased by decreasing concentration of KCl to zero. Rotenone was present in all cases.

osmotically active space because it may be bound to the membrane. Measurement of the amount of glutamine taken up by the mitochondria as a function of the osmotic pressure of the medium enables one to distinguish transport from the binding process. Our data suggest that ^{14}C label, whether in glutamine or glutamate, is not significantly bound to the membrane but that it appears in the matrix space (Table 2). Preliminary experiments indicate that the same happens if PDG is inhibited by NEM.

CONCLUSION

Since the amount of mersalyl which completely inhibits PDG activity in intact mitochondria does not oxidize intramitochondrial GSH and it is therefore a non penetrant —SH reagent, this inhibition is probably the result of the inhibition of glutamine carrier rather than glutaminase. In addition the inhibition of PDG by NEM does not lead to the inhibition of glutamine transport.

The activity of PDG and its inhibition by mersalyl is greatly influenced by volume changes of the mitochondria. Swelling of the mitochondria induced by energization or by a hypotonic solution increases the activity of PDG probably due to the stimulation of glutamine transport. In the presence of mersalyl energized mitochondria shrink whereas deenergized mitochondria swell. It is very probable that swelling increases accessibility of the functional —SH groups of glutamine carrier to glutamine and mersalyl. For this reason the swelling increases glutamine transport and the inhibitory effect of mersalyl.

SUMMARY

Experiments carried out with rat kidney mitochondria showed a correlation between the amount of different —SH reagents and the inhibition of PDG activity in intact and lysed mitochondria. The amount of mersalyl which completely inhibits PDG does not penetrate the inner mitochondrial membrane since it does not oxidize intramitochondrial GSH. This suggests that mersalyl primarily inhibits glutamine carrier rather than the enzyme. The inhibition of PDG by NEM does not inhibit the influx of [^{14}C]glutamine indicating that the activity of the enzyme is not necessary for the transport of glutamine.

If the mitochondria swell in a hypotonic solution PDG activity is increased 2–3 times but the membrane is not freely permeable for glutamine since mersalyl inhibits influx of [^{14}C]glutamine. This suggests that transport of glutamine is the rate-limiting step in the enzyme activity and that swelling increases glutamine influx by a specific carrier-mediated process. Energized mitochondria do not swell in the presence of mersalyl even in a hypotonic solution indicating significant volume changes in the presence of this —SH reagent. These and other data suggest that swelling of the mitochondria leads to unmasking of the functional —SH groups of glutamine carrier resulting in the stimulation of its activity and the increase of the inhibitory effect of mersalyl.

REFERENCES

Azzone G. F. & Massari S. (1973) Active transport and binding in mitochondria. *Biochim. biophys. Acta* **301**, 195–226.

Chappell J. B. (1968) Systems Used for Transport of Substrates into mitochondria. *Br. Med. Bull.* **24**, 150–157.

Curthoys N. P. & Shapiro R. A. (1978) Effect of metabolic acidosis and of phosphate on the presence of glutamine within the matrix space of rat renal mitochondria during glutamine transport. *J. biol. Chem.* **235**, 63–68.

Jocelyn P. C. (1976) The reduction of diamide by rat liver mitochondria and the role of glutathione. *Biochem. J.* **176**, 449–664.

Kovačević Z., Breberina M., Pavlović M. & Bajin K. (1979) Molecular form and kinetic properties of phosphate-dependent glutaminase in the mitochondria isolated from the kidneys of normal acidotic rats. *Biochim. biophys. Acta* **567**, 216–224.

Kovačević Z. (1976) Importance of the flux of phosphate across the inner membrane of kidney mitochondria for the activation of glutaminase and the transport of glutamine. *Biochim. biophys. Acta* **430**, 399–412.

Kovačević Z., McGivan J. D. & Chappell J. B. (1970) Conditions for activity of glutaminase in kidney mitochondria. *Biochem. J.* **118**, 265–274.

Kvamme E., Svenneby G. & Tveit B. (1968) *Regulation of Enzyme Activity and Allosteric Interactions* (Edited by Kvamme E. & Pihl A. pp. 89–108, Universitetsforlaget, Oslo and Academic Press, London.

Tannen R. L. (1978) Ammonia metabolism. *Am. J. Physiol.* **235**, F265–F277.

SYMPOSIUM DISCUSSION

Jorgensen: At low concentrations of NEM and DTNB you found stimulation of enzyme activity, How do you explain this?

Kovacevic: I cannot.

Koepsell: You showed that the alterations in the osmolarity did not alter the inhibition by mersalyl and concluded that mersalyl acts on the carrier protein, but we have found, in studies with the Na-K-ATPase, that alteration of the osmolarity alters the degree of inhibition by SH-group reagents.

Kovacevic: But in this case, there is a membrane between glutaminase and the substrate and even after swelling, the membrane is still impermeable to glutamine, so that mersalyl may still be inhibiting transport.

Schoolwerth: I want to ask Dr Curthoys or Dr Kovacevic whether they have used chloroketone in the presence of mersalyl?

Curthoys: We have not done that experiment, however, our experiments with chloroketone suggest that even when you have limited the enzyme, transport continues, and you can still demonstrate movement across the membrane.

Kovacevic: That is a similar result to our finding with NEM.

Int. J. Biochem., Vol. 12, pp. 145 to 149
0020-711X/80/0701-0145$02.00/0

EFFECT OF AMINOOXYACETATE AND α-KETOGLUTARATE ON GLUTAMATE DEAMINATION BY RAT KIDNEY MITOCHONDRIA

ANTON C. SCHOOLWERTH, WANDA J. HOOVER, CATHERINE H. DANIEL and KATHRYN F. LANOUE

Departments of Medicine and Physiology, The Milton S. Hershey Medical Center, The Pennsylvania State University, Hershey, PA 17033, U.S.A.

Abstract—1. Glutamate dehydrogenase flux by rat kidney mitochondria incubated with 1 mM glutamine plus 2–3 mM glutamate was stimulated by aminooxyacetate. This effect was inhibited by α-ketoglutarate.

2. Studies with intact mitochondria and mitochondrial sonicates revealed a linear inverse relationship between glutamate deamination and α-ketoglutarate levels.

3. The data revealed that α-ketoglutarate is a competitive inhibitor of glutamate dehydrogenase with an apparent K_i of 0.6 mM.

4. The data suggest that aminooxyacetate stimulates glutamate deamination by a mechanism mediated by α-ketoglutarate.

INTRODUCTION

The mitochondria, which contain the major ammoniagenic enzymes, glutaminase and glutamate dehydrogenase, have recently become the focus for studies on the control of renal ammoniagenesis. These studies (Adam & Simpson, 1974; Simpson & Adam, 1975; Goldstein, 1975) have suggested that the mitochondrial transport and deamidation of glutamine are rate-limiting processes for the augmented ammonia production in chronic metabolic acidosis. Recent studies from our laboratory (Schoolwerth *et al.*, 1978) and others (Kunin & Tannen, 1979) have indicated that the mitochondrial transport and metabolism of glutamate may also play a major role in the accelerated ammonia synthesis in metabolic acidosis. These studies have demonstrated that external glutamate enters rat kidney mitochondria primarily by exchange with internal aspartate, a process linked to intramitochondrial transamination by glutamate oxalacetate transaminase. Glutamate entry on the glutamate-hydroxyl carrier is minimal and glutamate for deamination by glutamate dehydrogenase is generated inside the matrix space by the deamidation of transported glutamine. In the presence of physiological concentrations of glutamine and glutamate, mitochondrial glutamate utilization occurs almost exclusively by transamination, a reaction yielding no ammonia. Glutamate deamination under these conditions is negligible. However, in metabolic acidosis, flux through glutamate dehydrogenase is accelerated markedly and contributes one-half of the augmented ammonia synthesis.

The data suggested that competition for glutamate existed between glutamate dehydrogenase and glutamate oxalacetate transaminase. In mitochondria from control rats, the transaminase competed much more effectively for substrate. Although glutamate dehydrogenase competed ineffectively for substrate in control, it did so considerably more effectively in acidosis. To test the possibility that competition for glutamate existed between the two enzymes, studies were performed with aminooxyacetate, a potent transaminase inhibitor. It was reasoned that if competition for glutamate existed, inhibition of glutamate transamination should result in stimulation of glutamate deamination. The studies (Schoolwerth & LaNoue, 1980) demonstrated that in the presence of both glutamine and glutamate in the incubation medium, aminooxyacetate resulted in a stimulation of glutamate dehydrogenase flux by rat kidney mitochondria. Moreover, careful analysis of the data suggested the possibility that the effect of aminooxyacetate was mediated by α-ketoglutarate. To provide further insight into the stimulation of glutamate deamination resulting from aminooxyacetate, additional studies were performed which indicated that the effect of this inhibitor was indeed mediated by α-ketoglutarate.

MATERIALS AND METHODS

Chronic metabolic acidosis was induced in male Sprague–Dawley rats by providing 0.28 M ammonium chloride as the sole source of drinking water for 7 days. Renal cortical mitochondria from control and acidotic rats were isolated and purified as previously described (Schoolwerth *et al.*, 1978; Schoolwerth & LaNoue, 1980). Intact mitochondria (3–5 mg. ml^{-1}) were incubated at 28°C in a medium containing 120 mM KCl, 10 mM Tris–HCl, 20 mM KH_2PO_4, 20 mM MOPS, 5 mM $MgCl_2$, 0.1 mM malate, 0.2 mM ADP, 30 mM glucose, hexokinase (6 units ml^{-1}), 7% Dextran, 1 mM glutamine and 2–3 mM glutamate, pH 7.4. When utilized, aminooxyacetate was present in a concentration of 2 mM. α-Ketoglutarate was added as indicated in the text. Following a 4 min period, the medium and mitochondrial pellet were separated by silicone oil filtration (Schoolwerth *et al.*, 1978). The changes in medium ammonia (Nazar & Schoolwerth, 1979), glutamate and aspartate were measured enzymatically, allowing calculation of enzyme fluxes in the intact mitochondria as previously described (Schoolwerth *et al.*, 1978). When aspartate was measured in the presence of aminooxyacetate, 5 mM distilled acetaldehyde was included in the assay mixture. Glutamate was measured in mitochondrial pellets

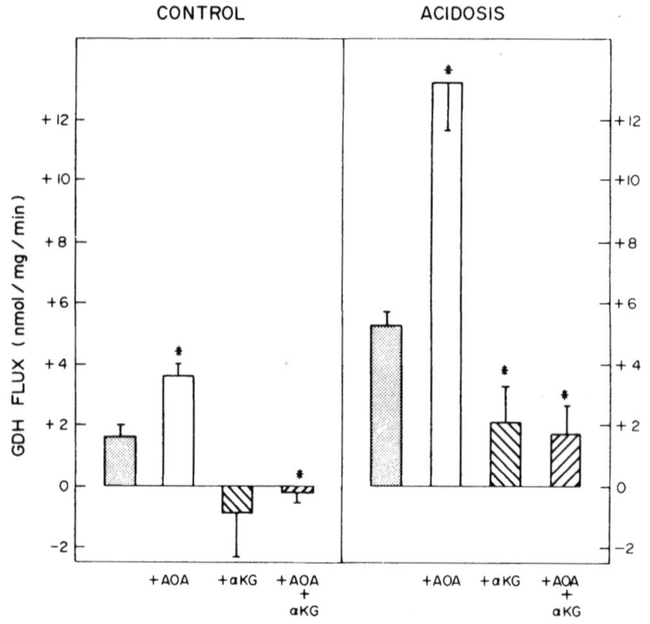

Fig. 1. Effect of aminooxyacetate and α-ketoglutarate on glutamate dehydrogenase flux by intact rat kidney mitochondria. Mitochondria from control and acidotic rats were incubated with 1 mM glutamine + 3 mM glutamate + additions listed at the bottom of the figure. When added, aminooxyacetate (AOA) and α-ketoglutarate (αKG) were present in concentrations of 2 mM and 1 mM, respectively. Changes in medium ammonia, glutamate and aspartate were measured allowing calculations of glutamate dehydrogenase (GDH) flux. The data are presented as mean ± SE for 8–12 observations. *, significantly different from data without additions (dark bars) in each group, $P < 0.02$.

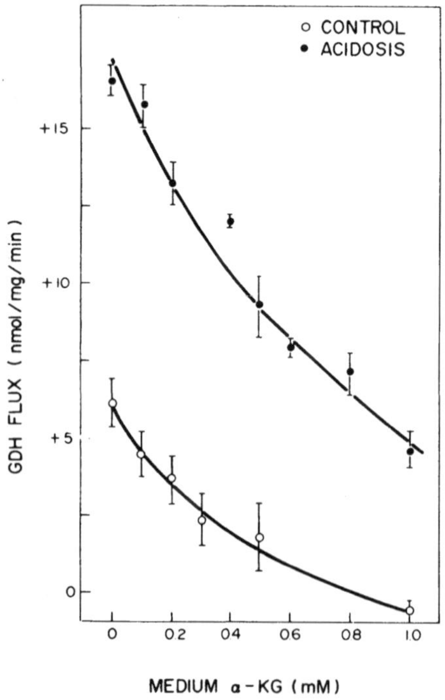

Fig. 2. Effect of α-ketoglutarate (αKG) on glutamate dehydrogenase (GDH) flux. Mitochondria from control (○) and acidotic (●) rats were incubated with 1 mM glutamine + 2 mM glutamate + 2 mM aminooxyacetate in the absence and presence of added αKG, in concentrations listed on the ordinate. Mean ± SE GDH flux was plotted as a function of medium αKG concentration. $n = 4$.

and matrix glutamate concentrations were calculated on the basis of mitochondrial spaces. Glutamate dehydrogenase activity in mitochondrial sonicates was determined spectrophotometrically in the direction of glutamate deamination by a modification of the method of McGivan *et al.* (1974) as previously described (Schoolwerth *et al.*, 1978; Schoolwerth & LaNoue, 1980).

RESULTS

To investigate the possibility that aminooxyacetate may stimulate glutamate dehydrogenase flux by

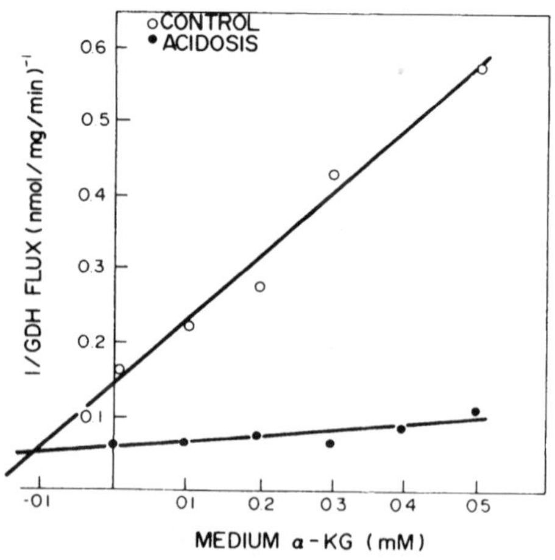

Fig. 3. The data from Figure 2 were linearized by plotting the reciprocal of mean glutamate dehydrogenase (GDH) flux versus medium α-ketoglutarate (αKG) concentration.

reducing α-ketoglutarate formation, experiments were performed in which mitochondria were incubated with added α-ketoglutarate. The data are shown in Fig. 1. Mitochondria from control and acidotic rats were incubated with 1 mM glutamine plus 3 mM glutamate. Addition to the medium of aminooxyacetate resulted in a stimulation of glutamate dehydrogenase flux. This stimulation was completely abolished by the addition of 1 mM α-ketoglutarate. An inhibitory effect of added α-ketoglutarate was evident both in the presence and absence of aminooxyacetate. Of note is the fact that glutamate dehydrogenase flux was inhibited by α-ketoglutarate to a greater degree in mitochondria from control rats. Analysis of additional data obtained in these experiments (not shown) revealed that the changes in glutaminase flux paralleled those of glutamate dehydrogenase. Moreover, a linear inverse relationship between glutaminase flux and matrix glutamate levels was noted, particularly in mitochondria from acidotic rats.

Further studies were performed utilizing physiological concentrations of α-ketoglutarate. In this series of experiments (Fig. 2), mitochondria were incubated with 1 mM glutamine + 2 mM glutamate + 2 mM aminooxyacetate. α-Ketoglutarate was added to the medium in concentrations ranging from 0.1 to 1.0 mM. The data indicate a concentration dependent inhibition by α-ketoglutarate of glutamate dehydrogenase flux with significant inhibition apparent at low levels of the ketoacid. When data from these experiments were replotted (Fig. 3), a linear inverse relationship between glutamate dehydrogenase flux and medium α-ketoglutarate was apparent in mitochondria from both control and acidotic rats. One would expect plots of this sort to be linear if the α-ketoglutarate is directly proportional to matrix α-ketoglutarate levels and if the supply of substrate is constant for a given line. We have not yet completed studies with this experimental protocol measuring matrix α-ketoglutarate levels but have no reason to doubt that these levels will be proportional to medium concentrations under these conditions. Matrix glutamate levels varied only slightly with each group of rats, 0.96 ± 0.06 and 2.00 ± 0.11 nmol. mg protein^{-1} in control and acidosis, respectively. The data suggest that α-ketoglutarate inhibits glutamate dehydrogenase, possibly competitively, in the physiologic range. Since V_{max} of glutamate dehydrogenase may not be a constant in these two preparations, the value of I (α-ketoglutarate) at the point of intersection of the two lines has no special significance. However, the fact that the slope of the line drawn is much steeper in the case of the control data than the acidotic data is significant and suggested the possibility that the K_i might be different in the two preparations. Further experiments were thus conducted with mitochondrial sonicates where the environment of the enzyme could be more stringently controlled.

To assess the effect of α-ketoglutarate directly and to obtain a K_i for α-ketoglutarate in both control and acidosis, glutamate dehydrogenase activity was measured in sonicates with various concentrations of substrate and inhibitor. The data were analyzed by Dixon plots and are shown in Fig. 4. Since initial rates were measured at a time when ammonia levels were negligible, the effects of α-ketoglutarate do not represent increased activity of glutamate dehydrogenase in the reverse direction but rather a direct effect on the enzyme. The data show that α-ketoglutarate is a competitive inhibitor of the enzyme. The apparent inhibitory constant, K_i was 0.6 mM in both control and acidosis.

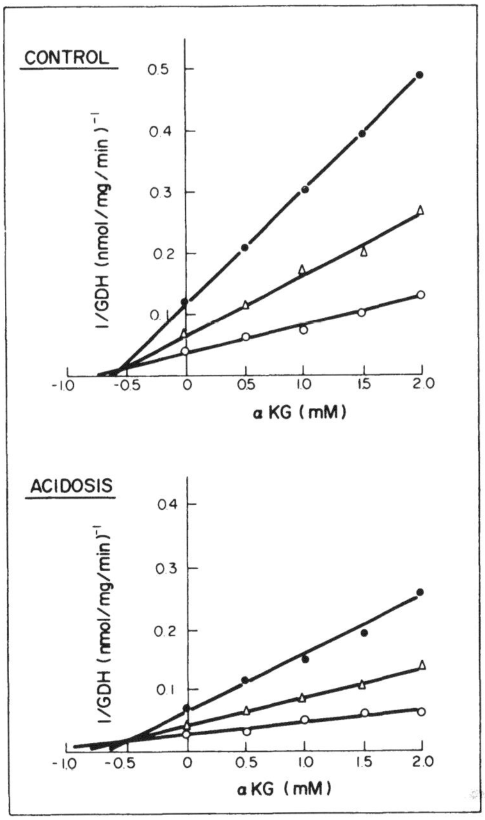

Fig. 4. Effect of α-ketoglutarate on glutamate dehydrogenase (GDH) activity in mitochondrial sonicates. Mitochondrial sonicates from kidneys of control and acidotic rats were prepared as previously described (Schoolwerth *et al.*, 1978). GDH activity was measured spectrophotometrically with different glutamate concentrations in the absence and presence of α-ketoglutarate (αKG) in a medium containing 120 mM KCl, 10 mM Tris-HCl, 1 mM NAD^+, 2 mM ADP, 1 mM EDTA and 1 μg/mg^{-1} protein rotenone at pH 7.2 and 25°C. The initial rate of increase in absorbance at 340 nm on addition of enzyme was recorded. Glutamate concentrations utilized were 5 mM (●), 10 mM (Δ) and 25 mM (O). The data are plotted as a Dixon plot. The apparent K_i for αKG in both control and acidosis was 0.6 mM.

When the kinetic parameters of glutamate dehydrogenase were measured in the sonicates in the absence of α-ketoglutarate it was found that the K_m was 14 mM in both the control and acidotic preparations, but that the V_{max} was 64.6 nmol. mg^{-1}. min in control and 114 nmol. mg.$^{-1}$ min in acidosis. From further comparison of control and acidotic data it is apparent that the slope of the line relating glutamate dehydrogenase flux to inhibitor concentration for any given substrate concentration is higher in controls than acidotic mitochondrial sonicates. In the sonicates this is due solely to the fact that the V_{max} of the dehydrogenase is higher in acidosis than in the controls. However, the large difference in slope of the lines relating flux to inhibitor concentration in the intact mitochondria (Fig. 3) cannot be explained entirely by the differences in V_{max} and the matrix glutamate levels.

DISCUSSION

Previous studies from our laboratory (Schoolwerth & LaNoue, 1980) have demonstrated that the addition of glutamate to the medium of mitochondria incubated with glutamine resulted in a decrease in glutamate dehydrogenase flux. However, in the presence of aminooxyacetate, the addition of external glutamate resulted in a simulation of flux through glutamate dehydrogenase. With 2–3 mM glutamate in the medium, the addition of aminooxyacetate to control mitochondria resulted in a stimulation of flux similar to that observed in mitochondria from acidotic rats incubated without aminooxyacetate. The data thus suggested that aminooxyacetate, a transaminase inhibitor, could simulate the effects of metabolic acidosis on glutamate deamination by rat kidney mitochondria. Moreover, since a linear inverse correlation was noted between glutamate dehydrogenase flux and α-ketoglutarate production, calculated as the sum of glutamate transamination and deamination, it was suggested that the effect of aminooxyacetate was mediated by α-ketoglutarate.

The present studies provide more direct evidence that α-ketoglutarate is a competitive inhibitor of glutamate dehydrogenase in rat kidney. α-Ketoglutarate inhibited glutamate dehydrogenase flux and completely abolished the stimulatory effect of aminooxyacetate on glutamate deamination. Moreover, this effect was evident at low levels of α-ketoglutarate, providing suggestive evidence for the physiological significance of this effect. It was possible to calculate an apparent inhibitory constant for α-ketoglutarate utilizing mitochondrial sonicates. These data indicated that α-ketoglutarate is a competitive inhibitor of the enzyme with a K_i of 0.6 mM.

It is interesting that in intact mitochondria, but not in sonicates, α-ketoglutarate appears to be a much less effective inhibitor in acidosis compared to controls. It has been noted in our laboratory previously (Schoolwerth & LaNoue, 1980) that glutamate formed from glutaminase in mitochondria from acidotic rats appears to have better access to glutamate dehydrogenase than the glutamate similarly formed in control mitochondria. We have proposed that channeling of glutamate to its dehydrogenase occurs in intact mitochondria and that the efficiency of this channeling is increased in acidosis. The improved access of glutamate to glutamate dehydrogenase in acidosis would account for the diminished inhibitory effect of α-ketoglutarate in acidosis.

A variety of data have suggested an important physiological role for α-ketoglutarate in renal ammoniagenesis. α-Ketoglutarate levels in renal tissue have been shown to decrease markedly in metabolic acidosis (Hems & Brosnan, 1971). Moreover, α-ketoglutarate has been shown to inhibit renal ammonia formation *in vivo* and *in vitro* (Balagura-Baruch *et al.*, 1970; Goldstein, 1976; Goldstein & Boylan, 1978). The data of Goldstein (1976) suggested that α-ketoglutarate inhibited glutamine transport and/or deamidation directly. In the present studies, glutaminase flux paralleled the changes in glutamate dehydrogenase flux and was inversely related to matrix glutamate concentration. These findings suggest that the inhibition of glutamate dehydrogenase flux by α-ketoglutarate may increase matrix glutamate levels which in turn inhibit glutaminase. These studies therefore suggest that enhanced flux through glutamate dehydrogenase, and glutaminase, may relate in part to reduced tissue α-ketoglutarate levels which occur in metabolic acidosis *in vivo*.

Acknowledgements—The assistance of Sandra Flowers in the preparation of the manuscript is kindly appreciated. This research was supported by Grant AM- 19714 from the National Institutes of Health and by Grant PCM78-23163 from the National Science Foundation.

REFERENCES

ADAM W. & SIMPSON D. P. (1974) Glutamine transport in rat kidney mitochondria in metabolic acidosis. *J. clin. Invest.* **54,** 165–174.

BALAGURA-BARUCH S., SHURLAND L. M. & WELBOURNE T. C. (1970) Effects of α-ketoglutarate on renal ammonia release in the intact dog. *Am. J. Physiol.* **218,** 1070–1075.

GOLDSTEIN L. (1975) Glutamine transport by mitochondria isolated from normal and acidotic rats. *Am. J. Physiol.* **229,** 1027–1033.

GOLDSTEIN L. (1976) α-Ketoglutarate regulation of glutamine transport and deamidation by renal mitochondria. *Biochem. biophys. Res. Commun.* **70,** 1136–1141.

GOLDSTEIN L. & BOYLAN J. M. (1978) Renal mitochondrial glutamine transport and metabolism: studies with a rapid-mixing, rapid-filtration technique. *Am. J. Physiol.* **234,** F514–F521 or *Am. J. Physiol.*: Renal Fluid Electrolyte Physiology **3,** F514–F521.

HEMS D. A. & BROSNAN J. T. (1971) Effects of metabolic acidosis and starvation on the content of intermediary metabolites in rat kidney. *Biochem. J.* **123,** 391–397.

KUNIN A. S. & TANNEN R. L. (1979) Regulation of glutamate metabolism by renal cortical mitochondria. *Am. J. Physiol.* **237,** F55–F62 or *Am. J. Physiol.*: *Renal Fluid Electrolyte Physiology* **6,** F55–F62.

MCGIVAN J. D., BRADFORD N. M. & CHAPPELL J. B. (1974) Adaptive changes in the capacity of systems used for the synthesis of citrulline in rat liver mitochondria in response to high- and low-protein diets. *Biochem. J.* **142,** 359–364.

NAZAR B. L. & SCHOOLWERTH A. C. (1979) An improved microfluorometric enzymatic assay for the determination of ammonia. *Analyt. Biochem.* **95,** 507–511.

SCHOOLWERTH A. C., NAZAR B. L. & LANOUE K. F. (1978) Glutamate dehydrogenase activation and ammonia formation by rat kidney mitochondria. *J. biol. Chem.* **253,** 6177–6183.

SCHOOLWERTH A. C. & LANOUE K. F. (1980) The role of microcompartmentation in the regulation of glutamate metabolism by rat kidney mitochondria. *J. biol. Chem.* In press.

SIMPSON D. P. & ADAM W. (1975) Glutamine transport and metabolism by mitochondria from dog renal cortex. *J. biol. Chem.* **350,** 8148–8158.

SYMPOSIUM DISCUSSION

Bogusky: Your data convinced me, Dr Schoolwerth, that glutamate dehydrogenase may not be an equilibrium enzyme in kidney as it is in liver.

Lemieux: Did you measure the concentration of aspartate before and after the addition of AOA?

Schoolwerth: Yes, aspartate can be measured enzymatically if acetaldehyde is added to the incubation medium. We found that aminooxyacetate completely inhibited aspartate formation in isolated mitochondria.

Int. J. Biochem., Vol. 12, pp. 151 to 155
© Pergamon Press Ltd 1980. Printed in Great Britain

0020-711X/80/0701-0151$02.00/0

EFFECT OF pH ON METABOLISM OF THE GLUTAMINE CARBON SKELETON BY RENAL CORTICAL MITOCHONDRIA

ARTHUR S. KUNIN
Department of Medicine, University of Vermont College of Medicine, Burlington, VT 05401, U.S.A.

and

RICHARD L. TANNEN
Department of Medicine, University of Michigan Medical School, Ann Arbor, MI 48109, U.S.A.

Abstract—1. To determine the effect of altered acid–base homeostasis on the intramitochondrial metabolism of the glutamine carbon skeleton $^{14}CO_2$ production from [U-^{14}C]glutamine by isolated rat renal cortical mitochondria was measured.

2. Mitochondria from rats with chronic metabolic acidosis either showed no change or diminished $^{14}CO_2$ production in comparison with pair fed controls.

3. By contrast, when the pH of the medium incubating mitochondria from normal rats was manipulated (pH 7.0, 7.4, 7.7), $^{14}CO_2$ production was clearly altered, but the direction and magnitude of the change depended on the glutamine concentration used (0.5 or 10.0 mM).

4. Mitochondria produced significant quantities of $^{14}CO_2$ when [1,4 ^{14}C]succinate was used as substrate, indicating that $^{14}CO_2$ production from glutamine does not originate solely from the decarboxylation of α KG.

5. Thus chronic acidosis and pH, per se, affect intramitochondrial glutamine carbon skeleton metabolism in different fashions, but the specific mechanism cannot be elucidated using $^{14}CO_2$ production from [U-^{14}C]glutamine.

6. Additional studies directly quantitating the metabolic products of glutamine have confirmed these findings and more precisely defined the sites of metabolic alteration.

INTRODUCTION

Conversion of the carbon skeleton of glutamine to glucose by rat renal cortex is accelerated in chronic metabolic acidosis, presumably due to an increase in activity of the rate limiting cytoplasmic enzyme phosphoenolpyruvate carboxykinase (Alleyne & Scullard, 1969; Flores & Alleyne, 1971). Incubation of renal tissue at low pH also stimulates glucose formation, but the mechanism is unknown (Goodman *et al.*, 1966; Alleyne *et al.*, 1973; Irias & Greenberg, 1972; Kamm *et al.*, 1967; Nagata & Rasmussen, 1970; Preuss, 1971). The direct influence, if any, of acid–base perturbations on the intramitochondrial metabolism of the carbon skeleton of glutamine is unclear. In one previous report $^{14}CO_2$ formation from [U-^{14}C]glutamine by isolated renal cortical mitochondria was unaltered by metabolic acidosis but stimulated by incubation at a low pH (Simpson & Sherrard, 1969). However, in studies from another laboratory a decrease in $^{14}CO_2$ formation at a low pH was observed (Kurokawa & Rasmussen, 1973). In view of these conflicting results and observations with intact renal tissue indicating that tracer methodology might lead to spurious conclusions (Vinay *et al.*, 1978), we reinvestigated this issue.

MATERIALS AND METHODS

Renal cortical mitochondria isolated from male Sprague–Dawley rats were incubated as described previously (Tannen & Kunin, 1976a,b; Kunin & Tannen, 1979a] with 0.5 to 10 mM L-[U-^{14}C]glutamine (New England Nuclear Corporation). In some studies, tracer amounts of [1,4-^{14}C]succinate (New England Nuclear Corporation) were added to flasks containing 0.5 mM succinate. After incubation for 10–20 min, 0.3 ml of Hyamine hydroxide, 10 × (Packard) was injected through the serum stoppers into a suspended plastic center well, followed immediately by the rapid injection of 1 ml of 1 M perchloric acid into the incubation mixtures to stop the reaction and release CO_2. Shaking was resumed for 30 min to allow complete diffusion of $^{14}CO_2$ into the Hyamine. The plastic center wells containing Hyamine were then transferred into counting vials, 10 ml of a toluene phosphor system added and radioactivity assayed with a Packard Tricarb Liquid Scintillation Spectrometer. The phosphor system contained 0.3% 2,5-diphenyloxazole and 0.01% p-bis (5-phenyloxozolyl-2) benzene in toluene. Counting efficiency was consistently between 80–82%. Mitochondrial protein was determined by the biuret reaction.

Studies utilizing intact renal cortical mitochondria isolated from rats with chronic metabolic acidosis or potassium deficiency, as well as incubations with mitochondria from normal rats at different media pHs (7.0, 7.4 and 7.7, achieved by equimolar manipulation of bicarbonate and chloride concentration), were carried out in paired fashion as described previously (Tannen & Kunin, 1976a,b).

These data are reported as nmol $CO_2 . min^{-1} . mg^{-1}$ mitochondrial protein. Statistics were performed using paired or non-paired Student's *t*-test.

RESULTS

Preliminary studies confirmed that $^{14}CO_2$ production was linear during the period of incubation chosen.

Table 1. Effect of chronic metabolic acidosis or potassium depletion on mitochondrial $^{14}CO_2$ production from [U-^{14}C]glutamine

	1.0 mM Gln		10.0 mM Gln	
	nmol CO_2/mg^{-1}·min^{-1}			
	Normal	Acidotic	Normal	Acidotic
Mean	37.4	32.4	48.1	36.1
SE	+3.3	±1.7	±4.4	±3.5
n	7		7	
P	NS		<0.01	
	Normal	K^+ Dep.	Normal	K^+ Dep.
Mean	31.6	30.4	37.6	32.6
SE	±1.2	±2.3	±2.7	±2.4
n	7		7	
P	NS		<0.05	

The effect of either chronic metabolic acidosis or potassium deficiency on $^{14}CO_2$ formation from glutamine is shown in Table 1. With both conditions $^{14}CO_2$ production is unchanged with 1.0 mM glutamine as substrate and significantly decreased in comparison with pair fed controls when 10 mM glutamine is used.

The results of experiments in which mitochondria from normal rats were incubated at three different medium pHs are shown in Table 2. The results are dependent on the concentration of media glutamine used. With 0.5 mM glutamine $^{14}CO_2$ production from [U-^{14}C]glutamine is lowest at pH 7.7; while with 10 mM glutamine $^{14}CO_2$ production is lowest at pH 7.0.

To determine whether $^{14}CO_2$ formation from [U-^{14}C]glutamine resulted solely from decarboxylation of alpha ketoglutarate to succinate, mitochondria from normal animals were incubated at pH 7.4 with 0.5 mM, 1,4-^{14}C-labeled succinate. Preliminary studies indicated that $^{14}CO_2$ production was negligible with 2,3-^{14}C-labeled succinate. In seven studies $^{14}CO_2$ production from [1,4 ^{14}C]succinate averaged 6.0 ± 0.8 nmol.min^{-1}.mg^{-1}. Thus a significant fraction of the $^{14}CO_2$ produced during incubations with glutamine originates from substrate decarboxylation subsequent to succinate, in spite of the absence of any 2 carbon donor added to the incubation medium.

In a series of separate studies performed under identical conditions intramitochondrial metabolism of alpha ketoglutarate was quantitated by measuring the key nitrogen and carbon metabolites of glutamine (Kunin & Tannen, 1979a,b). A comparison of these data with the experiments measuring $^{14}CO_2$ generation yielded reasonable similarity.

Table 2. Effect of alterations in medium pH on mitochondrial $^{14}CO_2$ production from [U-^{14}C]glutamine

	0.5 mM Gln			10 mM Gln		
pH	7.0	7.4	7.7	7.0	7.4	7.7
Mean	27.8	28.5	20.1	29.0	37.1	41.9
SE	±2.1	±2.5	±1.8	±2.0	±2.0	±2.3
n	6	6	6	10	9	8
P		NS	<0.01		<0.01	NS

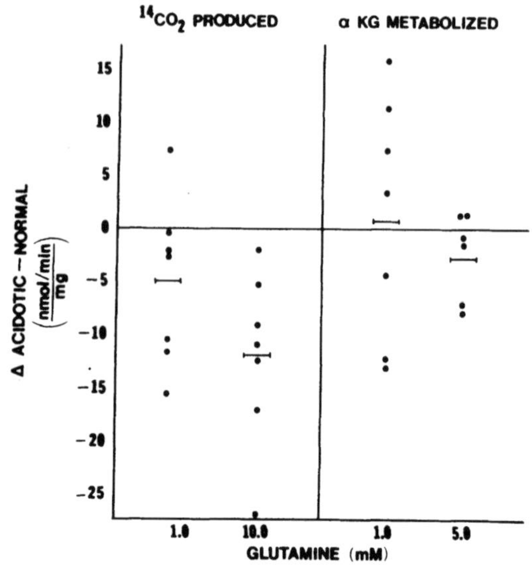

Fig. 1. Effect of chronic acidosis on metabolism of the glutamine carbon skeleton. Each point represents a comparison between mitochondria from a rat with chronic metabolic acidosis and a pair fed control, and the horizontal bar the mean change for the entire group. In this and subsequent figures, the left panel depicts changes in $^{14}CO_2$ production from [U-^{14}C]glutamine, and the right panel changes in directly quantitated αKG metabolized. $^{14}CO_2$ production is unchanged by acidosis at 1.0 mM glutamine and decreased significantly ($P < 0.01$) at 10 mM. αKG metabolized is unchanged at both substrate concentrations.

As shown in Fig. 1, αKG metabolism was unaltered by chronic acidosis using both low and high concentrations of glutamine; $^{14}CO_2$ production was not significantly changed at 1 mM glutamine and was decreased with higher levels of substrate.

Manipulations of pH *in vitro* are shown in Figs 2 and 3. A high pH significantly depresses both $^{14}CO_2$ production and calculated αKG metabolized at low glutamine concentrations, but not at higher substrate levels (i.e. 5 or 10 mM) (Fig. 2). A low pH significantly diminishes both $^{14}CO_2$ production and αKG metabolized at high substrate concentrations, and significantly stimulates αKG metabolized ($P < 0.05$) at 0.5 mM glutamine (Fig. 3). Thus the pattern of response is similar with direct measurement of αKG metabolized and with an indirect assessment utilizing $^{14}CO_2$ production. Although the isotopic technique does not provide a quantitative measure of the decarboxylation of αKG to succinate, it does appear to qualitatively reflect changes in this intramitochondrial process.

DISCUSSION

Since renal ammoniagenesis can be influenced by the metabolism of the glutamine carbon skeleton, metabolic regulation of this process could play an important role in modulating ammonia production (Tannen, 1978). In chronic acidosis the increase in PEPCK activity directly alters metabolism of the carbon products of glutamine in the cytoplasm and may indirectly influence intramitochondrial events. Whether acidosis, or pH per se, directly modifies the

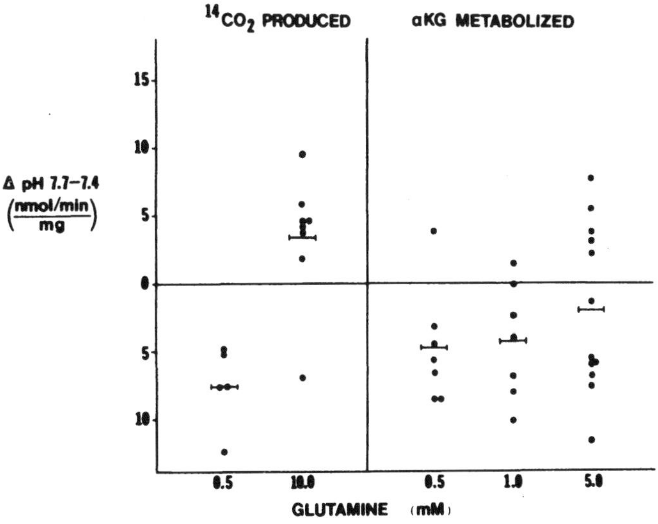

Fig. 2. Effect on an alkaline pH on metabolism of the glutamine carbon skeleton. The data represent a comparison between normal mitochondrial incubated at pH 7.7 and 7.4. $^{14}CO_2$ production is diminished significantly ($P < 0.01$) at 0.5 mM glutamine but unchanged at 10 mM. αKG metabolized is decreased significantly at 0.5 mM ($P < 0.05$) and 1.0 mM ($P < 0.05$), and unchanged at 5 mM.

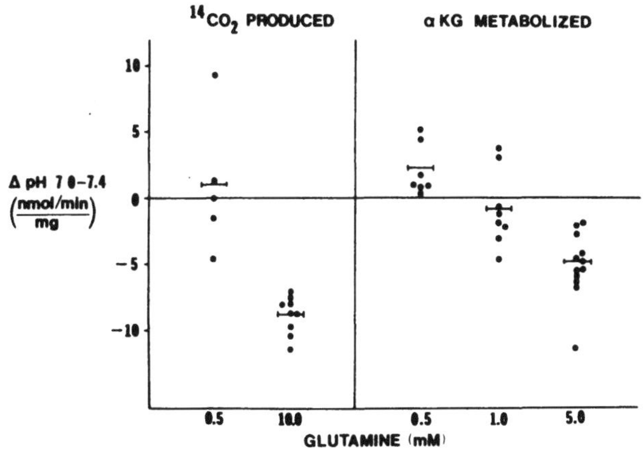

Fig. 3. Effect of an acid pH on metabolism of the glutamine carbon skeleton. The data represent a comparison between normal mitochondria incubated at pH 7.0 and 7.4. $^{14}CO_2$ production is unchanged at 0.5 mM glutamine and decreased significantly ($P < 0.01$) at 10 mM. αKG metabolized is increased significantly at 0.5 mM ($P < 0.05$), unchanged at 1.0 mM, and decreased significantly ($P < 0.001$) at 5 mM glutamine.

intramitochondrial metabolism of the glutamine carbon skeleton is undefined.

Consistent with the prior observation of Simpson & Sherrard (1969) using dogs, our studies of $^{14}CO_2$ generation from [U-^{14}C]glutamine by rat kidney mitochondria suggest that chronic acidosis either has

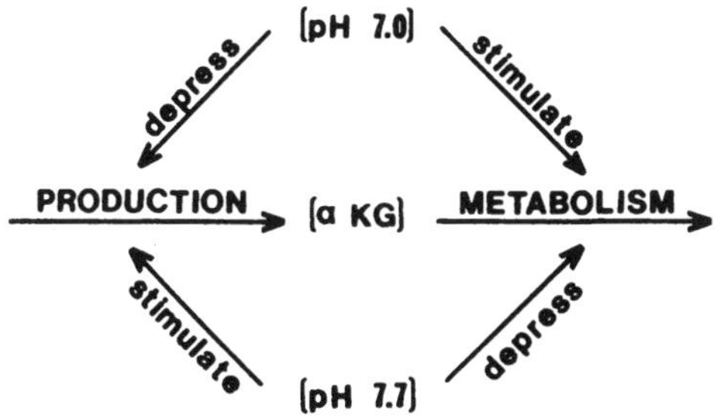

Fig. 4. The influence of pH on intramitochondrial αKG metabolism.

no effect or diminishes intramitochondrial metabolism of the glutamine carbon skeleton. By contrast, pH manipulations of the medium incubating normal mitochondria indicate that pH, *per se*, directly affects mitochondrial glutamine carbon metabolism. The response of $^{14}CO_2$ production to pH manipulations *in vitro* is highly dependent on the glutamine concentration employed, which appears to account for the conflicting findings reported by previous investigators. Simpson and Sherrard, utilizing 0.5 mM glutamine found more $^{14}CO_2$ produced at lower media pHs (Simpson & Sherrard, 1969); while Kurokawa & Rasmussen (1973), utilizing 2 mM glutamine, found a 17% decrease in $^{14}CO_2$ production at a media pH of 7.0 compared with 7.4. Our results, which indicate that a low pH stimulates $^{14}CO_2$ production with low glutamine concentrations but inhibits at high substrate levels, appear to resolve the discrepancy between these earlier reports.

Under the conditions utilized in our experiments, the mitochondria produce significant quantities of $^{14}CO_2$ from labeled succinate, indicating that isotopic CO_2 generation from uniformly labeled glutamine does not solely reflect the decarboxylation of αKG to succinate. With this complexity, as well as the substrate dependence of the response, it is impossible to interpret these observations with $^{14}CO_2$ production in a mechanistic fashion. Nevertheless, they do suggest that chronic acidosis and pH, per se, affect intramitochondrial glutamine carbon skeleton metabolism in a different fashion.

A comparison with studies from our laboratory that assess carbon skeleton metabolism more directly, confirms the qualitative implications of the findings with $^{14}CO_2$ production and clarifies the mechanism responsible for the confusing substrate dependence of the pH response.

In a series of separate studies performed under identical conditions the intramitochondrial metabolism of αKG was quantitated by measuring the key nitrogen and carbon metabolites of glutamine (Kunin & Tannen, 1979a,b). The findings with this approach were reasonably similar to those using $^{14}CO_2$ generation. Both the direct assessment of αKG metabolism as well as the measurement of $^{14}CO_2$ production indicate that chronic acidosis does not directly stimulate the intramitochondrial metabolism of αKG. On the other hand, when pH is manipulated *in vitro*, significant changes are observed with both techniques, but, as shown in Figs 2 and 3, the response is highly dependent on the glutamine concentration used. An acid incubation medium stimulates αKG metabolism at low glutamine concentrations and diminishes it at high substrate levels; while the response to an alkaline pH is the converse, with inhibition at a low glutamine concentrations and no significant change at higher glutamine levels.

Since these studies are carried out with glutamine as substrate the net amount of αKG converted to succinate is dependent on all the factors that influence this enzymatic process, including the amount of substrate available for metabolism. Previous experiments from our laboratory have shown that pH affects the production of αKG from glutamine by isolated mitochondria (Kunin & Tannen, 1979a). When the effect of pH on αKG production and metabolism are considered simultaneously, the data indicate that a low pH depresses production but stimulates the subsequent metabolism of αKG; while a high pH acts in the opposite fashion (Fig. 4). The overall response at a given glutamine concentration depends on which effect predominates, but it seems clear that a low pH favors while a high pH inhibits the intramitochondrial conversion of αKG to succinate.

Thus pH, *per se*, can alter the intramitochondrial metabolism of the glutamine carbon skeleton while chronic acidosis appears to directly modify the cytoplasmic portion of the metabolic pathway. These different sites of action may provide increased flexibility for the regulation of ammonia production during alterations in acid–base homeostasis.

Acknowledgements—These studies were supported by U.S. Public Health Service Grants R01-18251, R01-AM 14225, and R01-AM 25248. A portion of this work was done by Dr Tannen during the tenure of an Established Investigatorship of the American Heart Association. The excellent technical assistance of Mrs P. McHugo and Mr W. Barnes is gratefully acknowledged.

A portion of this work appeared as an abstract in *Clin. Res.* **23,** 367, 1975.

REFERENCES

ALLEYNE G. A. O., FLORES H. & ROOBOL A. (1973) The interrelationship of the concentration of hydrogen ions, bicarbonate ions, carbon dioxide and calcium ions in the regulation of renal gluconeogenesis in the rat. *Biochem. J.* **136,** 445–453.

ALLEYNE G. A. O. & SCULLARD G. H. (1969) Renal metabolic response to acid-base changes. I. Enzymatic control of ammoniagenesis in the rat. *J. clin. Invest.* **48,** 364–370.

FLORES H. & ALLEYNE G. A. (1971) Phosphoenolpyruvate carboxykinase of kidney. Subcellular distribution and response to acid–base changes. *Biochem. J.* **123,** 35–39.

GOODMAN A. D., FUISZ R. E. & CAHILL G. F. (1966) Renal gluconeogenesis in acidosis, alkalosis and potassium deficiency: Its possible role in regulation of renal ammonia production. *J. clin. Invest.* **45,** 612–619.

IRIAS J. J. & GREENBERG R. E. (1972) Relationship of renal gluconeogenesis to control of ammonia production. *Am. J. Physiol.* **223,** 750–755.

KAMM D. E., FUISZ R. E., GOODMAN A. D. & CAHILL G. F. JR (1967) Acid–base alterations and renal gluconeogenesis: Effect of pH, bicarbonate concentration, and pCO_2. *J. clin. Invest.* **46,** 1172–1177.

KUNIN A. S. & TANNEN R. L. (1979a) Regulation of glutamate metabolism by renal cortical mitochondria. *Am. J. Physiol.* **237,** F55–F62.

KUNIN A. S. & TANNEN R. L. (1979b) The effect of H^+ on α-ketoglutarate metabolism by renal cortical mitochondria. *Clin. Res.* **27,** 500A.

KUROKAWA K. & RASMUSSEN H. (1973) Ionic control of renal gluconeogenesis: I. The interrelated effect of calcium and hydrogen ions. *Biochim. biophys. Acta* **313,** 17–31.

NAGATA N. & RASMUSSEN H. (1970) Renal gluconeogenesis: Effects of Ca^{++} and H^+. *Biochim. biophys. Acta* **215,** 1–16.

PREUSS H. G. (1971) Ammonia production from glutamine and glutamate in isolated dog renal tubules. *Am. J. Physiol.* **220,** 54–58.

SIMPSON D. P. & SHERRARD D. J. (1969) Regulation of glutamine metabolism *in vitro* by bicarbonate ion and pH. *J. clin. Invest.* **48,** 1088–1096.

TANNEN R. L. (1978) Ammonia metabolism. *Am. J. Physiol.* **235,** F265–F277.

TANNEN R. L. & KUNIN A. S. (1976a) Effect of potassium on ammoniagenesis by renal mitochondria. *Am. J. Physiol.* **231,** 44–51.

TANNEN R. L. & KUNIN A. S. (1976b) Effect of pH on ammonia production by renal mitochondria. *Am. J. Physiol.* **231,** 1631–1637.

VINAY P., MAPES, J. P. & KREBS H. A. (1978) Fate of glutamine carbon in renal metabolism. *Am. J. Physiol.* **234,** F123–F129.

SYMPOSIUM DISCUSSION

Schoolwerth: We have obtained somewhat different results from experiments in which glutamine alone or glutamine plus physiological concentrations of glutamate were used. When mitochondria were incubated with 1 mM [U-^{14}C]glutamine plus 2 mM cold glutamate, α-ketoglutarate production, measured indirectly by the same method you described, was similar in control and acidosis. However, the specific activity of α-ketoglutarate was two-fold higher in acidosis compared to control. These findings indicate an alteration in the intramitochondrial metabolism of the carbon skeletons of both glutamine and glutamate in acidosis.

Tannen: Our observations focus on metabolism of the α-ketoglutarate formed. There is no reason to suspect that the metabolism of α-ketoglutarate is influenced by its source.

Vinay: Are your results compatible with the increase in glutaminase activity in acidosis?

Tannen: Yes, in acidotic rats. Addition of acid to isolated mitochondria does not evoke the response that is seen in tubules or in isolated perfused kidney. Thus, part of the response may require the presence of cytosol, or even the whole organ, but I don't think that is the whole answer.

Alleyne: How soon do you see the effects of pH on CO_2 production? The fall in α-ketoglutarate concentration in response to acidosis is very rapid, within minutes (see Lowry, discussion to paper by Vinay *et al.*, p. 97, this volume.

Tannen: We see a fall in intramitochondrial 2-oxoglutarate within 2 minutes in response to acidosis in isolated mitochondria, but have not measured the CO_2 production as early as that.

Alleyne: Is the reduction of intracellular pH which Dr Radda reports (p. 277, this volume) in acidosis, 0.2–0.3 pH units, sufficient to explain the fall in 2-oxoglutarate concentration that you see?

Schoolwerth: We find a ΔpH of about 0.4 units between the medium and mitochondrial matrix.

Vinay: How do you explain the persistently low 2-oxoglutarate concentration in kidneys from chronic acidotic rats, in which the pH is almost back to normal?

Alleyne: The key word there is "almost".

Weiner: Since your incubations are carried out without added ADP, could some of the changes be due simply to an effect of pH on respiratory rate?

Tannen: Dr Simpson, who has looked at this, never saw changes in respiratory rate in response to change in pH, except at very low pH's.

Schoolwerth: I agree that it is not necessary to assume that the same factors which initiate response to acidosis are those which maintain it.

Tannen: Dr Brosnan reported an increase in CO_2 production from [1-^{14}C]glutamine in acidotic mitochondria, in contrast to our own studies. The major difference in technique was that Dr Brosnan's study was performed at room temperature, and in the presence of ADP rather than ATP, as in our study. The kinetics of the metabolic pathway may differ at 37°C and room temperature.

Baverel: What do you see as the role of aspartate in regulation of ammonia production?

Tannen: The role of the transaminase reaction in the intact cell is controversial. The purine nucleotide cycle is one of the possible alternatives.

Int. J. Biochem., Vol. 12, pp. 157 to 161
© Pergamon Press Ltd 1980. Printed in Great Britain

0020-711X/80/0701-0157$02.00/0

TRIACYLGLYCEROL METABOLISM IN KIDNEY CORTEX AND OUTER MEDULLA

GABRIELE WIRTHENSOHN, MARGIT GERL and WALTER G. GUDER
Klinisch-chemisches Institut, Städtisches Krankenhaus, München-Schwabing, Kölner Platz 1, 8000 München 40, Federal Republic of Germany

Abstract—1. Triacylglycerol (TAG) metabolism was studied with a fully enzymic method, in tubule fragments from rat kidney cortex and outer medulla isolated by collagenase treatment.

2. TAG content of freshly prepared cortical tubules correlated well with plasma fatty acid levels of the rats.

3. Presence of fatty acids in the incubation medium led to a net synthesis of TAG, whereas TAG content decreased in the absence of fatty acids.

4. Gluconeogenic substrates stimulated TAG synthesis from oleate in cortical tubules. Glucose, which was not stimulatory in the cortex, provided glycerol moieties in the outer medulla.

5. Label from newly formed TAG preincubated with [^{14}C]-oleate was quantitatively recovered in $^{14}CO_2$, indicating oxidative breakdown as the metabolic fate of tubular TAG.

INTRODUCTION

Oxidation of fatty acids has been discussed as an important energy source in kidney cortex. This is indicated by a low respiratory quotient of 0.75 in renal cortex which increases towards the papilla (Hohenegger, 1976). Weidemann & Krebs (1969) provided evidence that fatty acids derived from endogenous triacylglycerols are the main fuel of respiration when no exogenous fatty acids are available.

A decrease in endogenous TAG content without added oleate was found by Huang *et al.* (1971) in the perfused dog kidney and by Hohenegger (1976) in rat kidney cortex slices. On the other hand exogenous fatty acids taken up by the kidney are not completely oxidized (Gold & Spitzer, 1964; Barac-Nieto & Cohen, 1968). Isotope experiments revealed that a major fraction of labeled fatty acids were incorporated in triacylglycerols (Tinker & Hanahan, 1966; Barac-Nieto, 1976). This observation stimulated us to study renal triacylglycerol metabolism with a newly developed fully-enzymic method (Guder & Wirthensohn, 1979) for cellular triacylglycerol.

MATERIALS AND METHODS

Kidney cortex and outer medulla from fed and 24 hr starved male Sprague–Dawley rats (Ivanovas, Kisslegg, F.R.G.) were treated with collagenase to prepare isolated tubule fragments (Guder, 1979). Tubules corresponding to 1–2 mg of protein were incubated in 1 ml Krebs–Henseleit bicarbonate buffer in 20 ml vessels. The NaCl content of the medium was doubled when medullary tubules were incubated (Abodeely & Lee, 1971). Samples were gassed with 95% O_2–5% CO_2 and incubated for 30 or 60 min at 37°C. L-lactate (Serva, Heidelberg, F.R.G.), L-glutamine (C. Roth, Karlsruhe, F.R.G.) and glucose (Merck, Darmstadt, F.R.G.) were added as freshly prepared neutral solutions. Oleate (C. Roth, Karlsruhe, F.R.G.) was bound to albumin (Fraction V, Serva, Heidelberg, F.R.G.) which was purified according to Chen (1967). In all experiments using the oleate–albumin complex, albumin was added to the controls.

Incubation was stopped on ice. After transferring samples into Eppendorf cups tubules were separated from medium by a 5 sec centrifugation at 10,000 *g*. Substrate changes were measured either directly or after deproteinization from the supernatant medium (Wirthensohn & Guder, 1980). The tubule sediments were heated for 3 min at 100°C to destroy endogenous lipases. A lipase–esterase mixture was added to one of two identical samples and glycerol was determined enzymatically (Guder & Wirthensohn, 1979). The difference in glycerol content between lipase-treated sample and control was taken as glyceride-glycerol. The results were nearly identical with those obtained after organic solvent extraction and alkaline hydrolysis (Wirthensohn & Guder, 1980).

In isotope experiments [1-^{14}C]oleate, [2-^{14}C]lactate and [U-^{14}C]glucose (Radiochemical Centre, Amersham, England) were added to the incubation medium in the specific activities indicated in the legends to Table 2 and Fig. 3. In these experiments lipids were extracted with organic solvents and separated by thin layer chromatography. The visualized spots of triacylglycerols and fatty acids were transferred into counting vials and radioactivity was determined in a Packard Tri Carb liquid scintillation counter. $^{14}CO_2$ was collected in 400 μl 2-phenylethylamine (Fluka, Buchs, Switzerland) after addition of sulfuric acid to the samples and a further 60 min incubation at 37°C and counted in a Packard Tri Carb liquid scintillation counter. Diabetic animals and their insulin treated controls were those described in the paper of Le Hir *et al.* (1980).

RESULTS

Freshly prepared tubules from kidney cortex contained different TAG contents which were dependent on the metabolic state of the animal and correlated linearly to plasma fatty acid concentrations (Table 1). Addition of 0.8 mM oleate led to a steady increase in TAG content, whereas endogenous triacylglycerols decreased in the absence of fatty acids (Guder & Wirthensohn 1979, Wirthensohn & Guder 1980). The rate of triacylglycerol synthesis was not significantly different between tubules from fed and starved rats (fed: 21.3 μmols per g protein per hr; starved: 27.1 μmols per g protein per hr).

Metabolic substrates like glutamine, lactate or glucose did not prevent the decrease in endogenous triacylglycerol content (Fig. 1). In the presence of oleate,

Table 1. Triacylglycerol (TAG) content of rat kidney cortex tubules and plasma fatty acid (FA) concentration in different metabolic states

Condition	TAG content (μmols·g protein^{-1})	FA in plasma (μmols·l^{-1})
Fed	9.8 ± 1.1 (8)	268 ± 62 (8)
Starved 24 hr	22.7 ± 1.1 (27)	513 ± 52 (3)
Diabetic (ketotic)	87 (1)	1084 ± 79 (5)
Diabetic + insulin	15 (1)	277 ± 15 (3)

Triacylglycerols were measured enzymatically in freshly prepared tubules as described in the methods section. Plasma fatty acid concentration was determined as described elsewhere (Guder & Wirthensohn, 1979). Diabetic animals and their insulin treated controls were those described in the paper of LeHir *et al.* (1980). Results are given as means ± SEM. The number of tubule preparations tested (TAG determination) or number of rats (plasma fatty acids) is given in parentheses. The TAG content of tubules from diabetic and insulin-treated diabetic rats was measured from a cell pool prepared from 5 and 3 rats respectively.

however, glutamine, lactate and all gluconeogenic substrates tested stimulated triacylglycerol synthesis from oleate significantly. Interestingly, glucose did not show this stimulatory effect. Therefore, we also tested the effect of glucose on triacylglycerol synthesis in tubules from the outer medulla, where higher activities of glycolytic enzymes are present. (Guder & Schmidt, 1976).

As can be seen from Fig. 2 endogenous triacylglycerol content was similar in cortical and outer medullary tubules from fed rats. Oleate stimulated TAG synthesis only slightly in the outer medulla compared to cortex. As expected, glucose stimulated TAG formation in tubules from outer medulla. Lactate had a small stimulatory effect as well. This could be due to the presence of proximal straight tubules in the tubule preparations from outer medulla.

Similar results were obtained when tubules from cortex and outer medulla were incubated with labelled lactate and glucose in the presence of oleate (Table 2). Lactate-label was recovered to a significantly greater extent from TAG of kidney cortex compared to medullary tubules. In contrast glucose was incorporated to a greater extent into TAG of outer medullary cells. After incubation of tubules with lipase the label in the TAG-fraction of medulla and cortex completely disappeared. Lipase treatment did not increase label in the fatty acid fraction.

To examine the fate of the newly formed triacylglycerols we prelabelled cortex tubule triacylglycerols with [1-^{14}C]oleate (Fig. 3). On a second incubation TAG label decreased by about 40% in 60 min in parallel to net TAG decrease. Nearly the same amount of label was recovered as $^{14}CO_2$ in the absence of fatty acids. Addition of unlabelled oleate inhibited the decrease in labelled TAG and labelled $^{14}CO_2$-formation to the same degree.

DISCUSSION

Our results indicate that the kidney is able to synthesize triacylglyceols from exogenous fatty acids and endogenous α-glycerophosphate. The parallelism between endogenous TAG content of tubules and plasma fatty acid levels *in vivo* indicates, that arterial fatty acid concentrations may regulate renal triacylglycerol levels (see also Hohenegger & Schuh, 1980). This is further supported by the fact that net triacylglycerol synthesis is linearly dependent on fatty acid concentrations in the medium (Wirthensohn & Guder, 1980). Earlier findings of Gold & Spitzer 1964), Barac-Nieto & Cohen (1968) and Dies *et al.* (1970) show that fatty acid uptake increases with arterial fatty acid concentrations.

The finding that all gluconeogenic substrates stimulated reesterification rates from oleate in kidney cortex led us to the suggestion that these gluconeogenic substrates may provide the glycerol moiety of the lipids via the gluconeogenic pathway. Since phosphoenol-pyruvate-carboxykinase, EC 4.1.1.32—the rate limiting enzyme in gluconeogenesis—has been found to be exclusively located in the proximal tubule, the glyceroneogenesis from gluconeogenic

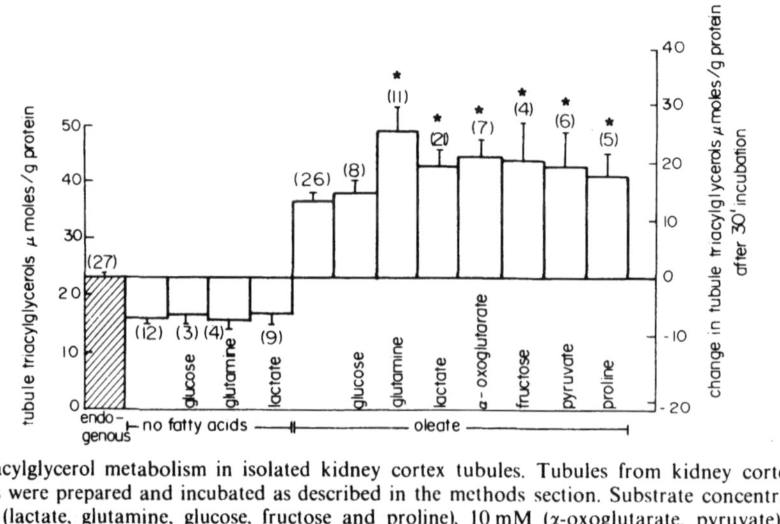

Fig. 1. Triacylglycerol metabolism in isolated kidney cortex tubules. Tubules from kidney cortex of starved rats were prepared and incubated as described in the methods section. Substrate concentration was 5 mM (lactate, glutamine, glucose, fructose and proline), 10 mM (α-oxoglutarate, pyruvate) and 0.8 mM (oleate). Results are given as means with the number of tubule preparations in parentheses. The bars represent SEM. Significance of changes due to added substrates were tested by paired data *t*-test. * $P < 0.01$ vs oleate.

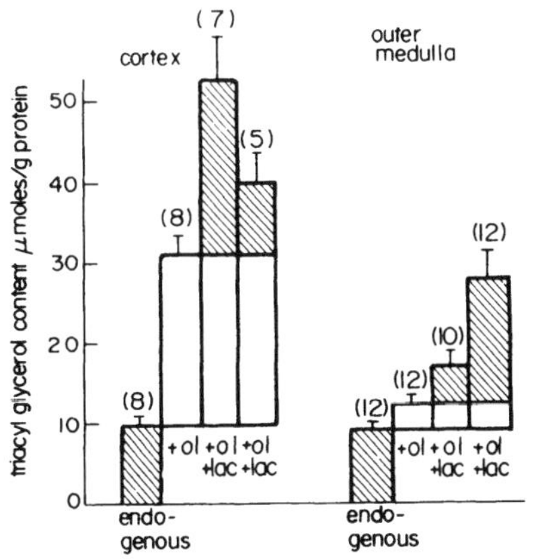

Fig. 2. Comparison of triacylglycerol metabolism in tubules from kidney cortex and outer medulla. Tubules from kidney cortex and outer medulla of fed rats were prepared and incubated as described in the methods section. Substrates added were oleate (0.8 mM), L-lactate (5 mM) and glucose (5 mM). Incubation time was 60 min. Results are given as means with the number of tubule preparations in parentheses. The bars represent SEM.

substrates should also be restricted to this nephron structure.

In contrast, glucose seems to contribute the α-glycerophosphate in the medulla, which is in line with the higher activity of glycolytic enzymes in this part of the kidney (Guder & Schmidt, 1976).

The lack of incorporation of label from [^{14}C]lactate and [^{14}C]glucose into the fatty acid moiety indicates that fatty acid synthesis does not contribute to the increased TAG synthesis observed. This is also supported by the finding that lipogenic enzyme activities (ATP citrate lyase (EC 4.1.3.8.), acetyl-CoA carboxylase (EC 6.4.1.2.) (Fig. 4) and ^3H_2O incorporation into lipids (Hohenegger & Schuh, 1980) is very low. The finding that for every four fatty acids taken up three were recovered in triacylglycerols (Guder & Wirthensohn, 1979) may explain, why under *in vivo* conditions the kidney takes up more fatty acids than can be accounted for by oxidation. In spite of this fact, our findings do not permit any conclusion about the physiological significance of renal triacylglycerols. Barac-Nieto & Cohen (1971) and Hohenegger *et al.* (1978) provided evidence for renal triacylglycerol release into blood stream.

Table 2. Incorporation of labelled precursors in the glycerol-moiety of triacylglycerols (TAG)

	Cortex				Outer medulla			
Labelled precursor	lactate		glucose		lactate		glucose	
Lipid fraction	TAG	FA	TAG	FA	TAG	FA	TAG	FA
cpm incorporated	7620	80	1965	110	885	190	3910	280
After lipase treatment cpm incorporated	165	100	35	50	110	160	110	140

Tubules from cortex and outer medulla of starved rats were incubated with either [2-^{14}C]lactate (5 mM, 1.8 × 10^6 cpm per tube) or [U-^{14}C]glucose (5 mM, 2.4 × 10^6 cpm per tube) in presence of 0.8 mM oleate. Incubation time was 60 min. Incorporation of label in triacylglycerols and fatty acids was measured after extraction and separation of TLC (see method). Results are given as cpm incorporated of a representative experiment.

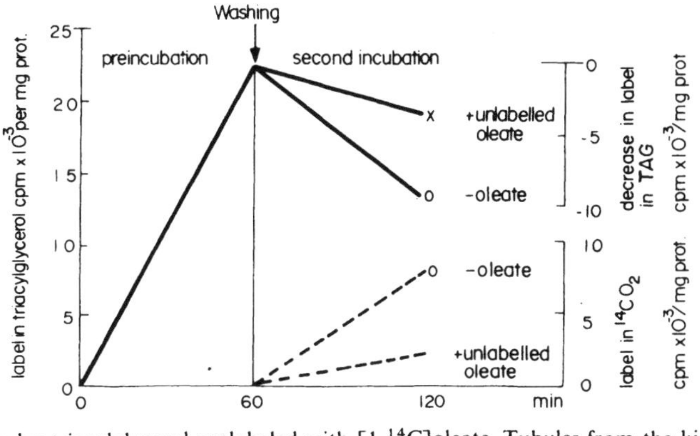

Fig. 3. Fate of tubular triacylglycerol prelabeled with [1-^{14}C]oleate. Tubules from the kidney cortex of starved rats were prepared as described in the methods section and preincubated for 60 min with 0.8 mM [1-^{14}C]oleate (sp.act. 0.125 μCi μmol^{-1}) and 5 mM glutamine. After washing of the tubules a second 60 min incubation was performed. $^{14}CO_2$ was determined as described in the methods section. Labelled triacylglycerols were measured after extraction with organic solvents and separation on TLC in a Tri-Carb liquid scintillation counter. Results are means of 2 experiments.

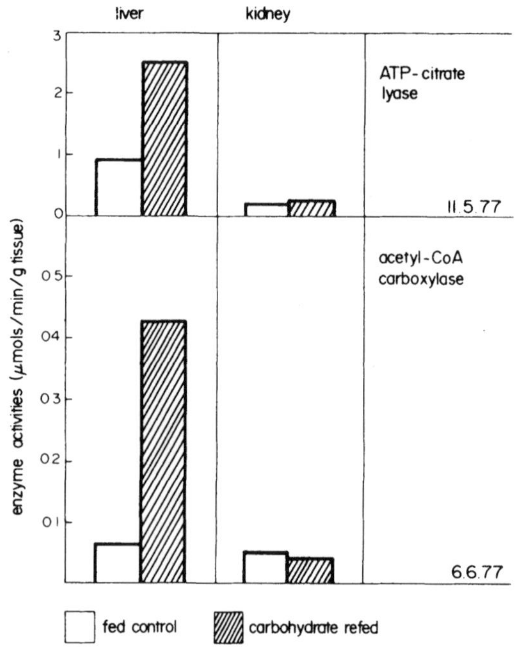

Fig. 4. Enzymes of fatty acid synthesis in rat liver and kidney.

Under our *in vitro* conditions no triacylglycerols could be detected in the medium. On the other hand, TAG fatty acids are thought to be the major fuel of kidney cortex (Weidemann & Krebs, 1969) and outer medulla (Hohenegger, 1976). Since no fatty acids were recovered from the medium when tubular triacylglycerols decreased, they were probably oxidized. The recovery of label from TAG in $^{14}CO_2$ also supports the concept that renal TAG are used as a metabolic fuel to cover tubular energy needs.

Acknowledgements—This work was supported by the Deutsche Forschungsgemeinschaft (project C 41 of the Sonderforschungsbereich 51, München). The help of Mrs H. Kuhn, Mrs E. Rausch and Mrs D. Lehmeier during preparation of this manuscript is gratefully acknowledged.

REFERENCES

ABODEELY D. A. & LEE J. B. (1971) Fuel of respiration of outer renal medulla. *Am. J. Physiol.* **220,** 1693–1700.

BARAC-NIETO M. & COHEN J. J. (1968) Nonesterified fatty acid uptake by dog kidney: effects of probenecid and chlorothiazide. *Am. J. Physiol.* **215,** 98–107.

BARAC-NIETO M. & COHEN J. J. (1971) The metabolic fates of palmitate in the dog kidney. *Nephron* **8,** 488–499.

BARAC-NIETO M. (1976) Effects of lactate and glutamine on palmitate metabolism in rat kidney cortex. *Am. J. Physiol.* **231,** 14–19.

CHEN R. F. (1967) Removal of fatty acids from serum albumin by charcoal treatment. *J. biol. Chem.* **242,** 173–181.

DIES F., HERRERRA J., MATOS M., AVELAR E. & RAMOS G. (1970) Substrate uptake by the dog kidney *in vivo*. *Am. J. Physiol.* **218,** 405–410.

GOLD M. & SPITZER J. J. (1964) Metabolism of free fatty acids by myocardium and kidney. *Am. J. Physiol.* **206,** 153–158.

GUDER W. G. (1979) Stimulation of renal gluconeogenesis by angiotensin II. *Biochim. biophys. Acta* **584,** 507–519.

GUDER W. G. & SCHMIDT U. (1976) In *Proceedings of the Sixth International Congress of Nephrology*. Florence 1975 (Edited by GIOVANNETTI S., BONOMINI V. & D'AMICO G.) pp. 187–195. Karger, Basel.

GUDER W. G. & WIRTHENSOHN G. (1979) Metabolism of isolated kidney tubules. Interactions between lactate, glutamine and oleate metabolism. *Eur. J. Biochem.* **99,** 577–584.

LE HIR M., DUBACH U. C. & GUDER W. G. (1980) Distribution of acid hydrolases in the nephron of normal and diabetic rats. *Int. J. Biochem.* **12,** 41–45 (this volume).

HOHENEGGER M. (1976) In Renal metabolism in Relation to Renal Function (Edited by SCHMIDT U. & DUBACH U. C.) pp. 99–107. Huber, Bern.

HOHENEGGER M., RABERGER G., MÜLLER M. M., SCHULZ W. & KÜPPER M. (1978) In *Biochemical Nephrology* (Edited by GUDER W. G. & SCHMIDT U.) pp. 397–404. Huber, Bern.

HOHENEGGER M. & SCHUH H. (1980) Fatty acid uptake and synthesis by the kidney. *Int. J. Biochem.* **12,** 169–172 (this volume).

HUANG J. S., DOWNES G. L. & BELZER F. O. (1971) Utilization of fatty acids in perfused hypothermic dog kidney. *J. Lipid Res.* **12,** 622–627.

TINKER D. O. & HANAHAN D. J. (1966) Phospholipid metabolism in kidney. III. Biosynthesis of phospholipids from radioactive precursors in rabbit renal cortex slices. *Biochemistry* **5,** 423–435.

WEIDEMANN M. J. & KREBS H. A. (1969) The fuel of respiration of rat kidney cortex. *Biochem. J.* **112,** 149–166.

WIRTHENSOHN G. & GUDER W. G. (1980) Triacylglycerol metabolism in isolated rat kidney cortex tubules. *Biochem. J.* **186,** 317–324.

SYMPOSIUM DISCUSSION

Baverel: Have you checked whether incorporation of labelled lactate into triglycerides by outer medulla was due to contamination with cortical material, for example by using an inhibitor of PEPCK?

Wirthensohn: Yes, we used mercaptopicolinic acid, but only in cortical tubules. We found a decrease in triglyceride synthesis and a similar decrease occurred when we incubated only with oleate. Thus provision of endogenous α-glycerophosphate may be inhibited, too. Since gluconeogenesis was not totally inhibited, sufficient activity may remain for triglyceride formation. In the same experiment performed with labelled and unlabelled lactate, we found an apparently greater inhibition of incorporation of lactate label than of net triglyceride synthesis. (Wirthensohn & Guder, 1980).

Saggerson: I notice you have very little incorporation into fatty acids.

Wirthensohn: We see no incorporation in tubules from fed and fasted rats.

Guder: We have now measured ATP-citrate lyase and acetyl CoAcarboxylase in kidney, and found that these enzymes did not respond to lipogenic diet. So we would agree that the source of fatty acid for renal triglyceride synthesis must be plasma fatty acids. (Fig. 4).

Lemieux: Have you omitted lactate and incubated only with glutamine?

Wirthensohn: Gluconeogenic substrates, in the absence of fatty acids, always led to a decrease.

Ross: What is the rate of lactate incorporation into triglyceride, compared with the rate of gluconeogenesis?

Wirthensohn: When 300 μmols glucose were formed from lactate about 20 μmols TAG were found.

Baverel: What is the yield of tissue in your outer-medullary preparation?

Guder: We start with 2–3 g from 20 rats, and have 3 ml suspension of 10 mg ml^{-1} protein.

Hohenegger: Can you correlate the decrease in triglyceride that you observe, with oxygen consumption?

Wirthensohn: We didn't measure oxygen consumption.

Ross: Dr Hohenegger and I have so far been unable to detect net triglyceride synthesis in the perfused kidney, using the conditions you have found to be effective in tubules. This may still be a technical problem of lipid analysis, but may also indicate that there are differences when the kidney is transporting sodium and oxidising fatty acids.

Guder: We have looked *in vivo*, where we find net TG synthesis. There is also an old finding of increased lipid levels in the kidneys of patients dying with diabetes.

Williamson: If you give an anti-diabetic drug, how rapidly does it go down? The most important thing is how quickly is triglyceride turning over?

Guder: That has still to be measured.

Int. J. Biochem., Vol. 12, pp. 163 to 168
© Pergamon Press Ltd 1980. Printed in Great Britain

0020-711X/80/0701-0163$02.00/0

LACTATE AND PYRUVATE METABOLISM IN DOG RENAL OUTER MEDULLA. EFFECTS OF OLEATE AND KETONE BODIES

GABRIEL BAVEREL, MARTINE FORISSIER and MICHEL PELLET
Laboratoire de Physiologie Renale et Metabolique, Faculte de Medicine Alexis Carrel, 69008 Lyon, France

Abstract—1. The removal of L-lactate and pyruvate (1 or 5 mM) by tubular fragments isolated from the dog renal outer medulla and incubated in Krebs–Henseleit medium with 95% O_2–5% CO_2, is concentration-dependent and linear over a 60 min period.

2. The release of $^{14}CO_2$ from [1-^{14}C]lactate or [1-^{14}C]pyruvate showed that the major fraction of the lactate and pyruvate removed was metabolized via pyruvate dehydrogenase.

3. Oleate inhibited lactate utilization and lactate conversion into pyruvate, as well as the release of $^{14}CO_2$ from [1-^{14}C]lactate.

4. Oleate and ketone bodies (which were removed by the tubular fragments) decreased pyruvate utilization and the release of $^{14}CO_2$ from [1-^{14}C]pyruvate, but increased the conversion of pyruvate into lactate.

INTRODUCTION

It is well known that lactate is taken up from the blood by the intact functional dog kidney (Levy, 1962; Dies *et al.*, 1970; Leal-Pinto *et al.*, 1973). *In vitro* studies have shown that the dog kidney cortex produces glucose, carbon dioxide and alanine from lactate (Pashley & Cohen, 1973; Baverel *et al.*, 1978). In the renal medulla, lactate is generally not regarded as a possible substrate, but, rather, as an end-product of the metabolism of glucose, which is considered to be an important source of energy in the counter-current mechanism of urine concentration (Kean *et al.*, 1961; McCann, 1962; Lee *et al.*, 1962; Lee *et al.*, 1964; Bernanke & Epstein, 1965; Lee & Peter, 1969; Abodeely & Lee, 1971).

In the present study, it is shown that lactate and pyruvate are utilized by tubular fragments isolated from the dog renal outer medulla, and the fates of both lactate and pyruvate are determined. In addition, it is demonstrated that oleate and ketone bodies greatly alter the metabolism of lactate and pyruvate in this renal zone.

MATERIALS AND METHODS

Dogs

We used adult mongrel dogs, of either sex, weighing 13–25 kg. The dogs were fed according to a standard diet (U.A.R., Villemoisson-sur-Orge, France).

Preparation of isolated fragments from the renal outer medulla

After the dogs were anesthetized with i.v. sodium penthiobarbital (25 mg/kg body wt^{-1}), both kidneys were excised through a midline abdominal incision and placed in ice-cold isotonic saline. After the capsule was removed, the cooled kidneys were longitudinally hemisected and the outer (red) medulla was carefully separated from the cortex and the inner medulla by scissor dissection. Then, slices of the outer medulla, made with a Stadie–Riggs microtome, were incubated for 90 min in Krebs–Henseleit medium (Krebs & Henseleit, 1932), containing collagenase (0.3%, w/v) and hyalurodinase (0.3%, w/v). After the homogenate obtained was filtered and centrifuged, the tubular fragments were washed, centrifuged, and resuspended as is described for the preparation of cortical tubular fragments (Baverel *et al.*, 1978).

Incubation procedures

Incubations were carried out at 37°C in a shaking water bath in 25 ml stoppered Erlenmeyer flasks in an atmosphere of 95% O_2–5% CO_2. In all experiments, the tubular fragments obtained were incubated with or without substrates (1 or 5 mM) in 4 ml of Krebs–Henseleit medium. In some experiments, the medium also contained fatty acid-free bovine serum albumin (2.5%, w/v). Bovine serum albumin (fraction V) was dialyzed according to the procedure of Krebs *et al.* (1974). Incubations were terminated by adding perchloric acid (2% final concentration) to each flask.

In all experiments, zero-time flasks, with and without substrates, were prepared by adding perchloric acid before the tubules. After removing the denatured protein by centrifugation, the supernatant was neutralized with 20% KOH before performing assays of metabolites.

In experiments where [1-^{14}C]pyruvate, or [1-^{14}C]L-lactate, or [2-^{14}C]pyruvate were used as substrates, incubations were carried out in 25 ml Erlenmeyer flasks having a centre well and sealed with Subaseal stoppers. At the end of the incubation, 1 ml N NaOH was introduced into the centre well and 0.2 ml 40% $HClO_4$ into the main compartment with long-needled syringes. The flasks were shaken for an additional 2 hr at room temperature, in order to quantitatively collect the $^{14}CO_2$. The contents of the centre well were thoroughly mixed, removed, and centrifuged, and 0.1 ml was counted by liquid scintillation in a 3255 Packard model liquid scintillation spectrometer. The medium was then treated for metabolite assays as described above. When incorporation of [2-^{14}C]pyruvate into lipid was to be determined, separate flasks were incubated and lipids were extracted as described by Folch *et al.* (1957) and their radioactivity counted.

Analytical methods

Lactate, pyruvate, glucose, alanine, aspartate, citrate, 2-oxoglutarate, fumarate, malate, glutamate, as well as the dry weight of the amount of tubules added to the flasks, were determined as previously described (Baverel *et al.*,

1978). Glutamine was measured by the method of Lund (1974) and ammonia by the method of Kun & Kearney (1974). Glycogen was measured by the method of Keppler & Decker (1974). Acetoacetate and D-3-hydroxybutyrate were determined as described by Williamson *et al.* (1962). For comparison with results obtained with isolated kidney-cortex tubules, the dry weight of outer medulla was also determined by drying pieces of outer medulla at 100°C to constant weight. The fresh weight to dry weight ratio averaged 5.17 ± 0.15 ($\bar{X}$ ± SEM; 16 observations). Thus, tubule dry weights were multiplied by 5.17 to convert to wet weights.

Measurement of enzyme activities

Pieces of cortex and outer medulla (from the same kidneys) were rapidly excised, weighed, and homogenized in 10 vol of ice-cold distilled water in a Potter–Elvehjem glass homogenizer with a motor-driven Teflon pestle. The homogenates were frozen in liquid nitrogen and thawed 3 times, and then centrifuged at 30,000 *g* for 30 min at 4°C. The supernatant was immediately used for measurements of enzyme activities. Glutamate dehydrogenase activity (EC.1.4.1.2) was measured by the method of Schmidt (1974) and alanine aminotransferase activity (EC 2.6.1.2) as described by Pollak *et al.* (1965). All measurements of enzyme activity were carried out at 25°C. A unit of enzyme activity is defined as the amount of enzyme that transforms 1 μmol of substrate per min at 25°C.

Calculations

Net substrate utilization and product formation were calculated as the difference between the total flask contents (tissue + medium) at the start (zero-time flasks) and after the period of incubation. The metabolic rates are expressed in micromoles of substances removed or produced per gram dry weight of tubular fragments per unit time. They are reported as mean ± SEM.

Reagents

Bovine serum albumin, amino acids and glutaminase (grade V) were from Sigma Chemical Co. (St. Louis, MO, U.S.A.); oleate was bought from Matheson, Coleman and Bell (Nordwood, OH, U.S.A.). L-lactate, pyruvate, DL-3-hydroxybutyrate, other enzymes and coenzymes were products of Boehringer Mannheim GmbH (Mannheim, Germany). The ethylacetoacetate used for acetoacetate synthesis by the method of Krebs & Eggleston (1945) was from BDH Chemicals Ltd (Poole, England). [1-^{14}C]pyruvate (10.7 mCi/mmol^{-1}) and [2-^{14}C]pyruvate (9.67 mCi/mmol^{-1}) were obtained from the Radiochemical Centre (Amersham, England) and [1-^{14}C]L-lactate from NEN Chemicals GmbH (Dreieich, Germany). The remainder of the chemicals used were of analytical grade.

RESULTS

Time–courses of the metabolism of lactate and pyruvate at low (1 mM) and high (5 mM) concentrations

Figure 1 shows the time sequence of lactate and pyruvate metabolism in tubular fragments isolated from dog renal outer medulla. When incubated with 5 mM, or with 1 and 5 mM pyruvate, the tubules utilized lactate and pyruvate in a roughly linear manner over a 60 min period. With 1 mM lactate, substrate utilization became linear after 15 min (Fig. 1). The utilization of both lactate and pyruvate increased, when the substrate concentration was raised from 1 to 5 mM. At equimolecular concentration, the utilization of pyruvate was higher than that of lactate. With lactate as substrate, pyruvate accumulation was not linear with time, and pyruvate re-utilization was observed after 30 min with 1 mM lactate.

When pyruvate was the substrate, the rate of lactate synthesis was found to be constant with time, and lactate synthesis almost doubled when pyruvate was used at 5 mM instead of 1 mM.

As expected, owing to the exclusive localization in the cortex of key gluconeogenic enzymes (Szepesi *et al.*, 1970; Guder & Schmidt, 1974; Schmidt & Guder, 1976; Schmidt *et al.*, 1978; Burch *et al.*, 1978) glucose and glycogen were not synthetized from lactate and pyruvate. With 1 and 5 mM lactate and pyruvate, no accumulation of tricarboxylic acid cycle intermediates, glutamate, glutamine or aspartate was observed. No significant synthesis of alanine was noted with lactate or pyruvate alone, or in combination with 1 mM glutamate or glutamine. This is consistent with the very low activity of alanine aminotransferase found in the outer medulla (0.72 ± 0.22 μmol/g fresh wt^{-1}·min; $\bar{X}$ ± SEM; $n = 4$) as compared to that found in the cortex (12.81 ± 2.51). Although much lower than that found in the cortex (37.56 ± 1.38 μmol/g fresh wt^{-1}·min; $\bar{X}$ ± SEM; $n = 4$), significant activity of glutamate dehydrogenase was found in the outer medulla (13.62 ± 2.54). However, no accumulation of glutamate was observed, when 1 or 5 mM NH_4Cl was added to the incubation medium containing 1 or 5 mM lactate or pyruvate, and no ammonia was removed.

Figure 1 shows that the fraction of lactate or pyruvate removed and not accounted for (by the accumulation of pyruvate or lactate, respectively) is linear with time. Table 1 shows that the lactate and pyruvate "not accounted for" was in close accordance with the release of $^{14}CO_2$ from 1 mM [1-^{14}C]lactate or [1-^{14}C]pyruvate. This was also true for 5 mM [1-^{14}C]lactate and [1-^{14}C]pyruvate ($n = 4$). The release of $^{14}CO_2$ was linear over a 60 min incubation period. From these data, it is, therefore, clear that the lactate not found as pyruvate, and the pyruvate not converted into lactate were metabolized via pyruvate dehydrogenase. With 1 or 5 mM lactate or pyruvate, no accumulation of ketone bodies or incorporation of 5 mM [2-^{14}C]pyruvate into lipids was observed. Thus, it is likely that, following the pyruvate dehydrogenase step, carbon skeletons of lactate and pyruvate were completely oxidized to CO_2.

In the absence of added substrate, none of the substances measured were found to be formed or removed in net amounts.

Effects of oleate and ketone bodies on the metabolism of lactate and pyruvate

Table 1 shows that albumin-bound oleate (1 mM) greatly altered the metabolism of both lactate and pyruvate used at 1 mM concentration. The removal of lactate was inhibited by 48%, and that of pyruvate by 24%. Oleate increased the formation of lactate from pyruvate by 36.4%, whereas it reduced the accumulation of pyruvate from lactate by 38%. With both substrates, oleate caused a 40–45% inhibition of the flux through pyruvate dehydrogenase. With lactate as substrate, the lactate:pyruvate ratio, which reflects the redox state of the cytosolic nicotinamide adenine dinucleotide couple was shifted to a more reduced

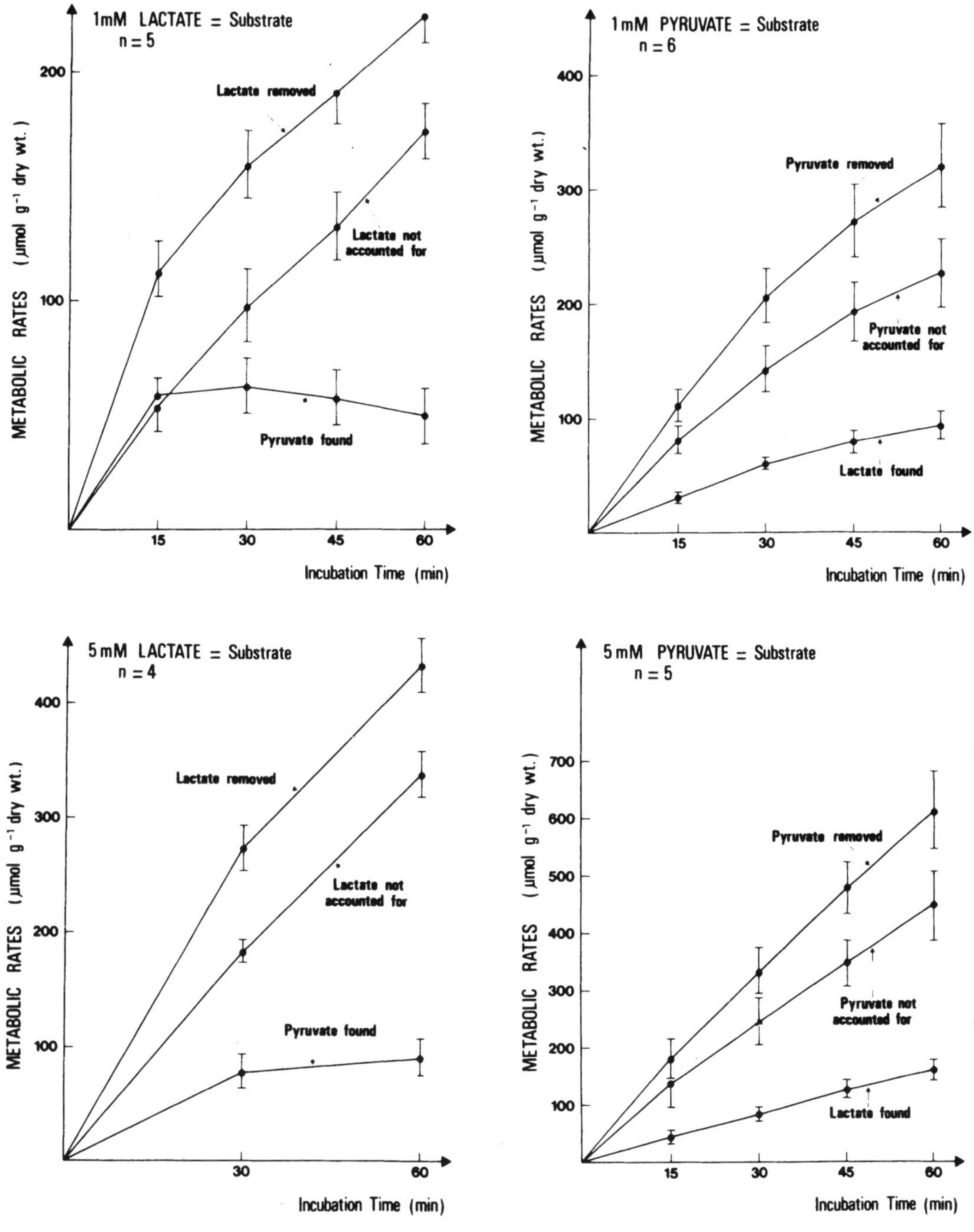

Fig. 1. Time–course of L-lactate and pyruvate metabolism in tubular fragments isolated from dog renal outer medulla. Incubations occurred in 4 ml of Krebs–Henseleit medium. Values are given as means, and vertical lines represent $\pm$SEM. Each flask contained 10.0 ± 1.2 and 14.8 ± 2.6 mg dry wt tissue in the 1 mM and 5 mM lactate series, respectively. Each flask contained 7.8 ± 1.1 and 6.6 ± 0.8 mg dry wt tissue in the 1 and 5 mM pyruvate series, respectively.

state in the presence of oleate. (The ratio increased from 3.3 ± 0.3 under control conditions to 8.0 ± 1.0 in the presence of oleate).

Table 1 also shows that addition of albumin to the incubation medium did not increase the ability of the tubular fragments to use lactate or pyruvate, indicating that albumin is useful only when the effect of long-chain fatty acids has to be studied.

The effects of acetoacetate and DL-3-hydroxybutyrate on the metabolism of pyruvate are also shown in Table 1. In the presence of pyruvate, the removal of acetoacetate was 166.1 ± 3.8 μmol·g dry wt^{-1}·hr^{-1} and that of D-3-hydroxybutyrate was 194.0 ± 8.5 μmol/g dry wt^{-1} hr^{-1}. Addition of acetoacetate and 3-hydroxybutyrate caused only a slight inhibition of the removal of pyruvate. As in the case

Table 1. Effect of oleate and ketone bodies on the metabolism of [1-^{14}C]L-lactate and [1-^{14}C]pyruvate in tubular fragments isolated from dog renal outer medulla

Additions	Lactate removed or found	Pyruvate removed or found	$^{14}CO_2$ found	Lactate or Pyruvate not accounted for
1 mM Lactate	−228.0 ± 7.6	61.3 ± 12.1	156.4 ± 5.0	166.7 ± 10.9
1 mM Lactate +2.5% Albumin	−223.4 ± 2.0	61.7 ± 10.3	150.7 ± 7.6	161.8 ± 9.7
1 mM Lactate +2.5% Albumin +1 mM Oleate	−115.3 ± 6.0	38.0 ± 10.7	83.1 ± 4.6	77.3 ± 9.0
1 mM Pyruvate	87.3 ± 8.3	−315.3 ± 29.6	203.4 ± 17.1	228.1 ± 21.8
1 mM Pyruvate +2.5% Albumin	82.8 ± 6.9	−312.9 ± 35.5	213.0 ± 18.8	230.1 ± 28.8
1 mM Pyruvate +2.5% Albumin +1 mM Oleate	112.9 ± 3.5	−238.2 ± 26.0	125.0 ± 14.5	125.2 ± 26.9
1 mM Pyruvate	90.8 ± 21.4	−343.7 ± 22.0	230.6 ± 13.7	252.9 ± 15.1
1 mM Pyruvate +2 mM DL-3-hydroxybutyrate	123.5 ± 11.2	−303.4 ± 22.5	166.5 ± 13.5	180.0 ± 19.0
1 mM Pyruvate +1 mM Acetoacetate	129.8 ± 9.2	−295.7 ± 20.1	161.1 ± 11.9	165.9 ± 18.6

Results are means ± SEM of 4 experiments for the "lactate + oleate" series, 4 experiments for the "pyruvate + oleate" series, and 5 experiments for the "pyruvate + ketone bodies" series. Values are expressed as μmol/g dry wt^{-1} hr^{-1}. Incubations occurred for 60 min in 4 ml of Krebs–Henseleit buffer—the flasks contained 10.5 ± 1.4, 8.3 ± 0.9, and 8.8 ± 0.6 mg dry wt of tubular fragments in the first, second, and third experimental series, respectively. Removal of substrates is indicated by the − sign.

of addition of oleate, addition of ketone bodies increased the conversion of pyruvate into lactate and reduced its metabolism via pyruvate dehydrogenase.

DISCUSSION

The present study demonstrates that lactate and pyruvate are removed linearly over a 60 min incubation period by tubular fragments isolated from the dog renal outer medulla in a concentration-dependent manner. Such linearity implies that the tubular fragments employed were metabolically viable. Thus, tubular fragments from the renal outer medulla can be considered as a useful tool for metabolic studies. This was further emphasized by the observation that, on a fresh weight basis, tubular fragments from dog outer medulla used 5 to 6 times more glucose than did slices prepared from the same tissue of the same kidneys and incubated under identical conditions ($n = 2$).

It should be noted that, at 5 mM concentration, the utilization of lactate and pyruvate was in the same range as that of glucose (in C_3-units), which was 494.9 ± 53.5 μmol/g dry wt^{-1}·hr ($\bar{X}$ ± SEM; $n = 5$). Thus, lactate which is at a concentration of about 1 to 2 mM in the dog outer medulla (Dell & Winters, 1967), appears to be a potential substrate of this tissue. This could also be true of pyruvate, which is removed by the dog kidney *in vivo*, when its blood concentration is raised by i.v. infusion (Levy, 1962). Using a fresh weight:dry weight ratio of 4.67 for the cortex and 5.17 for the outer medulla, it can be calculated that tubular fragments obtained from dog renal cortex (Baverel *et al.*, 1978) remove 1.3–1.8 times more lactate and pyruvate (at equimolar concentration) than do tubular fragments from the outer medulla. For this reason, and taking into account the fact that the outer medulla represents only a small fraction of the kidney, it is likely that the outer medulla removes little lactate or pyruvate from the blood in relation to the rest of the intact functioning dog kidney.

The kinetics of pyruvate accumulation imply that, in order for the lactate dehydrogenase reaction to reach near-equilibrium, the pyruvate concentration has to be adjusted to that of lactate according to the equation: pyruvate = K [Lactate][NAD^+]/[NADH] (Krebs, 1969). This suggests that pyruvate accumulation from lactate in the outer medulla is only an *in vitro* phenomenon and does not occur *in vivo*.

The linearity of lactate formation from pyruvate indicates that the transport of reducing equivalents from the mitochondria to the cytosol is constant with time. The fact that lactate formation increases with pyruvate concentration also reveals that this transport increases with pyruvate concentration. It is considered that the reducing equivalents necessary for lactate formation from pyruvate in the renal cortex are transported in the form of malate (Krebs *et al.*, 1967; Rognstad & Katz, 1970), and this transport is inhibited by 2-*n*-butylmalonate (Saggerson, 1978). In the present study, lactate formation from 1 mM pyruvate was almost insensitive to the addition of 40 mM 2-*n*-butylmalonate, suggesting that malate is not involved in the transport of the needed reducing equivalents. However, failure of 2-*n*-butylmalonate to alter the formation of lactate might be due to a cellular or mitochondrial impermeability to this compound. Thus, further study is required to elucidate this question.

The absence of alanine formation from lactate and

pyruvate, in the presence of nitrogen sources such as ammonia, glutamate, and glutamine (which were not removed by the tubular fragments), contrasts with the formation of alanine found in isolated kidney-cortex tubules under identical conditions (Baverel *et al.*, 1978). This suggests that the lactate, pyruvate and glucose possibly metabolized by the dog renal outer medulla do not provide the carbon skeleton of the alanine released by the dog kidney *in vivo* (Shalhoub *et al.*, 1963).

The carbon balance calculations and the release of $^{14}CO_2$ from [1-^{14}C]lactate and [1-^{14}C]pyruvate indicate that, under control conditions, the major portion of the lactate and pyruvate used was metabolized via pyruvate dehydrogenase. The absence of accumulation of TCA cycle intermediates, ketone bodies and amino acids, and of lipid formation from pyruvate strongly suggests that, after the pyruvate dehydrogenase step, lactate and pyruvate are completely oxidized to CO_2 and H_2O. These data, as well as the demonstration by Lee & Peter (1969) of oxidation of pyruvate in the rabbit renal outer medulla, suggest that lactate and pyruvate are potential sources of energy in this renal zone. When 5 mM glucose was the substrate, the formation of lactate and pyruvate were 201.6 ± 50.1 and 67.9 ± 10.3 μmol·g dry wt^{-1} hr^{-1}, respectively. The carbon balance shows that the maximum amount of glucose (in C_3-units) completely oxidized was 225.4 ± 31.8 μmol/g dry wt^{-1} hr^{-1}. This value is slightly higher than the corresponding value found with 1 mM lactate as substrate, and lower than that found with 5 mM lactate. These results imply that, at physiological concentrations and under identical conditions, lactate might be as efficient as glucose for supplying energy to the renal outer medulla.

In view of the demonstration by Guder & Schmidt (1976) that the active portion of pyruvate dehydrogenase measured in the cortex is higher than that in the outer medulla of kidneys removed from starved dogs, the flux of lactate and pyruvate carbon skeletons through pyruvate dehydrogenase (taken as the lactate and pyruvate not accounted for by the non-volatile carbon products measured) was compared in tubular fragments isolated from the dog renal cortex (Baverel *et al.*, 1978) and from the outer medulla. The calculations show that this flux is in the same range in the cortex and in the outer medulla, when lactate and pyruvate are the substrates under identical conditions. Thus, lactate and pyruvate might be as good potential energy-suppliers for the reabsorptive work in the outer medulla as they are in the cortex.

The present study demonstrates that oleate, which is probably removed and partly oxidized by the dog renal outer medulla as palmitate is by the rat outer medulla (Dalheim & Hohenegger, 1972), greatly affects the metabolism of lactate and pyruvate in the outer medulla. It inhibits the removal of lactate and pyruvate and the flux through pyruvate dehydrogenase. Similar effects of fatty acids on pyruvate dehydrogenase have been demonstrated in rat renal cortex (Guder & Wieland, 1974). Increased lactate formation from pyruvate induced by the addition of oleate probably results from an increased concentration of free NADH in the cytosol, due to an enhanced delivery of reducing equivalents from the mitochondria to the cytosol secondary to fatty acids oxidation. A shift to a more reduced state of the cytosolic NAD^+/NADH couple induced by oleate is also suggested by the increased lactate:pyruvate ratio.

Our results also demonstrate that ketone bodies are removed by the dog renal outer medulla. Ketone bodies have similar effects to oleate on the metabolism of pyruvate without greatly inhibiting pyruvate utilization. Thus, fatty acids and ketone bodies, which are substrates of the dog kidney *in vivo* (Hohenleitner & Spitzer, 1961; Barac-Nieto & Cohen, 1968; Dies *et al.*, 1970; Little & Spitzer, 1971) are potential *in vivo* regulators of lactate and pyruvate metabolism in dog renal outer medulla.

Finally, it should be noted that all the comparisons made in the present study between the cortex and the outer medulla on the one hand, and between the metabolism of lactate, pyruvate and glucose in the outer medulla on the other hand, remain true under identical conditions of oxigenation and osmolality. In view of the fact that the pO_2 in the outer medulla (Leichtweiss *et al.*, 1969) is lower, and the osmolality higher than in the cortex, the extent to which this can be extrapolated to the *in vivo* situation remains to be established.

Acknowledgement—This work was supported by grant No. 002 ATP 62.78.94 from INSERM.

REFERENCES

ABODEELY D. A. & LEE J. B. (1971) Fuel of respiration of outer renal medulla. *Am. J. Physiol.* **220,** 1693–1700.

BARAC-NIETO M. & COHEN J. J. (1968) Nonesterified fatty acid uptake by dog kidney: effects of probenecid and chlorothiazide. *Am. J. Physiol.* **215,** 98–107.

BAVEREL G., BONNARD M., D'ARMAGNAC DE CASTANET E. & PELLET M. (1978) Lactate and pyruvate metabolism in isolated renal tubules of normal dogs. *Kidney Int.* **14,** 567–575.

BERNANKE D. & EPSTEIN F. H. (1965) Metabolism of the renal medulla. *Am. J. Physiol.* **208,** 541–545.

BURCH H. B., NARINS R. G., CHU C., FAGIOLI S., CHOI S., MCCARTHY W. & LOWRY O. H. (1978) Distribution along the rat nephron of three enzymes of gluconeogenesis in acidosis and starvation. *Am. J. Physiol.* **235,** F246–F253.

DALHEIM H. & HOHENEGGER M. (1972) Palmitate oxidation by slices from cortex, outer and inner medulla of the rat kidney. In *Biochemische Aspekte der Nierenfunktion* (Edited by HOHENEGGER M.) pp. 173–180. Goldmann, München.

DELL R. B. & WINTERS R. W. (1967) Lactate gradients in the kidney of the dog. *Am. J. Physiol.* **213,** 301–307.

DIES F., HERRERA J., MATOS M., AVELAR E. & RAMOS G. (1970) Substrate uptake by the dog kidney *in vivo*. *Am. J. Physiol.* **218,** 405–410.

FOLCH J., LEES M. & SLOANE-STANLEY G. H. (1957) A simple method for the isolation and purification of total lipids from animal tissues. *J. biol. Chem.* **226,** 497–509.

GUDER W. G., WIELAND O. H. & STUKOWSKI B. (1974) Metabolism of isolated kidney tubules. Regulation of pyruvate dehydrogenase by metabolic substrates. *Eur. J. Biochem.* **42,** 529–538.

GUDER W. & SCHMIDT U. (1974) The localization of gluconeogenesis in rat nephron. *Hoppe-Seyler's Z. physiol. Chem.* **355,** 273–278.

GUDER W. G. & SCHMIDT U. (1976) Substrate and oxygen

dependence of renal metabolism. *Kidney Int.* **10,** S32–S38.

HOHENLEITNER F. J. & SPITZER J. J. (1961) Changes in plasma free fatty acid concentrations on passage through the dog kidney. *Am. J. Physiol.* **200,** 1095–1098.

KEAN E. L., ADAMS P. H., WINTERS R. W. & DAVIES R. E. (1961) Energy metabolism of the renal medulla. *Biochim. biophys. Acta* **54,** 474–478.

KEPPLER D. & DECKER K. (1974) Glycogen. Determination with amyloglucosidase. In *Methods of Enzymatic Analysis* (Edited by BERGMEYER H. U.) Vol. 3, pp. 1127–1131 Academic Press, New York.

KREBS H. A. & HENSELEIT K. (1932) Untersuchungen über die Harnstoffbildung im TierKörper. *Hoppe-Seyler's Z. physiol. Chem.* **210,** 33–66.

KREBS H. A. & EGGLESTON L. V. (1945) Metabolism of acetoacetate in animal tissues. *Biochem J.* **39,** 408–419.

KREBS H. A., GASCOYNE T. & NOTTON B. M. (1967) Generation of extramitochondrial reducing power in gluconeogenesis. *Biochem. J.* **102,** 275–282.

KREBS H. A. (1969) The role of equilibria in the regulation of metabolism. In *Current Topics in Cellular Regulation* (Edited by HORECKER B. L. & STADMAN E. R.) Vol. 1, pp. 45–55. Academic Press, New York.

KREBS H. A., CORNELL N. W., LUND P. & HEMS R. (1974) Isolated liver cells as experimental material. In *Regulation of Hepatic Metabolism.* Alfred Benzon Symposium (Edited by LUNDQUIST F. & TYGSTRUP N.) Vol. 6, pp. 726–750. Munksgaard, Copenhagen.

KUN E. & KEARNEY E. B. (1974) Ammonia. In *Methods of Enzymatic Analysis* (Edited by BERGMEYER H. U.) Vol. 4, 1802–1806. Academic Press, New York.

LEAL-PINTO E., PARK H. C., KING F., MACLEOD M. & PITTS R. F. (1973) Metabolism of lactate by the intact functioning kidney of the dog. *Am. J. Physiol.* **224,** 1463–1467.

LEE J. B., VANCE V. K. & CAHILL G. F. (1962) Metabolism of C^{14}-labelled substrates by rabbit kidney cortex and medulla. *Am. J. Physiol.* **203,** 27–36.

LEE J. B., VANCE V. K. & CAHILL G. F. (1964) Effect of osmolality on glucose metabolism in rabbit kidney cortex and medulla *in vitro. Am. J. Physiol.* **207,** 473–482.

LEE J. B. & PETER H. M. (1969) Effect of oxygen tension on glucose metabolism in rabbit kidney cortex and medulla. *Am. J. Physiol.* **217,** 1464–1471.

LEICHTWEISS H. P., LUBBERS D. W., WEISS C., BAUMGARTL H. & RESCHKE W. (1969) The oxygen supply of the rat kidney: measurements of intrarenal PO_2. *Pflügers Arch. ges. Physiol.* **309,** 328–349.

LEVY M. N. (1962) Uptake of lactate and pyruvate by intact kidney of the dog. *Am. J. Physiol.* **202,** 302–308.

LITTLE J. R. & SPITZER J. J. (1961) Uptake of ketone bodies by dog kidney *in vivo. Am. J. Physiol.* **221,** 679–683.

LUND P. (1974) L-Glutamine. Determination with glutaminase and glutamate dehydrogenase. In *Methods of Enzymatic Analysis* (Edited by BERGMEYER H. U.) Vol. 4, pp. 1719–1722. Academic Press, New York.

MCCANN W. P. (1962) Renal glucose production and uptake in separate sites, and its significance. *Am. J. Physiol.* **203,** 572–576.

PASHLEY D. H. & COHEN J. J. (1973) Substrate interconversion in dog kidney cortex slices: Regulation by ECF-pH. *Am. J. Physiol.* **225,** 1519–1528.

POLLAK V. E., MATTENHEIMER H., DEBRUIN H. & WEINMAN K. J. (1965) Experimental metabolic acidosis: The enzymatic basis of ammonia production by the dog kidney. *J. Clin. Invest.* **44,** 169–181.

ROGNSTAD R. & KATZ J. (1970) Gluconeogenesis in the kidney cortex. Effects of D-malate and amino-oxyacetate. *Biochem. J.* **116,** 483–491.

SCHMID H., SCHOLZ M., MALL A., SCHMIDT U. & GUDER W. G. (1978) Carbohydrate metabolism in rat kidney: heterogeneous distribution of glycolytic and gluconeogenic key enzymes, In *Current Problems in Clinical Biochemistry* (Edited by GUDER W. G. & SCHMIDT U.) Vol. 8, pp. 282–289. Huber, Bern.

SAGGERSON E. D. (1978) A study of regulation of gluconeogenesis and the supply of cytosolic reducing equivalents for lactate formation in rat kidney-cortical-tubule fragments incubated with pyruvate. *Biochem. J.* **174,** 131–142.

SCHMIDT E. (1974) Glutamate dehydrogenase. UV-Assay. In *Methods of Enzymatic Analysis* (Edited by BERGMEYER H. U.) Vol. 2, pp. 650–656. Academic Press, New York.

SCHMIDT U. & GUDER W. G. (1976) Sites of enzyme activity along the nephron. *Kidney Int.* **9,** 233–242.

SHALHOUB R., WEBER W., GLABMAN S., CANESSA-FISCHER M., KLEIN J., DEHAAS J. & PITTS R. F. (1963) Extraction of amino acids from and their addition to renal blood plasma. *Am. J. Physiol.* **204,** 181–186.

SZEPESI B., AVERY E. H. & FREEDLAND R. A. (1970) Role of kidney in gluconeogenesis and amino acid catabolism. *Am. J. Physiol.* **219,** 1627–1631.

WILLIAMSON D. H., MELLANBY J. & KREBS H. A. (1962) Enzymic determination of D(–)-β-hydroxybutyric acid and acetoacetic acid in blood. *Biochem. J.* **82,** 90–98.

SYMPOSIUM DISCUSSION

Vinay: Have you looked for alanine production from lactate plus glutamine or glutamate, and excluded the possibility that you are looking at proximal tubule metabolism?

Baverel: We did that. There is no alanine formation and no glucose or glycogen synthesis in this preparation.

Guder: Dr Julius Cohen postulated at the last meeting that lactate was the best substrate for the thick ascending limb and supports sodium transport in that part of the nephron. This is in contrast to the findings of Ross *et al.* (*Am. J. Physiol.* **225** 1165–1171, 1973) who found glucose to be the best substrate, but these views could be reconciled if there was competition between lactate and glucose as fuels in this part of the nephron. Did you find competition between these 2 substrates?

Baverel: I have not done that experiment, which anyway would be difficult because lactate would be formed from glucose and the removal of lactate under-estimated.

Kovacevic: What is your explanation for the effect of oleate on pyruvate and lactate flux through pyruvate dehydrogenase? Is it an effect on the redox state of pyridine nucleotides of the mitochondria?

Baverel: Possibly. There is certainly an increased conversion of pyruvate to lactate under these circumstances, indicating an increased delivery of reducing equivalents from the mitochondrion to the cytosol, possibly as a direct effect of oleate oxidation.

Kurokawa: In experiments with tubule fragments, we found that the medullary thick ascending limb of Henle oxidizes glucose and lactate very well. On the other hand, the proximal convolution does not oxidise glucose, and lactate is relatively poorly oxidized.

Baverel: We must remember that there may be some influence of osmolarity in the medulla, and extrapolation to the *in vivo* situation has yet to be established.

Guder: We have measured pyruvate dehydrogenase in dog kidney, and found, as in the rat that the proportion of "active" pyruvate dehydrogenase is the same in the outer medulla as in the cortex. With reference to Kovacevic's question, it seems PDH is mainly regulated by the AcCoA:CoA ratio.

Weiner: I wonder if the results you obtained with oleate indicate that it is fatty acid which is the preferred fuel in this region, not pyruvate, lactate or glucose?

Baverel: We have not measured the rate of removal or oxidation of oleate; Dalheim & Hohenegger (1972) have shown that the rate of oxidation of palmitate is higher in the rat renal outer medulla than in the cortex.

Int. J. Biochem., Vol. 12, pp. 169 to 172
0020-711X/80/0701-0169$02.00/0

UPTAKE AND FATTY ACID SYNTHESIS BY THE RAT KIDNEY*

M. HOHENEGGER and H. SCHUH
Institute for General and Experimental Pathology, University of Vienna, Vienna, Austria

Abstract—1. In the state of starvation the kidney takes up more fatty acids (free fatty acids and triacylglycerol) than can be utilized.

2. In the fed state fatty acids are released. This results in higher levels of triacylglycerol in kidney cortex during starvation.

3. Lipoprotein lipase activity is present in all zones of the kidney. It is independent of the nutritional state.

4. *De novo* synthesis of fatty acids is very low in all zones of the kidney. Refeeding after fasting does not stimulate it.

5. The exact part played by fatty acids in the energy metabolism of the kidney *in vivo* is still not clear.

INTRODUCTION

In the previous symposium on "Biochemical Nephrology" (Hohenegger *et al.*, 1978) we reported on uptake or release of fatty acids by the dog kidney. Uptake of free fatty acids (FFA) and fatty acids (FA) bound to glycerol was shown after a 12 hr period of starvation. FA esterified with cholesterol or bound to phospholipids did not show any specific trend. After glucose infusion, FFA and triacylglycerol were released by the kidney. The amount of FA taken up during starvation (calculated from arterio-venous differences × renal plasma flow) was greater than could be utilized on the basis of the known oxygen consumption of the kidney. It must, therefore, be assumed that FA concentration of kidney tissue will change according to the nutritional state. The present investigations were undertaken to test the validity of this hypothesis. For practical reasons, rats were employed for this study.

MATERIALS AND METHODS

Male Sprague–Dawley rats were used. They were kept at a room temperature of 23–24°C and had free access to water. The following series of experiments were performed:

Experiment 1

Rats weighing 300 g (average) were anesthetized with nembutal (50 mg·kg body wt^{-1}, given intraperitoneally). The abdomen was opened. The left renal vein was clamped and immediately afterwards renal venous blood was collected by inserting a catheter. Blood was collected simultaneously in a similar way from the abdominal aorta. After centrifuging the blood in heparinized tubes plasma was obtained and analyzed for free and total glycerol (Eggstein & Kreutz, 1966), total and free cholesterol (Röschlau *et al.*, 1974), phospholipids (Zilversmit & Davis, 1950) and total FA (Albrink, 1959).

The experiments were performed between 8 and 10 a.m. Rats which had unrestricted access to food or animals starved for 24 hr were investigated.

Experiment 2

Rats with similar average weight were sacrificed by cervical dislocation in the morning; the night before they had free access to food. Other rats were deprived of food for 12 or 24 hr respectively. The experiment was started at 8 a.m. The kidneys were removed immediately and dissected into cortex, outer and inner medulla. Pieces of 40–150 mg were placed for at least 8 hrs in a 19-fold volume of chloroform–methanol (2:1, v/v). Aliquots of dried extracts were analyzed for total glycerol employing the method of Eggstein & Kreutz (1966). Triacylglycerol content of the tissue was calculated, neglecting free glycerol levels. These are very low and of the order of less than 10% of total glycerol (unpublished results obtained by employing freeze clamping technique and extraction with 0.6 N perchloric acid). Kidneys of rats fed normally and of those starved for 24 hr were also analyzed for lipoprotein lipase activity (LA). Tissues were homogenized in Krebs–phosphate buffer, pH 7.4, employing a Potter–Elvehjem apparatus (1 g tissue per 9 ml buffer). Practically the whole cortex of one kidney was taken for one assay. For measurements on outer and inner medulla the tissue from 5–10 rats was pooled. To the homogenates (1.5 ml) 0.4 ml of a fat emulsion (Intralipid 20%®) in plasma from rats starved for 48 hrs 1;4, v/v) and 0.1 ml Tris buffer, pH 8.4, were added. The release of FFA per 1 g dry tissue per hour was calculated by measuring the FFA content in the samples before and after incubation for 120 min at 30°C. Extraction and microtitration of FFA was performed as mentioned by Dole & Meinertz (1960). In some incubation experiments 0.6 M NaCl or 1 mM sodium deoxycholate respectively, were added and their inhibitory effect on FFA release calculated.

Experiment 3

In this experiment rats weighing 100–200 g were used. They were starved for 24 hr (8 a.m.–8 a.m.). At the end of this period one group of rats was given 2 mCi ^3H_2O in 1 ml 0.9% solution of NaCl per 100 g body wt intraperitoneally. An hour after the injection the animals were sacrificed by cervical dislocation and liver and kidneys were removed. After a period of starvation as mentioned above, a second group of rats was given 20 g of a standard diet enriched with 40% glucose at 6 p.m. on the two following days. At 8 a.m. of the third day after starvation 5 ml of a 50% glucose solution (per 100 g body wt) was given per stomach tube. Two hours later these rats were given ^3H_2O and also treated as the starved rats mentioned above.

Tissue samples (about 2 × 300 mg of liver and kidney cortex and about 100 mg of outer medulla from each rat, about 100 mg of inner medulla from the kidneys of 2 rats) were homogenized in a 5–10 fold volume of 0.9% solution of NaCl. After saponification and FA extraction (see Lowenstein, 1971) the radioactivity was determined in the

* Supported by Eisner-Stiftung, Austria.

Table 1. Lipid concentrations (μM/l) of arterial and renal venous plasma in fed rats and after 24 hr of starvation (means ± SD of 8 rats in each group)

	Arterial	Renal venous	Art. − Ven.	P
A. Free glycerol	154 ± 24	172 ± 21	−18 ± 17	<0.01
Esterified glycerol	1118 ± 104	1178 ± 103	−71 ± 25	<0.01
Esterified cholesterol	1403 ± 215	1349 ± 277	55 ± 351	N.S.
Phospholipids	2227 ± 671	2347 ± 609	−120 ± 428	N.S.
Total fatty acids	8137 ± 629	8410 ± 622	−273 ± 97	<0.01
B. Free glycerol	246 ± 34	225 ± 34	22 ± 5	<0.01
Esterified glycerol	703 ± 54	614 ± 42	88 ± 17	<0.01
Esterified cholesterol	1273 ± 168	1193 ± 136	81 ± 94	N.S.
Phospholipids	2370 ± 560	2416 ± 658	−46 ± 132	N.S.
Total fatty acids	7046 ± 922	6756 ± 869	290 ± 60	<0.01

A = Fed rats B = After 24 hr of starvation.

extracts by employing a liquid scintillation counter of the Beckmann type.

Naphthalene 60.0 g, PPO 4.0 g, POPOP 0.2 g, methanol 100 ml, ethylenglycol 20 ml, dioxan ad 1000 ml were used as scintillation liquid. FA synthesis is expressed in nmol ^3H_2O incorporated into FA of 1 g dry tissue per hour. Dry weight and water content of tissues used in experiments 2 and 3 were determined by keeping the samples for 24 hr at 100°C and measuring the change in weight.

Paired and unpaired *t*-tests were employed for statistical evaluation of the results.

RESULTS

In Table 1 the renal arterio-venous concentration differences for various lipid fractions are presented. In the state of starvation an uptake of FFA and total FA is observed, in fed rats a release is found. It may be seen that the balance of total FA is mainly dependent on uptake or release of FA from triacylglycerol. On the other hand FA bound to cholesterol and phospholipids show no significant trend in either nutritional states. In Table 2 the kidney tissue triacylglycerol levels are given. After starvation, these are higher in kidney cortex, showing a two-fold increase after 24 hr. The triacylglycerol levels of outer and inner medulla remain unaltered in different states of nutrition.

It is evident from Table 3 that in all zones of the kidney a lipoprotein lipase-like activity is present with the highest activity in the outer medulla. The enzyme activities are independent of the nutritional state.

The presence of 0.6 M NaCl in the essay results in an inhibition of 60 ± 21% ($n = 6$) in cortex, 62 ± 9% ($n = 3$) in outer medulla and 79 ± 2% ($n = 3$) in the inner medulla. When 1 mM sodium deoxycholate is present an inhibition of 46 ± 20 ($n = 4$) is found in cortex, 48 ± 17% ($n = 3$) in outer and 51 ± 8% ($n = 3$) in inner medulla.

In Table 4 the results of measurements of lipid synthesis are given. In the state of starvation lipid synthesis is very low in the liver as well as in all zones of the kidney. Refeeding after fasting results in an increased synthesis in the liver tissue only whereas, in all zones of the kidney the rate of FA synthesis remains low.

DISCUSSION

For many years increasing attention has been payed to FFA metabolism of the kidney. Practically all investigations (see Hohenegger *et al.*, 1978) reported an uptake in the state of starvation. A good accord was observed between the absolute amount of FFA taken up and the oxygen consumption of the kidney and it has been speculated that FFA might be a main fuel of respiration. Experiments employing labelled FA have shown that the exogenous FA account only a part of oxygen consumption of the kidney *in vivo* and *in vitro* (Weidemann & Krebs 1969; Hohenegger *et al.*, 1973; Park *et al.*, 1974). Dzurik & Chorvathova (1972) reported that FFA and esterified FA are assimilated by the kidney in the state of starvation whereas, in fed rats FFA and esterified FA are released. Our results on rats and dogs are in

Table 3. Lipoproteinlipase activity in the rat kidney (μM free fatty acids released by 1 g of dry tissue per hr) (means ± SD, number of experiments in parentheses)

	Fed rats	24 hr starvation
Cortex	141 ± 21 (10)	146 ± 18 (5)
Outer medulla	241 ± 48 (5)*	230 ± 19 (3)*
Inner medulla	179 ± 34 (3)†	181 ± 21 (3)†

* Each sample consists of pooled tissue from 5 rats.
† Each sample consists of pooled tissue from 10 rats.

Table 2. Levels of triacylglycerol in cortex, outer and inner medulla of the rat kidney (% of dry wt) (Means ± SD, number of experiments in parentheses)

	Cortex	Outer medulla	Inner medulla
Fed rats	2.40 ± 0.88 (14)	2.57 ± 0.47 (6)	3.56 ± 0.75 (6)
12 hrs starvation	3.69 ± 0.94 (8)*	2.45 ± 0.53 (8)	3.72 ± 1.07 (8)
24 hrs starvation	4.89 ± 1.15 (11)*	2.98 ± 0.86 (7)	3.78 ± 1.07 (6)

* $P < 0.01$ for differences between fed and starving rats.

Table 4. Lipid synthesis in rat liver and kidney (nmol ^3H_2O incorporated into fatty acids of 1 g dry tissue per hr) (means ± SD, number of experiments in parentheses)

	Liver	Kidney Cortex	Kidney Outer med.	Kidney Inner med.
24 hr starvation	247 ± 149 (7)	88 ± 40 (4)	65 ± 5 (6)	142 ± 136 (4)
After 2 days refeeding	2849 ± 543 (7)	93 ± 35 (8)	109 ± 30 (8)	221 ± 45 (7)

accordance with the results of Dzurik & Chorvatova (1972). Furthermore our present results point out that a major fraction of FA taken up under starvation and released in the fed state is triacylglycerol. No such behavior is observed with regard to cholesterol and phospholipids.

The differences in renal arterial and venous plasma for FFA and esterified FA are of the order of about 10%. As the renal plasma flow is quite high this results in significant amounts taken up during starvation. Taking the renal plasma flow to be about $1.5\,ml \cdot g\ kidney^{-1} \cdot min$ (estimated from hematocrit and outflow from the renal venous catheter) more FA are taken up than can be utilized when the normal oxygen consumption of the kidney is assumed. The above conclusions are corroborated by the fact that during starvation the triacylglycerol content of kidney cortex is increased. Outer and inner medulla, however, do not seem to take any part in this process. No definite conclusions can be drawn regarding the final amount of FA utilized by the kidney when longer periods (24 hr) are considered. The activity of lipoprotein lipase, the enzyme involved in triacylglycerol uptake, is present in all zones of the kidney and has its maximum in the outer medulla. The activity is of the same order in the heart muscle (Chohan & Cryer, 1978) and in the kidney found previously by Hollenberg & Horowitz (1962). These authors, however, did not separate outer and inner medulla. Whereas the LA in the kidney is independent of the nutritional state, FFA and triacylglycerol metabolism is particularly dependent on it. The reasons for this behaviour are not clear. It may be mentioned that the amount of *de novo* FA synthesis (chain elongation) in the kidney is very low and cannot be stimulated by refeeding after fasting, the determining stimulus for FA synthesis in the liver.

REFERENCES

ALBRINK M. J. (1959) The microtitration of total fatty acids of serum, with notes on the estimation of triglycerides. *J. Lipid Res.* **1,** 53–59.

CHOHAN P. & CRYER A. (1978) The lipoprotein lipase (clearing-factor lipase) activity of cells isolated from rat cardiac muscle. *Biochem. J.* **174,** 663–666.

DOLE V. P. & MEINERTZ H. (1960) Microdetermination of long-chain fatty acids in plasma and tissues. *J. biol. Chem.* **235,** 2595–2599.

DZURIK R. & CHORVATHOVA V. (1972) Relation between the uptake of glucose and fatty acids by the rat kidney *in vivo. Physiol. bohem.* **21,** 361–365.

EGGSTEIN M. & KREUTZ F. H. (1966) Eine neue Bestimmung der Neutralfette im Blutserum und Gewebe. *Klin. Wschr.* **44,** 262–273.

HOHENEGGER M., WITTMANN G. & DAHLHEIM H. (1973) Oxidation of fatty acids by different zones of the rat kidney. *Pflügers Arch. Eur. J. Physiol.* **341,** 105–112.

HOHENEGGER M., RABERGER G., MÜLLER M. M., SCHÜTZ W. & KÜPPER M. (1978) On the renal balances for different lipid fractions in dog. In *Biochemical Nephrology,* (Edited by GUDER G. W. & SCHMIDT U.) pp. 397–404. Huber, Bern.

HOLLENBERG C. H. & HOROWITZ I. (1962) The lipolytic activity of rat kidney cortex and medulla. *J. Lipid Res.* **3,** 445–447.

LOWENSTEIN J. M. (1971) Effect of (−)-hydroxycitrate on fatty acid synthesis by rat liver *in vivo. J. biol. Chem.* **246,** 629–632.

PARK H. C., LEAL PINTO E., MACLEOD M. B. & PITTS R. F. (1974) CO_2 production from plasma free fatty acids by the intact functioning kidney of the dog. *Am. J. Physiol.* **227,** 1192–1198.

RÖSCHLAU P., BERNT E. & GRUBER W. (1974) Enzymatische Bestimmung des Gesamtcholesterins im Serum. *Ztschr. Klin. Chem.* **12,** 403–407.

WEIDEMANN M. J. & KREBS H. A. (1969) The fuel of respiration of rat kidney cortex. *Biochem. J.* **112,** 149–166.

ZILVERSMIT D. B. & DAVIS A. K. (1950) Microdetermination of plasma phospholipids by trichloracetic acid precipitation. *J. Lab. clin. Med.* **35,** 155–160.

SYMPOSIUM DISCUSSION

Saggerson: What substrate did you use for the assay of lipoprotein lipase? Did you have to add an activator and was it affected by salt or protamine?

Hohenegger: Either intralipid or trioleate suspended in gum arabic. No activator was required and the inhibitors had the expected effects.

Weiner: What regulates uptake or release of fatty acid by the kidney? Is there some signal between liver and kidney which regulates the process?

Hohenegger: In the case of free fatty acid, but not for triglyceride, it appears to be simply a matter of the concentration in the blood circulating through the kidney.

Angielski: In what form is triglyceride deposited in the kidney? In other tissues, an apo-lipoprotein is required for triglyceride deposition. I would propose that you add apolipoprotein in your perfusion system, thereby providing a trapping system which should promote synthesis and accumulation of triglyceride.

Guder: Dr Hohenegger's findings open possibilities to examine the hyperlipidaemias of renal failure. We have methods available for the separation of different lipoproteins and if you repeat the experiments of Barac-Nieto & Cohen, (1971) it should be possible to precisely identify the product of renal triglyceride secretion. These specific lipoproteins may be the "language" between liver and kidney that Dr Weiner asked about. Have you measured lipoprotein lipase in diseased kidney?

Hohenegger: No, but to the Barac-Nieto and Cohen experiments, they were conducted for a very short time; no recirculation and no equilibrium so they would be very difficult to interpret.

Dzurik: I have data on the inhibition of lipoprotein lipase in renal disease. We have studied the effect of incubation in uraemic serum on the uptake of added labelled fatty acids. In muscle, we found—surprisingly—an increase in fatty acid oxidation, and unchanged or slightly increased incorporation into triglycerides. In the liver, on the other hand, there is a decrease in oxidation and increase in TG incorporation. The kidney showed no changes whatever.

Saggerson: Is it known into which compartments the smaller lipoproteins can partition themselves?

Hohenegger: No.

Trimble: May I comment on the experiment with uraemic serum? It is important to note the binding of fatty acids to albumin under these conditions. The binding may change due to other substances in uraemic serum.

Tannen: Does the difference in osmolarity of medulla and cortex tissue alter the interpretation of lipid incorporation data?

Hohenegger: I don't think that it influences these results.

Int. J. Biochem., Vol. 12, pp. 173 to 176
© Pergamon Press Ltd 1980. Printed in Great Britain

0020-711X/80/0701-0173$02.00/0

UPTAKE AND UTILIZATION OF LONG CHAIN AND MEDIUM CHAIN FATTY ACIDS BY THE PERFUSED RAT KIDNEY

MARY ELLEN TRIMBLE
Veterans Administration Hospital and Department of Physiology,
SUNY Upstate Medical Center, Syracuse, NY 13210, U.S.A.

Abstract—1. The apparent transport maximum (T_m) for renal peritubular uptake of the long chain fatty acid, palmitate, is 2.4 μmols·20 min^{-1}·g^{-1}. This value is similar to that observed for peritubular uptake of the medium chain fatty acid, octanoate (2.1 μmols·20 min^{-1}·g^{-1}).

2. Maximum palmitate uptake is not changed by altering fatty acid metabolism through inhibition of fatty acid oxidation or by prior starvation.

3. It is possible to inhibit [^{14}C]palmitate uptake with a conventional inhibitor of the organic acid transport system (probenecid) only when palmitate is present in trace amounts.

INTRODUCTION

In many tissues such as liver (Heimberg *et al.*, 1978), kidney (Dies *et al.*, 1970; Barac-Nieto & Cohen, 1968) and Ehrlich ascites tumor cells (Spector *et al.*, 1965), the uptake of free fatty acids (FFA) has been shown to be proportional to the extracellular FFA concentration. In addition, the uptake appears to be independent of metabolic energy in many systems. These observations are consistent with uptake occurring by simple diffusion. However, in the kidney, there is also much evidence to suggest that a transport system for fatty acids is linked to the general transport system for organic acids. Substances transported by this system characteristically show a tubular transport maximum (T_m) and their transport can be competitively inhibited by certain other organic acids. Most studies have demonstrated that FFA inhibit transport of substances known to be transported by the organic acid system such as para-aminohippurate (PAH) or probenecid (Cohen & Barac-Nieto, 1973; Sheikh & Stahl, 1977). Only in a limited number of studies has the reverse been shown, in that α-ketoglutarate, probenecid and chlorothiazide inhibited uptake of FFA by the intact dog kidney (Barac-Nieto & Cohen, 1968).

Relatively little is known of the transport of individual fatty acids by the kidney. The present studies were done to determine the characteristics of transport of the long chain fatty acid, palmitate, by the perfused rat kidney. Comparisons were made with transport of the medium chain fatty acid, octanoate. The extent to which alterations in fatty acid metabolism might affect observed rates of fatty acid uptake was also examined.

MATERIALS AND METHODS

Kidneys from male Charles River rats (325–425 g) were perfused according to previously described techniques (Bowman & Maack, 1972; Trimble, 1979). Perfusate contained 1% defatted albumin (Chen, 1967) in Krebs bicarbonate buffer with 0.1–2.0 mM palmitate (added as the potassium salt) and 0.12–0.25 μCi [U-^{14}C]palmitate (Amersham/Searle, S.A. 928 mCi·mmol^{-1}. Measurements involving octanoate have been described previously (Trimble, 1979). Aliquots of perfusate were acidified to drive off $^{14}CO_2$ and then assayed for ^{14}C radioactivity by liquid scintillation counting. The radioactivity remaining in perfusate is referred to subsequently as Non-CO_2 ^{14}C. FFA were extracted from a second aliquot (Dole, 1956; Trout *et al.*, 1960). The extracts were analyzed for FFA by titration (Albrink, 1959) and for ^{14}C radioactivity present as FFA. When unlabelled palmitate was added to perfusate, ^{14}C radioactivity at the end of an experiment was present only as FFA. When only trace amounts of ^{14}C palmitate were used, approximately 94 ± 2% of ^{14}C radioactivity was present as FFA.

Uptake of fatty acid was determined as the loss of fatty acid from perfusate with time. Both unlabelled and ^{14}C FFA were measured in initial and terminal perfusate samples. When clearance measurements were made, the amount of fatty acid removed in perfusate samples could not be determined chemically since the quantity of FFA was too small. In these cases, the amount of fatty acid removed was determined from the amount of Non-CO_2 ^{14}C removed. The amount of Non-CO_2 ^{14}C label excreted in the urine represented less than 0.5% of the total ^{14}C label removed (see Table 1). This amount and the amount taken in perfusate sampling were added back prior to determination of net loss of label from the system.

Kidneys were generally perfused for 60 min in a recirculating system. Uptake has been reported in terms of μmols·20 min^{-1}·g kidney^{-1} in order to make comparisons with previous experiments (Trimble, 1979). In some experiments, kidneys were initially perfused for 30 min with 0.4 mM α-bromopalmitate. This procedure has been shown to inhibit fatty acid oxidation in this system (Trimble & Bowman, 1973). Kidneys were then transferred, without interruption of perfusion, to a second chamber for 60 min perfusion in the presence of palmitate and [^{14}C]palmitate. Fatty acid uptake was measured during the 60 min period. Control kidneys were treated similarly except that α-bromopalmitate (α-BP) was omitted from perfusate. In other experiments, kidneys were obtained from rats which had been maintained with water *ad libitum* but without food for 48 hr (starved).

RESULTS

Filtration and excretion of palmitate

Since long chain fatty acids are insoluble in water, perfusate contained 1% defatted albumin added as a carrier. As a result of extensive binding to albumin,

Table 1. Filtration and excretion of palmitate and ^{14}C label derived from [U-^{14}C]palmitate

	Palmitate concentration 0.4 mM	0.1 mM
1. Percentage of palmitate bound to 1% defatted albumin	99.6%	99.6*
2. Total initial amount of perfusate palmitate (μmols)	16	4
3. Filtered palmitate (μmols)	$0.77 \pm 0.14 \times 10^{-3}$†	$0.33 \pm 0.03 \times 10^{-3}$†
4. Non-CO_2 ^{14}C dpm excreted		
(a) % of initial total dpm	0.19 ± 0.03	0.21 ± 0.03
(b) % of total dpm removed from perfusate	0.40 ± 0.09	ND
5. Percentage of terminal non-CO_2 ^{14}C present as FFA	97.5 ± 1.5	—
6. Number of kidneys	4	4

* 3 determinations.

† Based on amount of free palmitate. Kidneys were perfused for 60 min (0.4 mM) or 30 min (0.1 mM). ND = a net decrease in ^{14}C dpm was not detectable at a significant level. FFA = free fatty acid.

very little palmitate was available for filtration (Table 1). Maximum possible reabsorption would be in terms of nmols·min^{-1}. In contrast, the measured rate of uptake, to be reported subsequently, is in terms of μmoles. Consequently, reabsorptive uptake can be considered a negligible factor and the measured uptake represents essentially peritubular uptake. Excretion of ^{14}C radioactivity in the urine is also negligible (Table 1). In this particular experiment, Non-CO_2 ^{14}C radioactivity in perfusate was present entirely as FFA. In some experiments, with 0.4 mM palmitate or less, we have observed a decrease in final specific activity (^{14}C dpm·μmol fatty acid^{-1}) indicating release of endogenous fatty acid. This was not uniformly observed, however, and the maximum calculated release was 0.17 μmols·20 min^{-1}·g^{-1}.

Fatty acid uptake

Peritubular uptake of palmitate reached an apparent transport maximum (T_m) of approximately 2.4 μmols·20 min^{-1}·g^{-1} at concentrations of palmitate greater than 1 mM (Fig. 1A).

In previous experiments, uptake of the medium chain fatty acid, octanoate, was studied (Trimble, 1979). Octanoate is water soluble and less extensively bound to albumin than is palmitate. To measure peritubular octanoate uptake, a non-filtering kidney was used (10% Dextran, 50 mm Hg perfusion pressure). Perfusate flow rate was comparable to that observed in the filtering kidney. Since filtration and reabsorption from the tubular lumen were eliminated, uptake of octanoate under these conditions must have occurred from the peritubular side. Maximum peritubular uptake was approximately 2.1 μmols·20 min^{-1}·g^{-1}, a value similar to that observed for palmitate (Fig. 1).

There is an "apparent T_m" of 2–2.5 μmols·20 min^{-1}·g^{-1} for peritubular uptake of both long chain and medium chain fatty acids. This T_m could reflect a limit to the capacity of the kidney to metabolize fatty acids or saturation of a membrane transport system. In an attempt to distinguish between these two possibilities, kidneys were perfused first with α-BP, an inhibitor of fatty acid oxidation, and then switched to new perfusion medium containing 1.2 mM palmitate and [^{14}C]palmitate. Fractional sodium reabsorption was reduced from 50 ± 6% in controls to 31 ± 6% in α-BP treated kidneys by the end of the second perfusion. Also, analysis of ^{14}C compounds in renal tissue indicated that water soluble metabolites of fatty acid oxidation were reduced

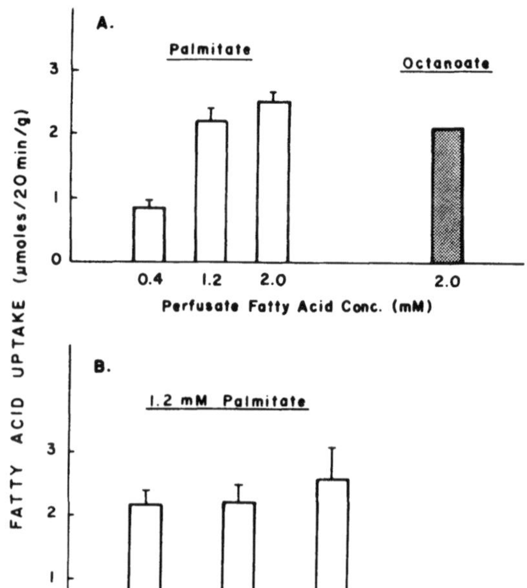

Fig. 1A. Peritubular uptake of fatty acids at various perfusate fatty acid concentrations. Each bar represents Mean ± SE of 4–7 kidneys.

Fig. 1B. Lack of effect of changes in fatty acid metabolism on maximum peritubular palmitate uptake. Each bar represents Mean ± SE of 4–7 kidneys.

by 66% in α-BP treated kidneys. Although metabolism of fatty acids was depressed, this was not reflected in the rate of fatty acid uptake (Fig. 1B) which did not differ significantly from controls.

It has previously been reported that uptake of fatty acids is stimulated in kidneys isolated from fasted rats (Ross *et al.*, 1973). It was thought that perhaps the "T_m" observed in the present experiments could be increased by prior starvation of the rats for 48 hr. Under conditions of these experiments, however, no increase in maximum fatty acid uptake could be observed (Fig. 1B).

If fatty acids are indeed transported by way of an organic acid transport system, one might expect to be able to demonstrate inhibition of their transport by such inhibitors as probenecid or PAH. We have shown previously that when trace [^{14}C]palmitate was added to perfusate, the removal of ^{14}C label from perfusate was inhibited by 1 mM probencid (Trimble *et al.*, 1978). However, the label was not specifically identified as FFA. These experiments have been repeated and in one experiment, after 20 min perfusion, 1 mM probencid had decreased removal of [^{14}C]palmitate from perfusate from 23.4 ± 3.7% in controls ($n = 4$) to 10.9 ± 3.2% with probenecid ($n = 4$). However, it should be noted that in a second similar experiment ($n = 1$ each) no inhibition was observed. In a series of experiments with 1–2 mM probenecid or 10–20 mM PAH, it has been impossible to demonstrate any inhibition of peritubular fatty acid uptake.

DISCUSSION

It has been demonstrated that an apparent T_m exists for fatty acid transport across the peritubular or antiluminal membrane of the renal tubular cell. It is of interest that the T_m values for both medium chain and long chain fatty acids are similar, between 2.0–2.5 μmols·20 min^{-1}·g^{-1}. This would tend to suggest that the T_m does not reflect a mitochondrial transport step since palmitate requires carnitine for mitochondrial transport while octanoate does not. Exogenous carnitine was not present in the perfusion medium.

An apparent T_m for palmitate uptake has also been demonstrated in the perfused rat heart (Oram *et al.*, 1975). At a perfusion pressure of 50 mm Hg, this T_m was approx 12 μmols·20 min^{-1}·g^{-1}. However, these investigators presented evidence that the T_m was a reflection of palmitate metabolism in that acetyl CoA oxidation was limited. Also, it was possible to increase the maximum fatty acid uptake through acceleration of the citric acid cycle brought about by increasing cardiac work (perfusion pressure 100 mm Hg). In the present experiments, rather than increasing renal work, an attempt was made to decrease fatty acid metabolism by prior perfusion with an inhibitor of fatty acid oxidation, α-BP. This was without demonstrable effect on peritubular palmitate uptake. It is possible, however, that the degree of inhibition of fatty acid oxidation was insufficient or that simultaneous increases in esterification occurred.

In contrast to the findings of others (Ross *et al.*, 1973), prior starvation produced no changes in renal fatty acid uptake. However, in the present experiments, only possible effects on maximal uptake were examined. McGarry *et al.* (1973) have observed that in the perfused liver, for example, starvation does not change the total amount of fatty acid taken up but the metabolic fate of the fatty acid is altered.

It has been possible to inhibit palmitate uptake by probenecid, a competitive inhibitor of the organic acid transport system, only when palmitate is present in trace amounts (Trimble *et al.*, 1978; present experiments). In a previous study of medium chain fatty acid transport (Trimble, 1979), we also found that when exogenous octanoic acid was added to perfusate in greater than trace amounts, inhibitors of organic acid transport such as probenecid or PAH were ineffective in inhibiting uptake of the fatty acid. Although these experiments with the perfused kidney represent non-steady state conditions, it is possible to show inhibition of other organic acid transport in this system. For example, probenecid will inhibit PAH transport (Trimble, 1979). It is possible that the affinity of the fatty acids for a postulated carrier molecule exceeds that of other organic acids. However, more experiments are necessary to rule out possible metabolic limitations.

Acknowledgement—This research was supported by the Veterans Administration.

REFERENCES

ALBRINK M. J. (1959) The microtitration of total fatty acids of serum with notes on the estimation of triglycerides. *J. Lipid Res.* **1**, 53–59.

BARAC-NIETO M. & COHEN J. J. (1968) Nonesterified fatty acid uptake by dog kidney: effects of probenecid and chlorothiazide. *Am. J. Physiol.* **215**, 98–107.

BOWMAN R. H. & MAACK T. (1972) Glucose transport by the isolated perfused rat kidney. *Am. J. Physiol.* **222**, 1499–1504.

CHEN R. F. (1967) Removal of fatty acids from serum albumin by charcoal treatment. *J. biol. Chem.* **242**, 173–181.

COHEN J. J. & BARAC-NIETO M. (1973) Renal metabolism of substrates in relation to renal function. In *Handbook of Physiology, Sect. 8, Renal Physiology* (Edited by ORLOFF J. & BERLINER R.), Am. Physiol. Soc., Washington DC.

DIES F., HERRERA J., MATAS M., AVELAR E. & RAMOS G. (1970) Substrate uptake by the dog kidney *in vivo*. *Am. J. Physiol.* **218**, 405–410.

DOLE V. P. (1956) A relation between nonesterified fatty acids in plasma and the metabolism of glucose. *J. clin. Invest.* **35**, 150–154.

HEIMBERG M., GOH E. H., KLAUSNER H. A., SOLER-ARGILAGA C., WEINSTEIN I. & WILCOX H. G. (1978) Regulation of hepatic metabolism of free fatty acids: interrelationships among secretion of very-low-density lipoproteins, ketogenesis and cholesterologenesis. In *Disturbances in Lipid and Lipoprotein Metabolism* (Edited by DIETSCHY J., GOTTO A. M. JR & ONTKO J. A.) pp. 251–267. Am. Physiol. Soc., Bethesda, MD.

MCGARRY J. D., MEIER J. M. & FOSTER D. W. (1973) The effects of starvation and refeeding on carbohydrate and lipid metabolism *in vivo* and in the perfused rat liver. The relationship between fatty acid oxidation and esterification in the regulation of ketogenesis. *J. biol. Chem.* **248**, 270–278.

ORAM J. F., BENNETCH S. I. & NEELY J. R. (1973) Regulation of fatty acid utilization in isolated perfused rat hearts. *J. biol. Chem.* **248**, 5299–5309.

ROSS B. D., EPSTEIN F. H. & LEAF A. (1973) Sodium reabsorption in the perfused rat kidney. *Am. J. Physiol.* **225**, 1165–1171.

SHEIKH M. I. & STAHL M. (1977) Characteristics of accumulation of probenecid by rabbit kidney cortical slices. *Am. J. Physiol.* **232**, F513–F523.

SPECTOR A. A., STEINBERG D. D. & TANAKA A. (1965) Uptake of free fatty acids by Ehrlich ascites tumor cells. *J. biol. Chem.* **240**, 1032–1041.

TRIMBLE M. E. & BOWMAN R. H. (1973) Renal Na^+ and K^+ transport: effects of glucose, palmitate and α-bromopalmitate. *Am. J. Physiol.* **225**, 1057–1062.

TRIMBLE M. E., HARRINGTON W. W. JR & BOWMAN R. H. (1978) Fatty acid transport and metabolism in the isolated perfused rat kidney. In: *Current Problems in Clinical Biochemistry*, Vol. 8, *Biochemical Nephrology* (Edited by GUDER W. W. & SCHMIDT U.) pp. 362–370. Huber, Bern.

TRIMBLE M. E. (1979) Transport and metabolism of octanoate by the perfused rat kidney. *Am. J. Physiol.* In press.

TROUT D. L., ESTES H. & FRIEDBERG S. J. (1960) Titration of free fatty acids of plasma: a study of current methods and a new modification. *J. Lipid Res.* **1**, 199–202.

SYMPOSIUM DISCUSSION

Saggerson: Have you done any experiments where you put in mono-, di-, or tri-unsaturated fatty acids? I ask because some of the uptake must be for phospholipid synthesis, and the palmitate uptake may be reduced if the optimum conditions for phospholipid synthesis are not present.

Trimble: I have not tried any such combinations.

Ross: Does bromopalmitate inhibit fatty acid oxidation in perfused kidney?

Trimble: Yes, $^{14}CO_2$ production from palmitate is inhibited within 30–40 min by 40%.

Guder: In the tubule system bromopalmitate acts like a fatty acid: it is oxidized, stimulates gluconeogenesis, and decreases pyruvate dehydrogenase, so some of what you describe as inhibition, we would interpret as dilution. If there really was an inhibitory effect, CoA levels would fall, and triacyl glycerol formation would be inhibited. Have you measured that?

Trimble: When we perfused with palmitate and bromopalmitate simultanesouly, about half of the ^{14}C label from [^{14}C]palmitate was found as free fatty acid compared to about 10% when only palmitate was present. Radioactivity in phospholipids was decreased from 70 to 35%. We concluded that bromopalmitate was inhibiting esterification although incorporation into neutral lipids was unaffected. (Trimble *et al.*, Fatty acid transport and metabolism in the isolated perfused rat kidney. In *Current Problems in Clinical Biochemistry* (Edited by GUDER W. G. & SCHMIDT U. Vol. 8, pp. 362–370. Huber, Bern, 1978). Conversely, when you perfuse first with bromopalmitate and then change to palmitate, label in free fatty acids is only slightly increased but that in triacyl glycerol almost doubles. This suggests that oxidation of fatty acids released from triacyl glycerol is being inhibited. With respect to oxidation of bromopalmitate, Pande *et al.* (*Biochim. biophys. Acta* **248**, 156–166, 1971) have reported that the rate of bromopalmitate activation is only 5–6% that of palmitate activation.

Franke: What was the GFR during bromopalmitate infusion, and have you looked at the effects of hypoxia?

Trimble: These experiments were performed with a non-filtering kidney, but from previous experiments, we know that it lowers GFR. (Trimble & Bowman, *Am. J. Physiol.* **225**, 1057–1062, 1973). Substitution of nitrogen for oxygen inhibits the uptake of octanoate.

Tannen: Have you looked at the effects of an energy source other than fatty acids in your perfusions?

Trimble: No.

Schurek: You used only 1 g% albumin?

Trimble: In all the experiments with octanoate transport in non-filtering kidneys, 10% dextran was used. 1 g% albumin was added as a carrier for long chain fatty acids (palmitate).

Chapter 3

Biochemistry of filtration and reabsorption; glomeruli and brush border

Int. J. Biochem., Vol. 12, pp. 177 to 180
© Pergamon Press Ltd 1980. Printed in Great Britain

0020-711X/80/0701-0177$02.00/0

INTRODUCTION

VARIATIONS IN GLOMERULAR FUNCTION DUE TO CHANGE IN GLOMERULAR MEMBRANE CHARACTERISTICS

CHRISTINE BAYLIS
Department of Physiology, Manchester University, Manchester, M13 9PT, U.K.

Abstract—1. Experiments using physiological techniques have indicated that the transport of water, electrolytes and large molecules may be influenced by local variations in the characteristics of the glomerular membrane.

2. It is beyond the scope of such experiments, however, to define the mechanisms involved in reduction of the water ultrafiltration coefficient seen in various conditions and in development of proteinurias due to loss of glomerular polyanion.

3. Application of biochemical methods to these problems will certainly yield considerable insight into our understanding of glomerular function in both health and disease.

Physiological studies on glomerular function have been advanced by the discovery of the Munich–Wistar rat—a strain possessing superficial glomeruli which are accessible to direct puncture. Micropuncture studies in these rats have indicated that, in the superficial single nephron population, filtration may be controlled, acutely, by changes in the characteristics of the glomerular membrane (permeability/surface area) as well as by alterations in pre- and post-glomerular arteriolar resistances.

According to the Starling equation the rate of ultrafiltration for a single glomerulus is given by:

$$\begin{aligned} \text{SNGFR} &= (\Delta P - \Delta\pi).k.S. \\ &= [(P_{GC} - P_T) - (\pi_{GC} - \pi_T)]\,k_f \qquad (1) \end{aligned}$$

where single nephron glomerular filtration rate, SNGFR, is determined by the hydrostatic and oncotic pressure differences acting across the glomerular wall (ΔP and $\Delta\pi$ respectively) as well as by the water permeability (k) and available surface area (S) of the glomerular membrane. The transglomerular hydrostatic pressure difference is measured by direct determination of glomerular capillary (P_{GC}) and proximal tubule (P_T) hydrostatic pressure. The pre- and post-glomerular oncotic pressures may be calculated from the measured protein concentrations at these sites, which gives an estimate of the mean oncotic pressure within the glomerular capillary (π_{GC}); since protein concentration within the tubule is extremely low the proximal tubular oncotic pressure (π_T) may be ignored (see Baylis *et al.*, 1978a).

Although not appearing specifically in equation (1), the glomerular plasma flow rate will also influence filtration rate by affecting the rate of change of oncotic pressure along the glomerular capillary network (Baylis *et al.*, 1978a); glomerular plasma flow rate may be calculated from the measured single nephron GFR (the single nephron inulin clearance determined from tubular fluid samples obtained by micropuncture) and the single nephron filtration fraction (calculated from pre- and post-glomerular protein concentrations).

Since it is possible to directly determine all the pressures and flows which govern glomerular ultrafiltration in the Munich–Wistar rat, it is theoretically possible to calculate the remaining unknown in equation (1), the glomerular capillary ultrafiltration coefficient, k_f (the product of glomerular water permeability and surface area). Calculation of this variable is, however, complicated for the following reasons: micropuncture studies in the Munich–Wistar rat have indicated that under the control conditions of hydropenia and euvolemia, filtration pressure equilibrium obtains in the superficial nephron population (Baylis *et al.*, 1978a; Ichikawa *et al.*, 1978a). In filtration pressure equilibrium, formation of protein-free ultrafiltrate has caused the oncotic pressure within the glomerular capillary to rise to a value equal (and in opposition) to the transglomerular hydrostatic pressure gradient before blood has reached the efferent end of the glomerulus. Thus, at the equilibrium point (when $\pi_{GC} = \Delta P$) filtration must cease since there is no longer a net driving pressure. As discussed elsewhere it is impossible to calculate a unique value of the glomerular ultrafiltration coefficient in an animal at filtration pressure equilibrium and only a minimum value may be determined (see Baylis *et al.*, 1978a). Furthermore, in an animal at equilibrium, *increases* in ultrafiltration coefficient will have a negligible effect on single nephron GFR, since an increase in glomerular ultrafiltration coefficient will simply displace the equilibrium point towards the afferent end of the capillary i.e. ~ the same quantity of fluid will be filtered over a shorter length of the capillary network. Reductions in the ultrafiltration coefficient will displace the equilibrium point towards the efferent end of the glomerulus and, if of sufficient magnitude, the fall in ultrafiltration coefficient will result in filtration pressure *disequilibrium*. In the disequilibrium condition a positive net driving pressure exists even at the efferent end of the glomerular capillary. Also, in this condition alterations in either water permeability or surface area will exert marked effects on the filtration rate; further, the product of permeability and surface area,

Table 1. Summary of some agents which acutely reduce the glomerular capillary ultrafiltration coefficient (k_f)

Agent	Reference
Prostaglandin E_1	Baylis *et al.*, 1976; Ichikawa *et al.*, 1978b
Acetylcholine	Baylis *et al.*, 1976
Bradykinin	Baylis *et al.*, 1976
Papaverine	Deen *et al.*, 1974
Histamine	Ichikawa *et al.*, 1978c
Angiotensin II	Blantz *et al.*, 1976; Baylis *et al.*, 1978b; Ichikawa *et al.*, 1978b
Antidiuretic hormone	Ichikawa *et al.*, 1977
Dibutyryl cyclic AMP	Ichikawa *et al.*, 1977
Parathyroid hormone	Ichikawa *et al.*, 1978d
High plasma [Ca^{2+}]	Humes *et al.*, 1978
Low plasma [protein]	Baylis *et al.*, 1977a; Schurek *et al.*, 1978

the ultrafiltration coefficient (k_f) may be calculated uniquely (see Baylis *et al.*, 1978a).

For the reasons discussed above, glomerular micropuncture studies have tended to define agents or circumstances which *reduce* glomerular capillary ultrafiltration coefficient, rather than those which increase this variable. Table 1 summarizes some of the agents which have been shown to evoke an acute reduction in glomerular ultrafiltration coefficient. In most of the studies cited here the actions of pharmacological doses of hormonal agents have been studied. Angiotensin II, the antidiuretic and parathyroid hormones have, however, been observed to reduce ultrafiltration coefficient at, or around the physiological concentrations of these substances (Blantz *et al.*, 1976; Ichikawa *et al.*, 1977, 1978d).

As well as being acute in onset, the reductions in ultrafiltration coefficient due to some of the agents listed in Table 1 have been shown to be rapidly reversible. The angiotensin II and prostaglandin E_1-induced reductions in ultrafiltration coefficient are reversed by antagonism of transcellular calcium transport with the drug verapamil, or with manganese (Ichikawa *et al.*, 1978b). Furthermore, the fall seen in ultrafiltration coefficient during acute reduction in plasma protein concentration may be rapidly reversed by infusion of concentrated, homologous rat plasma which restores plasma protein concentration to the normal value (Baylis *et al.*, 1977a).

The mechanisms by which ultrafiltration coefficient is reduced are unknown at present although possible mediating roles for calcium and cyclic nucleotides have been suggested (Humes *et al.*, 1978; Ichikawa *et al.*, 1977, 1978b, 1978d). It should be emphasised, however, that conventional micropuncture techniques cannot define whether falls in membrane permeability or filtration surface area are responsible when a reduction in the ultrafiltration coefficient occurs.

As well as varying acutely, the ultrafiltration coefficient has been found to be reduced in several chronic conditions including daily administration of the antibiotic gentamicin, administration of puromycin aminonucleoside (a drug which induces a lesion resembling the minimal change nephrotic syndrome) and in experimental glomerulonephritis (Baylis *et al.*, 1977b; Bohrer *et al.*, 1977, 1978). The lesions associated with puromycin aminonucleoside administration and experimental glomerulonephritis are also characterised by proteinuria of glomerular origin (see Bohrer *et al.*, 1977, 1978). The classical explanation for this type of proteinuria is that increased glomerular permeability to protein occurs; however this suggestion is difficult to reconcile with the reduction in water ultrafiltration coefficient which also occurs in both of these lesions. It is well known that in the normal animal the transglomerular transport of large circulating molecules, such as the plasma proteins, is progressively restricted with increasing molecular size (Renkin & Gilmore, 1973). It is possible to investigate the glomerular permeability to large molecules in normal and proteinuric animals by comparison of whole kidney clearance of large molecules, of varying sizes, with the simultaneous clearance of inulin (Renkin & Gilmore, 1973); examples of such studies in the Munich–Wistar rat are given in Fig. 1. Here, the clearance of dextran is compared to that of inulin (giving a fractional clearance value) over a range of dextran radii. A fractional clearance of 1.0 indicates that dextran traverses the glomerular wall as freely as does inulin (and therefore water), while fractional clearance values < 1.0 indicate that dextran transport is restricted relative to water transport. The use of whole kidney clearance methods to assess the glomerular handling of large circulating molecules relies on the assumption that the macromolecule employed is not handled within the renal tubule. This assumption has been verified for large molecular weight dextrans in the Munich–Wistar rat, by analysis of fluid obtained directly from Bowman's space. Previous studies using these techniques have indicated that in proteinuric rats with experimental nephrotoxic serum nephritis or puromycin aminonucleoside-induced nephrosis, the transglomerular transport of electrically neutral dextrans is significantly reduced compared to normals, over most of the range of molecular size studied (Bennett *et al.*, 1976; Bohrer *et al.*, 1977). These findings indicate an apparent reduction in glomerular permeability to dextran in nephritic rats, observations which accord well with the fall in the ultrafiltration coefficient for water also seen in these lesions, but which completely fail to explain the concomitant proteinuria.

Histochemical and function studies have indicated that in addition to the permeability properties of the glomerular membrane, the transport of circulating, anionic plasma proteins are also influenced by the

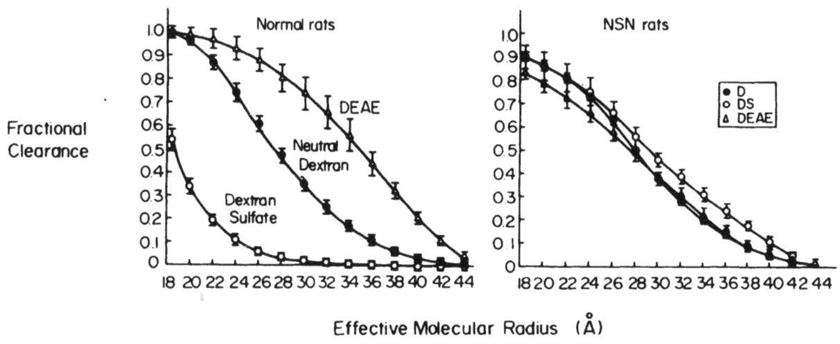

Fig. 1. Fractional clearances of anionic dextran sulphate, neutral dextran and cationic diethylaminoethyl dextran, plotted as a function of effective molecular radius in normal rats and in rats with nephrotoxic serum nephritis (NSN). Values are expressed as means ± 1 SEM. Reproduced with permission from Bohrer *et al.*, 1978.

presence of fixed negative charges on the wall of the glomerular capillary (see Brenner *et al.*, 1977). In normal rats the fractional clearance of an anionic dextran species, dextran sulphate, is markedly reduced compared to that of neutral dextran over the entire range of molecular radii studied (Fig. 1). Further, a cationic dextran species, diethylaminoethyl dextran, exhibits enhanced fractional clearances relative to neutral dextran (Fig. 1). These findings are consistent with the existence of an electronegative barrier within the wall of the glomerulus.

In contrast, observations in rats with nephrotoxic serum nephritis and rats pre-treated with puromycin aminonucleoside have demonstrated markedly enhanced fractional clearances of anionic dextran sulphate in these proteinuric animals, relative to normals (Bennett *et al.*, 1976; Bohrer *et al.*, 1977). Indeed, as shown in Fig. 1, the fractional clearance profiles for both anionic and cationic dextran polymers (dextran sulphate and diethylaminoethyl dextran respectively) approached that seen for neutral dextran in rats with nephrotoxic serum nephritis (Bohrer *et al.*, 1978). These functional studies, together with histochemical investigations (see Brenner *et al.*, 1977) have indicated that loss of fixed glomerular negative charge in rats with experimental glomerulonephritis causes the glomerular capillary to handle the anionic and cationic dextrans as if they were electrically neutral (Fig. 1). Reduction in glomerular polyanion together with falls in the glomerular ultrafiltration coefficient will have the net effect of reducing transglomerular transport of neutral and cationic macromolecules while enhancing transport of anionic macromolecules (such as protein) in nephritic rats, relative to normals, thus providing an explanation for the proteinuria of experimental glomerulonephritis. It is likely that puromycin aminonucleoside-induced proteinuria is the result of similar changes in glomerular membrane function.

Acknowledgements—I thank the Wellcome Trust for their support. The secretarial assistance of Mrs Anne Mogie is gratefully acknowledged.

REFERENCES

Baylis C., Deen W. M., Myers B. D. & Brenner B. M. (1976) Effects of some vasodilator drugs on transcapillary fluid exchange in renal cortex. *Am. J. Physiol.* **230,** 1148–1158.

Baylis C., Ichikawa I., Willis W. T., Wilson C. B. & Brenner B. M. (1977a) Dynamics of glomerular ultrafiltration IX. Effects of plasma protein concentration. *Am. J. Physiol.* **232,** F58–F71.

Baylis C., Rennke H. R. & Brenner B. M. (1977b). Mechanism of the defect in glomerular ultrafiltration associated with gentamicin administration. *Kidney Int.* **12,** 344–353.

Baylis C. & Brenner B. M. (1978a) The physiological determinants of glomerular ultrafiltration. *Rev. Physiol. Biochem. Pharmac.* **80,** 1–46.

Baylis C. & Brenner B. M. (1978b) Modulation by prostaglandin synthesis inhibitors of the action of exogenous angiotensin II on glomerular ultrafiltration in the rat. *Circ. Res.* **43,** 889–898.

Bennett C. M., Glassock R. J., Chang R. L. S., Deen W. M., Robertson C. R. & Brenner B. M. (1976) Permselectivity of the glomerular capillary wall. Studies of experimental glomerulonephritis in the rat using dextran sulphate. *J. clin. Invest.* **57,** 1287–1294.

Blantz R. C., Konnen K. S. & Tucker B. J. (1976) Angiotensin II effects upon the glomerular microcirculation and ultrafiltration coefficient of the rat. *J. clin. Invest.* **57,** 419–434.

Bohrer M. P., Baylis C., Robertson C. R. & Brenner B. M. (1977) Mechanisms of the puromycin-induced defect in the transglomerular passage of water and macromolecules. *J. clin. Invest.* **60,** 152–161.

Bohrer M. P., Baylis C., Humes H. D., Glassock R. J., Robertson C. R. & Brenner B. M. (1978). Permselectivity of the glomerular capillary wall. Facilitated filtration of circulating polycations. *J. clin. Invest.* **61,** 72–78.

Brenner B. M., Bohrer M. P., Baylis C. & Deen W. M. (1977) Determinants of glomerular permselectivity: Insights derived from observations *in vivo*. *Kidney Int.* **12,** 229–237.

Deen W. M., Robertson C. R. & Brenner B. M. (1974) Glomerular ultrafiltration. *Fedn Proc. Fedn Am. Soc. exp. Biol.* **33,** 14–20.

Humes H. D., Ichikawa I., Troy J. L. & Brenner B. M. (1978). Evidence for a parathyroid hormone-dependent influence of calcium on the glomerular ultrafiltration coefficient. *J. clin. Invest.* **61,** 32–40.

Ichikawa I. & Brenner B. M. (1977) Evidence for glomerular actions of ADH and dibutyryl cyclic AMP in the rat. *Am. J. Physiol.* **233,** F102–F117.

Ichikawa I., Maddox D. A., Cogan M. G. & Brenner B. M. (1978a). Dynamics of glomerular ultrafiltration in euvolemic Munich-Wistar rats. *Renal Physiol.* **1,** 121–131.

Ichikawa I. & Brenner B. M. (1978b) Role of calcium on the glomerular actions of angiotensin II (AII) and prostaglandin *in vivo*. Abst. VII Int. Congr. Nephrol. F-8.

ICHIKAWA I., TORRES V. E., DOUSA T. P. & BRENNER B. M. (1978c) Influences of histamine (H) on glomeruli *in vivo* and *in vitro*. Abst. VII Int. Congr. Nephrol. K-16.

ICHIKAWA I., HUMES H. D., DOUSA T. P. & BRENNER B. M. (1978d) Influence of parathyroid hormone on glomerular ultrafiltration in the rat. *Am. J. Physiol.* **234,** F393–F401.

RENKIN E. M. & GILMORE J. P. (1973) Handbook of Physiology. Section 8—Renal Physiology. pp. 185–248. American Physiological Society, Washington DC.

SCHUREK H. J., SCHWIETZER G., ALT J. & STOLTE H. (1978) Albumin filtration and effective filtration pressure in cortical nephrons in the isolated perfused rat kidney. Abst. VII Int. Congr. Nephrol. X-4.

SYMPOSIUM DISCUSSION

Osswald: Maybe there has been some change in the available surface for glomerular filtration in your puromycin poisoned rats, so that you have loss of the fixed charge but also reduction of surface area.

Baylis: There was certainly a reduction in either surface area or water permeability in those animals, but we have no indication of which of those two it was.

Osswald: What do you see morphologically in the sections through the glomerulae? Do the glomerulae and the endothelium of the capillary look different?

Baylis: In the glomerulae there is a retraction of foot processes and loss of foot process organisation in the epithilial cells. By transmission electron microscopy, the endothelial cells look grossly normal.

Morgensen: I would like to ask, whether it is possible to distinguish between alteration in surface area and glomerular permeability in your acute studies?

Baylis: No, not directly using micropuncture techniques, although there is a study by Ichikawa (Ichikawa *et al.*, *Kidney Int.* **16,** 137, 1979) using the drug verapamil which inhibits trans-cellular calcium transport. He has investigated the effect of verapamil in animals receiving infusions of angiotensin and prostaglandins and has found in both cases, that verapamil reverses the fall in ultrafiltration coefficient seen with those two hormones. He interprets that as suggesting that both of those substances either directly or indirectly evoke constriction of mesangial cells within the glomerulus thus reducing filtration surface area, and that the verapamil is preventing mesangial constriction.

Kiil: Do your experiments permit the conclusion that all nephrons, or most of them, are contributing to proteinuria, not only a few of them?

Baylis: Yes, we may assume that the changes in whole kidney handling of neutral, anionic and cationic dextran in rats with experimentally induced nephrotoxic serum nephritis, relative to normals, are the result of fairly uniform glomerular injuries. It is unlikely that an effect as marked as that seen at the whole-kidney level could be due to impaired glomerular barrier function in just a few nephrons. In addition, histological studies of this lesion have indicated that the glomerular injury is fairly uniform throughout the kidney. (Maddox *et al.*, *J. clin. Invest.* **55,** 305, 1975).

Alleyne: You indicated that levels of serum protein may influence the ultra-filtration co-efficient. Do you have any data on the effect of raising the plasma protein in your rats, or of the effect on dextran clearances of increasing plasma proteins?

Baylis: No, there are studies in the rat and dog (Blantz *et al.*, *Kidney Int.* **6,** 209, 1974; Thomas *et al.*, *Kidney Int.* **15** 502, 1979), on the effect of raising protein concentration on water ultrafiltration coefficient, and it goes up with increasing protein concentration. But we have not looked at the effects of protein-overload proteinuria.

Int. J. Biochem., Vol. 12, pp. 181 to 184
© Pergamon Press Ltd 1980. Printed in Great Britain

0020-711X/80/0701-0181$02.00/0

RENAL PROTEIN HANDLING IN MAN, MODIFIED BY INSULIN ADMINISTRATION, STRESS SITUATIONS AND HYPERTENSION

C. E. MOGENSEN[1], C. K. CHRISTENSEN[1], N. J. CHRISTENSEN[2], H. J. GUNDERSEN[3] and P. GJODE[4]

[1]Medical Department I and [4]Department of Surgery, Århus Amtssygehus, Medical Department M, Århus Kommunehospital, and [3]Institute of Experimental Clinical Research, University of Arhus, [2]Arhus and Department of Internal Medicine and Endocrinology, Herlev Hospital, Copenhagen, Denmark.

Abstract—1. The aim of the study was to clarify the effect on glomerular function of various factors found to modify the cardiovascular system generally.

2. Insulin: intravenous injection of insulin resulted in an increased albumin excretion and a rise in heart rate and in plasma noradrenaline in diabetics in whom blood glucose was maintained at unchanged levels after insulin by glucose infusion. In patients where insulin was given alone both GFR and RPF decreased. Thus insulin has a marked effect on glomerular function.

3. Stress situations: in surgeons performing intraabdominal operations we found a marked increase in urinary albumin excretion whereas creatinine excretion was unchanged. A marked increase in pulse rate is also seen, indicating a systemic cardiovascular response.

4. Hypertension: we found greatly elevated albumin excretion in newly diagnosed severe hypertension before treatment. The abnormal albumin excretion was very rapidly but not completely reversible by conventional treatment and subsequent fall in blood pressure, clearly indicating the pressure dependency.

5. The glomerulus thus in these situations closely responds to changes in the systemic circulation.

INTRODUCTION

The introduction and the systematic use of sensitive methods for measuring urinary proteins have revealed that a great number of factors are able to modify the renal excretion of plasma proteins in man (Mogensen, 1980). Thus protein excretion is a much more dynamic function than hitherto believed.

Two main processes in the kidney determine the protein pattern in the final urine, the glomerular filtration of plasma proteins and, subsequently, tubular reabsorption. We have two radioimmunoassays for measuring these two separate functions, namely assays for measuring albumin and β-2-microglobulin (Miles *et al.*, 1970; Evrin *et al.*, 1971). Albumin is a marker of enhanced glomerular transport of proteins, whereas the small protein molecule β-2-microglobulin, is a marker of decreased tubular uptake. It is normally freely filtered in the glomerulus and thereafter almost completely reabsorbed by the tubule (Mogensen & Sølling, 1977). On the other hand, albumin is normally largely retained by the glomerular capillaries (Mogensen, 1980).

The aim of the present study was to examine the possible effect on the glomerular capillaries of some factors, namely insulin administration, stress situations and hypertension, all of which are known to modify the cardiovascular system generally.

Urinary albumin excretion was measured to examine changes of the passage rate over the glomerular membrane of a rather large plasma protein and, in order to clarify possible modifying effects from the tubular cells, β-2-microglobulin excretion was determined in addition.

INTRAVENOUS INSULIN ADMINISTRATION AND ALBUMIN EXCRETION

It is now well established that insulin, apart from its effect on metabolism and ion fluxes has a marked effect on the cardiovascular system (Page *et al.*, 1976; Gundersen & Christensen, 1977). Insulin, at least when injected intravenously, also markedly affects renal function (Mogensen *et al.*, 1978). Glomerular filtration rate (GFR) and in particular renal plasma flow are reduced as well as urine flow rate and excretion of several electrolytes. A marked effect is also seen on urinary protein excretion.

Excretion of albumin is enhanced whereas the excretion of β-2-microglobulin decreases, suggesting that insulin, directly or indirectly, stimulates both glomerular passage and tubular reabsorption (Mogensen *et al.*, 1978).

In the present study we examined if the acute renal effects of insulin are modified when blood glucose concentration after intravenous insulin is kept constant by glucose infusion.

Patients and procedures

Five young male juvenile diabetic outpatients were studied. The duration of diabetes averaged 8 yr. They were all treated with insulin twice a day and had their last dose of insulin 24 hr before the investigation.

The patients were examined in the morning after overnight fasting. They rested in the supine position, standing up only to void. They drank 20 ml of water every 20 min starting 1 hr before the experiment and during the whole experimental period.

Following a resting period of 1.5 hr glomerular filtration rate, renal blood flow, urinary albumin and β-2-microglobulin excretion were measured in three 45 min periods before and three 45 min periods after insulin. Seven or eight i.u. of insulin (Actrapid®, Novo) were given intravenously as a 1 min bolus injection. At the same time an infusion of 50% glucose was started at a rate of about 1.2 ml·min^{-1} throughout the subsequent 3 periods.

GFR and RPF were measured by constant infusion techniques using [^{125}I]iothalamate as filtration marker and the clearance of [^{131}I]hippuran for measuring plasma flow (Mogensen, 1971).

Results

In Fig. 1 are shown results of measurements of urinary albumin and β-2-microglobulin excretion before and after insulin injection. Results are given for experiments both without and with glucose infusion; (mean of 3 periods are given in all cases, with the exception of β-2-microglobulin excretion after insulin where only the two periods immediately after injection are used for calculation. In the third period after insulin there was a tendency for excretion to rise again).

We found a significant and almost identical increase in albumin excretion both with and without glucose. The percentage rise was 92 and 94% respectively.

After insulin injection alone β-2-microglobulin excretion decreased significantly by 59%. In the experiments with glucose infusion mean β-2-microglobulin excretion decreased in 4 of the 5 patients but the difference was not significant.

There was a tendency for plasma glucose to increase when insulin injection was followed by glucose infusion (mean 10.7 mM to 12.2 mM). After insulin alone plasma glucose fell, but importantly, not to hypoglycemic values (mean 13.9 mM to 6.5 mM).

There was no significant changes in glomerular filtration rate and in renal plasma flow after insulin followed by glucose-infusion. Urine flow decreased, however, significantly and averaged in the three post-insulin periods only 55% of pre-insulin values.

Comments

The magnitude of the increase in albumin excretion after insulin in the present study was very similar to that in a previously reported study in which blood glucose was allowed to decline after insulin (Mogensen *et al.*, 1978).

Therefore the fall in plasma glucose cannot be operative in producing this increase.

The increased urinary albumin excretion after insulin is most likely due to an increased transglomerular escape rate of albumin. The decrease in β-2-microglobulin excretion after insulin suggests that tubular reabsorption of proteins could even be increased.

Thus insulin stimulates both glomerular passage and tubular uptake of plasma proteins.

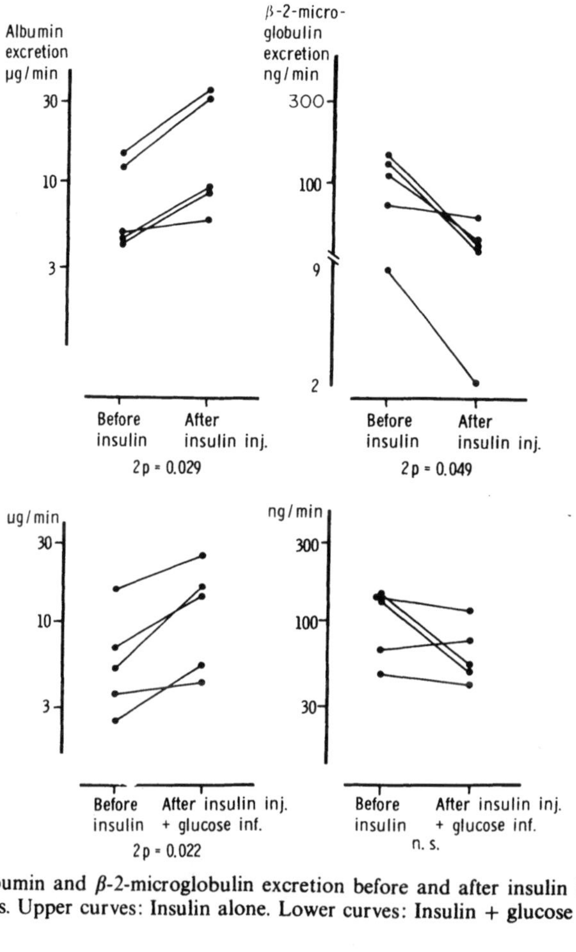

Fig. 1. Urinary albumin and β-2-microglobulin excretion before and after insulin injection in juvenile diabetics. Upper curves: Insulin alone. Lower curves: Insulin + glucose infusion.

The effect of insulin on urinary albumin excretion may be due to a direct effect of insulin on glomerular permeability or mediated via the autonomic nervous system since plasma noradrenaline also increases after insulin (Gundersen & Christensen, 1977). Insulin has been shown to increase the number of micropinocytotic vesicles in muscle capillary endothelial cells in rats (Osterby *et al.*, 1978). This finding may suggest that effects of insulin on albumin excretion may be due to a direct effect of insulin on glomerular capillary endothelial and epithelial cells.

The recently obtained evidence of insulin receptors on glomerular cells may favour this view (Kurokawa *et al.*, 1980).

ALBUMIN EXCRETION IN A STRESS SITUATION: SURGEONS PERFORMING OPERATIONS

It has earlier been suggested that a stress situation may provoke proteinuria but we know of no convincing study documenting an increase in protein excretion during stress. Prompted by a report from Foster *et al.* (1978) that surgeons doing intra-abdominal operations consistently had high heartrates (mean 121 beats$\cdot$min^{-1}, mean peak value 137 beats$\cdot$min^{-1}) we have been exploring vascular permeability in stress by measuring urinary albumin excretion in surgical colleagues.

Six surgeons collected timed urine samples before, during, and after five major intra-abdominal operations and one vaginal hysterectomy. Fig. 2 shows that urinary albumin excretion increased from $5.8 \pm 3.3\ \mu g \cdot min^{-1}$ (SD) before surgery to $15.2 \pm 11.2\ \mu g \cdot min^{-1}$ during the operation ($2P = 0.011$). No changes were seen when the surgeons worked in the outpatient clinic as also seen on the figure. No significant change in urinary β_2-microglobulin excretion was seen, indicating undisturbed tubular protein reabsorption. Also creatinine clearance was unchanged.

Thus the increase in albumin excretion in stress seems to be of glomerular origin, due to increased glomerular permeability. These studies clearly indicate that at least one kind of a stress situation leads to increased protein excretion. The mechanism involved may be increased blood pressure, which is known to increase albumin excretion as mentioned below.

SEVERE, UNTREATED HYPERTENSION AND PROTEIN EXCRETION

Examination of the effect of acute alterations in arterial blood pressure level on protein excretion is not easily feasible in normal man. However, it is possible to go the other way around, namely to examine the relationship between pressure levels and protein excretion in patients being treated intensively for acute, newly diagnosed severe hypertension. Earlier studies have shown that albumin excretion is increased in patients with insufficiently treated hypertension (Parving *et al.*, 1974; Pedersen & Mogensen, 1976).

Five young patients with a mean arterial blood pressure of 165 mm Hg (diastolic pressure plus 1/3 pulse pressure) were studied before and during intensive antihypertensive treatment for a mean of 3 days as shown on Fig. 3. Albumin excretion was very high and dropped considerably during treatment, clearly indicating pressure dependency. Abnormal structure

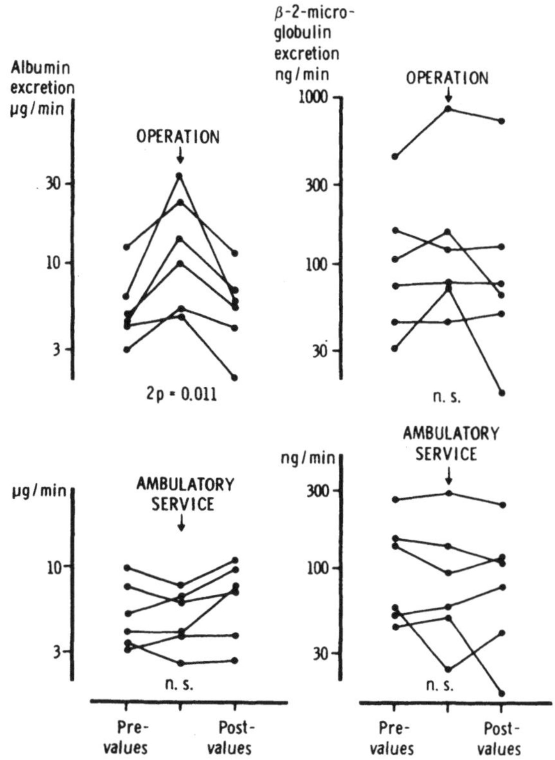

Fig. 2. Urinary albumin and β-2-microglobulin excretion in operating surgeons (upper curves) and in surgeons in the out patient clinic (lower curves).

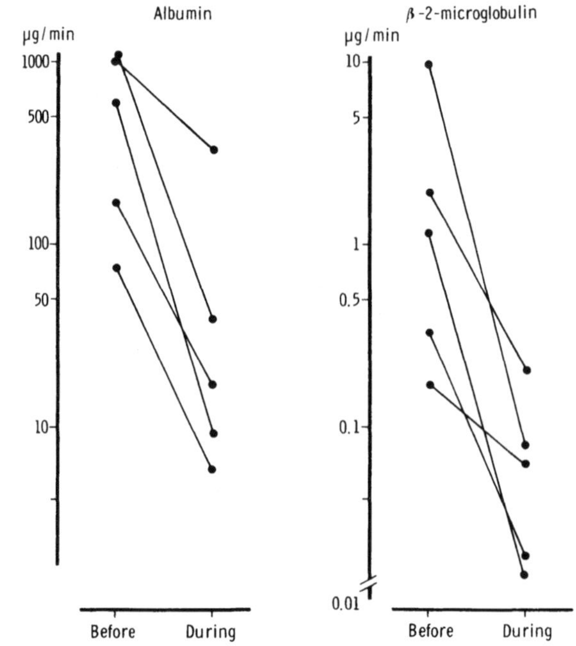

Fig. 3. Urinary albumin and β-2-microglobulin excretion before and during treatment of severe hypertension for in mean 3 days. (Mean arterial pressure 165 → 124 mm Hg).

is probably also involved to some extent since excretion was not normalized in all patients. However, the major cause of the increase in albumin excretion in newly diagnosed untreated patients is very likely increased pressure, since hypertensive vascular damage would not tend to be so rapidly reversible.

β_2-microglobulin excretion was considerably increased before treatment and dropped along with the fall in albumin excretion. The high excretion of the freely filtered β_2-microglobulin must be due to inhibition of reabsorption, the mechanism probably being competition in the reabsorption process from other plasma protein, e.g. albumin, filtered due to the increased blood pressure. Renal ischemia may also play a role.

CONCLUSIONS

It can be concluded that the three factors investigated, intravenous insulin injection, a stress situation of undertaking a surgical operation, and hypertension all have considerable influence on glomerular function, inducing increased glomerular escape of albumin. The pattern of total renal protein handling in the three situation are, however, different. Insulin stimulates protein reabsorption in the tubules, whereas no change is seen when a surgeon is operating. In the case of severe hypertension very high albumin excretion rates are associated with impairment of tubular protein reabsorption, probably due to competition for the reabsorption process due to large amounts of filtered proteins.

REFERENCES

EVRIN P. E., PETERSON P. A., WIDE L. & BERGGARD J. (1971) Radioimmunoassay of β-2-microglobulin in human biological fluids. *Scand. J. clin. lab. Invest.* **28,** 439–444.

FOSTER G. E., EVANS D. F. & HARDCASTLE J. D. (1978) Heart-rates of surgeons during operations and other clinical activities and their modification by oxprenolol. *Lancet* **I,** 1323–1325.

GUNDERSEN H. J. G. & CHRISTENSEN J. J. (1977) Intravenous insulin causing loss of intravascular water and albumin and increased adrenergic nervous activity in diabetics. *Diabetes* **26,** 551–557.

KUROKAWA K., SILVERBLATT F. J. & KLEIN K. L. (1980) Insulin receptors of isolated glomeruli. *Int. J. Biochem.* **12,** 185–190 (this volume).

MILES D. W., MOGENSEN C. E. & GUNDERSEN H. J. G. (1970) Radioimmunoassay for urinary albumin using a single antibody. *Scand. J. clin. lab. Invest.* **26,** 5–11.

MOGENSEN C. E. (1971) Glomerular filtration rate and renal plasma flow in short-term and long-term juvenile diabetes. *Scand. J. clin. lab. Invest.* **28,** 91–100.

MOGENSEN C. E. & SØLLING K. (1977) Studies on renal tubular protein reabsorption: Partial and near complete inhibition by certain amino acids. *Scand. J. clin. lab. Invest.* **37,** 477–486.

MOGENSEN C. E., CHRISTENSEN N. J. & GUNDERSEN H. J. G. (1978) The acute effect of insulin on renal haemodynamics and protein excretion in diabetics. *Diabetologia* **15,** 153–157.

MOGENSEN C. E. (1980) Mechanism of glomerular filtration and tubular uptake of plasma proteins in health and disease. In Proceedings from the International Symposium: *Correlation of Renal Ultrastructure and Function* (Edited by MAUNSHBACH, OLSEN & CHRISTENSEN I.). Academic Press, London. (In press).

OSTERBY R., GUNDERSEN H. J. G. & CHRISTENSEN N. S. (1978) The acute effect of insulin on capillary endothelial cells. *Diabetes* **27,** 745–749.

PAGE M. MCB., SMITH R. B. W. & WATKINS P. J. (1976) Cardiovascular effects of insulin. *Br. Med. J.* **I,** 430–432.

PARVING H. H., JENSEN H. Æ., MOGENSEN C. E. & EVRIN P. E. (1974) Increased urinary albumin excretion rate in benign essential hypertension. *Lancet* **I,** 1190–1192.

PEDERSEN E. B. & MOGENSEN C. E. (1976) Effect of antihypertensive treatment on urinary albumin excretion, glomerular filtration rate and renal plasma flow in patients with essential hypertension. *Scand. J. clin. lab. Invest.* **36,** 231–237.

Int. J. Biochem. Vol. 12, pp. 185 to 190
Pergamon Press Ltd 1980. Printed in Great Britain

INSULIN RECEPTORS OF ISOLATED GLOMERULI

KIYOSHI KUROKAWA[1], FREDERIC J. SILVERBLATT[2] and KEITH L. KLEIN[1]
[1]Nephrology Section, Medical and Research Services, Veterans Administration Wadsworth Medical Center;
[2]Infectious Disease Section, Medical Service,
Sepulveda Veterans Administration Hospital and the
Department of Medicine, the University of California, Los Angeles, CA 90073, U.S.A.

Abstract—1. To investigate a possible action of insulin on the glomerulus, the binding of [^{125}I]insulin to isolated glomeruli prepared from rat kidney was examined. When incubated at 22°C, [^{125}I]insulin binding proceeded with time and reached a steady state at 45 min at which time non-specific binding was less than 25% of total binding.

2. This binding was specific to insulin in that other hormonal agents known to act on the glomerulus were without effects on the binding. Increasing concentrations of non-labelled insulin displaced [^{125}I]insulin binding in a dose-dependent fashion. Scatchard plot of data was curvilinear.

3. The addition of excess non-labeled insulin to the glomeruli preincubated with [^{125}I]insulin resulted in a rapid dissociation of approx 70% of bound [^{125}I]insulin.

4. Insulin decreased the increments in glomerular cyclic AMP levels by epinephrine and by prostaglandin E_2, but not those by histamine.

5. The autoradiographic studies demonstrated the presence of insulin binding primarily on the surface of the endothelium and epithelium.

6. These data showed the presence of specific insulin receptors in the glomeruli, probably in the endothelium and epithelium, and that insulin action may be, at least in part, through modulation of glomerular cyclic AMP concentrations.

7. Such action of insulin may underlie the alteration in glomerular ultrafiltration and the development of characteristic glomerular lesions in diabetes mellitus, a disease in which insulin deficiency or tissue resistance to insulin exists.

INTRODUCTION

Several lines of evidence suggest that insulin may have biological actions on glomerular function and metabolism. First, characteristic glomerular lesions develop with distinct alterations in basement membrane collagen composition (Spiro, 1973). Second, the glomerular filtration rate (GFR) becomes higher than normal early in the course of juvenile onset diabetes mellitus while renal plasma flow remains normal, resulting in an elevation of the filtration fraction. (Stalder & Schmid, 1959; Ditzel & Schwartz, 1967; Mogensen, 1971a). Since diabetes mellitus is a condition in which deficiency of insulin or tissue resistance to insulin exists, insulin may play some role in the regulation of glomerular function and metabolism. It has been well established that insulin actions are initiated by the binding of insulin to its specific receptors on plasma membrane of target cells (Roth, 1973; Cuatrecasas, 1974). Therefore insulin receptors will exist in the glomerulus if insulin is to have direct actions on glomerular cells.

MATERIALS AND METHODS

Wistar male rats, weighing 200–250 g, were used. Isolated glomeruli were prepared using the methods of Staer *et al.* (1974a) and Norgaard (1976) with minor modifications. Details of the experimental procedures have been reported from our laboratory (Kurokawa *et al.*, 1979).

For the autoradiography study, isolated glomeruli were incubated for 45 min at 22°C in the same incubation medium as used for the binding study, but with 5 nM [^{125}I]insulin and with or without 17 μM non-labeled insulin. After the incubation glomeruli were washed in phosphate buffer and fixed for 2 hr in Karnovsky's fixative (Karnovsky, 1965) mixed 1:1 with the phosphate buffer at 4°C. The glomeruli were then post-fixed for 1 hr in 1% osmium tetroxide in 0.1 M S-collide buffer, pH 7.2, dehydrated in a graded series of ethanol and propylene oxide, and embedded in Maroglas epoxy resin. Sections 1–2 μm were cut with glass knives and imprinted, precoated with gelatin and chrome alum on glass slides. The sections were coated with NTB2 nuclear emulsion diluted 1:1 with distilled water (Eastman Kodak, Rochester, NY). After 1–4 weeks exposure the autoradiographs were developed in Dektol and the sections were lightly stained with toluidine blue.

RESULTS

The specific binding of insulin, i.e. the difference between the total insulin binding minus the non-specific binding, reached a steady-state at 45 min of incubation at 22°C.

There was a linear relation between glomerular protein concentrations of 150–250 μg per incubation and percent intact insulin bound.

None of the peptide hormones tested including parathyroid hormone, calcitonin, angiotensin II, vasopressin, glucagon, except insulin had any significant effect on the binding of [^{125}I]insulin. When the glomeruli were incubated with 0.5 nM [^{125}I]insulin together with increasing concentrations of non-labeled insulin at 22°C for 45 min, the competitive displacement of [^{125}I]insulin binding to the glomeruli was observed as shown in Fig. 1. The Scatchard plot of the data based on the assumption that the binding was in a steady state was curvilinear (Fig. 2), consistent with two classes of receptor sites, i.e. high affinity–low capacity and low affinity–high capacity receptor sites. The association constant and binding

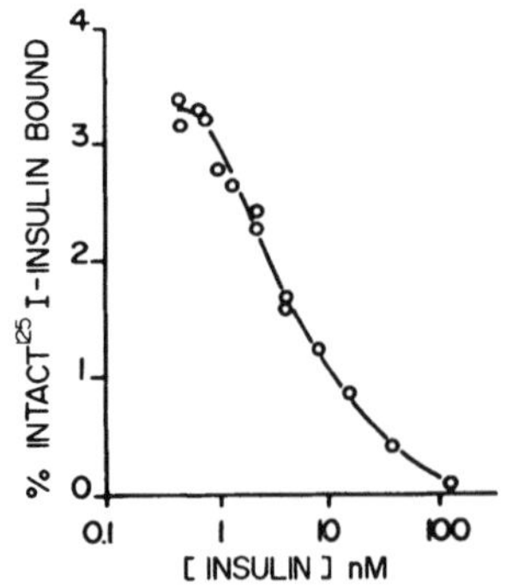

Fig. 1. Competitive displacement of [^{125}I]insulin binding to the glomeruli by non-labeled insulin. The isolated glomeruli (170 μg protein) were incubated with 0.5 nM [^{125}I]insulin with varying concentrations of non-labeled insulin at 22°C for 45 min. Each point represents a single incubation.

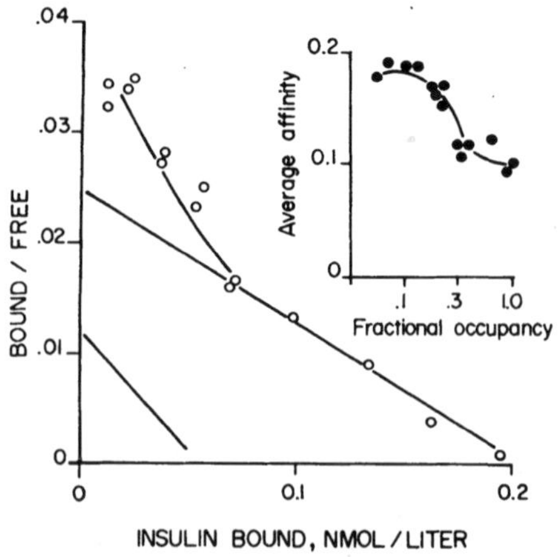

Fig. 2. Scatchard analysis and the average affinity of the insulin binding. Data were calculated from Fig. 1. For Scatchard analysis a least-squares straight line was drawn to fit the low affinity site using the data from insulin concentrations from 4.2–195 nM. The contribution of this site was subtracted from the points obtained at lower insulin concentrations and the resultant points were fitted by a second least squares line. The average affinity, calculated as (B/F) ÷ (Ro − B), is plotted as a function of log B/Ro based on the data in Fig. 1 and the Scatchard analysis.

capacity for high affinity-low capacity sites, were 1.8×10^8 l. mol^{-1} and 0.06 pmol. mg protein^{-1}, respectively, and for low affinity-high capacity sites 1.0×10^8 l. mol^{-1} and 0.18 pmol. mg protein^{-1}, respectively. The "average affinity" was consistent with the presence of a class of receptors of negative cooperative type (DeMeyts & Roth, 1975) (Fig. 2).

The addition of excess non-labeled insulin, 1.7 μM, to the incubation medium after 45 min incubation of the glomeruli with 0.5 nM [^{125}I]insulin resulted in a rapid dissociation of bound radioactivity. This dissociation was not complete leaving approximately 30% of bound radioactivity remaining with the glomeruli.

As shown in Table 1 insulin itself had little effect on cyclic AMP levels in glomeruli. However, insulin attenuated the rises in cyclic AMP levels induced by epinephrine and prostaglandin E_2 while it was without effect on the rises in cyclic AMP induced by histamine. Insulin had no effect on cyclic GMP concentrations in the glomeruli with or without these agonists (data not shown).

Localization of insulin binding by the autoradiographs

Glomeruli incubated with 5 nM [^{125}I]insulin at 22°C for 45 min demonstrated autoradiographic grains predominantly but not exclusively on the surface of the epithelial and endothelial cells (Fig. 3A). Because the width of the capillary wall was smaller than the grain diameter, it was not possible to ascertain whether the radioactivity was associated with plasma membranes of the epithelial and endothelial cells, or with the basement membranes. Large mesangial areas were virtually devoid of grains.

Radiolabeling was significantly decreased when excess non-labeled insulin (17 nM) was added to the incubation mixture (Fig. 3B). Radiolabeling was virtually absent when the incubation was carried out at 4°C for 45 min.

DISCUSSION

The present results demonstrate the presence of insulin binding and degradation in the isolated glomeruli of rat kidney. Increasing concentrations of unlabeled insulin resulted in a dose-dependent displacement of [^{125}I]insulin binding to the glomeruli. The

Table 1. Effects of insulin, epinephrine, prostaglandin E_2 and histamine on cyclic AMP levels in the isolated glomeruli

Experiment	Additions	Cyclic AMP (pmol. mg protein^{-1})
1.	None	14.1 ± 1.6
	Insulin, 3.4 μM	11.8 ± 1.8
	Epinephrine, 1.0 μM	27.4 ± 0.6
	Epinephrine + insulin	20.9 ± 1.9*
2.	None	25.2 ± 2.8
	Insulin, 2.0 μM	23.8 ± 1.1
	Prostaglandin E_2, 1.0 μM	48.3 ± 3.4
	Prostaglandin E_2 + insulin	36.5 ± 2.5*
	Histamine, 1.5 μM	39.7 ± 2.4
	Histamine + insulin	38.3 ± 0.7

Values are the mean ± SD of quadruplicate incubations. See text for details.
* Significantly ($P < 0.01$) different from values with each hormone alone.

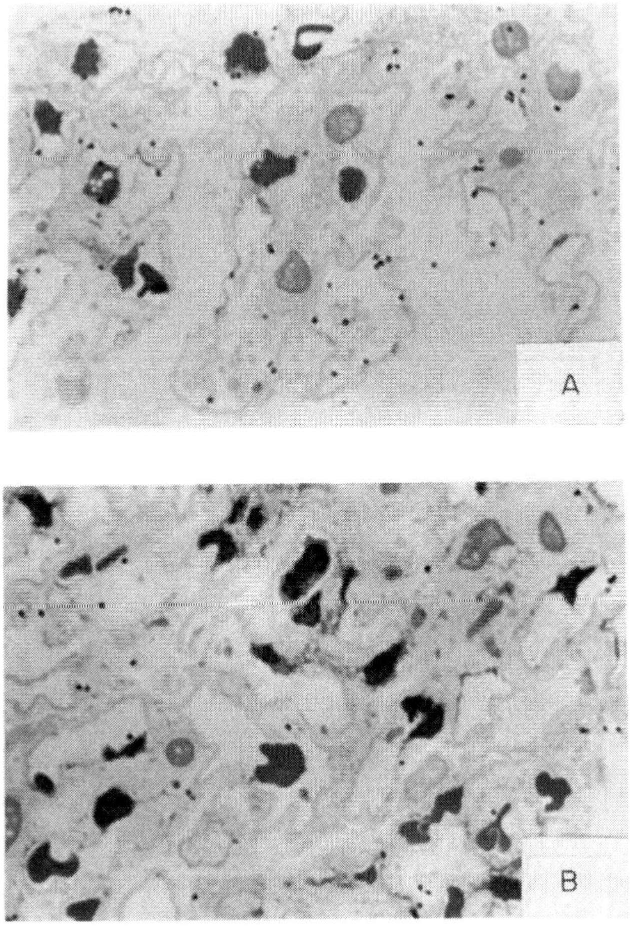

Fig. 3. Autoradiographs of [^{125}I]insulin binding to the isolated glomeruli. Isolated glomeruli were incubated with 5 nM [^{125}I]insulin at 22°C for 45 min. (A). Dense grains of radioactivity are associated with predominantly but not exclusively on the surface of the epithelium and the endothelium. Mesangial areas were virtually devoid of the grains. The incubation of the glomeruli with [^{125}I]insulin together with 17 μM non-labeled insulin resulted in a reduction in the number of grains as shown in B. Magnification of the pictures is A = 1400 ×, and B = 1400 ×.

Scatchard plot of data was curvilinear and was consistent with two classes of binding sites of high affinity–low capacity and low affinity–high capacity and/or a negative cooperative type of hormone-receptor interaction.

The addition of excess non-labeled insulin to the glomeruli which were in equilibrium with [^{125}I]insulin resulted in a rapid dissociation of [^{125}I]insulin from the glomeruli, suggesting that the majority ($\simeq 70\%$) of [^{125}I]insulin was bound in a reversible fashion on the surface of glomerular cells, probably to its receptors in the plasma membranes. The fraction of bound radioactivity not dissociated by the subsequent addition of excess non-labeled insulin may represent [^{125}I]insulin bound irreversibly to the plasma membranes or located intracellularly, either as an intact hormone or as degradation products.

The glomerulus is composed of three major cell types; epithelium, endothelium and mesangium. The autoradiographic studies showed the insulin binding to the surface of the epithelium and the endothelium. These data suggest a possible role of insulin to regulate metabolism and function of glomerular epithelium and endothelium through the binding to the receptors on the plasma membranes, and cyclic AMP may be involved as a mechanism. In diabetes mellitus, a condition in which deficiency of insulin or tissue resistance to insulin exists, the presence of abnormalities in the glomerular basement membrane collagen biosynthesis has been demonstrated in both man and in experimental animals. Thus, the glomerular basement membrane collagen in diabetes is characterized by an increased hydroxylysine content with increased glucosyl-transferase and lysyl-hydroxylase activities (Spiro & Spiro, 1971; Khalita & Cohen, 1975). These abnormalities in glomerular basement membrane collagen biosynthesis can be prevented by insulin treatment in experimental diabetic animals, even in the absence of complete correction of hyperglycemia, suggesting the role of insulin on the regulation of basement membrane collagen biosynthesis (Cohen & Khalifa, 1977). If the glomerular epithelium is the primary cell type responsible for the production of basement membrane collagen (Kurtz & Goldman, 1962) the presence of insulin binding to the epithelium shown in the autoradiographic studies is consistent with a possible role of insulin on the epithelial cell function and collagen biosynthesis. Mechanisms of insulin action on the glomerular epithelium and on the regulation of basement collagen biosynthesis are not known and must await further investigation.

Early in the course of diabetes mellitus in man a greater than normal GFR with normal renal blood flow and, thus, an elevated filtration fraction have been reported (Stalder & Schmid 1959; Ditzel & Schwartz, 1967; Mogensen, 1971a). Although the exact mechanisms responsible for the elevated GFR and filtration fraction have not been elucidated, elevated plasma levels of growth hormone and glucose have been proposed as possible mechanisms (Mogensen, 1971b). That the growth hormone tends to increase both GFR and renal blood flow and that hyperglycemia by glucose infusion in normal and diabetic patients increases GFR only minimally but not to the extent seen in untreated early diabetic patients suggest roles played by elevated plasma growth hormone levels and hyperglycemia are of minor significance (Mogensen, 1971a). Insulin administration to these diabetic patients with high GFR and high filtration fraction results in a fall in GFR and filtration fraction toward normal within 1–2 weeks, an observation demonstrating the reversible nature of the abnormal glomerular functions in these patients (Mogensen, 1971). What cell types are responsible for the elevated GFR and filtration fraction and how such changes are induced in diabetes are not known.

It has been demonstrated that various hormonal agents such as parathyroid hormone, vasopressin, prostaglandins, catecholamines, and histamine stimulate glomerular adenylate cyclase, probably through the binding to their specific receptors, and increase glomerular cyclic AMP levels (Sraer *et al.*, 1974a,b; Imbert *et al.*, 1974; Dousa *et al.*, 1977; Sraer *et al.*, 1978; Schlondorff *et al.*, 1978; Torres *et al.*, 1978). Brenner and his associate using micropuncture techniques demonstrated that these hormonal agonists may affect GFR accompanied by changes in the glomerular capillary ultrafiltration coefficient (K_f) and suggested that their effects on K_f may be mediated by cyclic AMP (Baylis *et al.*, 1976; Ichikawa & Brenner, 1977; Ichikawa *et al.*, 1978). The determinants of glomerular ultrafiltration other than K_f may also change with these hormonal agents and therefore the fall in K_f may not necessarily be accompanied by the reduction in GFR. As shown in the present study, insulin does attenuate the epinephrine- and PGE_2-induced rises in cyclic AMP levels in the glomeruli. This observation is of importance in two respects; on the one hand, the data demonstrate a possible biological significance of insulin receptors in the glomeruli, and on the other, the data imply a possible role of insulin in the regulation of GFR. It is of note that both clearance and micropuncture studies failed to show the effect of both exogenous and endogenous hyperinsulinemia on GFR in normal humans and in dogs (De Fronzo *et al.*, 1975, 1976). The circulating and local (intraglomerular) concentrations of catecholamines and prostaglandins may be different in normal and disease states such as diabetes mellitus. Thus, it is possible that insulin may affect GFR by modulating the effects of catecholamines and prostaglandins on the determinants of glomerular ultrafiltration, and as such insulin effects on GFR may become apparent only in certain conditions such as diabetes mellitus.

Acknowledgements—This work was supported in part by grants from the United States Public Health Service, AM-21351 and AM-18657, from American Diabetes Association, Inc., and from Veterans Administration Medical Research Funding. Dr Keith L. Klein is a Research Associate of the Veterans Administration.

REFERENCES

Baylis C., Deen W. M., Myers B. D. & Brenner B. M. (1976) Effects of some vasodilator drugs on transcapillary fluid exchange in the renal cortex. *Am. J. Physiol.* **230,** 1148–1158.

Cohne M. P. & Khalifa A. (1977) Effect of diabetes and insulin on rat renal glomerular protocollagen hydroxylase activities. *Biochim. biophys. Acta* **496,** 88–94.

Cuatrecases P. (1974) Membrane receptors *A. Rev. Biochem* **43,** 169–214.

DE FRONZO R. A., COOKE C. R., ANDRES R., FALOONA G. R. & DAVIS P. J. (1975) The effect of insulin on renal handling of sodium, potassium, calcium, and phosphate in man. *J. clin. Invest.* **55,** 845–855.

DE FRONZO R. A., GOLDBERG M. & AGUS Z. S. (1976) The effects of glucose and insulin on renal electrolyte transport. *J. clin. Invest.* **58,** 83–90.

DEMEYTS P. & ROTH J. (1975) Cooperativity in ligand binding: A new graphic analysis. *Biochem. biophys. Res. Commun.* **66,** 1118–1125.

DITZEL J. & SCHWARTZ M. (1967) Abnormally increased glomerular filtration rate in short-term insulin-treated diabetic subjects. *Diabetes* **16,** 264–267.

DOUSA T. P., BARNES L. D., ONG S. H. & STEINER A. L. (1977) Immunohistochemical localization of 3′,5′-cyclic AMP and 3′,5′-cyclic GMP in rat renal cortex: Effect of parathyroid hormone. *Proc. Natn. Acad. Sci. U.S.A.* **74,** 3569–3573.

ICHIKAWA I. & BRENNER B. M. (1977) Evidence for glomerular actions of ADH and dibutyryl cyclic AMP in the rat. *Am. J. Physiol.* **233,** F102–F117.

ICHIKAWA I., HUMES H. D., DOUSA T. P. & BRENNER B. M. (1978) Influence of parathyroid hormone on glomerular ultrafiltration in the rat. *Am. J. Physiol.* **234,** F393–F401.

IMBERT M., CHABARDES D. & MOREL F. (1974) Hormone-sensitive adenylate cyclase in isolated rabbit glomeruli. *Mol. cell. Endocr.* **1,** 295–304.

KHALITA A. & COHEN M. P. (1975) Glomerular protocollagen lysylhydroxylase activity in streptozotocin diabetes. *Biochim. biophys. Acta* **386,** 332–339.

KUROKAWA K., SILVERBLATT F. J., KLEIN K. L., WANG M-S. & LERNER R. L. (1979) Binding of [^{125}I]insulin to the isolated glomeruli of rat kidney. *J. clin. Invest.,* **64,** 1357–1364.

KURTZ S. M. & GOLDMAN J. D. (1962) Experimental studies of the formation of the glomerular basement membrane. *J. Ultrastruct. Res.* **6,** 19–27.

KARNOVSKY M. J. (1965) A formaldehyde-glutaldehyde fixation of high osmolality for use in electron microscopy. *J. Cell Biol.* **27,** 137A–138A.

MOGENSEN C. E. (1971a) Kidney function and glomerular permeability to macro-molecules in early juvenile diabetes. *Scand. J. clin. lab. Invest.* **28,** 79–90.

MOGENSEN C. E. (1971b) Glomerular filtration rate and renal plasma flow in normal and diabetic man during elevation of blood sugar levels. *Scand. J. clin. lab. Invest.* **28,** 177–182.

NORGAARD J. O. R. (1976) A new method for the isolation of ultrastructurally preserved glomeruli. *Kidney Int.* **9,** 278–285.

ROTH J. (1973) Peptide hormone binding to receptors: A review of direct studies *in vitro*. *Metabolism* **22,** 1059–1073.

SCHLONDORFF D., YOO P. & ALPERT B. E. (1978) Stimulation of adenylate cyclase in isolated rat glomeruli by prostaglandins. *Am. J. Physiol.* **235,** F458–464.

SPIRO R. G. (1973) Biochemistry of the renal glomerular basement membrane and its alterations in diabetes mellitus. *New Engl. J. Med.* **288,** 1337–1342.

SPIRO R. G. & SPIRO M. J. (1971) Effect of diabetes on the biosynthesis of the renal glomerular basement membrane. Studies on the glucosyltransferase. *Diabetes* **20,** 641–648.

SRAER J. D., SRAER J., ARDAILLOU R. & MIMOUNE O. (1974(a)) Evidence for renal glomerular receptors for angiotensin II. *Kidney Int.* **6,** 241–246.

SRAER J., ARDAILLOU R., LOREAU N. & SRAER J. D. (1974(b)) Evidence for parathyroid hormone sensitive adenylate cyclase in rat glomeruli. *Mol. cell. Endocr.* **1,** 285–294.

SRAER J., SRAER J. D., CHANSEL D., JUEPPNER H., HESCH R. D. & ARDAILLOU R. (1978) Evidence for glomerular receptors for parathyroid hormone. *Am. J. Physiol.* **235,** F96–F103.

STALDER G. & SCHMID R. (1959) Severe functional disorders of glomerular capillaries and renal haemodynamics in treated diabetes mellitus during childhood. *Ann. Paediat.* **193,** 129–138.

TORRES, V. E., NORTHRUP T. E., EDWARDS R. M., SHAH S. V. & DOUSA T. P. (1978) Modulation of cyclic nucleotides in isolated rat glomeruli. *J. clin. Invest.* **62,** 1334–1343.

SYMPOSIUM DISCUSSION

Lemieux: Do you have any evidence that insulin modifies glomerular permeability?

Kurokawa: I think that question should be directed to Dr Mogenson. At the last American Society of Nephrology Meeting Hostetter *et al.* (*Kidney Int.* **14,** 725, 1978) examined the effect of insulin on GFR and K_f but the experimental model was not appropriate. At least in normal humans and normal dogs, insulin infusion has no effect on GFR (DeFronzo *et al.*, *J. clin. Invest.* **55,** 845, 1975; *J. clin. Invest.* **58,** 83, 1976).

Mogenson: When we inject insulin 8 i.u. intravenously in diabetic patients, you can see an increase in urinary albumin excretion, indicating an increase in glomerular permeability to albumin. At the same time we observe a decrease in β_2 microglobulin excretion, indicating also that tubular protein reabsorption is enhanced. So insulin acts in 2 ways on the protein excretion mechanism. Furthermore, in these studies, we found a decrease in GFR of about 10%, and a decrease in renal plasma flow of about 13% (Mogensen *et al. Diabetologia*, **15,** 153–157, 1978).

Saggerson: What was the affinity of binding of insulin compared with that seen in other systems?

Kurokawa: With this Scatchard transformation, high affinity site K_a was about 10^8 l. mol^{-1}, which is slightly lower than the value observed in liver membranes or fat cells. Explanation for this lower K_a was the limited specific activity of the tracer we used and the smaller volume of incubation in the present study. There may therefore be higher affinity binding sites (Kurokawa *et al.*, *J. clin. Invest.* **64,** 1357, 1979).

Epstein: Insulin receptors on other cells, like monocytes are altered by fasting and feeding. I wonder if you have looked at that?

Kurokawa: No, this study was done in fed animals, and we have not looked at the effect of fasting.

Franke: Did you show that the increase of cAMP could be antagonised by insulin? Did you find binding of insulin to adenylate cyclase?

Kurokawa: Insulin antagonizes the increase in cAMP by epinephrine, prostaglandin E_2 or parathyroid hormone in intact glomeruli. We did not examine the insulin binding in the adenylate cyclase preparation.

Guder: In other tissues, the specificity of the insulin antagonism to other hormones was established by excluding an effect on fluoride sensitive cyclase. Have you done this?

Kurokawa: No.

Int. J. Biochem., Vol. 12, pp. 191 to 194
© Pergamon Press Ltd 1980. Printed in Great Britain

0020-711X/80/0701-0191$02.00/0

THE EFFECTS OF PROTEINASES ON THE FILTRATION PROPERTIES OF ISOLATED BASEMENT MEMBRANES

THOMAS G. COTTER and GARTH B. ROBINSON
Department of Biochemistry, South Parks Road, Oxford OX1 3QU, U.K.

Abstract—1. The filtration properties of proteinase digested renal basement membranes were examined using *in vitro* filtration methods.

2. Trypsin digestion rendered films of the basement membranes more permeable to proteins as compared with untreated membranes.

3. Digestion with proteinase-containing extracts of the granule membranes from rabbit polymorphonuclear leucocytes at neutral pH, and with a proteinase purified from the extract, resulted in films of the membranes becoming more permeable to serum proteins.

INTRODUCTION

In an earlier (unpublished) paper in this symposium Newsholme has drawn attention to the importance of "flux generating steps" in regulating flux through pathways. In excretion the flux generating step is glomerular filtration which produces a remarkably constant flux of ultrafiltrate from the plasma. In glomerular disease the characteristics of filtration alter and increased amounts of plasma proteins escape the filter barrier to appear in the urine. The reasons for this increase in the escape of protein across the glomerular barrier are not known but the proteinuria of nephrotoxic serum nephritis can be prevented by depletion of the polymorphonuclear leucocyte population (Kniker & Cochrane, 1965; Cochrane *et al.*, 1965) and polymorph infiltration is seen in some forms of human glomerular disease (Dunnill, 1976). The granules of the polymorphs contain proteinases capable of degrading connective tissue components (Goldstein, 1976) and it is tempting to assume that polymorph proteinases may damage the glomerular basement membrane so inducing proteinuria. Here we attempt to test the hypothesis directly.

Previously we have shown that isolated basement membranes can be used to prepare ultrafiltration films *in vitro* (Cotter & Robinson, 1978; Robinson & Cotter, 1979). In this study we have used proteinases to digest basement membranes and then have examined the filtration properties of films prepared from the digested membranes. The effects on filtration of both trypsin, and of proteinases from rabbit polymorphonuclear leucocytes, have been examined.

MATERIALS AND METHODS

Renal basement membranes were isolated by a detergent procedure (Ligler & Robinson, 1977) from the kidney cortices of rabbits (New Zealand White, 2–2.5 kg, Oxford University Farm). The preparations were a mixture of glomerular and tubular basement membrane.

Filtration studies were conducted as described (Cotter & Robinson, 1978). In brief, suspensions containing known amounts of basement membrane protein were placed in pressure filtration cells (Amicon Ltd, High Wycombe, Bucks.) assembled with cellulose acetate membranes (Millipore (U.K.) Ltd., London, 0.45 μm exclusion) as the filter barrier. The suspension was forced through the filter at 200 kPa pressure using nitrogen gas to compact the basement membrane fragments into coherent films on the surface of the cellulose acetate membrane. This film forms a filtration barrier capable of excluding macromolecules and filtrations of solutions of proteins were conducted at a filtration pressure of 150 kPa, with magnetic stirring of the contents of the chambers at a stirrer speed of 1000 r.p.m. The basement membranes were digested with proteinases prior to forming the filtration films and were washed centrifugally with 0.15 M NaCl in 0.01 M Tris–HCl buffer pH 7.4 before use. Filtration experiments were conducted either with pure proteins dissolved in buffered saline or with rabbit serum.

When trypsin was used for digestion, basement membranes (5 mg) were incubated with pure trypsin (Sigma (London) Chemical Co. Ltd, U.K.) 2.8×10^3 units of activity (measured against *n*-benzoyl-1-arginine ethyl ester) in 0.05 M Tris–HCl buffer pH 7.4 at 37°C with shaking.

In some experiments extracts of membranes from the granules of rabbit polymorphs were used to digest the membranes. Granules were isolated from peritoneal polymorphonuclear leucocytes as described by Cohn & Hirsch (1960). The granules were lysed by freezing and thawing three times in 0,1 M sodium phosphate buffer pH 7.4 and were then centrifuged at 30,000 *g* for 20 min to yield a pellet of granule membranes. This pellet was extracted further with 1.0 M NaCl containing 0.1% Triton X-100 (v/v) and 0.01 M sodium phosphate buffer pH 7.4. Solubilized protein was collected after centrifuging as described above, and this extract contained proteinases active against basement membrane; the extract also catalysed the hydrolysis of *p*-nitrophenol-*n*-tertbutoxycarbonyl-1-alaninate (NBA) at pH 6.5. Basement membranes (6 mg) were incubated with extract containing 100 units of activity against NBA, where 1 unit was taken as the hydrolysis of 1 μmol of NBA per min at pH 6.5. Incubations were carried out in 0.5 M NaCl containing 0.01 M Tris–HCl, pH 7.4 and 37°C with constant shaking. A proteinase active against NBA and basement membrane was isolated from this extract (Cotter & Robinson, to be published) and was used for digesting the basement membranes under the same conditions.

Protein concentrations were determined by A_{280} measurements when solutions of single proteins were filtered, and by the Lowry procedure (Lowry *et al.*, 1951) when serum was filtered. The latter procedure was also used to measure basement membrane protein except that dried basement membrane was used as the standard rather than bovine serum albumin. Hydroxyproline was determined using the method of Blumenkrantz & Asboe-Hansen (1975). Polyacrylamide gel electrophoresis in the presence of sodium dodecyl sulphate was conducted as described earlier (Ligler & Robinson, 1977).

RESULTS

Digestion of the basement membranes with trypsin was allowed to proceed and samples of membranes were removed at different times for analysis. There was a gradual loss of protein from the membranes with time as judged by the Lowry procedure. After 6 hr digestion 23% of the protein had been lost but no loss of OH-proline was found to have occurred. Analysis of the membranes after 6 hr digestion by polyacrylamide gel electrophoresis showed complex changes in the gel patterns. Notably bands at 230,000 and 65,000 mol.wt disappeared and bands at 175,000 and 92,000 increased in intensity. The number of bands in the range 40,000 to 90,000 also increased.

In filtration studies, membrane films were prepared from digested membranes using amounts of membrane that were equivalent to the amounts of undigested membranes used in the control films. That is proportionately less digested membrane protein was used to prepare the films as digestion proceeded. When the fluxes of cytochrome c, bovine serum albumin and IgG were measured it was found that films of the digested membranes showed an increasing flux for all proteins as digestion times lengthened. (Fig. 1a). When rabbit serum was filtered samples were collected progressively from the start of filtration since the flux of protein was high in the first few minutes of filtration and then declined with time; the results of these experiments are shown in Fig. 1b. It was found that as digestion time lengthened the initial flux of protein through the films increased but this initial flux rapidly declined to steady state values that were little different from the controls except in the case of membranes digested for the longest period (6 hr).

When granule extract was used to hydrolyse the membranes there was a progressive loss of both protein and hydroxyproline with 18 and 23% removal respectively after 36 hr digestion. Again complex changes were seen in the gel electrophoresis patterns of the digested membranes, most obviously apparent in the mol. wt. range 120,000–175,000. Filtration of serum through films prepared from membranes digested for 36 hr showed a marked increase in both the initial and steady state fluxes as compared with normal membranes (Fig. 2a).

A proteinase isolated from the granule extract was shown to have activity against collagen and azo-albumin as well as against basement membrane. This enzyme was shown to be a serine proteinase as judged by inhibitor studies and was active against NBA a substrate used for the assay of elastases though the enzyme exhibited no activity against elastin as such (Cotter & Robinson, to be published). This enzyme was used to digest the basement membranes and after incubation for 36 hr 12% of the membrane protein and 15% of the OH-proline had been released. Gel electrophoresis of the digested membranes showed changes similar to those seen with the granule extract. The flux of serum proteins through films prepared from these digested membranes again showed increased protein flux both during the initial period of filtration and when steady state was reached (Fig. 2b).

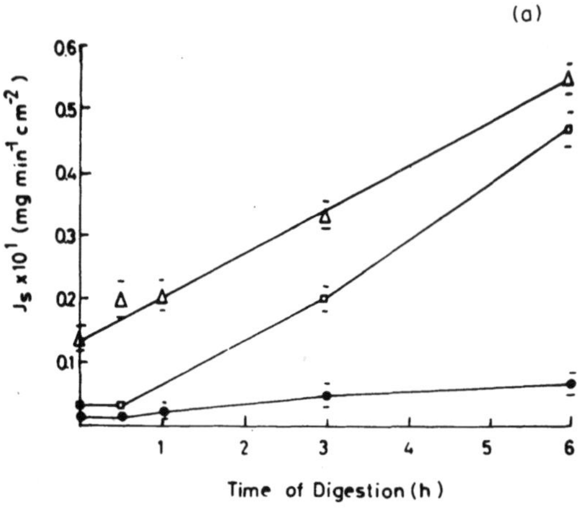

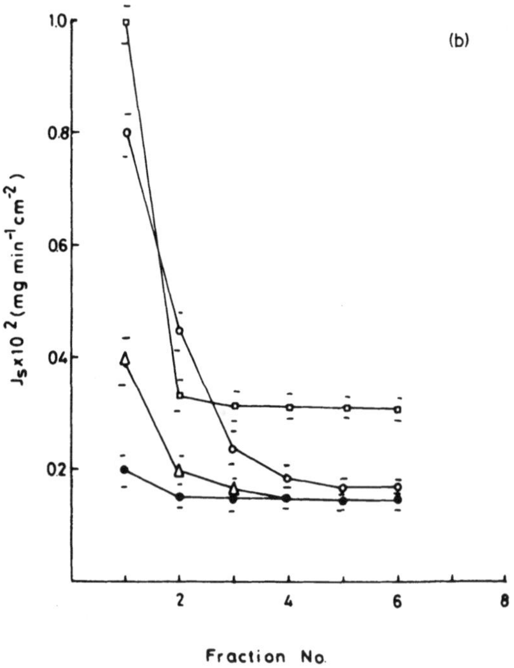

Fig. 1a. Filtration of solutions of proteins through films prepared from basement membranes digested for increasing times with trypsin. Each result is the mean of three observations on each of three films ±1 SD. Films were prepared using 0.11 mg of undigested basement membrane protein per cm^2 of filtration surface for the zero time point and for other times proportionate amounts of membrane protein were used depending upon the degree of digestion. Filtration was conducted at 150 kPa pressure with stirring at 1000 rpm. △ cytochrome c; □ bovine serum albumin; ● horse IgG; all at 0.5 mg per ml.

Fig. 1b. Filtration of serum across films of basement membranes after digestion of the membranes with trypsin for different times. Filtrate was collected in 3 ml fractions from the start of filtration. Films were prepared as described for Fig. 1a and operated under the same conditions. Digestion times: ● zero; △ 1.5 hr; ○ 3 hr; □ 6 hr.

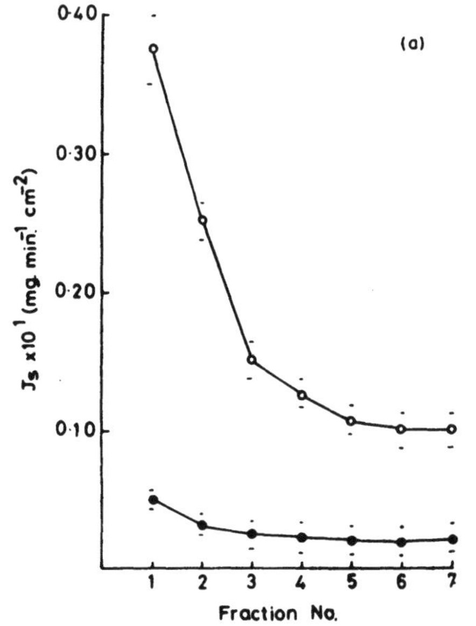

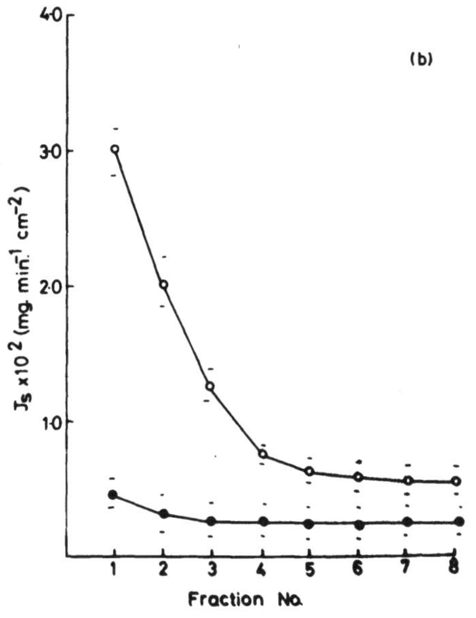

Fig. 2a. Filtration of serum across films prepared from basement membranes digested for 36 hr with an extract of polymorph granule membranes (see Methods). The results are the mean results from six separate filters with filtrate collected as 3 ml fractions from the start of filtration. Filtration conditions were as for Fig. 1a. ● normal membranes ○ digested membranes.

Fig. 2b. As for Fig. 2a except that purified NBA esterase was used for digestion for 36 hr. ● normal membranes; ○ digested membranes.

DISCUSSION

The results reported here demonstrate that changes in the filtration properties of basement membranes can be detected using a model filtration system *in vitro*. Further, the studies with enzymes from polymorphonuclear leucocyte granules show that proteinases present in these cells alter the filtration characteristics of the membranes. In considering these results it is pertinent to mention that filtration behaviour of filter films is determined by the thickness of the films. Hence were digestion to destroy some membranes entirely leaving other fragments unscathed then using proportionately less protein to prepare films of digested membranes would mean that these films would be thinner and so would give higher protein fluxes. Counts of the membrane fragments before and after digestion showed that the numbers of fragments remained unchanged, hence films would contain the same numbers of fragments and so would have the same number of layers of fragments as compared with the controls. It is possible that the membranes themselves become thinner as a result of digestion accounting for the changed filtration behaviour but presumably this might happen *in vivo* and indeed thinning has been reported to occur in aminonucleoside nephritis (Caulfield *et al.*, 1976). More detailed studies are needed to establish whether proteinase treatment merely makes the membranes thinner so altering the filtration characteristics of the films or whether the intrinsic permeabilities of the membranes are altered as a consequence of proteinase action.

One interesting feature which emerges from the experiments with serum filtration was the finding that the flux of serum proteins diminished markedly as filtration proceeded when digested membrane films were used. This suggests that the membranes may become plugged with proteins so reducing loss into the filtrate. Thus the membranes might be "self-sealing" after proteinase damage so providing protection against loss of protein. However the sealing is not completely effective since the steady state fluxes were still higher than those seen with control membranes.

These experiments provide support for the idea that proteinase damage of basement membranes may promote proteinuria and that polymorphs possess proteinases capable of effecting such damage at neutral pH.

REFERENCES

Blumenkrantz N. & Asboe-Hansen N. G. (1975) An assay for hydroxyproline and proline or one sample and a simplified method for hydroxyproline. *Analyt. Biochem.* **63**, 331–340.

Caulfield J. P., Reid J. J. & Farquhar M. G. (1976) Alterations of the glomerular epithelium in acute aminonucleoside nephrosis. *Lab. Invest.* **34**, 43–59.

Cochrane C. G., Unanue E. R. & Dixon F. J. (1965) A role of polymorphonuclear leucocytes and complement in nephrotoxic nephritis. *J. exp. Med.* **122**, 99–116.

Cohn Z. A. & Hirsch J. G. (1960) The isolation of properties of specific cytoplasmic granules of rabbit polymorphonuclear leucocytes. *J. exp. Med.* **112**, 983–1004.

Cotter T. G. & Robinson G. B. (1978) Effects of concentration polarisation on filtration of proteins through filters constructed from isolated renal basement membranes. *Clin. Sci. mol. Med.* **55**, 113–119.

Dunnill M. S. (1976) Pathological Basis of Renal Disease. Saunders, London.

Goldstein I. M. (1976) Polymorphonuclear leucocyte lysosomes and immune tissue injury. *Prog. Allergy* **20**, 310–340.

Kniker W. T. & Cochrane C. G. (1965) Pathogenic factors in vascular lesions of experimental serum sickness. *J. exp. Med.* **122**, 83–98.

LIGLER F. S. & ROBINSON G. B. (1977) A new method for the isolation of renal basement membrane. *Biochim. biophys. Acta* **468,** 327–340.

LOWRY O. H., ROSEBROUGH N. J., FARR A. L. & RANDALL R. J. (1951) Protein measurement with the Folin phenol reagent. *J. biol. Chem.* **193,** 265–275.

ROBINSON G. B. & COTTER T. G. (1979) Studies on the filtration properties of isolated renal basement membrane. *Biochim. biophys. Acta* **551,** 85–94.

SYMPOSIUM DISCUSSION

Weiner: Shouldn't you look to see how much cytochrome *c* is left in your membranes?

Robinson: In those experiments we have filtered whole serum and we suspect that it is the large macro-molecules in the serum that actually have the "plugging" effect. From a few other experiments that we have done, for example, using trypsin and then filtering cytochrome *c*, we don't see that kind of a plugging.

Weiner: How do you maintain uniformity and thickness of the protein content from one experimental day to the other, or is there variation?

Robinson: Thickness is precisely determined because we add a precisely measured amount of protein to each filtration chamber and blow it down into the uniform film. What we cannot control is the thinness of the film across the whole of the millipore membrane but EM studies indicate that it is quite an even deposition.

Lowenstein: Are these experiments done only on extracted membranes? Proteins from the serum that are plugging up the holes may rapidly disappear from your initial preparation.

Robinson: We extract the membranes with detergent treating the cortex so as to destroy all the cells.

Lowenstein: So that you are leaving naked membranes without the proteins, I thought you might be studying proteins different from those expected on the filter?

Robinson: We could be getting artefactual problems of that sort; we have looked at enzyme levels in the basement membrane to see if we are getting contamination and we find virtually no enzymes at all. Of course, there may be proteins there that we are not able to measure, and it is reported that isolated basement membranes do contain serum proteins (ref.: Westberg & Michael, *Biochemistry*, **9,** 3837–3846, 1970). We haven't actually looked for them in our preparations but I suspect they may be there.

Osswald: Do your membranes have selectivity to the charge of the molecules you send through?

Robinson: That is something we are currently investigating. We do in fact see the sort of effects with dextran which Dr Baylis was reporting but if you look at compact molecules, such as proteins, the effects are less obvious. We think that proteins will go through the membranes more readily when they are at their iso-electric point rather than when they are charged, either positively or negatively. This, of course, would make sense because if you have a charge-barrier, then a molecule of opposite charge will tend to enter the barrier but will tend not to leave it; it will tend to anchor there. A protein of opposite charge will tend not to go in. An electrically neutral molecule won't experience a barrier and won't be held within the barrier and so will tend to go through more readily.

Int. J. Biochem., Vol. 12, p. 195
© Pergamon Press Ltd 1980. Printed in Great Britain

0020-711X/80/0701-0195$02.00/0

DISCUSSION OF PAPER "THE GLOMERULAR PERMEABILITY FOR WATER AND ALBUMIN IN THE ISOLATED PERFUSED RAT KIDNEY"

H. J. SCHUREK *et al.*

INTRODUCTION

A paper given by Dr H-J Schurek, entitled "The glomerular permeability for water and albumin in the isolated perfused rat kidney" (Hans-Joachim Schurek, Gerd Schwietzer, Jeannette M. Alt and Hilmar Stolte) has been published elsewhere, (*Kidney International* **16**, 377–384, 1979). The discussion follows.

SYMPOSIUM DISCUSSION

Baylis: You would expect there to be an increase in permeability *per se* wouldn't you?

Schurek: We don't know exactly whether the high flow rate which causes a high transport of albumin through the filtering area may have any influence on this high proteinuria.

Baylis: Well, the high rate of perfusion would certainly increase the absolute flux but it would also decrease the fractional clearance; you haven't measured that?

Schurek: We did both, measurements of the whole kidney albumin clearance and direct estimations of the sieving coefficient by micropuncture methods. On the other hand, we have ideal conditions concerning the exposure of the whole filtering area with a very low filtration fraction so that the whole filtering area is exposed to the same physical conditions. That is the difference from the *in vivo* state.

Weiner: I wonder whether you have more leaky glomerulae in the perfused kidney. You are comparing the excretion of protein *in vivo* when the kidney is filtering its own endogenous albumin, which is probably loaded with fatty acids and other things, with the isolated perfused kidney in which a rat kidney is being perfused with defatted bovine albumin. It is possible that just simply the molecular size of the de-fatted albumin is less than the molecular size of the albumin *in vivo* and there may be species differences in terms of albumin size that might affect the permeability. Unless you actually determine the molecular radius of the two albumin fractions, it is not quite fair to say that you have increased the permeability of the glomerulus to protein.

Schurek: You may be right, and we will speculate on the point that other proteins and let us say polarised molecules, such as phospholipids or something like that will influence the normal pattern of filtration of albumin, because we have no indication that the normal scatter of negative charges are changing under these conditions, because the pattern is the same as *in vivo*.

Weiner: You could simply test my point by measuring the molecular radius of rat albumin and bovine defatted albumin and see if they are equivalent.

Int. J. Biochem., Vol. 12, pp. 197 to 202
0020-711X/80/0701-0197$02.00/0

TISSUE CULTURE OF NORMAL RAT GLOMERULI

BASEMENT MEMBRANE BIOSYNTHESIS BY HOMOGENEOUS EPITHELIAL AND MESANGIAL CELL LINES

JACQUELINE B. FOIDART, CHRISTINE H. DUBOIS, JEAN-MICHEL FOIDART, CHARLES A. DECHENNE and PHILIPPE MAHIEU
Department of Medicine, State University of Liège, Liège, Belgium

Abstract—1. The biosynthesis of basement membrane polypeptides by confluent cultures of normal rat glomerular epithelial or mesangial cells has been studied by immunological and biochemical techniques.

2. The epithelial cells synthesize and secrete GBM polypeptides, sharing some antigenic determinants with type IV collagen, into the culture medium.

3. On the contrary, the mesangial cells synthesize and secrete GBM polypeptides different from type IV collagen into the culture medium.

INTRODUCTION

Basement membranes are specialized forms of connective tissue which are widely distributed in nature and which play a role of supporting structure and filtration (Kefalides, 1973). The glomerular basement membrane (GBM) represents an important example of these extracellular membranes. It has been shown indeed that the GBM is one of the major determinants of glomerular permeability, at least for the largest serum proteins (Karnowsky & Ainsworth, 1972). In diseases such as diabetes mellitus or glomerulonephritis, morphological changes are observed in the GBM, which appear particularly as diffuse or localized thickenings (Kimmelstiel *et al.*, 1962; Vernier *et al.*, 1960), the glomerular permeability being increased (Hardwicke, 1972). Biochemical analyses of "diseased" GBM are generally performed using a material isolated from hyalinized glomeruli. It remains difficult therefore to correlate the biochemical modifications observed in "diseased" GBM with their morphological and functional alterations.

We have described a method allowing the propagation of homogeneous cell lines derived from normal rat glomeruli (Foidart *et al.*, 1979), showing that pure epithelial and mesangial cell lines can be cultivated and subcultivated up to five times without any appreciable morphological alteration. In the present work, the biosynthesis of GBM polypeptides by confluent cultures of normal epithelial or mesangial cells has been studied by immunological and biochemical techniques. Some properties of the GBM polypeptides synthesized by each type of glomerular cells have been determined and compared. These data will subsequently be used as a basis for comparison with those obtained from glomerular cells cultured from pathological rat kidneys.

MATERIALS AND METHODS

Materials

Insoluble GBM, GBM soluble antigens and anti-GBM antibodies were prepared as previously described (Mahieu & Winand, 1973a; Mahieu *et al.*, 1974). Procollagen and α chains of type I collagen were a gift from Professor C. M. Lapière (Liège). Rabbit anti-type IV collagen antiserum was kindly provided by Dr N. A. Kefalides (Philadelphia, PA); type IV collagen and rabbit anti-type IV procollagen antibodies were also prepared according to the method of Gunson & Kefalides (1976). Sheep anti-rabbit Ig antiserum was purchased from Organon (OSS), [^{14}C]proline (42 mCi·mmol^{-1}) and [^{14}C]lysine (25 mCi·mmol^{-1}) from the Radiochemical Center (Amersham, Bucks), RPMI medium and fetal bovine serum from Flow Laboratories (Irvine, Ayrshire), cycloheximide from Sigma Chemical Co (London, SW6), 2,2′-bipyridyl from Calbiochem (Los Angeles, CA), and highly purified collagenase from Worthington (Freehold, NJ). All other chemicals were of analytical grade.

Methods

Cultures and subcultures of rat glomerular epithelial and mesangial cells were prepared as previously described (Foidart *et al.*, 1979). Immunological and biochemical studies were always performed at complete confluency. The density at cell saturation, evaluated by counting the cells with an hemocytometer, was about 1×10^4 cells·cm^{-2} for the epithelial cells and 0.5×10^4 cells·cm^{-2} for the mesangial cells. Incorporation experiments were performed during 2, 4, 6 or 8 hr. The RPMI medium was then supplemented with 10 to 50 μCi of the radioactive precursors, with freshly prepared ascorbate (50 μg·ml^{-1}) and with β-aminopropionitrile (50 μg·ml^{-1}). The incubations were stopped by adding 2 μmol each of cycloheximide and 2,2′-bipyridyl, in a volume of 0.2 ml, to inhibit further protein synthesis and hydroxylation during the immediate post-incubational period (Cohen & Vogt, 1975). To prevent non-specific proteolysis of newly synthesized macromolecules, phenylmethane-sulfonylfluoride (1.7 mM), N-ethylmaleimide (10 mM) and EDTA (25 mM) were also added to the incubation mixture. Collected media were chilled to 4°C, exhaustively dialyzed against distilled water and lyophilized. Lyophilized supernatants were chromatographed on Sephadex G-100 columns as previously described (Foidart *et al.*, 1975), and the presence of cross-reactive GBM or type IV collagen antigenic material in the chromatographic fractions was searched for by radioimmunoassay (Mahieu *et al.*, 1974; Foidart *et al.*, 1975).

The molecular size of GBM polypeptides was evaluated by gel filtration on columns of 6% Agarose (Bio-Gel,

A-5 m, 200–400 mesh), equilibrated and eluted with 0.1% dodecylsulfate in 0.1 M sodium phosphate buffer, pH 7.4 (Foidart *et al.*, 1975). The production of hydroxy [^{14}C]proline *in vitro* was taken as an index of GBM collagenous polypeptide biosynthesis. The 4-hydroxy [^{14}C]proline content was assayed by the method of Juva & Prockop (1966), and the 3-hydroxy [^{14}C]proline content was determined by the method of Grant *et al.* (1972). The extent of glycosylation of hydroxylysine was determined using GBM polypeptides obtained after incubation of the cultivated cells with [^{14}C]lysine. Peaks of radioactivity corresponding to the elution positions of standards of glucosyl-galactosylhydroxylysine, galactosyl-hydroxylysine and hydroxylysine were obtained as previously described (Mahieu *et al.*, 1973b).

RESULTS

Synthesis of hydroxy [^{14}C]proline and of glycosylated hydroxy [^{14}C]lysine by the epithelial and mesangial cells in culture

The incorporation rate of [^{14}C]proline into extracellular non-dialysable peptide material was found to be linear for up to 8 hr, for both epithelial and mesangial cells (Fig. 1). Moreover, the presence of 4-hydroxy [^{14}C]proline in this material demonstrated that some of the ^{14}C-labelled polypeptides synthesized by these cells were collagenous in nature. About 14% of the total hydroxy [^{14}C]proline synthesized by the epithelial cells was the 3-isomer, while only 4% of the total hydroxy [^{14}C]proline synthesized by the mesangial cells was the 3-isomer. These data indicated that both cell types synthesized and secreted basement membrane collagenous polypeptides into the culture medium.

Glomerular cells were incubated with 50 μCi [^{14}C]lysine and the proportions of hydroxy [^{14}C]lysine, galactosyl-hydroxy [^{14}C]lysine, and glucosyl-galactosyl-hydroxy [^{14}C]lysine were determined after a 6 hr incubation. About 90% of the hydroxy [^{14}C]lysine synthesized by the epithelial cells were glycosylated, and about 80% of the glycosylated hydroxy [^{14}C]lysine were found as glucosyl-galactosyl-hydroxy-[^{14}C]lysine units. For the mesangial cells, the extent of the glycosylation of hydroxy [^{14}C]lysine was only 55% and about 50% of the glycosylated hydroxy [^{14}C]lysine were present as disaccharide units.

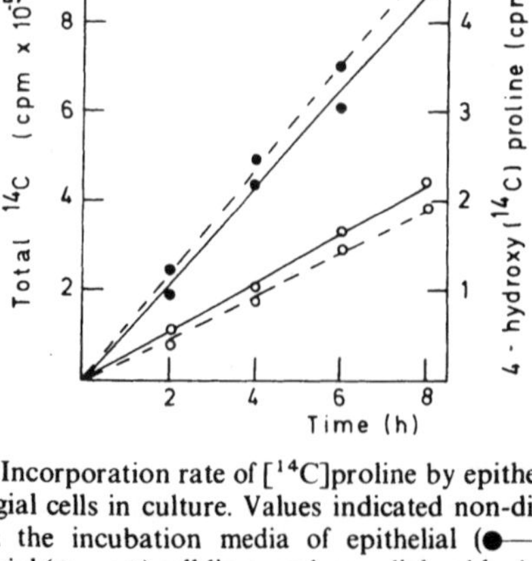

Fig. 1. Incorporation rate of [^{14}C]proline by epithelial and mesangial cells in culture. Values indicated non-dialysable ^{14}C in the incubation media of epithelial (●——●) or mesangial (●- - -●) cell lines, and non-dialysable 4-hydroxy[^{14}C]proline in the incubation media of epithelial (○——○) or mesangial (○- - -○) cell lines.

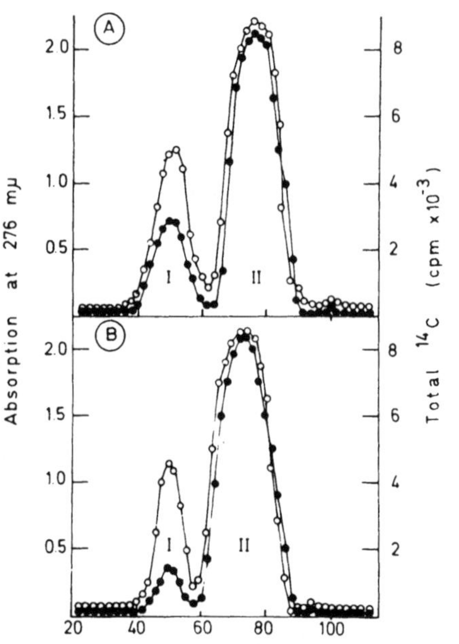

Fig. 2. Elution diagrams from Sephadex G-100 columns of culture media of epithelial (A) or mesangial (B) cell lines incubated with [^{14}C] proline. Columns were eluted, at room temperature, with 0.1 M phosphate buffer, pH 7.2; 2.4 ml per tube were collected and the samples were characterized by their absorption at 276 nm (●——●), or by their ^{14}C (○——○) content. Tubes number 40 to 57 (fraction I) and 64 to 85 (fraction II) were pooled, exhaustively dialysed against distilled water and lyophilized. They were tested by radioimmunoassay using specific anti-GBM antibodies (Fig. 3).

Purification and characterization of basement membrane polypeptides synthesized by the cultivated cells

A. Gel filtration on Sephadex G-100 columns. Confluent cultures of epithelial and mesangial cells were incubated for 6 hr with 10 μCi [^{14}C]proline. At that time, the incubation media were exhaustively dialysed against distilled water and lyophilized. Gel filtration of lyophilized supernatants on Sephadex G-100 columns is presented in Fig. 2. Two fractions (called I and II), characterized by their radioactivity and their absorption at 276 nm, were eluted using the incubation media of mesangial or epithelial cells. After dialysis and lyophilization, the presence of cross-reactive GBM or type IV collagen antigenic material in fractions I and II was searched for by radioimmunoassay, using specific anti-GBM and anti-type IV collagen antibodies.

B. Characterization of the protein material of fractions I and II. It has been shown (Mahieu *et al.*, 1974) that rabbit anti-GBM antibodies can be detected by radioimmunoassay, using soluble GBM antigens labelled with ^{125}Iodine. Indeed, less than 10% of the labelled antigens are precipitated in presence of normal rabbit serum (NRS) diluted 20 times, by a 20% polyethylene glycol (PEG) solution.

Conversely, more than 80% of the same antigens are precipitated in presence of NRS containing 100 μg of anti-GBM IgG, by the same PEG solution (Mahieu *et al.*, 1974). The specificity of the radioimmunoassay has been demonstrated by the inhibition of binding of labelled antigens to anti-GBM antibodies in presence of increasing amounts of unlabelled GBM antigens. On the contrary, increasing amounts of procollagen or α chains of type I collagen do not significantly reduce the specific precipitation (Mahieu *et al.*, 1974).

In order to characterize the protein material eluted from Sephadex G-100 columns, similar inhibition experiments were performed with fractions I and II obtained from either epithelial or mesangial cell culture media.

Increasing amounts (1–1000 μg) of fractions I and II were added to a solution of rabbit anti-GBM antibodies diluted 1000 times and binding specifically 60% of labelled GBM antigens. The results are shown in Fig. 3. One hundred μg of fraction I strongly reduced the binding of 50 ng of labelled membrane antigens to antibodies, whereas 100 μg of fraction II reduced the specific precipitation by only 15%. These results demonstrate the presence of an antigenic material immunologically related to GBM in both fractions I.

In order to further characterize the GBM material of fractions I, similar experiments were performed using a specific anti-type IV collagen antiserum. The radioimmunoassay was performed according to the method of Gunson & Kefalides (1976). The antiserum was diluted with 10% normal rabbit serum in phosphate-buffered saline up to a final dilution of 1:1000. One hundred μl of antiserum were used and added to 10 μg of fractions I contained in 100 μl phosphate-buffered saline solution. The mixtures were incubated at 4°C for 3 hr, after which 200 μl of sheep anti-rabbit Ig antiserum were added. After overnight incubation at 4°C, the tubes were centrifuged at 1000 ***g*** for 20 min, the supernatant was discarded, and the precipitate counted as previously described (Mahieu *et al.*, 1974). It should be stressed that (a) in the presence of 10 μg of the fraction I obtained from epithelial cell culture media, the specific precipitation of ^{14}C-labelled polypeptides reached 12.4%; (b) in presence of similar amounts of the fraction I obtained from mesangial cell culture media, the specific precipitations was only 0.8%; (c) in presence of 100 ng of ^{125}I-labelled type IV collagen prepared according to the method of Gunson and Kefalides (1976), the specific precipitation was about 70%. These results clearly show that cross-reactive type IV collagen antigenic material is present only in the fraction I obtained from the culture medium of epithelial cells.

Molecular size of the hydroxy [^{14}C]proline-containing polypeptides. The ^{14}C-labelled polypeptides of fractions I were chromatographed on a dodecylsulfate-agarose column. The elution diagrams of labelled polypeptides are represented in Fig. 4. After reduction and denaturation with 2-mercaptoethanol and sodium dodecylsulfate (Foidart *et al.*, 1975), one major fraction, characterized by its 4-hydroxy [^{14}C]proline content, was eluted just ahead of the internal procollagen marker. Using various standard proteins, the molecular weight was evaluated to be about 140,000. No major difference was observed in the molecular weight of 4-hydroxy [^{14}C]proline-containing polypeptides purified from the epithelial or mesangial cell culture media. After incubation of labelled GBM polypeptides with purified collagenase, most of the 4-hydroxy [^{14}C]proline was recovered in small peptide fragments (Fig. 4), thus confirming the collagenous nature of these polypeptides. Samples (0.2 ml) from fractions 30 to 33, 34 to 36 and 37 to 40 (Fig. 4) were pooled, exhaustively dialyzed against distilled water and lyophilized. They were then tested by radioimmunoassay using anti-GBM antibodies. It was found that significant amounts of cross-reactive GBM antigenic material was present in fractions 34 to 36 from both epithelial or mesangial cell culture media. However, only the fractions 34–36 from the epithelial cell culture media reacted with the anti-type IV collagen antiserum by radioimmunoassay.

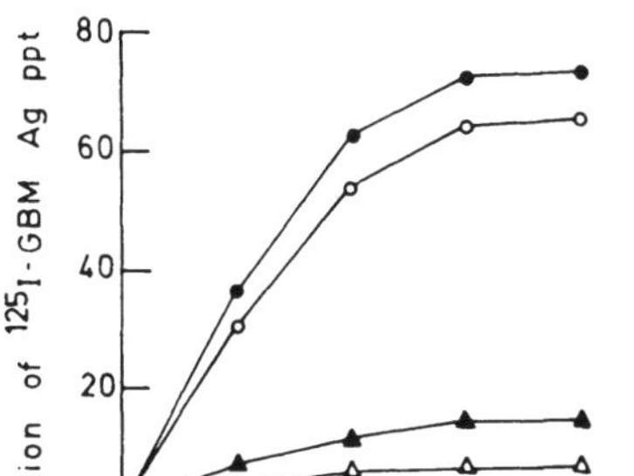

Fig. 3. Inhibition of binding of labelled GBM antigens to anti-GBM antibodies by fractions I and II obtained by gel filtration on Sephadex columns. Increasing amounts (1–1000 μg) of fractions I obtained from glomerular epithelial (●——●) or mesangial (○——○) cells, and of fractions II obtained from epithelial (▲——▲) or mesangial cell (△——△) culture media were added to a solution of anti-GBM antibodies binding specifically 60% of ^{125}I-labelled GBM antigens. The protein content was measured by the method of Lowry *et al.* (1951), using bovine serum albumin as a standard.

DISCUSSION

It is generally admitted that glomerular basement membranes (GBM) are composed of distinctive collagen molecules associated with one or more non-collagenous glycoprotein moieties (Kefalides, 1973). In an attempt to study the specific functions of glomerular cells, new methods have been developed for the cultivation and subcultivation of homogeneous epithelial and mesangial cell lines (Foidart *et al.*, 1979). In the present work, the biosynthesis of GBM polypeptides by both types of cells was studied by radio-labelled amino acid analyses and radioimmunoassay.

When the epithelial and mesangial cells were incubated in RPMI medium with [^{14}C]proline, the incorporation rate of the isotopic labelled precursor into non-dialysable extracellular polypeptides was found to be linear for up to 8 hr. Moreover, the synthesis of 4-hydroxy [^{14}C]proline and of hydroxy [^{14}C]lysine by both epithelial and mesangial cells may be used as an argument in favor of the presence of collagenous polypeptides in the newly synthesized protein ma-

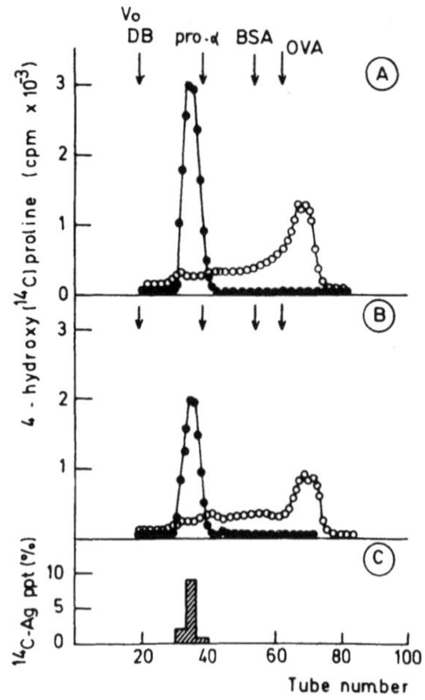

Fig. 4. Gel filtration on dodecylsulfate-agarose of ^{14}C-labelled fractions I synthesized by epithelial (A) or mesangial (B) cells in culture. After reduction and denaturation with 2-mercaptoethanol and sodium dodecylsulfate (Foidart-Willems *et al.*, 1975), labelled polypeptides were chromatographed on biogel A-5 m columns equilibrated and eluted with 0.1 M sodium phosphate buffer, pH 7.4, containing 0.1% sodium dodecylsulfate. The void volumn (V_0) was in fraction 20 and the total volume was in fraction 82. Fractions of 2 ml were collected and aliquots were used for detection of 4-hydroxy [^{14}C]proline (●——●) by the method of Juva and Prockop (1966). The position of the markers used for calibrating the columns prior to the run are indicated (↓): D.B.: dextran blue 2000, excluded from the column (V_0); pro-α: pro-α-chains of the type I procollagen; BSA, bovine serum albumin and OVA, ovalbumin. In control experiments, 4-hydroxy [^{14}C]proline (○——○) was measured after enzymatic digestion of ^{14}C-labelled polypeptides by purified collagenase, prior to reduction, denaturation and gel filtration of the samples as described above. Samples (0.2 ml) of fractions 30 to 33, 34 to 36 and 37 to 40 were pooled, exhaustively dialyzed against distilled water and lyophilized. The presence of cross-reactive GBM antigenic material in these samples was searched for by radioimmunoassay, using sheep anti-rabbit Ig antiserum (C).

terial. These results support those reported by Grant *et al.* (1975), using whole rat glomeruli.

The hydroxy [^{14}C]proline-containing component synthesized by the epithelial cells *in vitro* exhibits some chemical and antigenic properties similar to those of type IV collagen, since we have shown that: (a) the 3-hydroxyproline to total hydroxyproline ratio is about 14%; (b) over 80% of the total hydroxylysine is recovered as glucosyl-galactosyl-hydroxylysine units; (c) the molecular weight of the hydroxy [^{14}C]proline-containing polypeptides, determined by gel filtration on dodecylsulfate-agarose, is about 140,000. Not withstanding the fact that this determination can only be regarded as an approximation (Reynolds & Tanford, 1970), the value obtained corresponds to the molecular size of type IV collagen synthesized by embryonic chick lenses (Grant *et al.*, 1972), by cells of the embryonic rat parietal yolk sac (Clark *et al.*, 1975), or by whole rat glomeruli (Grant *et al.*, 1975), and to that of some collagenous polypeptides isolated from pepsin digests of GBM (Daniels & Hao Chu, 1975); (d) this component binds specifically to anti-type IV collagen antibodies.

Some of the ^{14}C-labelled polypeptides synthesized by the mesangial cells *in vitro* correspond to GBM collagenous polypeptides for the following reasons: (a) about 50% of the total hydroxylysine is recovered as glucosyl-galactosyl-hydroxylysine units; (b) they contain 3- and 4-hydroxyproline and, after digestion with purified collagenase, most of the 4-hydroxyproline is recovered into small peptide fragments; (c) the molecular weight of the 4-hydroxy [^{14}C]proline-containing polypeptides is about 140,000. It has been previously suggested (Grant *et al.*, 1972), that the higher molecular weight of the basement membrane (type IV) collagen precursor may be accounted for by its more extensive hydroxylation and glycosylation than the type I collagen precursor. The extent of glycosylation of GBM collagenous polypeptides synthesized by the mesangial cells is lower than that of GBM collagenous polypeptides synthesized by the epithelial cells. Since both collagenous polypeptides exhibit approximately the same molecular weight, it is therefore reasonable to suggest that the collagenous material synthesized by the mesangial cells may comprise a longer polypeptide chain than that synthesized by the epithelial cells; (d) these polypeptides bind specifically to anti-GBM antibodies. These findings therefore suggest that the epithelial and mesangial cells synthesize and secrete different types of collagenous polypeptides into the culture medium.

The amount of GBM antigenic material synthesized by each cell line during 6 hr has been found to be very low. This finding is consistent with studies performed *in vivo* on rat GBM synthesis (Grant *et al.*, 1975), and *in vitro* on embryonic chick lens basement membrane synthesis (Grant *et al.*, 1972), both studies indicating that only a small percentage of the incorporated [^{14}C]proline is present as 4-hydroxy [^{14}C]proline.

These studies show that both epithelial and mesangial cells in culture are able to synthesize a large molecular-weight collagenous component of the GBM. These components however show differences according to their origin. The mechanisms by which these GBM collagenous polypeptides interact with the non-collagenous material of the membrane remain unknown, but it seems reasonable to suggest that these interactions must take place extracellularly. Further, the techniques and results described in this work can be used to analyse more precisely the biosynthesis of the same membrane material in diseases such as glomerulonephritis or diabetes mellitus.

SUMMARY

Confluent cultures of epithelial or mesangial cells were incubated with [^{14}C]proline. The incorporation rate of the radioactive precursor was found to be linear for up to 8 hr. The synthesis and secretion of GBM collagenous polypeptides was demonstrated by the presence in the culture media of non-dialysable 3- and 4-hydroxy-[^{14}C]proline. After incubation with [^{14}C]lysine, it was shown that over 80% of the total hydroxy [^{14}C]lysine synthesized by the epithelial cells were recovered as glucosyl-galactosyl-hydroxy [^{14}C]lysine, while only 50% of the total hydroxy [^{14}C]lysine synthesized by the mesangial cells were recovered as glucosyl-galactosyl-hydroxy [^{14}C]lysine. After gel filtration of the culture media on Sephadex G-100 columns, GBM and type IV collagen polypeptides were searched for in the chromatographic fractions, using specific anti-GBM and anti-type IV collagen antibodies. Cross-reactive type IV collagen antigenic material was observed in the culture media of epithelial cells only, while cross-reactive GBM antigenic material was identified in the culture media of both epithelial and mesangial cells. The GBM collagenous polypeptides exhibited a molecular size of about 140,000, for both epithelial and mesangial cells. The synthesis of collagenous polypeptides represented about 10% of total proteins synthesized by each cellular line, as demonstrated by radioimmunoassay.

The data show that both cell lines synthesize GBM collagenous polypeptides *in vitro*. However, the GBM collagenous material synthesized by the epithelial or by the mesangial cells were dissimilar with respect to some of their biochemical and antigenic properties.

Acknowledgements—This work was supported in part by a grant from the "Délégation Générale à la Recherche Scientifique et Technique Française". We are indebted to Dr J. Deheneffe for his help in the evaluation of this work, and to Miss Y. Pirard and Mrs C. Flamand for their skilfull technical assistance.

REFERENCES

CLARK C. C., TOMICHEK E. A., KOSZALKA T. R., MINOR R. R. & KEFALIDES N. A. (1975) The embryonic rat parietal yolk sac. The role of the parietal endoderm in the biosynthesis of basement membrane collagen and glycoprotein *in vitro*. *J. biol. Chem.* **250**, 5259–5268.

COHEN M. P. & VOGT C. A. (1975) Collagen synthesis and secretion by isolated rat renal glomeruli. *Biochem. biophys. Acta* **393**, 78–87.

DANIELS J. R. & HAO CHU G. (1975) Basement membrane collagen of renal glomerulus. *J. biol. Chem.* **250**, 3531–3537.

FOIDART-WILLEMS J., DECHENNE C. & MAHIEU P. (1975) Biosynthesis of basement membrane collagen in cultures of renal glomerular and tubular epithelial cells. *Diabète Métab., Paris* **1**, 227–234.

FOIDART J. B., DECHENNE C. A., MAHIEU P. R., CREUTZ C. E. & DE MEY J. (1979) Tissue culture of normal rat glomeruli. Isolation and morphological characterization of two homogeneous cell lines. *Invest. Cell Pathol.* **2**, 15–26.

GRANT M. E., KEFALIDES N. A. & PROCKOP D. J. (1972) The biosynthesis of basement membrane collagen in embryonic chick lens. II. Synthesis of precursor form by matrix-free cells and a time-dependent conversion to α-chains in intact lens. *J. biol. Chem.* **247**, 3545–3551.

GRANT M. E., HARWOOD R. & WILLIAMS I. F. (1975) The biosynthesis of basement-membrane collagen by isolated rat glomeruli. *Eur. J. Biochem.* **54**, 531–540.

GUNSON D. E. & KEFALIDES N. A. (1976) The use of the radioimmunoassay in the characterization of antibodies to basement membrane collagen. *Immunology* **31**, 563–569.

HARDWICKE J. (1972) Glomerular filtration of macromolecules. In *Advances in Nephrology*, (Edited by HAMBURGER J., CROSNIER J. & MAXWELL M. D.) Vol. 2, pp. 61–74. Year Book Medical Publishers, Chicago.

JUVA K. & PROCKOP D. J. (1966) Modified procedure for the assay of ^{3}H or ^{14}C labelled hydroxyproline. *Analyt. Biochem.* **15**, 77–83.

KARNOVSKY M. J. & AINSWORTH S. K. (1972) The structural basis of glomerular filtration. In *Advances in Nephrology* (Edited by HAMBERGER J., CROSNIER J. & MAXWELL M. D.) Vol. 2, pp. 35–60. Year Book Medical Publishers, Chicago.

KEFALIDES N. A. (1973) Structure and biosynthesis of basement membranes. *Int. Rev. Connect. Tissue Res.* **6**, 63–107.

KIMMELSTIEL P., KIM O. J. & BERES J. (1962) Studies on renal biopsy specimens with the aid of the electron microscope. I. Glomeruli in diabetes. *Am. J. clin. Pathol.* **38**, 270–284.

LOWRY O. H., ROSEBROUGH N. J., FARR A. L & RANDALL R. J. (1951) Protein measurement with the folin phenol reagent. *J. biol. Chem.* **193**, 265–275.

MAHIEU P. & WINAND R. J. (1973a) Carbohydrate and amino-acid composition of human glomerular—basement—membrane fractions purified by affinity chromatography. *Eur. J. Biochem.* **37**, 157-163.

MAHIEU P., LAMBERT P. H. & MAGHUIN-ROGISTER G. (1973b) Primary structure of a small glycopeptide isolated from human glomerular basement membrane and carrying a major antigenic site. *Eur. J. Biochem.* **40**, 599–606.

MAHIEU P., LAMBERT P. H. & MIESCHER P. A. (1974) Detection of anti-glomerular basement membrane antibodies by a radioimmunological technique. Clinical application in human nephropathies. *J. clin. Invest.* **54**, 128–137.

REYNOLDS J. A. & TANFORD C. (1970) The gross conformation of protein–sodium dodecyl sulfate complexes. *J. biol. Chem.* **245**, 5161–5167.

VERNIER R. L., PAPERMASTER B. W., OLNESS K., BINET E. & GOOD R. A. (1960) Morphologic studies of the mechanism of proteinuria. *Am. J. Dis. Child.* **100**, 476–488.

SYMPOSIUM DISCUSSION

Horster: Could you expand on your last remark in which you refer to contractile activity in the B-cell type with angiotensin?

Mahieu: If you incubate the B-cells with 10^{-8} M angiotensin II for 10 min, in the presence of calcium and magnesium (each 2 mM), you observe a few seconds later a modification of the length of the cells, and more frequently, a modification in their shape, i.e. some evaginations are observed by light microscopy. The contraction reaches a maximum after 5–6 min, and is inhibited by saralasin.

Robinson: Do you also get continuous cultures of your A cells, or do they die out?

Mahieu: It is very easy to obtain sub-cultures of the B-cells. The B-cells represent on Day 22 almost 100% of the growing cells. For the A-cells, it is necessary to do subcultures 6 days after the glomerular explantation; at that time, these cells represent about 100% of the growing cells. In this case, it is necessary to use very low concentration of EDTA and trypsin (EDTA 5 mM and trypsin 0.0125%). The cells are incubated 5 sec in EDTA and thereafter 5 min in trypsin. If you use longer incubation times, the cells are destroyed. I should add that, if you put the glomeruli in distilled water for 3 min, you do not get any epithelial cells.

Horster: That isn't so strange. We observe in our work on epithelial cell cultures from individual nephron segments that epithelial cells have a natural disadvantage compared with fibroblasts; fibroblasts may rapidly outpopulate the cells displaying specific functions. Hence, we take great care not to transfer them from the organ into culture. This phenomenon is well recognized in many multi-type cell cultures (Sato *et al. Proc. Natn. Acad. Sci. U.S.A.* **46**, 963, 1960).

Mahieu: I do not think that the B-cells could be fibroblast cells. Indeed, if you stain fibroblasts with an anti-myosin antiserum, you never observe such prominent intracellular fibrillar structures; furthermore, the fibroblasts exhibit no contractile activity.

Robinson: Do your B-cells show phagocytic activity?

Mahieu: We have never observed that in the B-cells, but in glomerular explants, under normal conditions, you sometimes observe less than 1% of macrophages. I think that these cells come from the blood stream. In very old cultures, after 6 weeks at least, you may also observe a few macrophages. This may represent a macrophagic transformation of the cultivated cells.

Int. J. Biochem., Vol. 12, pp. 203 to 207
© Pergamon Press Ltd 1980. Printed in Great Britain
0020-711X/80/0701-0203$02.00/0

PROSTAGLANDIN SYNTHESIS BY RAT ISOLATED GLOMERULI AND GLOMERULAR CULTURED CELLS

J. SRAER[1], J. FOIDART[2], D. CHANSEL[1], P. MAHIEU[2] and R. ARDAILLOU[1]
[1]INSERM Research Unit 64, Hôpital Tenon, Paris, France, and
[2]Hôpital de Bavière, Liège, Belgium.

Abstract—1. PGE_2, $PGF_{2\alpha}$ and 6 keto-$PGF_{1\alpha}$ accumulated progressively with time in the incubation medium of glomeruli isolated from rat kidney cortex.

2. Synthesis of the three PGs was inhibited by indomethacin and stimulated by arachidonic acid.
3. Epithelial and mesangial glomerular cells were grown in homogenous monolayer cultures.
4. Synthesis by epithelial cells of the three PGs was low and fairly constant.
5. On the contrary, synthesis by mesangial cells of 6 keto-$PGF_{1\alpha}$ and mainly PGE_2 was maximum after 11 days of culture and greater than by epithelial cells.

INTRODUCTION

Synthesis of prostaglandins (PG) in the kidneys has been demonstrated by histochemical techniques in collecting ducts (Janszen *et al.*, 1971) and by tissue culture experiments in renal medullary interstitial cells (Muirhead *et al.*, 1972; Dunn *et al.*, 1976; Zusman & Keiser, 1977). PGs are also produced to a smaller extent in the renal cortex (Spector *et al.*, 1974; Whorton *et al.*, 1978) and several sites of production have been demonstrated: the arterial blood vessels (Terragno *et al.*, 1978; Smith *et al.*, 1978), the cortical collecting tubules (Smith *et al.*, 1978) and also the glomeruli: Smith *et al.* (1978) using immunohistochemical microscopy have found cyclooxygenase in ovine and bovine glomeruli. Folkert *et al.* (1979) and Hassid *et al.* (1979) have shown that [^{3}H]arachidonic acid in the presence of isolated glomeruli was converted into several PGs identified by thin layer chromatography. These studies left undefined the cellular localization within the glomerulus of PG synthesis. Using isolated glomeruli and glomerular epithelial and mesangial cultured cells, we have shown that PGE_2 was the major product synthesized by the rat glomerulus and that mesangial cells were the major site for its synthesis.

MATERIALS AND METHODS

Materials

PGE_2, $PGF_{2\alpha}$ and 6 keto-$PGF_{1\alpha}$ were gifts from Dr J. Pike (Upjohn Co., Kalamazoo, MI), indomethacin from Merck Sharp and Dohme (Paris) and angiotensin II (Asn^1, Val^5, A II) from Ciba-Geigy (Paris). Arachidonic acid (sodium salt) was obtained from Sigma (St Louis, MO); [^{3}H]PGE_2 and [^{3}H]$PGF_{2\alpha}$ (110–170 $Ci \cdot mmol^{-1}$) were purchased from the Radiochemical Center (Amersham, UK). 6 keto-$PGF_{1\alpha}$ was coupled to histamine using carbodiimide. The iodination with ^{125}I of this conjugate using the chloramine T procedure and the subsequent purification of the tracer were performed as previously described (Maclouf *et al.*, 1976). Anti-PGE_2, anti-$PGF_{2\alpha}$ and anti-6 keto-$PGF_{1\alpha}$ anti-serums were obtained from Institut Pasteur (Paris). These antibodies cross-react only slightly with other PGs and could be considered as specific (Dray *et al.*, 1975, 1978). All other chemicals were analytical grade.

Isolation and incubation of rat renal glomeruli

Renal glomeruli were isolated from Sprague–Dawley rats weighing 150–220 g according to a previously published technique (Sraer *et al.*, 1978). In short, cortex from four kidneys was dissected and minced to a paste-like consistency. The homogenate, suspended in 20 mM Tris–HCl buffer, pH 7.4, containing 5 mM glucose, 135 mM NaCl, 10 mM KCl and 10 mM $NaCH_3COO$, was pushed successively through a 106 μm-sieve which excluded the tubules and a 50 μm-sieve which retained the glomeruli. The suspension was then passed through a 25-gauge needle and centrifuged at 120 g for 90 sec. The supernatant was discarded, the pellet resuspended in the same buffer solution and passed again through the needle and centrifuged. This operation was repeated 5 times. Each individual preparation was checked for purity under light microscopy. Virtually no afferent and efferent arterioles could be detected. Tubular fragments were always below 2% of the total number of glomeruli. Isolated glomeruli (500–1000 $\mu g \cdot ml^{-1}$ of glomerular protein) were incubated at 37°C in room atmosphere under continuous agitation (100 1.6 Hz) in 200 μl of buffer similar to that employed in the purification procedure. After 60 min incubation, the preparation was centrifuged at 3000 g for 10 min and the supernatant collected.

Cell cultures

Rat glomerular mesangial and epithelial cells characterized by immunofluorescent microscopy using antimyosin antiserum and by transmission electron microscopy were isolated and grown in homogenous monolayer cultures according to previously described methods (Foidart *et al.*, 1979; Mahieu *et al.*, 1979). In short, glomeruli isolated as stated here above were cultured at 37°C in plastic flasks containing 5 ml of RPMI medium (Flow laboratories, Irvine, U.K.) supplemented with 10% decomplemented fetal bovine serum, and buffered with 20 mM N-2 hydroxyethylpiperazine-N'-2 ethanesulphonic acid (Hepes), pH 7.2. Epithelial cells grow rapidly with a peak of cell division on day 6 whereas mesangial cells grow at a slower rate with a maximum of cell division on day 22. These two cell lines were thus separated by performing subcultures at these two different times. The conditions of these subcultures were identical to those used for isolated glomeruli. Culture media were changed every 2 days as a rule. Samples were frozen and stored for further PG determinations.

Prostaglandin assays

The concentrations of PGE_2, $PGF_{2\alpha}$ and 6 keto-$PGF_{1\alpha}$

Table 1. Accumulation with time of PGE_2, $PGF_{2\alpha}$ and 6 keto-$PGF_{1\alpha}$ in the incubation medium of isolated glomeruli with ($2.5\ \mu g \cdot ml^{-1}$) or without arachidonic acid

Time (min)	PGE_2 ($ng \cdot mg^{-1}$) Basal	PGE_2 ($ng \cdot mg^{-1}$) With arachidonic acid	$PGF_{2\alpha}$ ($ng \cdot mg^{-1}$) Basal	$PGF_{2\alpha}$ ($ng \cdot mg^{-1}$) With arachidonic acid	6 keto-$PGF_{1\alpha}$ ($ng \cdot mg^{-1}$) Basal	6 keto-$PGF_{1\alpha}$ ($ng \cdot mg^{-1}$) With arachidonic acid
10	0.93 ± 0.02	4.29 ± 0.09	0.99 ± 0.09	1.39 ± 0.05	0.63 ± 0.07	1.44 ± 0.15
20	1.06 ± 0.09	5.15 ± 0.23	1.13 ± 0.07	1.65 ± 0.10	0.77 ± 0.15	1.78 ± 0.15
30	1.14 ± 0.15	5.16 ± 0.69	1.03 ± 0.04	1.84 ± 0.07	0.95 ± 0.06	2.04 ± 0.14
45	1.30 ± 0.08	6.76 ± 0.28	1.08 ± 0.08	1.80 ± 0.12	1.25 ± 0.03	2.26 ± 0.15
60	1.32 ± 0.11	6.48 ± 0.32	1.11 ± 0.06	1.83 ± 0.05	1.17 ± 0.19	2.77 ± 0.31
90	1.67 ± 0.04	7.27 ± 0.56	1.36 ± 0.11	1.93 ± 0.04	1.37 ± 0.13	2.35 ± 0.11
120	1.97 ± 0.09	7.29 ± 0.65	1.24 ± 0.10	2.03 ± 0.06	1.16 ± 0.10	2.88 ± 0.24

Each value is the mean ± SEM of six determinations performed at increasing dilutions of the incubation medium.

were determined on incubation mediums of isolated glomeruli immediately at the end of the incubation. These same PGs were also determined at the end of a given experiment on stored and frozen samples of culture mediums. After acidification to pH 3.5 and extraction with cyclohexane ethylacetate (1:1, v/v), PGE_2 and $PGF_{2\alpha}$ were separated by silicic acid chromatography and measured using specific radioimmunoassay (Dray *et al.*, 1975). 6 keto-$PGF_{1\alpha}$ was extracted according to the same procedure, but directly measured by radioimmunoassay without prior chromatography using [^{125}I] 6 keto-$PGF_{1\alpha}$ as a tracer and the corresponding specific antiserum at a final dilution of 1:30,000 (Dray *et al.*, 1978). In these conditions, 50% inhibition of binding for 6 keto-$PGF_{1\alpha}$, PGE_2 and $PGF_{2\alpha}$ occurred with 22 ng, 350 ng and 2000 ng per tube respectively. In each of the three radioimmunoassays a blank value obtained with the medium incubated in the absence of cells was subtracted. Each value of PG concentration given in the figure and the tables is the mean of six individual determinations performed at increasing dilutions of the culture medium. PG synthesis was currently expressed as ng per ml of incubation medium. In some experiments, PG production was related to the number of cells or to the protein content of the flask. Protein determinations were made according to Lowry *et al.* (1951).

RESULTS

Production of PGs by isolated glomeruli

Initial experiments indicated that PGE_2 and $PGF_{2\alpha}$ syntheses were linearly related to the concentrations of glomerular protein from 0 to $2\ mg \cdot ml^{-1}$ ($r = +0.99$ and $+0.97$ for each of these PGs respectively with 12 coupled values in both cases). PGE_2, $PGF_{2\alpha}$ and 6 keto-$PGF_{1\alpha}$ progressively accumulated as a function of time as shown in Table 1. When $2.5\ \mu g \cdot ml^{-1}$ of arachidonic acid was added, the production of the three PGs was clearly enhanced, but more markedly for PGE_2 (6 times the control value at 60 min) than for $PGF_{2\alpha}$ (1.5 times) and for 6 keto-$PGF_{1\alpha}$ (2.4 times). A plateau was rapidly reached for the three PGs in both experimental conditions. Addition of 1 mM indomethacin to the incubation medium strongly inhibited PGE_2 and $PGF_{2\alpha}$ productions whether or not arachidonic acid was present. PGE_2, $PGF_{2\alpha}$ and 6 keto-$PGF_{1\alpha}$ accumulations after 60 min incubation were stimulated in the presence of increasing doses of arachidonic acid. Maximum stimulation occurred above $5\ \mu g\ ml^{-1}$ for the first and represented approximately 4 and 2.5 times the basal value for PGE_2 and $PGF_{2\alpha}$ respectively. Concentrations corresponding to 50% of the maximum stimulations were close to $2\ \mu g \cdot ml^{-1}$ for both PGs. For 6 keto-$PGF_{1\alpha}$ the maximum rate of synthesis occurred above $2\ \mu g \cdot ml^{-1}$ arachidonic acid and represented slightly more than twice the basal value. The concentration corresponding to 50% of this maximum stimulation was $0.8\ \mu g \cdot ml^{-1}$. PGE_2 and $PGF_{2\alpha}$ production were temperature-dependent both in the presence and in the absence of arachidonic acid and were maximum in the range 30–37°C.

Production of PGs by glomerular cultured cells

PGE_2, $PGF_{2\alpha}$ and 6 keto-$PGF_{1\alpha}$ production rates by mesangial and epithelial cells respectively were measured on media which had been exposed to the cells for 48 hr. This 2 day incubation was started at various intervals of time from 0 to 39 days after subculture had been initiated (Table 2). Synthesis by epithelial cells of these three PGs was low but fairly constant whatever the time at which they were studied after subculture. On the contrary, synthesis by mesangial cells of PGE_2 and 6 keto-$PGF_{1\alpha}$ which was also very low when studied from 0 to 11 days after subculture increased markedly when measured from 11 to 24 days after, with a peak on day 15. At this time, the production rate was 30 and 20 times greater than with epithelial cells for PGE_2 and 6 keto-$PGF_{1\alpha}$ respectively. This was followed by a decreased synthesis of both PGs with return to base line levels on day 39. Synthesis of $PGF_{2\alpha}$ by mesangial cells increased earlier and reached its maximum on day 13. Difference with epithelial cells was not so striking and varied from day to day. When absolute values were considered, synthesis of PGE_2 by mesangial cells appeared markedly predominant since PGE_2 was synthesized by these cells in amounts 15–20 times greater than 6 keto-$PGF_{1\alpha}$ and $PGF_{2\alpha}$. Since the amount of PG synthesized per ml of incubation milieu depends both on the number of cells present in the flask and on the production per cell, interpretation of these results must take into account the rate of multiplication of the two lines of cells. Epithelial cells grow at a faster rate than mesangial cells. A homogenous monolayer made of confluent cells was obtained at day 8 and day 20 of the subculture for epithelial and mesangial cells respectively. Thus related to the number of cells, production of PGs by epithelial cells compared to that by mesangial cells must be much smaller initially than it appears from

Table 2. Production rates of PGE_2, $PGF_{2\alpha}$ and 6 keto-$PGF_{1\alpha}$ by cultured glomerular mesangial and epithelial cells at different times over a 40 day period. Each production rate was calculated over 2 days. The number of days elapsed from the start of the subculture is given

Time	PGE_2 ($pg \cdot ml^{-1} \cdot hr^{-1}$)		$PGF_{2\alpha}$ ($pg \cdot ml^{-1} \cdot hr$)		6 keto-$PGF_{1\alpha}$ ($pg \cdot ml^{-1} \cdot hr$)	
(day)	Epithelium	Mesangium	Epithelium	Mesangium	Epithelium	Mesangium
2	320	186	76	2	15	19
5	662	400	91	30	—	16
7	250	298	65	29	12	10
8	143	197	15	14	15	4
10	111	380	—	46	—	21
12	192	1735	77	48	16	101
13	89	2244	30	109	15	145
14	198	—	58	—	12	—
15	355	2971	28	66	—	165
19	—	2545	—	52	—	87
20	113	2545	56	55	18	160
21	—	1394	—	43	—	76
22	—	1852	—	50	—	93
23	188	1845	51	54	16	88
39	—	47	—	44	—	25

Each value is the mean of six determinations performed at increasing dilutions of the incubation medium.

Table 2. In order to confirm the marked differences observed from days 11–24 of the subculture, we compared PG production rates by the two lines of cells on day 20 of the subcultures when they were both confluent taking into account the number of cells and the amount of cell protein. The differences observed in Table 2 persisted. This demonstrated that PGE_2 and 6 keto-$PGF_{1\alpha}$ synthesis per cell was greater for mesangial than for epithelial cells whereas $PGF_{2\alpha}$ synthesis was in the same range. In order to establish that the extracellular accumulation of PGs reflected new synthesis by the cultured cells, either the precursor of this synthesis arachidonic acid, or a potent selective inhibitor indomethacin, was added to the culture medium at the start of a 3 hr incubation. PG synthesis was studied on days 12 and 7 of the subculture for mesangial and epithelial cells respectively when the rates of multiplication of both cell lines were maximum. Two flasks were used for each experiment. The culture medium of the 2 preceding days was removed and replaced by fresh serum-free medium with (experimental flask) or without (control flask) arachidonic acid. Fetal bovine serum was omitted in order to suppress any uncontrolled addition of arachidonic acid. After 3 hr incubation, mediums were collected and PG accumulation measured. Addition of arachidonic acid significantly stimulated the production by mesangial cells of the three PGs tested. The degree of stimulation was markedly greater for PGE_2 ($\times 12$) than for $PGF_{2\alpha}$ ($\times 3.5$) and 6 keto-$PGF_{1\alpha}$ ($\times 2$). Stimulation was also observed at a lesser degree with epithelial cells but only for PGE_2 ($\times 2$) and $PGF_{2\alpha}$ ($\times 2.5$). Addition of indomethacin (1 μM) resulted in inhibition at a similar degree ($\times 0.30$ to $\times 0.50$) of the synthesis by the two cell lines of the three PGs studied.

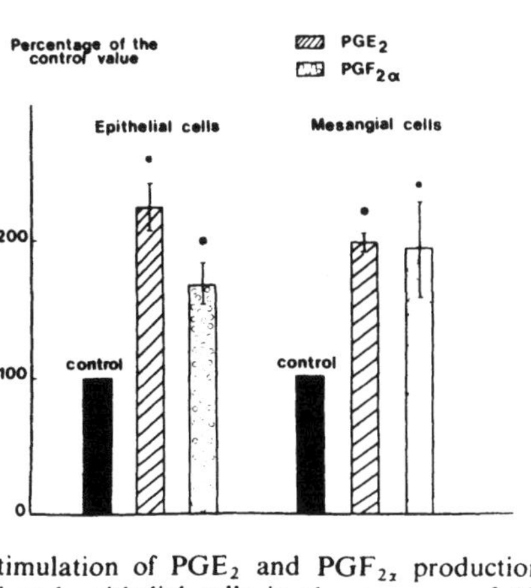

Fig. 1. Stimulation of PGE_2 and $PGF_{2\alpha}$ production by mesangial and epithelial cells in the presence of 10 nM Angiotensin II. Results are given as means $\pm$ SEM of six individual determinations performed at increasing dilutions of the incubation medium. They are expressed as percentages of the corresponding control values. Results of t-test between control and experimental values (expressed as $pg \cdot ml^{-1} \cdot hr^{-1}$) are given. * = $P < 0.05$.

The effect of angiotensin II was studied in the same conditions as for arachidonic acid but only on the production of PGE_2 and $PGF_{2\alpha}$. The degree of stimulation was close to 2 for the synthesis of these two PGs by both cell lines (Fig. 1).

DISCUSSION

Our data clearly indicate that glomeruli isolated from the rat kidney cortex synthesize PGE_2, $PGF_{2\alpha}$ and PGI_2. The two first prostaglandins were directly measured in the incubation medium of isolated glomeruli and cultured glomerular cells. The presence of the latter was demonstrated by the assay of its stable metabolic product, 6 keto-$PGF_{1\alpha}$. The extracellular accumulation of these three PGs reflects new synthesis rather than release of stored material since it was strongly enhanced by arachidonic acid and clearly inhibited by indomethacin. The amounts of PGs synthesized measured in the same conditions varied according to the day of the experiment. This may depend on the glomerular ability itself to produce PGs and also reflect variability in the incorporation into tissue phospholipids of arachidonic acid added. The maximum percentage conversions of arachidonic acid to PGE_2 and to $PGF_{2\alpha}$ were 0.20–0.25% per hr; the same parameter for 6 keto-$PGF_{1\alpha}$ was smaller, approx 0.12%. Zusman *et al.* (1977), using rabbit medullary interstitial cells in tissue culture, reported a similar value for PGE_2 but a clearly smaller one for $PGF_{2\alpha}$.

In the presence of 2.5 $\mu g \cdot ml^{-1}$ of arachidonic acid, stimulation of the basal production of PGE_2 was clearly greater than for $PGF_{2\alpha}$ and 6 keto-$PGF_{1\alpha}$ (Table 1). The plateaus obtained after 60 min incubation reflect the progressive degradation with time of the enzymes intervening in the syntheses, the decreased availability of arachidonic acid and/or equilibrium between PG formation and degradation. 6 keto-$PGF_{1\alpha}$ production by the renal cortex has recently been demonstrated (Whorton *et al.*, 1978; Terragno *et al.*, 1978). In these studies, the distribution of ^3H-radioactivity after incubation of renal tissue with [^3H]arachidonic acid only, was shown. This mode of expression allows comparison of the syntheses of the different PGs but does not provide the absolute values of PGs synthesized. 6 keto-$PGF_{1\alpha}$ was the principal arachidonic acid metabolite recovered from the cortical arteries (Terragno *et al.*, 1978) and was approximately equivalent to $PGF_{2\alpha}$ in microsomes prepared from rabbit renal cortex (Whorton *et al.*, 1978). This is different from our results with glomeruli in the presence of arachidonic acid which show a clear preponderance of PGE_2 and $PGF_{2\alpha}$ over 6 keto-$PGF_{1\alpha}$ when syntheses are expressed on a weight basis. More recently, Folkert *et al.* (1979) and Hassid *et al.* (1979) demonstrated PG production by isolated rat renal glomeruli. Their results differ from ours in several aspects. These authors used in most of their experiments thin layer chromatography to identify the PGs produced after incubation of the glomeruli with [^3H]arachidonic acid. This technique does not allow estimation of the amounts of PG produced and thus cannot provide precise studies of accumulation of PG with time, PG synthesis as a function of arachidonic acid concentration or of glomerular protein. Moreover the necessary presence of exogenous arachidonic acid in the medium prevents from studying the basal conditions. In contrast with these two studies, we observed a greater production of PGE_2 and not of $PGF_{2\alpha}$.

The present data clearly indicate that glomerular mesangial cells compared to epithelial cells are the major site for PGE_2 synthesis. The third cell line present in the glomerulus, endothelial cells, could not be studied due to the lack of a homogenous population of these cells. The particular pattern of the time-course of PGE_2 production by the mesangial cells can be related to the state of differentiation of these cells. Indeed, the initial percentage of contractile cells after exposure to angiotensin II was 5–12% whereas it reaches 33% after day 12 of the subculture (Mahieu *et al.*, 1979). Similarly, the fibrils of myosin detected by immunofluorescent microscopy were less obvious on the early days of the subculture than later (Foidart *et al.*, 1979). It can thus be considered that the high production rate of PGE_2 by mesangial cells from day 11 to day 24 corresponds to the recovery by these cells of their biological properties. The stimulating effect of angiotensin II on PG production by glomerular cultured cells is in agreement with the identical effect of this hormone observed with medullary cultured cells (Zusman *et al.*, 1977) and with the previously published demonstration by two of us (J.S. and R.A.) of glomerular receptors for angiotensin II (Sraer *et al.*, 1974).

PGE_2 and PGI_2 have been shown to stimulate glomerular adenylate cyclase (Schlondorff *et al.*, 1978). Since mesangial cells contain bundles of myosin filaments (Foidart *et al.*, 1979) and exhibit a contractile activity in the presence of angiotensin II (Mahieu *et al.*, 1979) the present data suggest that PGE_2 synthesis by the mesangial cells themselves in response to angiotensin II binding may regulate the role of these cells in glomerular vasoreactivity. Other effects of glomerular PGs, either directly or through cyclic AMP production could be the decrease in glomerular ultrafiltration coefficient (Baylis *et al.*, 1976; Ichikawa *et al.*, 1977) and the stimulation of renin production by the juxtaglomerular apparatus (Yun *et al.*, 1978). There could be a balance between the local productions of angiotensin II and PGs, each of them controlling the other.

SUMMARY

The PGE_2, $PGF_{2\alpha}$ and 6 keto-$PGF_{1\alpha}$ contents of the incubation medium of glomeruli isolated from rat kidney were measured at different times with or without addition of arachidonic acid. These prostaglandins accumulated progressively with time and reached equilibrium after 60–120 min incubation. Synthesis of the three PGs was inhibited when indomethacin was added whereas it was markedly enhanced, mainly for PGE_2, at increasing doses of arachidonic acid. Plateaus were reached above 5 $\mu g \cdot ml^{-1}$ and concentrations corresponding to 50% of the maximum values were 2 $\mu g \cdot ml^{-1}$ for PGE_2 and $PGF_{2\alpha}$, and 0.8 $\mu g \cdot ml^{-1}$ for 6 keto-$PGF_{1\alpha}$. There were strictly linear relationships between PGE_2 or $PGF_{2\alpha}$ productions and the concentration of glomerular protein. PGE_2 and $PGF_{2\alpha}$ syntheses with or without arachidonic acid were maximum at 30–37°C. PGE_2 glomerular content was almost undetectable initially and increased with time.

PGE_2, $PGF_{2\alpha}$ and 6 keto-$PGF_{1\alpha}$ were also measured in the incubation medium of cultured mesangial or epithelial cells. These cells were grown in homogenous monolayer cultures and characterized by electron microscopy and immunofluorescent microscopy. Synthesis by epithelial cells of these three PGs was low and fairly constant whatever the time after initiation of the culture. On the contrary, synthesis by mesangial cells of PGE_2 and 6 keto-$PGF_{1\alpha}$ increased markedly from day 11 with a peak on day 15. Production of PGE_2 by mesangial cells was 15–20 times greater than that of the other PGs by these cells and 30 times greater than that of PGE_2 by epithelial cells. These data demonstrate that PGE_2, $PGF_{2\alpha}$ and PGI_2, in order of decreasing abundance, are synthesized by the glomerular cells and that mesangial cells are the major site for PGE_2 synthesis.

Acknowledgments—This work was supported by grants from the "Délégation Générale à la Recherche Scientifique et Technique" (No. 76-7-1447) and from the "Institut National de la Santé et de la Recherche Médicale" (No. 447676). The authors are indebted to Mrs A. Morin for secretarial assistance.

REFERENCES

BAYLIS C., DEEN W. M., MYERS B. D. & BRENNER B. M. (1976) Effects of some vasodilator drugs on transcapillary fluid exchange in the renal cortex. *Am. J. Physiol.* **230,** 1148–1156.

DRAY F., CHARBONNEL B. & MACLOUF J. (1975) Radioimmunoassay of prostaglandins F_α, E_1 and E_2 in human plasma. *Eur. J. clin. Invest.* **5,** 311–318.

DRAY F., PRADELLES P., MACLOUF J., SORS H. & BRINGUIER A. (1978) Radioimmunoassay of \6 keto-$PGF_{1\alpha}$ using an iodinated tracer. *Prostaglandins* **15,** 715 (abstract).

DUNN M. J., STALEY R. S. & HARRISON M. (1976) Characterization of prostaglandin production in tissue culture of rat renal medullary cells. *Prostaglandins* **12,** 37–49.

FOIDART J. B., DECHENNE C. A., MAHIEU P., CREUTZ C. E. & DE MAY J. (1979) Tissue culture of normal rat glomeruli. Isolation and morphological characteristics of two homogenous cell lines. *Invest. cell. Pathol.* **2,** 15–26.

FOLKERT V. W. & SCHLONDORFF D. (1979) Prostaglandin synthesis in isolated glomeruli. *Prostaglandins* **17,** 79–86.

HASSID A., KONIECZKOWSKI M. & DUNN M. J. (1979) Prostaglandin synthesis in isolated rat kidney glomeruli. *Proc. natn. Acad. Sci. U.S.A.* **76,** 1155–1159.

ICHIKAWA I. & BRENNER B. M. (1977) Evidence for glomerular actions of ADH and dibutyryl cyclic AMP in the rat. *Am. J. Physiol.* **233,** F102–F117.

JANSZEN F. H. & NUGTEREN D. H. (1971) Histochemical localization of prostaglandin synthetase. *Histochemistry* **27,** 159–164.

LOWRY O. H., ROSEBROUGH N. J., FARR A. L. & RANDALL R. J. (1951) Protein measurement with the Folin phenol reagent. *J. biol. Chem.* **193,** 265–269.

MACLOUF J., PRADEL M., PRADELLES P. & DRAY F. (1976) ^{125}I derivatives of prostaglandins. A novel approach in prostaglandin analysis by radioimmunoassay. *Biochim. biophys. Acta* **431,** 139–146.

MAHIEU P., FOIDART J. B., DUBOIS C. H., DECHENNE C. A. & DEHENEFFE J. (1979) Effects of angiotensin II on cultivated glomerular cells. *Invest. cell. Pathol.* In press.

MUIRHEAD E. E., GERMAIN G., LEACH B. E., PITCOCK J. A., STEPHENSON P., BROOKS B., BROSIUS W. L., DANIELS F. G. & KINMAN J. W. (1972) Production of renomedullary prostaglandins by renomedullary interstitial cells grown in tissue culture. *Circ. Res.* **30–31,** suppl. II, 161–171.

SCHLONDORFF D., YOO P. & ALPERT B. E. (1978) Stimulation of adenylate cyclase in isolated rat glomeruli by prostaglandins. *Am. J. Physiol.* **235,** F458–F464.

SMITH W. L. & BELL T. G. (1978) Immunohistochemical localization of the prostaglandin-forming cyclooxygenase in renal cortex. *Am. J. Physiol.* **235,** F451–F457.

SPECTOR D., ZUSMAN R. M., CALDWELL B. V. & SPEROFF L. (1974) The distribution of prostaglandins A, E and F in the human kidney. *Prostaglandins* **6,** 263–270.

SRAER J., SRAER J. D., CHANSEL D., JUEPPNER H., HESCH R. D. & ARDAILLOU R. (1978) Evidence for glomerular receptors for parathyroid hormone. *Am. J. Physiol.* **235,** F96–F103.

SRAER J. D., SRAER J., ARDAILLOU R. & MIMOUNE O. (1974) Evidence for angiotensin II receptors in rat isolated glomeruli. *Kidney Int.* **6,** 241–246.

TERRAGNO N. A., TERRAGNO A., EARLY J. A., ROBERTS M. A. & MCGIFF J. C. (1978) Endogenous prostaglandin synthesis inhibitor in the renal cortex. Effects on production of prostacyclin by renal blood vessels. *Clin. Sci. mol. Med.* **55,** 199s–202s.

WHORTON A. R., SMIGEL M., OATES J. A. & FRÖLICH J. C. (1978) Regional differences in prostacyclin formation by the kidney. Prostacyclin is a major prostaglandin of renal cortex. *Biochim. biophys. Acta* **529,** 176–180.

YUN J. C. H., KELLY G. D., BARTTER F. C. & SMITH G. W. (1978) Role of prostaglandins in the control of renin secretion in the dog. *Life Sci.* **23,** 945–952.

ZUSMAN R. M. & KEISER H. R. (1977) Prostaglandin biosynthesis by rabbit renomedullary interstitial cells in tissue culture. Stimulation by angiotensin II, bradykinin and arginine vasopressin. *J. clin. Invest.* **60,** 215–223.

SYMPOSIUM DISCUSSION

Frohlich: Larsson & Anggard (*Eur. J. Pharmac.* **21,** 30, 1973) reported prostaglandin synthesis in the cortex in about 1976, and the work was done in tissue homogenates. We have subsequently investigated whether in addition to E_2 and $F_{2\alpha}$, which they described, another prostaglandin might be synthesized in the cortex. We used microsomes, to avoid the problem of the high rate of prostaglandin metabolism in whole cortex and found that PGI_2 was formed, in addition. It is, therefore, important to consider the possibility of prostaglandin degradation in any system in which whole cells are present. Have you looked at the rate of PG metabolism either in whole glomerulae or in your cell lines?

Sraer: I cannot answer that directly. We don't think that there is any degradation of prostaglandins in the medium in our studies. We can say that because when we take aliquots from the incubation at intervals during an incubation, the sum of PG which we find is the same as that in the total incubation at the end. How would you measure degradation?

Frohlich: I guess one way would be to add radio-tracer. It is somewhat strange that there should be no degradation, since the kidney cortex is one of the richest sources of 15-keto dehydrogenase and Δ13-reductase. It would mean that your cells are very different from normal cortex cells.

Guder: In terms of the function of prostaglandins, do you interpret the release of PG from mesangial cells as being the overflow of excess of the effector? Are the prostaglandins acting in the mesangial cell or acting on a distant cell?

Sraer: It seems to me likely that the prostaglandins released from one cell, in response to angiotensin, for example, could then act on another cell.

Hume (Oxford): I wonder if the production of prostaglandin from the mesangial cells is the reason for the death of the epithelial cells?

Horster: On the contrary, in our preliminary experiments, the addition of prostaglandin to culture medium with other hormones actually supports, rather than suppresses growth.

Int. J. Biochem., Vol. 12, pp. 209 to 214
© Pergamon Press Ltd 1980. Printed in Great Britain

0020-711X/80/0701-0209$02.00/0

DISTRIBUTION OF ENZYMES OF cGMP METABOLISM IN GLOMERULI AND TUBULES ISOLATED FROM NORMAL AND NEPHROTIC RAT KIDNEY CORTEX*

J. J. HELWIG†‡, A. N. K. YUSUFI, G. REBEL§, J. GEISERT, C. BOLLACK and P. MANDEL
Centre de Recherches Chirurgicales R. Leriche, Pavillon Poincaré, Hôpital Civil, and
Institut de Chimie Biologique, 11, rue Humann, 67085 Strasbourg Cedex, France

Abstract—1. Puromycin aminonucleoside (PA) nephrosis may constitute a good experimental model to investigate the involvement of the cGMP system in the regulation of several kidney functions and especially glomerular permeability.

2. After a single intravenous injection of PA we studied the evolution of the guanylate cyclase (GCase) and cGMP-phosphodiesterase (G-PDE) activities in pure preparations of glomeruli (Gl) and tubules (TU).

3. Both Gl and TU homogenates showed a strong increase of the GCase activity 12 days after PA injection.

4. In the presence of Triton X-100, TU homogenate GCase showed the same pattern as in absence of this detergent while the Gl enzyme decreased unexpectedly. On the other hand, the only G-PDE change was observed in the TU where this activity decreases progressively.

5. Gl pellets and TU supernatants showed similar changes as in total homogenates. But, compared to the total homogenate, both Gl and TU supernatant GCases were strongly activated and in the Gl these activation rates were not the same in normal and 12 days-nephrotic rats.

6. These results could be explained by the existence of a membrane bound GCase "effector" involved in the physiopathological evolution of the disease.

7. In conclusion it seems to be clear that the cGMP-system is involved in the evolution of PA-nephrosis. But the precise relation between variations in the cGMP-system and the disease remains unclear and needs further investigation.

INTRODUCTION

Since 1955 (Frank *et al.*, 1955) puromycin aminonucleoside (PA) has been used widely to induce nephrosis in rats. This experimental nephrotic syndrome is essentially characterized by high proteinuria and the perturbation of Gl permeability which has been shown by the loss of Gl polyanion (Michael *et al.*, 1970) and an increased permeability to dextran sulfate (Bohrer *et al.*, 1977a). Proteinuria may result from disruption of components of the Gl basement membrane (GBM) due to altered metabolism of Gl barrier cells, especially the epithelial cells (Andrews, 1977; Glasser *et al.*, 1977; Velosa *et al.*, 1977). These cells participate in the synthesis of the GBM (Kurtz & Feldman, 1962; Walter, 1973) and in the filtration process through pinocytosis of filtered proteins that may have leaked through the GMB (Farquhar, 1975). This is especially evident in PA induced nephrotic animals (Caufield & Farquhar, 1975). PA effect on the other Gl cells is unclear. However, recent work (Avasthi & Evan, 1979) suggests that the Gl ultrafiltration coefficient is reduced in PA-nephrotic rats due to the changes in the size and/or density of endothelial fenestrae. PA effects on the other parts of the nephron are still unknown.

The involvement of cyclic guanosine 3′5′-monophosphate (cGMP) in the regulation of several Gl functions has already been proposed. For example, the administration of agents such as parathyroid hormone (Ichikawa *et al.*, 1978) angiotensin (Blantz *et al.*, 1976; Bohrer *et al.*, 1977b), bradykinin, acetylcholine (Baylis *et al.*, 1976; Knox & Ott, 1976) and others (Brenner *et al.*, 1976) cause changes in Gl microcirculation and permeability properties of Gl membranes. Besides, it seems that not only cAMP, but also cGMP metabolism in Gl are controlled at least by humoral agents known to alter Gl functions *in vivo* (Torres *et al.*, 1978; Shah *et al.*, 1979). In addition, recent findings suggest that Gl isolated from rabbit kidney cortex contain a much higher guanylate cyclase activity than TU fragments isolated simultaneously from the same tissue (Helwig *et al.*, 1975) and that Gl have a higher content of immunoreactive cGMP than TU (Dousa *et al.*, 1977).

Therefore it seems that PA nephrosis may constitute a good experimental model for investigating the involvement of the cGMP-system in the regulation of kidney functions and especially Gl permeability. The present work reports the results obtained from the study of the evolution of the enzymes of cGMP metabolism in pure Gl and cortical TU isolated simultaneously from the same animal.

* This work was supported by a research grant from INSERM (ATP No. 62 78 94).

† Attaché de Recherches à l'INSERM, France.
‡ To whom reprint requests should be sent at: Centre de Recherches Chirurgicales R. Leriche, Pavillon Poincaré, Hôpital Civil, 67005 Strasbourg Cedex, France.
§ Chargé de Recherches au CNRS, France.

MATERIALS AND METHODS

Induction of the experimental nephrotic syndrome

August inbred male rats (200–250 g) were injected intravenously with a single dose of 2% PA in 0.9% NaCl (Sigma Chemical Co., St Louis, MO) into a tail vein (10 mg PA. 100 gm body weight^{-1}). Proteinuria was determined by the method of Lowry *et al.* (1951) on 24 urine collections in metabolic cages for 15 days after PA injections. The experiments were performed in groups of 5 rats 3, 6, 9, 12 and 15 days after PA injection and in groups without PA injection.

Fractionation of rat kidney cortex

After decapitation, the kidneys were rapidly removed and the cortices were dissected out and used for the preparation of Gl and TU as previously described in detail (Helwig *et al.*, 1974a) with some modifications. The cortices were forced through a tissue press and incubated for several 20 min intervals in 25 ml of modified Hanks solution (Imbert *et al.*, 1975) containing 0.05% collagenase. After each incubation period, the dissociated tissue was removed by filtering it through a nylon gauze and the residue was further digested by addition of fresh collagenase. The collagenase and lysed cells were eliminated by repeated washings in 10 mM Tris–HCl buffer (pH 7.4) containing 0.25 M sucrose. The washed dissociated tissue was resuspended in the latter buffer and placed on a three-step sucrose gradient (46, 57, 75%) containing the same buffer throughout. After allowing the gradients to stand for 10 min at 0°C, they were centrifuged for 10 min at 5000 *g*. The purified Gl sedimented on the 57–75% interphase, whereas the pure TU fragments were recovered from the 46–57% interphase. Both fractions were very pure, as judged from their morphology (Helwig *et al.*, 1974b) and from the distribution of alkaline phosphatase, which can be regarded as a TU marker enzyme.

Preparation of homogenates

Gl and TU suspensions recovered from the gradients were diluted with 2 ml of 10 mM Tris–HCl buffer (pH 7.4) and then centrifuged for 20 min at 5000 *g*. The Gl and TU thus obtained were suspended in 1 and 8 ml respectively of the above-mentioned buffer. Homogenates were prepared at 2–4°C using a Potter–Elvehjem homogenizer fitted with Teflon pestle in the same buffer with or without 3% of Triton X-100 as specified in the Results section.

Assay of enzymes

As a control, we have checked that the enzyme activities were the same in perfused and non perfused kidneys. Perfusion was performed *in situ* with NaCl 0.9% via the aorta until the kidneys were blanched. Since guanylate cyclase and cGMP-phosphodiesterase activities in normal and 12 days nephrotic kidneys were similar in both cases, subsequent experiments were performed without perfusion.

Guanylate cyclase. Guanylate cyclase (GCase) activity was determined as previously reported (Goridis & Reutter, 1975; Helwig *et al.*, 1975). Reaction mixtures (130 μl) contained: 15 mM phosphocreatine, 75 μg of creatine kinase, cyclic [^{3}H]GMP (5 mM, 5.7 × 10^4 dis/min), 8 mM $MnCl_2$, 0.1 mM IBMX, [α-^{32}P]GTP (0.185 mM, 1.45 × 10^6, 2.9 × 10^6 dis/min). 60 mM Tris-HCl (pH 7.5) and enzyme (80 and 200 μg of protein for Gl and TU respectively) and were incubated for 10 min at 37°C. The reaction was terminated by addition of unlabelled GTP (500 nmol) in 4 mM EDTA and immersion of the samples in a boiling water bath for 3 min. No measurable hydrolysis of added cGMP occurred in any fraction. cGMP was separated from other labelled compounds by successive chromatography on columns of alumina and Dowex 1 (× 2). After the boiling step, 0.1 ml of ice-cold 0.60 M Tris HCl buffer (pH 7.5) was added and the denatured protein was removed by centrifugation (45 min at 2000 *g*). Portions (200 μl) of the supernatants were transferred to columns (1.5 g of dry neutral alumina, column diameter 0.5 cm), the columns were washed with 2 ml of 0.06 M Tris–HCl and the cGMP was eluted with 2 ml of 0.6 M Tris–HCl (pH 7.5). Eluates from the alumina columns were transferred to columns (0.5 × 3.5 cm) of Dowex 1 (× 2; formate form). These columns were washed with 2 ml of water, followed by 8 ml of 0.5 M formic acid, cGMP was eluted with 3 ml of 8 M formic acid directly into counting vials containing 20 ml of Scintix (Isotec), and the radioactivity was determined in an Intertechnique SL 4000 Liquid-scintillation counting system using the preset ^{3}H/^{32}P double-radioisotope counting window. All results were corrected for recovery of [^{3}H]cGMP (60–70%). All determinations were performed with freshly prepared enzymes. Protein was determined by the method of Lowry *et al.* (1951), using bovine serum albumin as standard.

cGMP-phosphodiesterase. cGMP dependent phosphodiesterase (G-PDE) was determined as previously reported (Kin *et al.*, 1977) in the presence of 15 to 30 μg of protein and 1 μmol of [^{3}H]cGMP in a reaction mixture (200 μl) containing 80 mM Tris–HCl buffer (pH 8) and 2 mM $MgSO_4$. After 15 min incubation at 37°C the reaction was stopped by heating at 95°C for 3 min and the [^{3}H]-5′ nucleotide and [^{3}H]3′ nucleotide were converted to [^{3}H] nucleosides by addition of 0.5% of snake venom (Crotalus Atrox; Sigma Chemical Co., St Louis, MO) and incubation during 20 min at 37°C. The reaction was stopped by addition of 750 μl of 0.1 mM guanosine. Nucleotides were separated from nucleosides by QAE-Sephadex A-25 columns (Pharmacia, Uppsala, Sweden) in 20 mM ammonium formate buffer (pH 7.2), according to the procedure of Wells *et al.* (1975). The columns (0.5 × 5 cm) were successively washed with 2 ml of the same buffer and 10 ml of water. After absorption of the total reaction mixture (1 ml) the columns were eluted with 4 ml of ammonium formate buffer. 1 ml of eluates were counted in counting vials containing 9 ml of Scintigel (Roth, West Germany) and the radioactivity was determined in an Intertechnique SL-4000 liquid scintillation counting system. All results were corrected for recovery of guanosine determined spectrophotometrically at 260 nm: optical densities were determined before and after passage of the reaction volume throughout the columns and the obtained recovery rates were constant(86–89%).

In both cases, enzyme activity was measured in a constant range of protein concentrations and incubation times, where proportionality between the reaction rate and the amount of protein or incubation time was assured. Activities of both enzymes were expressed in pmol of cGMP formed or hydrolyzed per min, per mg of protein.

RESULTS

After a single intravenous injection of PA, proteinuria starts between day 5 and 6, reaches a maximum on day 12 and then declines to a normal value. Therefore the GCase and G-PDE activities were determined at 3, 6, 9, 12 and 15 days after PA injection. The light microscopic observations show few Gl lesions such as an enlargement of urinary space. Some TU occlusions and peritubular cellular infiltration were observed 10–12 days after PA injection.

The distribution of GCase and G-PDE specific activities in normal August rats are given in Table 1. Both enzymes are preferentially localized in the purified Gl where GCase and G-PDE specific activities are 2.6 and 1.7 times higher than in the pure cortical TU fraction. In the presence of 1% Triton X-100, the

Table 1. Distribution of GCase and G-PDE in the glomeruli and tubules isolated from normal rat kidneys

	Glomeruli (pmols cGMP·min^{-1}·mg^{-1})	Tubules	G/T
Guanylate cyclase (6)	4.87 ± 1.34	1.87 ± 0.40	2.60
Guanylate cyclase + 1% Triton X-100 (6)	220.87 ± 1.34	11.56 ± 0.72	19.1
cGMP-phosphodiesterase (10)	226.4 ± 40.22	132.54 ± 11.95	1.71

Results represent the mean ± SEM for the number of experiments in parentheses. Each experiment has been performed on groups of 10 mixed rat kidneys as described in Materials and Methods.

Gl GCase is much more activated than the TU enzyme.

Results concerning the evolution of the cGMP-system in the Gl and TU homogenates are shown in Figs. 1 and 2. GCase specific activity in the total Gl homogenate (Fig. 1) increases up to 300% 12 days after PA injection while the G-PDE specific activity shows no statistical change. Attention can be drawn to the fact that maximum proteinuria is also observed on day 12. In the presence of 1% Triton X-100 in the reaction mixture the Gl homogenate GCase specific activities determined on day 9, 12 and 15 decreases unexpectedly to 60% of the control value. In the tubular homogenate too (Fig. 2) the GCase specific activity increases up to 200% in 12 days PA-nephrotic rats but the variations observed are the same in the absence and presence of 1% Triton X-100. In addition, in this fraction the G-PDE specific activity increases statistically up to 135% of the normal value.

These results led us to study the GCase specific activity in 100,000 *g* pellets and supernatants of both Gl and TU fractions isolated from normal and 12 days PA-nephrotic rats. Gl and TU pellets and supernatants were prepared simultaneously by centrifugation of the homogenates at 30,000 rev/min for 1 hr in a rotor R30 (Beckman). The results of these experiments are presented in Table 2. It must be stressed that in both control and PA nephrotic Gl and TU, the specific activities are considerably enriched in the supernatants with an overall recovery of total activities from the homogenate much higher than 100%. Furthermore these specific activity enrichments in the supernatants are not the same in normal glomeruli (×25) as in 12 days PA-nephrotic Gl (×6) while the TU fraction shows a similar specific activity enrichment in both cases (×8). This variation in the supernatant specific activity enrichment between the nor-

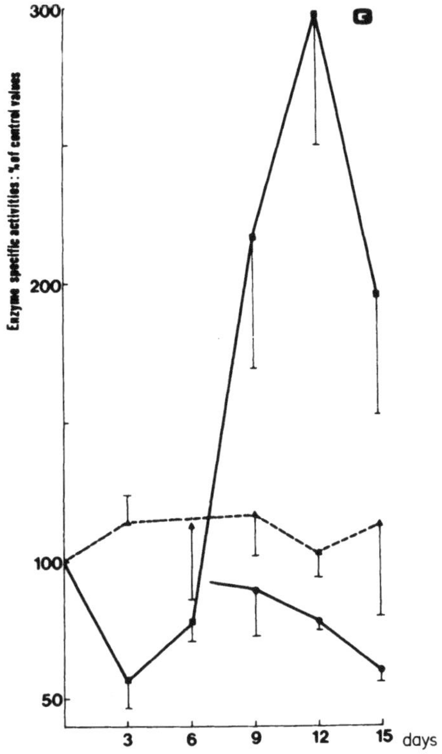

Fig. 1. Changes in enzymes of cGMP metabolism in isolated glomeruli of PAN rats. Each point represents the mean of ±SEM for 4 to 8 experiments. Each experiment was performed on groups of 10 mixed rat kidneys as described in the Material and Methods section. The control values of the enzyme specific activities are shown in Table 1. Guanylate cyclase specific activities determined in absence (■——■) and presence (●——●) of 1% Triton X-100, cGMP-phosphodiesterase (▲——▲).

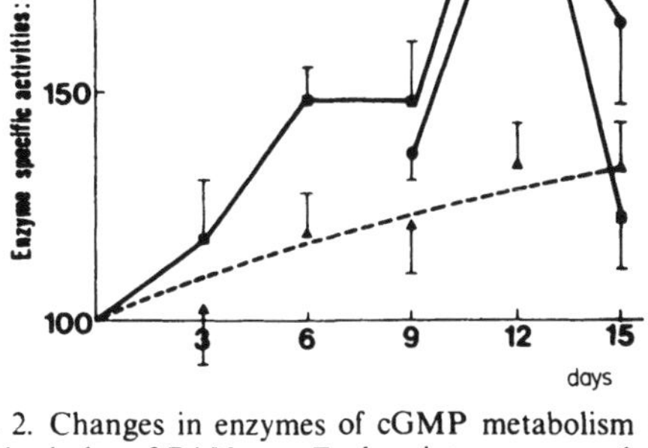

Fig. 2. Changes in enzymes of cGMP metabolism in isolated tubules of PAN rats. Each point represents the mean of ±SEM for 4 to 8 experiments. Each experiment was performed on groups of 10 mixed rat kidneys as described in Material and Methods section. The control values of the enzyme specific activities are shown in Table 1. Guanylate cyclase specific activities determined in absence (■——■) and presence (●——●) of 1% Triton X-100, cGMP-phosphodiesterase (▲——▲).

Table 2. Distribution of soluble and membrane bound-GCase in the glomeruli and tubules of normal and 12 days PA-nephrotic rats

	Controls		12 days PAN-rats	
	SA*	TA† (%)	SA	TA (%)
Glomeruli				
Homogenate	4.87 ± 1.34 (6)	100	14.50 ± 2.35 (4)	100
Pellet	2.79 ± 0.58 (4)	4.11	4.51 ± 0.70 (4)	22.3
Supernatant	123.55 ± 6.29 (4)	719	83.07 ± 9.06 (4)	162
Tubules				
Homogenate	1.87 ± 0.40 (6)	100	4.05 ± 0.44 (4)	100
Pellet	1.03 ± 0.06 (4)	32.8	1.10 ± 0.26 (4)	16.6
Supernatant	15.96 ± 0.71 (4)	345	33.10 ± 2.66 (4)	330

* SA: specific activity expressed in pmols cGMP. min^{-1} mg $protein^{-1}$; † TA: total activity expressed in pmols cGMP · min^{-1}. 71.7% of glomerular homogenate proteins and 59.6% of tubular homogenate proteins are to be found in the pellet. Results represent the mean ± SEM for the number of experiments in parentheses. Each experiment was performed on groups of 10 mixed rat kidneys as described in Materials and Methods.

mal and 12 days PA-nephrotic Gl is also shown by the total activity recovery rates compared with the corresponding total homogenates; the latter run from about 700% in the controls to 160% in 12 days PA-nephrotic rats. On the other hand, GCase total activity recoveries are the same in normal and 12 days PA-nephrotic TU supernatants (350%).

The 200% increase found in 12 days PA-nephrotic TU homogenate is observed again in the supernatant of this fraction. The 300% increase observed previously in the Gl homogenate is found to a lesser degree in the pellet of this fraction. But in this fraction a decrease in the supernatant activity is observed.

DISCUSSION

On fractionation of dissociated renal cortex of normal August rats both GCase and G-PDE activities are preferentially enriched in homogenates of pure Gl where their specific activities are respectively 2.6 and 1.7 times higher than that measured in pure TU fragments. But the rat Gl GCase enrichment rate is much lower than observed in rabbit cortex where the GCase specific activity of Gl homogenates is 40–50 times higher than in the simultaneously isolated TU homogenates (Helwig *et al.*, 1975). In the presence of 1% Triton X-100 the Gl GCase specific activity of the August rat is stimulated much more (× 45) than in the TU fraction (× 6). These Triton X-100 stimulation rates are also different from those observed in the rabbit kidney cortex. These interspecies differences between rabbit and rat glomerulo–tubular ratio could be explained either by a different role of cGMP in these species or by the existence of different GCases according to the species. In addition, our own recent studies performed on several rodent species show that only the rabbit exhibits such a high Gl enrichment (Yusufi *et al.*, 1979).

It is obvious that in our experimental conditions PA induced nephrosis modifies markedly the renal cGMP system. Parallel changes are found in the evolution of GCase activities in the homogenates of TU and Gl with proteinuria, both showing a maximum on day 12 in PA-nephrotic rats. The larger variations of GCase activity are found in the Gl homogenate. On the other hand, the changes observed in the G-PDE activity are not the same in the two fractions: in fact the TU enzyme increases while the Gl enzyme shows no statistical changes. From these results an accumulation of cGMP could be expected in the Gl. Another difference between Gl and TU homogenates is shown by the GCase activity determined in the presence of 1% Triton X-100. In these conditions the Gl GCase activity decreases unexpectedly while the TU homogenate exhibits the same pattern as in absence of Triton X-100.

In the TU a surprising GCase specific activity enrichment is observed in the control and 12 days PA-nephrotic supernatants with a recovery of total activity of about 350%. This result could be explained by the existence of a membrane bound "effector" discarded during the centrifugation. This component may be an humoral agent fixed on a membrane receptor. The action of such an "effector" on the TU supernatant GCase might be the same in normal and 12 days PA-nephrotic rats. The increase of the TU GCase specific activity in 12 days PA-nephrotic rats seems to be due to the increase of the soluble enzyme (Table 2).

At present, the results obtained for glomerular GCase development are difficult to explain. As in TU, Gl show a considerable enrichment of the supernatant GCase but, in this fraction the enrichment is not the same in 12 days PA-nephrotic rats as in the controls. Therefore, the above postulated membrane bound effector seems to play a role in the physiopathological evolution of the disease, at least in the glomeruli. In this fraction 12 days after PA injection, only the pellet exhibits an increase in GCase activity although this increase is smaller than that of total homogenate. In addition the supernatant enzyme decreases up to 30% of the control value. The above postulated difference in the action of a membrane bound "effector" between normal and nephrotic glomeruli could explain such a result. The most unexpected result concerns the decrease of GCase activity in 12 days PA-nephrotic Gl homogenate determined in the presence of 1% Triton X-100. The regulation which leads to the increase of GCase activity could be destroyed by the detergent. Further investigations are necessary, to determine the effect of other agents stimulating the GCase, such as sodium azide. Information about the cGMP levels in Gl and TU would also be helpful.

It is obvious that the cGMP system is considerably modified in the PA-nephrotic rat kidneys. The relations between the disease and these cGMP-system variations remain unclear and need further investigation. However it appears that the Gl cGMP-system does not play the same role in the physiopathological evolution of the PA-nephrosis as in the TU. In addition, as described in our earlier and present studies (Helwig *et al.*, 1974b, 1975) enzyme activities determined in total kidney do not reflect the enzyme contents of each nephron fraction especially the Gl and TU.

SUMMARY

Since the involvement of cGMP in several glomerular functions has been suggested, we studied the evolution of the cGMP-phosphodiesterase (G-PDE) and guanylate cyclase (GCase) activities, in purified glomeruli (Gl) and tubules (TU) for 15 days after a single intravenous injection of puromycin aminonucleoside (PA) in the rat.

In normal rats, G-PDE and GCase specific activities were higher in the Gl than in the TU (G:TU ratio— 2.6 for GCase, 19 for GCase in presence of 1% Triton X-100 and 1.7 for G-PDE). Twelve days after PA injection the GCase activity increased up to 300% in the Gl and up to 200% in TU homogenate. These GCase changes were similar to the progression of proteinuria which also showed a maximum 12 days after PA injection. The G-PDE activity remained stable in the Gl and increased up to 135% in the TU. In presence of 1% Triton X-100, the GCase activity in the TU showed the same pattern as in absence of Triton while in the Gl homogenate this activity decreased. GCase activity is preferentially localized in the Gl and TU 100,000 *g* supernatants. The GCase increase found in 12 days PA-nephrotic Gl and TU homogenates were again found in the TU supernatant and, in a lesser degree in the Gl pellet. But in this fraction, a decrease in the supernatant activity was also observed. Furthermore, in normal and PA-nephrotic rats, the GCase activities of both fractions were considerably enriched in the supernatants with overall recoveries up to 350–700% of homogenate total activities. In the Gl, these activation rates were not the same in normal and 12 days PA-nephrotic rats. This result could be explained by the existence of a cellular "effector" of the GCase activity, playing a role in the physiopathological evolution of the disease.

REFERENCES

ANDREWS P. M. (1977) A scanning and transmission electron microscopic comparison of puromycin aminonucleoside-induced nephrosis to hyperalbuninemia-induced proteinuria with emphasis on kidney podocyte pedical loss. *Lab. Invest.* **36,** 183–197.

AVASTHI P. S. & EVAN A. P. (1979) Glomerular permeability in aminonucleoside-induced nephrosis in rats. A proposed role of endothelial cells. *J. Lab. clin. Med.* **93,** 266–276.

BAYLIS C., DEEN W. M., MYERS B. D. & BRENNER B. M. (1976) Effects of some vasodilator drugs on transcapillary fluid exchange in renal cortex. *Am. J. Physiol.* **230,** 1148–1158.

BLANTZ R. C., KONNEN K. S. & TUCKER B. J. (1976) Angiotensin II effects upon the glomerular microcirculation and ultrafiltration coefficient of the rat. *J. clin. Invest.* **56,** 419–434.

BOHRER M. P., BAYLIS C., ROBERTSON C. R. & BRENNER B. M. (1977a) Mechanisms of the puromycin-induced defects in the transglomerular passage of water and macromolecules. *J. clin. Invest.* **60,** 152–161.

BOHRER M. P., DEEN W. M., ROBERTSON C. R. & BRENNER B. M. (1977b) Mechanism of angiotensin II-induced proteinuria in the rat. *Am. J. Physiol.* **233,** F13–F21.

BRENNER B. M., BAYLIS C. & DEEN W. M. (1976) Transport of molecules across renal glomerular capillaries. *Physiol. Rev.* **56,** 502–534.

CAUFIELD S. P. & FARQUHAR M. G. (1975) The permeability of glomerular capillaries of aminonucleoside-nephrotic rats to graded dextrans. *J. exp. Med.* **142,** 61–83.

DOUSA T. P., BARNES L. D., ONG S. H. & STEINER A. L. (1977) Immunohistochemical localization of 3',5'-cyclic AMP and 3'5'-cyclic GMP in rat renal cortex: effect of parathyroid hormone. *Proc. Natn. Acad. Sci. U.S.A.* **74,** 3569–3573.

FARQUHAR M. G. (1975) The primary glomerular filtration barrier-basement membrane or epithelial cells? *Kidney Int.* **8,** 197–211.

FRANK S., ANTONOWICZ J., CRAIG J. M. & METCOFF J. (1955) Experimental nephrotic syndrome induced in rats by aminonucleoside. Renal lesions and body electrolyte composition. *Proc. Soc. exp. Biol. Med.* **89,** 424–427.

GLASSER R. S., VELOSA J. A. & MICHAEL A. F. (1977) Experimental model of focal sclerosis—I. Relationship to protein excretion in aminonucleoside nephrosis. *Lab. Invest.* **36,** 519–526.

GORIDIS C. & REUTTER W. (1975) Plasma membrane-associated increase in guanylate cyclase activity in regenerating rat liver. *Nature, Lond.* **257,** 698–700.

HELWIG J. J., ZACHARY D. & BOLLACK C. (1974a) Isolation of glomeruli and tubular fragments from rabbit kidney. *Urol. Res.* **2,** 55–59.

HELWIG J. J., MANDEL P., BOLLACK C. (1974b) Distribution of some phosphohydrolases in glomerular and tubular fractions isolated from rabbit kidney. *Archs. Int. Physiol. Biochem.* **82,** 907–916.

HELWIG J. J., BOLLACK C., MANDEL P. & GORIDIS C. (1975) Renal cortex guanylate cyclase. Preferential enrichment in glomerular membranes. *Biochim. biophys. Acta* **377,** 463–472.

ICHIKAWA I., HUMES H. D., DOUSA T. P. & BRENNER B. M. (1978) Influence of parathyroid hormone on glomerular ultrafiltration in the rat. *Am. J. Physiol.* **234,** F393–F401.

IMBERT M., CHABARDES D., MONTEGUT M., CLIQUE A. & MOREL F. (1975) Adenylate cyclase activity along the rabbit nephron as measured in single isolated segments. *Pflügers Arch. ges Physiol.* **354,** 213–228.

KIN J. K., FRONHERT P. P., HUI Y. S. F., BARNES L. D., FARROW G. M. & DOUSA T. P. (1977) Enzymes of cyclic 3',5'-nucleotides metabolism in human renal cortex and renal adenocarcinoma. *Kidney Int.* **12,** 172–183.

KNOX F. G. & OTT C. E. (1976) Filtration pressure equilibrium in the dog glomerulus. *Proceedings of the 6th International Congress on Nephrology.* Florence, 1975, pp. 216–222, Karger, Basel.

KURTZ S. M. & FELDMAN I. D. (1962) Experimental studies on the formation of the glomerular basement membrane. *J. Ultrastruct. Res.* **6,** 19–27.

LOWRY O. H., & ROSEBROUGH N. J., FARR A. L. & RANDALL R. J. (1951) Protein measurement with the Folin phenol reagent. *J. biol. Chem.* **193,** 265–275.

MICHAEL A. F., BLAN E. & VERNIER R. L. (1970) Glomerular polyanions: alteration in aminonucleoside nephrosis. *Lab. Invest.* **23**, 649–657.

SHAH S. V., NORTHRUP T. E., HUI Y. S. F. & DOUSA T. P. (1979) Action of serotonin (5-hydroxytryptamine) on cyclic nucleotides in glomeruli of rat renal cortex. *Kidney Int.* **15**, 463–472.

TORRES V. E., NORTHRUP T. E., EDWARDS R. M., SHAH S. V. & DOUSA T. P. (1978) Modulation of cyclic nucleotides in isolated rat glomeruli: role of histamine, carbamylcholine, parathyroid hormone and angiotensin II. *J. clin. Invest.* **62**, 1334–1343.

VELOSA J. A., GLASSER R. J., NEVINS T. E. & MICHAEL A. F. (1977) Experimental model of focal sclerosis—II. Correlation with immunopathologic changes, macromolecular kinetics, and polyanion loss. *Lab. Invest.* **36**, 527–534.

WALTER F. (1973) The origin, turnover and removal of glomerular basement membrane. *J. Path.* **110**, 233–244.

WELLS J. N., BAIRD C. F., WU Y. J. & HARDMAN J. G. (1975) Cyclic nucleotide phosphodiesterase activities of pig coronary arteries. *Biochem. biophys. Acta* **384**, 430–442.

YUSUFI A. N. K., REBEL G., MANDEL P. & HELWIG J. J. (1979) Distribution of guanylate and adenylate cyclases in pure glomeruli of some rodents (Abstract). *Colloque: Structure and Function of the Glomerulus, Paris,* June 26–27.

SYMPOSIUM DISCUSSION

Robinson: Would you like to speculate on what the cyclic GMP is doing in proteinuria?

Helwig: I think that for the moment it is too early to answer this question but numerous hormonal agents which are known to modify glomerular permeability, change the cyclic GMP level of the glomerulae. This work has been done by Dousa (*J. Clin. Invest* **62**, 1334–1343, 1978; *Proc. Natn. Acad. Sci. U.S.A.* **74**, 3569–3573, 1977).

Robinson: Did you see changes in cell morphology that correlated with cyclic GMP levels?

Helwig: In this model, with a single intravenous injection of puromycin aminonucloside the glomerular lesions are very mild, but the tubules show peri-tubular infiltration.

Epstein: Do you know whether any other kind of glomerular injury, for example, nephrotoxic nephritis also produces these changes?

Helwig: Dousa has postulated that cGMP could play a role in some inflammatory diseases. Nephrotoxic nephritis would be a good model to test this idea.

Guder: From other tissues we know that guanylate cyclase and cGMP parallel the number of mitoses and regeneration. On the other hand, we know that thrombocytes, and probably leukocytes contain high activities. My question is: is what you are measuring a sign of regeneration of glomerular or tubular cells?

Helwig: You propose that there could be a correlation between glomerular cell proliferation and increasing cGMP level or guanyl cyclase activity? We have studied ^{3}H thymidine incorporation and saw no change between normal and nephrotic rats. However, this model, following a single intravenous injection may not be typical of chronic nephrotic syndrome.

Kurokawa: Do you have any data on adenylate cyclase?

Helwig: Preliminary experiments show that at 12 days, when there is an increase in guanylate cyclase there is a decrease in adenylate cyclase.

Int. J. Biochem., Vol. 12, pp. 215 to 217
© Pergamon Press Ltd 1980. Printed in Great Britain

0020-711X/80/0701-0215$02.00/0

PROTEINS OF THE KIDNEY MICROVILLAR MEMBRANE: TOPOLOGICAL CONSIDERATIONS

A. JOHN KENNY and ANDREW G. BOOTH
Department of Biochemistry, University of Leeds, 9 Hyde Terrace, Leeds LS2 9LS, U.K.

Abstract—1. A method for the asymmetric labelling of pig kidney microvillar membrane proteins is described.

2. The photo-activated reagent, 3,5-di[^{125}I]iodo-4-azido-benzene sulphonate, enabled four of the membrane peptidases to be characterized as transmembrane proteins.

INTRODUCTION

The proximal tubule cell is polarized in morphology, enzymology and function. The luminal pole is characterized by the presence of microvilli and is the major site in the nephron for the reabsorption of small solutes and of polypeptides and proteins. The former process depends on carrier-mediated transport systems; the latter involves pinocytosis in the pits between microvilli. Surprisingly, very little is known about the molecular events of either process. This lack of understanding about the proteins involved in absorptive functions contrasts with our fairly detailed knowledge of both the structural proteins of the microvillar core and the enzymes of the membrane (for a review see Kenny & Booth, 1978). In this paper we shall summarize some recent work in our laboratory concerning the topology of the membrane proteins.

MATERIALS AND METHODS

Vesicles were prepared by the Mg^{2+} precipitation method (Booth & Kenny, 1974) from fresh pig kidneys. The immunological methods were those previously described (Booth *et al.*, 1979). The labelling experiments using 3,5-di[^{125}I]iodo-4-azido-benzene sulphonate (DIABS) were performed as described by Booth & Kenny (1980).

RESULTS

Photolabelling of microvilli with 3,5-di[^{125}I]iodo-4-azido-benzene sulphonate ([^{125}I]DIABS)

Principle of the method. This novel photoreactive compound was synthesized from diazotized 3,5-di[^{125}I]iodosulphanilic acid. On exposure to light ($\lambda > 300$ nm) the azide group loses N_2 and generates a highly reactive nitrene which reacts with any C—H bond in its immediate vicinity. It therefore provides a method for covalently labelling membrane components, and, provided the disposition of the reagent before photolysis can be unequivocally established, the method has the potential to label at either the luminal or the cytoplasmic surface of the microvillar membrane. Clearly the interpretation of such experiments designed to establish the transmembrane nature of a protein depends crucially on the demonstration that neither intramembrane labelling (i.e. within the lipid bilayer) nor contramembrane labelling (i.e. labelling the surface opposite to the one intended) occurs to any significant extent. DIABS is a hydrophilic compound, by virtue of its charged sulphonate group, and hence is unlikely to partition into the lipids of the membrane. However, it is capable of crossing the membrane by a concentrative, Na^+-linked, carrier-mediated system. After photolysis the labelled proteins were resolved by crossed immunoelectrophoresis, in which the detergent-solubilized membrane components were run, in the second dimension, into rabbit antiserum raised to pig microvillar membrane. The immunoprecipitates of several enzymes have been identified by histochemical staining (Booth *et al.*, 1979). Radioautography permitted the identification of the radioactive antigens. The ability of proteinases, such as papain, to release many of the principal enzymes from the membrane provided a further check on the labelling method, since the immunoprecipitates after such treatment lack the part of the protein which served to anchor it to the membrane and which might also be exposed at the cytoplasmic surface. Hence if the label was located in this portion, the immunoprecipitate derived from the bulk of the protein (containing all the antigenic determinants) would no longer be radioactive if the photoreagent had been stationed at the cytoplasmic surface of the membrane.

Fidelity of labelling. When microvilli were photolysed with [^{125}I]DIABS, 22% of the radioactivity was found in the lipid fraction. Although this might suggest intramembrane labelling, the label was located in the polar head groups of the lipids and not in the hydrophobic fatty acid chains. Thus when the lipid fraction was subjected to methanolysis (Morrison & Smith, 1964) 92% of the label was in the polar fraction. Contramembrane labelling readily occurred when microvillar vesicles were incubated with [^{125}I]DIABS before photolysis. This suggested that the reagent could cross the membrane and, indeed, we observed that the uptake of DIABS is Na^+-dependent, the time curve showing a typical overshoot, which subsided as the Na^+ gradient dissipated. Since this transport system is temperature dependent, it was possible to position the reagent within vesicles by incubation at 37°C, after which they were cooled and washed before photolysing them with bovine serum albumin present in the suspension medium to provide a trap for any DIABS that might efflux during photolysis.

Transmembrane enzymes of the kidney microvillar membrane. Figure 1 (modified from Booth & Kenny,

1980) shows the results of one experiment in which vesicles were labelled from the luminal and cytoplasmic surfaces, solubilized by detergent (Emulphogen BC 720), part of which was further treated with papain. All four samples were examined by crossed immunoelectrophoresis. The precipitates were revealed by staining with Coomassie Blue and the radioactivity demonstrated by radioautography. The identities of the radioactive immunoprecipitates had earlier been established by histochemical staining (Booth *et al.*, 1979) and, in the case of aminopeptidase M (EC 3.4.11.2), by the use of a monospecific antibody preparation. The feature to be noted is that the externally labelled antigens are still demonstrable after papain treatment (although the mobilities may be changed) but the internally labelled antigens are, with one exception, no longer detectable as radioactive precipitates. This confirmed the absence of significant contramembrane labelling by DIABS in this procedure and established that aminopeptidase M, aminopeptidase A (EC 3.4.11.7) dipeptidyl peptidase IV (EC 3.4.14.—) are transmembrane even though the peptide chain containing the anchor region appears to be but a small proportion of the total (Macnair & Kenny, 1979). The one immunoprecipitate in which radioactivity persisted after papain treatment of the internally labelled membrane is neutral endopeptidase (EC 3.4.24.11), an enzyme which is not solubilized by papain (Booth *et al.*, 1979). Thus four peptidases, three of which are among the major proteins of the microvillar membrane, have been shown to be transmembrane proteins.

SUMMARY

Our knowledge of the enzymes of the microvillar membrane is now very detailed, particularly in respect of the complex group of peptidases. Some have not been characterized in molecular terms. The model that seems to typify this group is that of a large dimeric glycoprotein, the bulk of which is accessible at the luminal surface, anchored in the lipid bilayer by a relatively small domain which spans the membrane. The evidence supporting this model has been derived from studies on purified enzymes isolated after detergent solubilization and in part from the use of a novel photo-labelling reagent, 3,5-di[^{125}I]iodo-4-azido-benzene sulphonate.

Acknowledgement—This work has been generously supported by grants from the Medical Research Council.

REFERENCES

BOOTH A. G. & KENNY A. J. (1974) A rapid method for the preparation of microvilli from rabbit kidney. *Biochem. J.* **142,** 575–581.

BOOTH A. G. & KENNY A. J. (1980) Proteins of the kidney microvillar membrane. Asymmetric labelling of the membrane by lactoperoxide-catalysed radio-iodination and by photolysis of 3,5-di[^{125}I]iodo-4-azido-benzene sulphonate. *Biochem. J.* **187,** 31–44.

BOOTH A. G., HUBBARD L. M. L. & KENNY A. J. (1979) Proteins of the kidney microvillar membrane. Immunoelectrophoretic analysis of the membrane hydrolases: identification and resolution of the detergent- and proteinase-solubilized forms. *Biochem. J.* **179,** 397–405.

KENNY A. J. & BOOTH A. G. (1978) Microvilli: their ultrastructure, enzymology and molecular organization. *Essays Biochem.* **14,** 1–44.

MACNAIR R. D. C. & KENNY A. J. (1979) Proteins of the kidney microvillar membrane. The amphipathic form of dipeptidyl peptidase IV. *Biochem. J.* **179,** 379–395.

MORRISON W. R. & SMITH L. M. (1964) Preparation of fatty acid methyl esters and dimethylacetals from lipids with boron fluoride–methanol. *J. Lipid Res.* **5,** 600–608.

SYMPOSIUM DISCUSSION

Kinne: You have a small effect on sodium uptake, which is increased. Do you know anything about the potential? Were these measurements made under "gradient" conditions?

Kenny: The measurements were made under the same conditions as those used for leucine transport, except that we were using Na^{22} (100 mM outside, zero inside). We have not measured the potentials.

Alleyne: Is the inhibitition of the elastase-treated vesicles by phosphoramadon non-competitive?

Kenny: We have not looked at the kinetics in detail. With inhibitors the elastase-treated vesicles behave the same as the control, but I don't know whether the K_m for leucine has changed.

Kinne: Would you like to speculate about the action of the chelating agents on leucine transport? Is it on transport proper or on the size of the vesicles?

Kenny: The size of the vesicles doesn't seem to change. The transport of glucose and proline is inhibited by ortho-phenathrolene but it did not seem to change sodium conductance. EDTA and DTT did not inhibit glucose or proline uptake, so that may be a special characteristic. I don't wish to suggest that the endo-peptidase is the one and the same transport protein, but it does seem to have some similar properties and it may be homologous proteins.

Sacktor: I should like to comment that proteinases can be used successfully to differentiate transport systems. We reported (*Fedn Proc. Fedn Am. Socs exp. Biol.* **38,** 838, 1979) on the use of papain to inhibit Na-dependent phosphate transport yet the proteinase had no effect on glucose or proline transport.

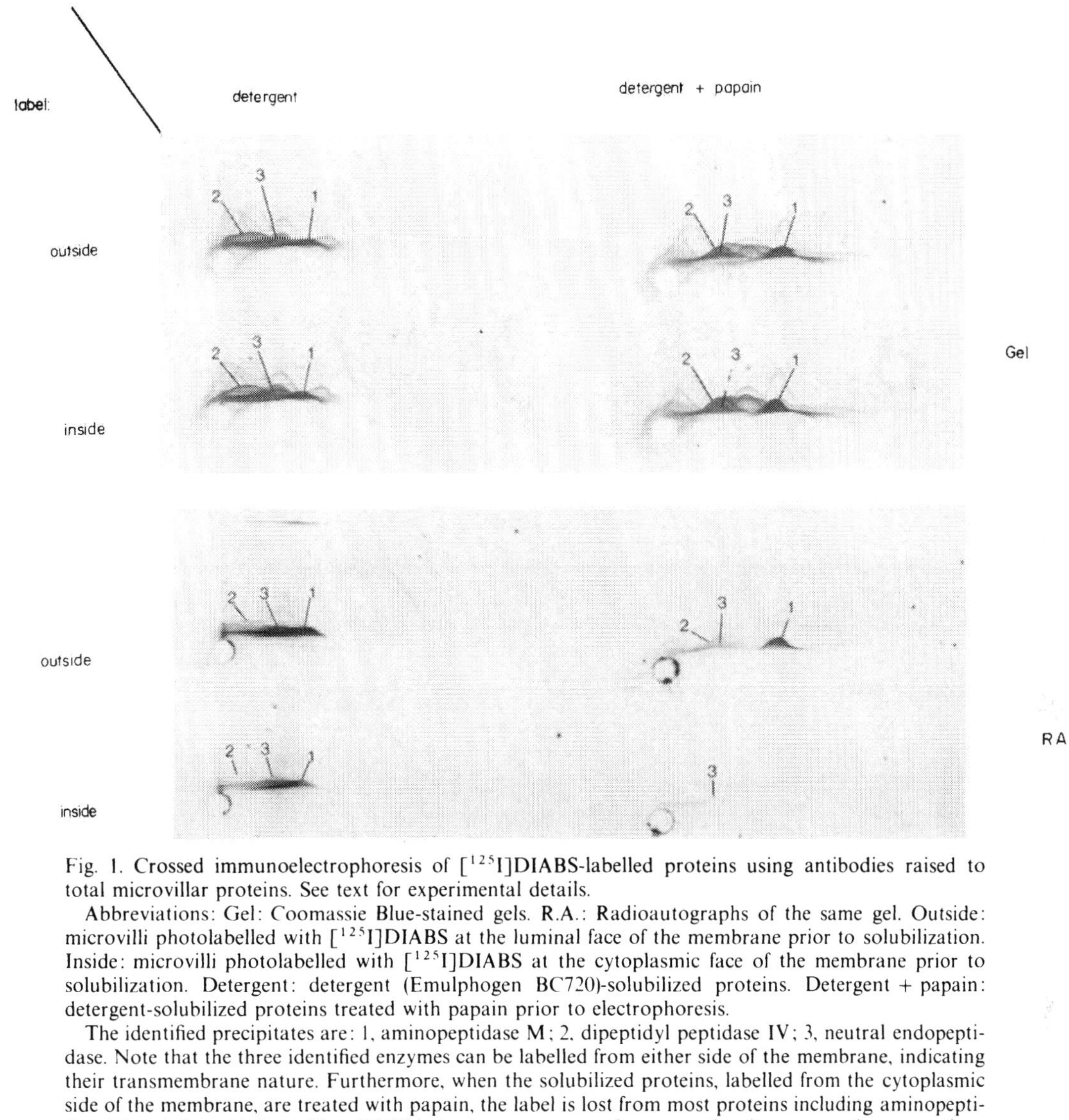

Fig. 1. Crossed immunoelectrophoresis of [^{125}I]DIABS-labelled proteins using antibodies raised to total microvillar proteins. See text for experimental details.

Abbreviations: Gel: Coomassie Blue-stained gels. R.A.: Radioautographs of the same gel. Outside: microvilli photolabelled with [^{125}I]DIABS at the luminal face of the membrane prior to solubilization. Inside: microvilli photolabelled with [^{125}I]DIABS at the cytoplasmic face of the membrane prior to solubilization. Detergent: detergent (Emulphogen BC720)-solubilized proteins. Detergent + papain: detergent-solubilized proteins treated with papain prior to electrophoresis.

The identified precipitates are: 1, aminopeptidase M; 2, dipeptidyl peptidase IV; 3, neutral endopeptidase. Note that the three identified enzymes can be labelled from either side of the membrane, indicating their transmembrane nature. Furthermore, when the solubilized proteins, labelled from the cytoplasmic side of the membrane, are treated with papain, the label is lost from most proteins including aminopeptidase M and dipeptidyl peptidase IV. This treatment removes the non-antigenic transmembrane portions of these proteins and confirms the lack of contramembrane labelling by this method. Neutral endopeptidase retains radioactivity after papain treatment because this enzyme is resistant to proteolytic attack by papain.

Int. J. Biochem., Vol. 12, pp. 219 to 222
© Pergamon Press Ltd 1980. Printed in Great Britain

0020-711X/80/0701-0219$02.00/0

MEMBRANE ASSOCIATION AND ORIENTATION OF RAT RENAL ACTIVITIES CAPABLE OF DEGRADING GLUTATHIONE

NORMAN P. CURTHOYS, BARBARA B. RANKIN and BETTY TSAO
Department of Biochemistry, University of Pittsburgh, School of Medicine, Pittsburgh, PA 15261, U.S.A.

Abstract—1. γ-Glutamyltranspeptidase and a peptidase which cleaves cysteinylglycine and its S-derivatives are localized within the brush border membrane of the proximal straight tubule.

2. The transpeptidase has previously been shown to be an amphipathic protein in which the membrane binding and catalytic domains are separated by a papain-sensitive sequence of amino acids.

3. The Triton-purified peptidase exhibits a higher apparent subunit molecular weight (150,000) than the papain-purified peptidase (135,000).

4. The presence of the papain-sensitive sequence of amino acids was required for the incorporation of the Triton-purified peptidase into lecithin vesicles.

5. Papain treatment of isolated brush border membrane vesicles results in 90–95% solubilization of transpeptidase and peptidase activities without altering the internal volume of the vesicles.

6. At least 92% of both activities associated with vesicles can be inactivated with specific Fab antibodies or precipitated by indirect immunoprecipitation.

7. The non-accessible γ-glutamyltranspeptidase and peptidase activities were shown to be associated with the internal surface of a unique population of inverted vesicles.

8. Therefore, the two activities are orientated exclusively on the outside of the brush border membrane, consistent with their proposed participation in the extracellular degradation of glutathione and mercapturic acid precursors.

INTRODUCTION

The turnover of glutathione appears to be an interorgan process (Curthoys & Hughey, 1979). Various isolated mammalian cells constantly release significant amounts of reduced glutathione to the extracellular medium. This implies that glutathione may normally be released from various tissues to the blood plasma. Such a process may be of particular importance to some tissues, such as liver, which do not contain appreciable γ-glutamyltranspeptidase activity but yet rapidly turnover their intracellular glutathione. The rate of efflux of glutathione from the isolated perfused liver has been found to closely approximate the rate of hepatic glutathione turnover (Bartoli & Sies, 1978). Although the plasma concentration of glutathione is only 3 to 5 μM, its turnover is extremely rapid (Hahn *et al.*, 1978) and more than 80% of this glutathione is removed by the kidney in a single pass (Bartoli *et al.*, 1978). Therefore, glutathione metabolism may be a process of intracellular synthesis and utilization, release from the cell, and degradation within the kidney.

The glutathionemia and glutathionuria observed in a patient deficient in γ-glutamyltranspeptidase (Schulman *et al.*, 1975) and in mice following specific inhibition of the transpeptidase (Griffith & Meister, 1979) indicates that this enzyme is responsible for catalyzing the initial reaction in glutathione degradation. Within rat kidney, γ-glutamyltranspeptidase and a peptidase activity, which cleaves cysteinylglycine and its S-derivatives, are localized on the brush border membrane of the proximal straight tubule (Hughey *et al.*, 1978). Together these activities could account for the complete hydrolysis of glutathione. γ-Glutamyltranspeptidase has been shown to be an amphipathic protein in which the membrane binding and catalytic domains are separated by a papain-sensitive sequence of amino acids (Hughey & Curthoys, 1976). In this paper, the ability of the isolated peptidase to reassociate with a lipid bilayer was also shown to be due to the presence of a small papain-sensitive sequence of amino acids. In addition, experiments with isolated brush border membrane vesicles established that both activities are exclusively orientated on the external or luminal surface of this membrane.

MATERIALS AND METHODS

The γ-glutamyltranspeptidase and peptidase activities were assayed as described previously (Hughey *et al.*, 1978) The peptidase was solubilized by either partial proteolysis or detergent extraction and purified by chromatography on DEAE-cellulose, Bio-Gel A5m and hydroxylapatite. Specific antibodies against the papain-purified forms of γ-glutamyltranspeptidase and the peptidase were prepared in rabbits. Goat anti-rabbit IgG Fab fragment antibodies were purchased from Miles Biochemicals. A cell wall fraction containing Protein A was prepared from *Staphylococcus aureus.*

Lecithin vesicles were prepared by the sodium cholate removal procedure of Brunner *et al.* (1976) using a mixture of egg lecithin and dipalmitoyl[^{14}C]lecithin (New England Nuclear). Brush border membrane vesicles were prepared by the procedure of Booth & Kenny (1974). The preparation exhibited a 10-fold increase in brush border membrane marker activities and was recovered with a 20% yield. The internal volume of the isolated vesicles was determined using a silicone-oil separation procedure (Ballas & Arion, 1977).

RESULTS AND DISCUSSION

The isolated peptidase is a glycoprotein. The

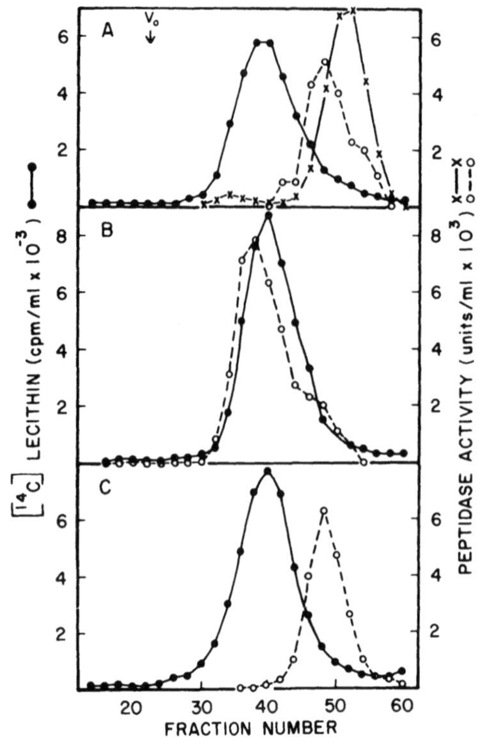

Fig. 1. Association of peptidase with [^{14}C]lecithin vesicles. Aliquots of vesicles and peptidase enzyme were chromatographed on a Sepharose 4B column. Fractions were collected and assayed for radioactivity and enzyme activity. Panel A: Vesicles prepared in the absence of protein (●), 100 μg Triton-purified (O) or 20 μg papain-purified (×) peptidase each chromatographed separately. Panel B: Vesicles prepared in the presence of 100 μg of freshly prepared Triton-purified peptidase. Panel C: Vesicles prepared as in Panel B and preincubated for 4 hr at 37°C with 75 units of papain.

papain-purified enzyme is soluble in aqueous buffers, whereas the Triton-purified form is insoluble in the absence of detergent. During sodium dodecyl sulfate polyacrylamide gel electrophoresis, the Triton-purified peptidase exhibits a higher apparent subunit molecular weight (150,000) than the papain-purified peptidase (135,000). The involvement of this additional peptide sequence in membrane association was determined by comparing the ability of the two isolated forms of the peptidase to be incorporated into lecithin vesicles.

Upon Sepharose 4B chromatography, the [^{14}C]lecithin vesicles produced the expected elution profile (Fig. 1A). Single layered vesicles were included in the column and eluted as a peak at fractions 39–40. The Triton purified peptidase eluted from the Sepharose 4B column with a peak at fraction 48, whereas the papain purified peptidase eluted later in the column profile (fraction 52). Chromatography of [^{14}C]lecithin vesicles prepared in the presence of the papain-purified peptidase produced a radioactivity and enzyme activity profile identical to that produced by the chromatography of either one alone. In contrast, the chromatography of [^{14}C]lecithin vesicles prepared in the presence of freshly prepared Triton-purified peptidase produced coincident peaks of enzyme activity and radioactivity (Fig. 1B). Following treatment of a sample of the enzyme-vesicle complex with papain, the peptidase was released from the vesicles and eluted from the Sepharose 4B column at fraction 48 (Fig. 1C). Therefore, the additional sequence of amino acids found in the Triton-purified enzyme contains the membrane binding domain of the peptidase.

Incubation of isolated brush border membrane vesicles with papain results in 90–95% solubilization of the peptidase and γ-glutamyltranspeptidase activities within 20 and 50 min, respectively (Fig. 2A). In contrast, the release of alkaline phosphatase activity was negligible even after a 1 hr incubation. Papain treatment did not alter the internal volume (6 $\mu l \cdot mg^{-1}$) of the vesicles. These observations clearly indicate that the catalytically important domains of the transpeptidase and peptidase are predominantly located on the external surface of the membrane. In order to determine if the papain-resistant activities were associated with inverted vesicles, the immuno reactivity of the γ-glutamyltranspeptidase and peptidase associated with untreated and papain-treated vesicles were compared.

The antibodies prepared against the γ-glutamyl-

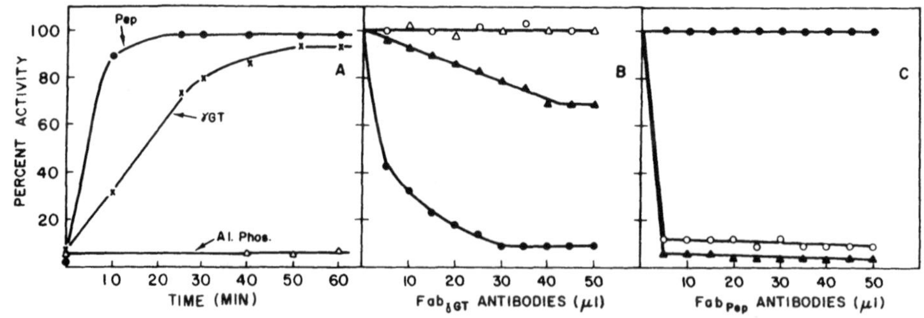

Fig. 2. Orientation of γ-glutamyltranspeptidase and the peptidase on isolated rat renal brush border membrane vesicles. Panel A: Release of transpeptidase (×, γGT), peptidase (●, Pep) and alkaline phosphatase (△, Al. Phos.) activities during incubation of 6 mg of vesicle protein with 0.6 mg papain at 37°C. Panel B: Inactivation (triangles) and indirect immunoprecipitation (circles) of γ-glutamyltranspeptidase activity associated with untreated (▲, ●) and with papain-treated (△, O) vesicles by Fab antibodies prepared against purified transpeptidase ($Fab_{\gamma GT}$). Panel C: Inactivation of peptidase activity associated with untreated (▲), with papain-treated (●) and with papain-treated, Triton-solubilized (O) vesicles by Fab antibodies prepared against purified peptidase (Fab_{Pep}).

transpeptidase were only partially inactivating. Incubation of papain-purified transpeptidase with increasing amounts of the Fab antibody resulted in only 37% inactivation. However, the subsequent addition of goat anti-rabbit IgG Fab fragment antibodies and Protein A resulted in 97% precipitation of the transpeptidase. When these procedures were applied to untreated vesicles, 31% of the transpeptidase activity was inactivated and 91% was precipitated (Fig. 2B). Therefore, at least 91% of the γ-glutamyltranspeptidase associated with isolated vesicles is externally orientated and accessible to interact with the Fab antibodies. In contrast, all of the transpeptidase activity associated with papain-treated vesicles was found to be resistant to both inactivation and indirect immunoprecipitation. Therefore, all of the papain-resistant transpeptidase activity is also non-accessible to interaction with antibodies. The binding of one Fab antibody per vesicle should be sufficient to cause its precipitation following indirect-immuno-complex formation. The resistant transpeptidase activity is therefore associated with a unique population of vesicles which have γ-glutamyltranspeptidase orientated internally.

The addition of Fab antibodies prepared against the purified peptidase inactivated 95% of the peptidase activity associated with untreated vesicles (Fig. 2C). In contrast, the peptidase activity associated with papain-treated vesicles was completely resistant to inactivation. Preincubation of papain-treated vesicles with 2% Triton X-100 permitted 91% of the papain-resistant peptidase activity to be inactivated by the Fab antibodies. The observed latency suggests that the resistant activity is located inside the vesicle membrane.

Similar experiments with crude kidney homogenates showed that 95% of the γ-glutamyltranspeptidase and peptidase activities can be solubilized by treatment with papain. In addition, 93% of the total peptidase activity in crude kidney homogenates can be inactivated with Fab antibodies. Therefore, the results obtained with the isolated fraction of the brush border membrane are indicative of the entire membrane.

All of these results are consistent with an absolute asymmetry in the orientation of the γ-glutamyltranspeptidase and peptidase activities and the location of the resistant enzyme molecules on the internal surface of inverted vesicles. The percentage (5–10%) of the γ-glutamyltranspeptidase and peptidase activities which are resistant to proteolysis and to interaction with antibodies is in close agreement with the previous estimation by freeze–fracture electron microscopy of the percentage (10–15%) of isolated brush border membrane vesicles which appear to be inverted (Haase *et al.*, 1978).

CONCLUSIONS

The absolute asymmetry of γ-glutamyltranspeptidase and peptidase activities observed with respect to the isolated vesicles implies that within the kidney, these activities are orientated exclusively on the external or lumenal surface of the brush border membrane. Therefore, these activities do not have direct access to intracellular renal glutathione. The degradation of renal glutathione would require its initial translocation to the tubular lumen. The recent demonstration that the transpeptidase can efficiently hydrolyze glutathione at the low concentration present within the lumen (McIntyre & Curthoys, 1979) is also consistent with the concept that hydrolysis of both renal and non-renal glutathione is an extracellular process which occurs primarily in the lumen of the proximal straight tubule.

REFERENCES

Ballas L. M. & Arion W. J. (1977) Measurement of glucose 6-phosphate penetration into liver microsomes. *J. biol. Chem.* **252,** 8512–8518.

Bartolli G. M., Häberle D. & Sies H. (1978) Glutathione efflux from perfused rat liver and its relation to glutathione uptake by the kidney. In *Functions of Glutathione in Liver and Kidney* (Edited by Sies H. & Wendel A.) pp. 27–31. Springer, Heidelberg.

Bartolli G. M. & Sies H. (1978) Reduced and oxidized glutathione efflux from liver. *FEBS Lett.* **86,** 89–91.

Booth A. G. & Kenny A. J. (1974) A rapid method for the preparation of microvilli from rabbit kidney. *Biochem. J.* **142,** 575–581.

Brunner J., Skrabel P. & Hauser H. (1976) Single bilayer vesicles prepared without sonication: physico-chemical properties. *Biochim. biophys. Acta* **445,** 322–331.

Curthoys N. P. & Hughey R. P. (1979) Characterization and physiological function of rat renal γ-glutamyltranspeptidase. *Enzyme,* **24,** 383–403.

Griffith O. W. & Meister A. (1979) Translocation of intracellular glutathione to membrane-bound γ-glutamyltranspeptidase as a discrete step in the γ-glutamyl cycle: Glutathionuria after inhibition of transpeptidase. *Proc. Natn. Acad. Sci. U.S.A.* **76,** 268–272.

Haase W., Schäfer A., Murer H. & Kinne R. (1978) Studies on the orientation of brush border membrane vesicles. *Biochem. J.* **172,** 57–62.

Hahn R., Wendel A. & Flohé L. (1978) The fate of extracellular glutathione in the rat. *Biochim. biophys. Acta* **539,** 324–337.

Hughey R. P. & Curthoys N. P. (1976) Comparison of the size and physical properties of γ-glutamyltranspeptidase purified from rat kidney following solubilization with papain or with Triton X-100. *J. biol. Chem.* **251,** 7863–7870.

Hughey R. P., Rankin B. B., Elce J. S. & Curthoys N. P. (1978) Specificity of a particulate rat renal peptidase and its localization along with other enzymes of mercapturic acid synthesis. *Archs Biochem. Biophys.* **186,** 211–217.

McIntyre T. M. & Curthoys N. P. (1979) Comparison of the hydrolytic and transfer activities of rat renal γ-glutamyltranspeptidase. *J. biol. Chem.* **254,** 6499–6504.

Schulman J. D., Goodman S. I., Mace J. W., Patrick A. D., Tietze F. & Butler E. J. (1975) Glutathionuria: Inborn error of metabolism due to tissue deficiency of gamma-glutamyltranspeptidase. *Biochem. biophys. Res. Commun.* **65,** 68–74.

SYMPOSIUM DISCUSSION

Lemieux: Are not your findings in contradiction with the Meister hypothesis?

Curthoys: Yes, I think they are. All of our characterizations of the enzyme, including its physical properties, its association with the membrane, its orientation, and its kinetics at plasma concentrations of substrates are inconsistent with the idea that the enzyme participates in amino acid transport.

Jorgensen: Your description of the enzyme in the lipid bi-layer seems to imply that the enzyme does not extend through the membrane whereas the model described by Dr Kenny assumes the protein extends to both membrane surfaces.

Curthoys: We are not yet sure if the transpeptidase extends through the membrane, but if it does, the portion of the protein which extends has no catalytic role. The catalytic portion of the enzyme is strongly hydrophylic, heavily glycosylated and it is unlikely that it would move across the membrane. So even if a small portion of the protein does penetrate the membrane, and is exposed to the internal surface, it is unlikely to be related to the catalytic function.

Kenny: I have 2 questions. Would you agree that cystinylglycine is hydrolysed by amino-peptidase M(EC3.4.11.2)? Secondly, do you know if there is an "anchor" on both sub-units of γ-glutamyl transpeptidase?

Curthoys: With the first, I agree! The anchor is associated only with the large subunit of γ-glutamyltranspeptidase.

Tannen: If glutathione was 80% cleared on one passage through the kidney, how do you explain that the enzyme activity was totally on the luminal surface?

Curthoys: It seems reasonable to accept that there is a selective γ-glutamyl transporter on the contra-luminal side of the cell. This is likely because the kidney also selectively extracts other γ-glutamyl derivatives. Such compounds would then have to be secreted into the lumen.

Kovacevic: How do you visualize metabolism of intracellular GSH?

Curthoys: It must involve secretion, but the only evidence for secretion comes from the one patient with γ-glutamyl transpeptidase deficiency, in whom the urine GSH exceeds the expected value from glomerular filtration alone.

Brosnan: Are oxidised and reduced glutatione equally good substrates for the enzyme, and what are their proportions in the plasma?

Curthoys: Plasma contains largely oxidised glutathione. In terms of hydrolytic activity both forms are equivalent as substrates.

Vinay: What is the intracellular glutathione concentration, and what is the evidence for its movement out of the cell?

Curthoys: 5 mM, and while there has been no demonstration of movement from kidney cells, other mammalian cells in tissue culture constantly release GSH into the medium.

Guder: Helmut Sies (Sies. *et al. FEBS lett.* **103,** 287–290, 1979) has shown glutathione release from the perfused liver into the bile. This was influenced by drugs. In human bile we found no glutathione, and concluded that this was the result of the presence of γ-glutamyl transpeptidase in human bile cannaliculae, and not in the rat. The similarity with kidney may be the drug metabolic-function of the tubule, and the degradation of glutathione by γ-glutamyl transpeptidase.

Anner: How do you explain your observation that even after reconstitution of the artificial membranes, your enzyme remains orientated?

Curthoys: I can only guess, but it is possible that the large degree of glycosylation, the charge on the protein and the fact that the majority of the protein is hydrophylic might be a sufficient driving force to orientate the protein on the external surface of the vesicle.

Alleyne: Are the liver and kidney enzyme immunologically identical; and would you say that it has the same purpose of degrading glutathione?

Curthoys: Inoue (Inoue *et al. Eur. J. Biochem.* **78,** 609–115, 1977) has shown that the liver and kidney enzyme are indeed immunologically identical.

Int. J. Biochem., Vol. 12, pp. 223 to 228

0020-711X/80/0701-0223$02.00/0

RECENT OBSERVATIONS ON THE PROXIMAL TUBULAR TRANSPORT OF ACIDIC AND BASIC AMINO ACIDS BY RAT RENAL PROXIMAL TUBULAR BRUSH BORDER VESICLES

HEINI MURER, ANJA LEOPOLDER, ROLF KINNE and GERHARD BURCKHARDT
Max-Planck-Institut für Biophysik, Kennedyallee 70, 6000 Frankfurt am Main, Federal Republic of Germany

Abstract—1. Transport of L-glutamic acid by rat renal brush border membrane vesicles is sodium-dependent.

2. Present at the inner membrane surface potassium stimulates sodium-dependent L-glutamic acid uptake.

3. Sodium stimulated L-glutamic acid uptake is potential-sensitive only in the presence of potassium.

4. Transport of L-ornithine can also be stimulated by a sodium gradient.

5. However, in the absence of sodium, L-ornithine seems to cross the membrane by facilitated diffusion.

INTRODUCTION

Renal amino acid transport has been studied in the past by various *in vivo* and *in vitro* techniques. Using electrophysiological as well as microperfusion methods different groups have documented that renal proximal tubular transport of L-amino acids is—at least in mammalian preparations (e.g. Ullrich, 1979)—sodium-dependent. By measuring the depolarization of the electrical potential difference across the brush border membrane after addition of different L-amino acids to the luminal perfusate it was demonstrated that sodium-dependent transport of L-amino acids across the brush border membrane of rat proximal tubule is accompanied by movement of positive charges indicating a potential-sensitive Na^+-symport of all the different L-amino acids. These electrophysiological studies suggested the presence of at least five* different systems for amino acids in the brush border membrane of rat proximal tubule (Samarzija, 1978).

Renal proximal tubular amino acid transport has also been studied with isolated brush border membrane vesicles (e.g. McNamara *et al.*, 1979; Evers *et al.*, 1976; Fass *et al.*, 1977; Weiss *et al.*, 1978; Hammerman & Sacktor, 1977; McNamara *et al.*, 1976; Goldmann *et al.*, 1979). The result obtained in these biochemical studies were in most cases in good agreement with the results obtained in experiments performed with intact epithelial preparations. The transport of neutral amino acids as well as of acidic amino acids into brush border membrane vesicles proceeds in cotransport with sodium (Evers *et al.*, 1976; McNamara *et al.*, 1976; Fass *et al.*, 1977; Hammerman & Sacktor, 1977). Also the potential-sensitivity of sodium-dependent uptake of neutral amino acids could be shown in the experiments with isolated brush border membrane vesicles (e.g. Evers *et al.*, 1976; Fass *et al.*, 1977; Hammerman & Sacktor, 1977). However, with respect to the transport of acidic amino acids and basic amino acids there are major differences between the results found in studies with the vesicles and the results obtained by electrophysiological methods as well as by microperfusion techniques. The experiments carried out with vesicles suggested that sodium-dependent transport of acidic amino acids is potential-insensitive and transport of L-arginine is not, or is only slightly, stimulated by sodium (Schneider *et al.*, 1978; Seeger *et al.*, 1979; Hammerman, 1975; Busse, 1979). These findings are clearly in contrast to the findings obtained from electrophysiological experiments and from micropuncture experiments on rat renal proximal tubular amino acid transport (Ullrich, 1979; Samarzija, 1978).

In the following we present experiments on the transport of L-glutamic acid and L-ornithine by rat renal brush border vesicles, which elucidate possible reasons for the apparent discrepancies concerning renal proximal tubular transport of acidic amino acids and basic amino acids.

* Taking all the data obtained thus far *in vivo* and *in vitro* including experiments with vesicles, one can assume that seven different systems for L-amino acid transport are present in the brush border membrane. This has recently been reviewed by Ullrich (1979).

MATERIALS AND METHODS

Brush border membranes were isolated by a calcium precipitation method as described in detail by Evers *et al.* (1978). Transport studies using radioactively labelled glutamic acid and glucose as well as the measurement of the changes in the transmembrane electrical potential difference by the fluorescent dye 3,3′-diethylthiadicarbocyanine iodide were carried out as described in detail by Burckhardt *et al.* (1980).

RESULTS AND DISCUSSION

Sodium-dependent glutamic acid transport

Earlier reports from the laboratories of Segal, and of Sacktor as well as from our own laboratory have

Table 1. The effect of K^+ on sodium-dependent L-glutamic acid and D-glucose uptake into brush border membrane vesicles from rat kidney cortex

K_o^+ or K_i^+ (mmol·l⁻¹)		L-Glutamic acid (%)	D-Glucose (%)
0	0	100	100
8	50	632	87
50	0	121	111
50	50	399	87

The uptake of L-glutamic acid and D-glucose was determined 20 sec after the addition of vesicles loaded with 200 mmol·l^{-1} mannitol, 20 mmol·l^{-1} Hepes–Tris, pH 7.4, 50 mmol·l^{-1} choline chloride or KCl, to incubation media containing 50 mmol·l^{-1} NaCl, 100 mmol·l^{-1} mannitol, 20 mmol·l^{-1} Hepes–Tris, pH 7.4 and 50 mmol·l^{-1} choline chloride or KCl. Glutamic acid concentration as well as D-glucose concentration was 0.1 mmol·l^{-1}. The uptake values in the absence of potassium are set to be 100.

shown that L-glutamic acid uptake by brush border membrane vesicles isolated from rat or rabbit kidney cortex is sodium-dependent (Seeger *et al.*, 1979; Schneider *et al.*, 1978; Weiss *et al.*, 1978). In two preliminary publications it was reported that sodium-dependent L-glutamic acid transport is potential-insensitive (Seeger *et al.*, 1979; Schneider *et al.*, 1978). Most interestingly it was found that sodium-dependent L-glutamic acid uptake is stimulated by an outwardly directed potassium gradient (Murer & Kinne, 1979; Kinne *et al.*, 1979; Burckhardt *et al.*, 1980; Schneider, 1979). As can be seen from the experiment presented in Table 1 an outwardly directed potassium gradient stimulates sodium-dependent L-glutamic acid uptake. Since this potassium effect is not observed for sodium-dependent transport of other solutes such as D-glucose (Table 1), L-phenylalanine (not shown) or L-ornithine (not shown) it seems most unlikely that potassium stimulation is due to a diffusion potential effect. The most likely explanation is a direct effect of potassium on sodium-dependent transport of L-glutamic acid. This is also supported by the finding that potassium stimulates sodium-dependent L-glutamic acid transport even in the absence of a potassium gradient, i.e. under conditions where no potassium diffusion potential exists. Furthermore, the potassium effect shows a strong sidedness. Potassium given from the outside is not able to stimulate sodium-dependent L-glutamic acid uptake. But with equal sodium concentrations at both sides of the vesicle membranes an outwardly directed potassium gradient is able to stimulate sodium-dependent L-glutamic acid transport (Schneider, 1979; Burckhardt *et al.*, 1980). These experiments clearly indicate sodium-dependent L-glutamic acid uptake too is driven by an outwardly directed potassium gradient. It is noteworthy that potassium (which can be replaced by rubidium and in part by cesium) can only exert its effect in the presence of sodium, whereas sodium can exert its stimulatory effect even in the absence of potassium (Burckhardt *et al.*, 1980).

The electrophysiological measurements indicating

Table 2. The effect of anion replacement on sodium-dependent L-glutamic acid uptake (20 sec) in the absence or presence of potassium

Anions added	Presence of potassium (%)	Absence of potassium (%)
Gluconate	100	100
Sulphate	113	121
Chloride	268	135
Thiocyanate	262	156
Nitrate	269	146

The incubation media contained one of the following anions: Gluconate, sulfate, chloride, thiocyanate, nitrate. The cations are 50 mmol·l^{-1} Na^+, no or 20 mM K^+, the osmolarity being kept constant with mannitol. The vesicles were preloaded with 100 mmol·l^{-1} mannitol, 20 mmol·l^{-1} Hepes–Tris, pH 7.4, 20 mmol·l^{-1} K^+ gluconate. For experiments in the absence of potassium, K^+ gluconate was replaced by mannitol. The uptake values observed for sodium-dependent L-glutamic acid transport in the presence of gluconate are set at 100.

Table 3. Effect of different amino acids on sodium-dependent L-glutamic acid transport

Additional amino acid (1 mmol·l⁻¹)	L-glutamic acid uptake (in pmols·20 sec⁻¹·mg protein⁻¹)	D-glucose uptake (in pmols·20 sec⁻¹·mg protein⁻¹)
Control	158	77
D-Glutamic acid	188	76
L-Aspartic, acid	30	67
L-Arginine	198	68
L-Lysine	201	69
L-Glutamine	177	70
Glycine	215	81
L-Proline	181	68
L-Histidine	191	77
L-Alanine	182	78
D-Glucose	162	50

Membranes were prepared in 100 mmol·l^{-1} mannitol, 20 mmol·l^{-1} Hepes–Tris at pH 7.4 and 5 mmol·l^{-1} KSCN. Uptake of L-glutamic acid and D-glucose was studied in an identical medium containing in addition 100 mmol·l^{-1} NaCl, 0.1 mmol·l^{-1} L-glutamic acid, 0.1 mmol·l^{-1} D-glucose, and 1 mmol·l^{-1} of the different substrates as indicated in the table. The experiments were performed in the presence of valinomycin.

potential sensitivity of sodium-dependent L-glutamic acid uptake in rat renal proximal tubule were performed under physiological conditions, i.e. in the presence of an inwardly directed sodium gradient and an outwardly directed potassium gradient. Previous experiments on the potential sensitivity of sodium-dependent L-glutamic acid transport were performed in the absence of potassium (Seeger *et al.*, 1979; Schneider *et al.*, 1978). Altering transmembrane diffusion potentials by anion replacement only showed minor effects on sodium-dependent L-glutamic acid uptake in the absence of potassium compared to the effects on sodium-dependent D-glucose uptake (Seeger *et al.*, 1979; Burckhardt *et al.*, 1980). In the presence of an outwardly directed potassium gradient, valinomycin showed only a slight stimulation of sodium-dependent L-glutamic acid uptake but a drastic stimulation of sodium-dependent D-glucose uptake. Although the stimulatory effect of valinomycin is small, it is significant and reproducible, suggesting partial potential sensitivity of Na^+-dependent L-glutamic acid transport. Since an outwardly directed potassium gradient is able directly to drive sodium-dependent L-glutamic acid uptake (Table 1), the results obtained on L-glutamic acid uptake in the presence of valinomycin may reflect a mixture of two separate effects which might cancel each other out. Firstly, sodium-dependent potential sensitive L-glutamic acid uptake in the presence of potassium can be stimulated by addition of valinomycin; secondly, potassium gradient dependent driving forces for a sodium and potassium dependent transport of L-glutamic acid can be diminished after the addition of valinomycin due to a faster dissipation of the potassium gradient. Therefore, we reinvestigated the question of potential sensitivity of sodium-dependent L-glutamic acid transport by considering the possible role of potassium.

Replacing rather impermeable anions such as gluconate or sulfate by more permeable anions such as chloride, nitrate or thiocyanate leads, in the presence of potassium to drastic stimulation of sodium-dependent L-glutamic acid uptake, whereas in the absence of potassium the anion replacement shows much smaller effects (Table 2). This result clearly shows that sodium-dependent L-glutamic acid transport in the presence of potassium can be stimulated by an inside more negative diffusion potential. Creating inside negative proton diffusion potentials by addition of the uncoupler FCCP in the presence of outwardly directed proton gradients leads to stimulation of sodium-dependent L-glutamic acid uptake only in the presence of potassium (Burckhardt *et al.*, 1970). Finally, potential sensitivity of sodium-dependent L-glutamic acid uptake in the presence of potassium was confirmed by following alterations of the transmembrane electrical potential difference by fluorometric methods using the dye 3,3′-diethylthiadicarbocyanine iodide. Increased inside positivity of the transmembrane potential difference after addition of L-glutamic acid could only be detected in the presence of potassium and sodium gradients but not in the presence of sodium alone, i.e. under conditions where addition of D-glucose provokes depolarization (Burckhardt *et al.*, 1980). Inhibition experiments showed that this sodium and potassium dependent transport system is very specific. Only the addition of L-aspartic acid but not other L-amino acids or D-glutamate caused inhibition (Table 3). The experiment was performed with 5 mmol·l^{-1} potassium on both sides of the membrane and in the presence of valinomycin, i.e. under conditions where indirect coupling effects of sodium-dependent transport processes should be minimized (Murer *et al.*, 1975). Furthermore, even 5 mmol·l^{-1} potassium leads to drastic stimulation of sodium-dependent L-glutamic acid transport (Burckhardt *et al.*, 1980).

Transport of ornithine

Based on electrophysiological experiments as well as on microperfusion experiments we know that the basic amino acids L-ornithine, L-arginine and L-lysine share a common sodium-dependent transport system (Samarzija, 1978). Experiments carried out with brush border membrane vesicles from rabbit kidney cortex could either not show any sodium-dependency (Hammerman, 1975) or sodium stimulation was very small (Busse, 1979). The experiments with vesicles were mostly performed in the presence of salt gradients, i.e. conditions which might exert a significant driving force for the uptake of an organic cation whose transport across the brush border membrane is not obligatorily coupled to the movement of sodium ions. As can be seen from the experiment presented in Fig. 1 a KSCN gradient is able to drive "overshooting" uptake of L-ornithine at concentrations of 0.1 mmol·l^{-1} but not at 1.0 mmol·l^{-1}. Since the uptake rates are significantly increased after preloading the vesicles with cold L-ornithine, we can assume that the uptake of L-ornithine in the absence of sodium is by facilitated diffusion. Sodium seems to exert only a minor stimulatory effect under conditions of anion gradients (compare conditions in the left panel with corresponding conditions in the right panel, Fig. 1). However, if the anion gradients across

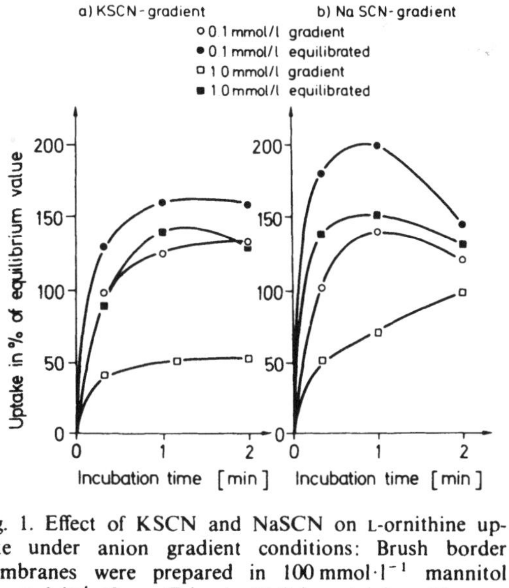

Fig. 1. Effect of KSCN and NaSCN on L-ornithine uptake under anion gradient conditions: Brush border membranes were prepared in 100 mmol·l^{-1} mannitol 20 mmol·l^{-1} Hepes–Tris at pH 7.4 containing either no L-ornithine, 0.1 mmol·l^{-1} L-ornithine or 1.0 mmol·l^{-1} L-orithine. Uptake of tracer L-ornithine was measured in a medium containing either 0.1 mmol·l^{-1} or 1.0 mmol·l^{-1} ornithine and 100 mmol·l^{-1} KSCN or NaSCN.

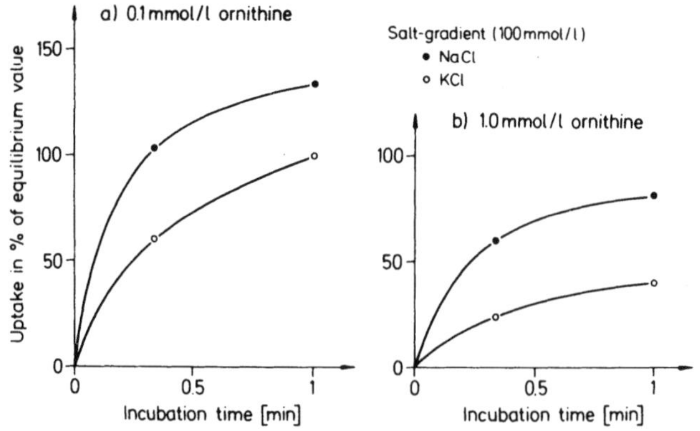

Fig. 2. Effect of sodium and potassium on L-ornithine uptake in the absence of anion gradients. Brush border membranes were prepared in 100 mmol·l⁻¹ mannitol, 20 mmol·l⁻¹ Hepes–Tris at pH 7.4 and 100 mmol·l⁻¹ choline chloride. Uptake of tracer L-ornithine was measured in an identical medium containing instead of choline-chloride either 100 mmol·l⁻¹ NaCl or KCl and 0.1 mmol·l⁻¹ or 1.0 mmol·l⁻¹ ornithine.

the membrane are abolished by preparing the membrane in 100 mmol·l⁻¹ choline chloride, sodium chloride in the incubation medium stimulates L-ornithine uptake as compared to its uptake in the presence of potassium chloride (Fig. 2). Recent experiments using valinomycin showed that sodium-dependent L-ornithine uptake is stimulated by increased inside negativity of the transmembrane electrical potential difference (Leopolder *et al.*, manuscript in preparation). Alterations in the membrane potential after addition of L-ornithine using the fluorescent dye clearly demonstrate potential-sensitivity of sodium-dependent L-ornithine uptake (Fig. 3). Since the fluorescence change is more pronounced at high sodium concentrations, where D-glucose addition also provokes depolarization, we can conclude from the experiment presented in Fig. 3 that L-ornithine is transported sodium-dependently. Furthermore, it seems, that at low sodium concentrations or even in the absence of sodium, L-ornithine flows slowly across the membrane carrying positive charges. This is in agreement with the tracer flux experiments.

CONCLUSIONS

The experiments presented in this contribution show that sodium-dependent transport of L-glutamic acid can be driven by an outwardly directed potassium gradient. Since, the transport of L-glutamic acid in the presence of sodium and potassium is potential-sensitive, the negative charge of the inwardly transported L-glutamic acid and the positive charge of the potassium transported in the opposite direction have to be overcompensated by sodium ions taken up during L-glutamic acid influx. Thereby one can assume cotransport of at least 3 sodium ions with one glutamic acid molecule coupled to the efflux of one potassium ion. This "specialization" in the driving forces for L-glutamic acid uptake, might explain the high accumulation ratio for acidic amino acids observed in renal cortical tissue. Sodium dependence of the transport of L-ornithine could also be demonstrated in studies with vesicles.

The experiments presented above demonstrate that discrepancies between observations obtained in

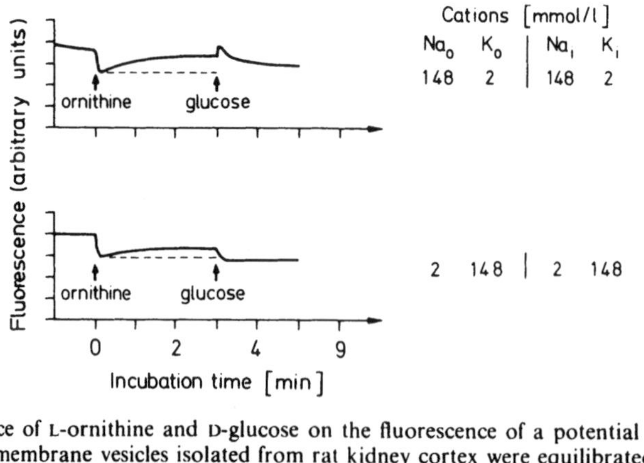

Fig. 3. The influence of L-ornithine and D-glucose on the fluorescence of a potential sensitive cyanine dye. Brush border membrane vesicles isolated from rat kidney cortex were equilibrated in 20 mmol·l⁻¹ Hepes–Tris buffers, pH 7.4 containing either 74 mmol·l⁻¹ Na_2SO_4, 1 mmol·l⁻¹ K_2SO_4 or 1 mmol·l⁻¹ Na_2SO_4, 74 mmol·l⁻¹ K_2SO_4. 3,3′-diethylthiadicarbocyanine iodide was added to the incubation medium to give a final concentration of 3 μmol·l⁻¹. At the times indicated L-ornithine and D-glucose were added (final concentrations 14 mmol·l⁻¹ and 4.8 mmol·l⁻¹, respectively).

studies with vesicles and data obtained in experiments with intact epithelia might be due to differences in the experimental conditions. In particular, one should try to mimick as closely as possible in experiments with vesicles the driving forces of the intact cell, at least with respect to ion gradients. As shown by the experiments on sodium-dependent L-glutamic acid transport the transport system behaves differently in the presence or absence of potassium. Furthermore, especially in the experiments on the transport of anions or cations, studies with vesicles have to consider "indirect coupling" effects due to diffusion potentials. An example of this is given in this paper in the effect of a KSCN gradient on overshooting L-ornithine uptake. Similarly, sodium stimulation of an anion flux across the brush border membrane does not necessarily imply sodium-dependent cotransport. Experiments with vesicles showing parallelism in the transport phenomena to studies performed on the intact epithelia offer the chance to analyze the system in more detail. Thus, it was possible in the case of glutamic acid transport to demonstrate a specific role of potassium. For L-ornithine as for proline (shown by McNamara *et al.*, 1979) experiments with vesicles demonstrate, that besides sodium-dependent transport, sodium-independent transport seem to occur across the brush border membrane.

SUMMARY

Transport of acidic and basic amino acids by brush border membrane vesicles isolated from rat kidney cortex was analyzed by tracer flux measurements or by measuring the accompanying alterations of the electrical potential difference by fluorescence of a cyanine dye.

L-glutamic acid and L-ornithine tracer uptake is stimulated in the presence of sodium as compared to the presence of other monovalent cations. Inside-negative transmembrane electrical potential differences stimulate the uptake of L-ornithine even in the absence of sodium. Therefore stimulation of L-ornithine uptake by sodium can be better observed in anion pre-equilibrated vesicles where anion diffusion potential effects are minimized.

Preloading of the vesicles with potassium leads to a specific stimulation of sodium-dependent L-glutamic acid transport. The potassium effect shows a strong sidedness, i.e. potassium is needed at the inner membrane surface. Furthermore, the enhancing effect of potassium is multiplied if potassium is present under gradient conditions ($K_i^+ > K_o^+$). Creating inside-more-negative anion diffusion potentials also leads to a marked stimulation of sodium-dependent L-glutamic acid uptake in potassium pre-equilibrated vesicles.

Measuring qualitatively the effect of amino acid translocation on the transmembrane electrical potential difference in sodium pre-equilibrated vesicles by use of the fluorescent dye, a polarization (inside positive) is found after the addition of L-ornithine. The addition of L-glutamic acid causes depolarization only in the presence of sodium and potassium.

The results show that like neutral amino acids transport of basic amino acids is driven by the electrochemical potential difference of sodium, whereas sodium-dependent transport of acidic amino acids can be driven in addition by an outwardly directed potassium gradient. Sodium/potassium-driven L-glutamic acid transport is also potential-sensitive.

Acknowledgements—We thank Professors Ullrich and Frömter for stimulating discussions, which enabled us to perform this study.

REFERENCES

Burckhardt G., Kinne R., Stange G. & Murer H. (1980) The effects of potassium and membrane potential on sodium-dependent glutamic acid uptake *Biochim. biophys. Acta* in press.

Busse D. (1978) Transport of L-arginine in brush border vesicles derived from rabbit kidney cortex. *Arch. Biochem. Biophys.* **191**, 551–560.

Evers J., Murer H. & Kinne R. (1976) Phenylalanine uptake in isolated renal brush border vesicles. *Biochim. biophys. Acta* **426**, 598–615.

Evers C., Haase W., Murer H. & Kinne R. (1978) Properties of brush border membrane vesicles isolated from rat kidney cortex by calcium precipitation. *Membr. Biochem.* **1**, 203–219.

Fass S. J., Hammerman M. R. & Sacktor B. (1977) Transport of amino acids in renal brush border membrane vesicles. Uptake of the neutral amino acid L-alanine. *J. biol. Chem.* **252**, 583–590.

Goldmann D. R., Roth K. S., Langfitt T. W. & Segal S. (1979) L-Proline transport by newborn rat kidney brush border vesicles. *Biochem. J.* **178**, 253–256.

Hammerman M. R. (1975) Transport of L-arginine by isolated renal cortex brush border membranes. *Fedn Proc. Fedn Am. Socs exp. Biol.* **34**, 309.

Hammerman M. R. & Sacktor B. (1977) Transport of amino acids in renal brush border vesicles. Uptake of L-proline. *J. biol. Chem.* **252**, 591–595.

Kinne R., Barac M. & Murer H. (1979) Sodium-cotransport systems in the proximal tubule. Current developments. *Curr. Topics Membr. Transp.* **13** In press.

McNamara P. D., Ozegovic B., Pepe L. M. & Segal S. (1976) Proline and glycine uptake by renal brush border vesicles. *Proc. natn. Acad. Sci. U.S.A.* **73**, 4521–4525.

McNamara P. D., Pepe L. M. & Segal S. (1979) Sodium gradient dependence of proline and glycine uptake in rat renal brush border membrane vesicles. *Biochim. biophys. Acta* **556**, 151–160.

Murer H. & Kinne R. (1979) The role of sodium in anion transport across renal and intestinal cells: studies with plasma membrane vesicles. *Fedn. Proc. Fedn Am. Socs. exp. Biol.* In press.

Samarzija J. (1978) Experimentelle Untersuchungen zum Aminosäure-Transport im proximalen Tubulus der Rattenniere. Ph.D.-Thesis, Universität Frankfurt, Fachbereich Biochemie und Pharmazie.

Seeger J., Stange G., Murer H. & Kinne R. (1979) Transport of L-glutamate by brush border membrane vesicles isolated from rat kidney cortex. *Pflugers Arch. ges. Physiol.* **379**, R 18.

Schneider E. G., Hammerman M. R. & Sacktor B. (1978) The Na^+-dependent transport of L-glutamic acid by renal brush border vesicles. Evidence for an electroneutral mechanism. *Fedn. Proc. Fedn. Am. Socs. exp. Biol.* **37**, 1295.

Schneider E. G. (1979) Effect of internal K^+ gradient ($K_i^+ > K_o^+$) on the Na^+ dependent transport of L-glutamate by rabbit renal brush border vesicles. *Fedn. Proc. Fedn. Am. Socs. exp. Biol.* **38**, 101.

ULLRICH K. J. (1979) Sugar, amino acid and Na^+ cotransport in the proximal tubule. *A. Rev. Physiol.* **41**, 181–195.

WEISS S. D., MCNAMARA P. D., PEPE L. M. & SEGAL S. (1978) Glutamine and glutamic acid uptake by rat renal brush border membrane vesicles. *J. Membr. Biol.* **43**, 91–105.

Int. J. Biochem., Vol. 12, pp. 229 to 234
Pergamon Press Ltd 1980. Printed in Great Britain

THE SINGULAR EFFECT OF AN INTERNAL K^+ GRADIENT ($K_i^+ > K_o^+$) ON THE Na^+ GRADIENT ($Na_o^+ > Na_i^+$)-DEPENDENT TRANSPORT OF L-GLUTAMATE IN RENAL BRUSH BORDER MEMBRANE VESICLES

BERTRAM SACKTOR* and E. GAYLE SCHNEIDER
Laboratory of Molecular Aging, National Institute on Aging, National Institutes of Health, Baltimore, MD 21224, U.S.A.

Abstract—1. A Na^+ gradient (extravesicular > intravesicular) energizes the concentrative uptake of L-glutamate into membrane vesicles.

2. In contrast to the uptakes of D-glucose and neutral amino acids, the uptake of the acidic amino acid is stimulated additionally, several-fold, by a K^+ (or Rb^+) gradient (intravesicular > extravesicular). This effect requires the presence of Na^+.

3. In the presence of Na^+, but in the absence of a Na^+ gradient, the internal K^+ gradient can drive the uphill transport of L-glutamate.

4. Membrane potential alterations, induced by permeant anions or developed by K^+ diffusion potentials in the presence of valinomycin, have no appreciable effect on the uptake of L-glutamate energized by either the Na^+ gradient, in the absence of K^+, or the K^+ gradient, in the absence of a Na^+ gradient.

5. In contrast, in parallel experiments the uptake of D-glucose, whose cotransport system is known to be electrogenic, is markedly increased by an internal negative membrane potential.

6. These findings provide evidence consistent with the view that the uphill uptake of L-glutamate in brush border membrane vesicles is an electroneutral transport system when energized by either the Na^+ or the K^+ gradient.

7. Several stoichiometric relationships for the cotransport of L-glutamate, Na^+ and K^+ are feasible in light of these observations.

INTRODUCTION

Previous studies of renal transport mechanisms using membrane vesicles isolated from the luminal (brush border) segment of the proximal tubular cell plasma membrane indicate that the concentrative uptake of neutral amino acids is mediated by electrogenic Na^+-amino acid cotransport systems (Fass *et al.*, 1977; Hammerman & Sacktor, 1977, 1978; Evers *et al.*, 1976; McNamara *et al.*, 1976; Rozen *et al.*, 1979; Segal *et al.*, 1977), analogous to that described for D-glucose (Kinne *et al.*, 1975; Aronson & Sacktor, 1975; Beck & Sacktor, 1975, 1978a, 1978b; Hilden & Sacktor, 1979). In contrast to D-glucose and the net neutrally charged amino acids, L-glutamate bears a net negative charge at physiological pH. Therefore, the transport mechanism for the acidic amino acid may be fundamentally different from the mechanisms of uptake of the neutral compounds. This hypothesis is examined in the present paper.

It was previously found that the uptake of L-glutamate into renal brush border membrane vesicles is stimulated by an extravesicular > intravesicular Na^+ gradient (Sacktor, 1977; Weiss *et al.*, 1978; Schneider *et al.*, 1978). We also reported earlier that the Na^+ gradient-dependent transport of L-glutamate is increased additionally by an intravesicular > extravesicular K^+ gradient (Schneider, 1979). In this paper, we describe evidence consistent with the view that the uphill uptake of L-glutamate in brush border membrane vesicles, energized by either a Na^+ gradient, in the absence of K^+, or a K^+ gradient, in the presence of Na^+, is an electroneutral transport system.

* To whom correspondence should be addressed, at: Gerontology Research Center, NIA, NIH, Baltimore City Hospitals, Baltimore, MD 21224, U.S.A.

MATERIALS AND METHODS

Rabbit renal brush border membrane vesicles were prepared by a previously described technique (Beck & Sacktor, 1978a). Uptakes of L-[^{3}H]glutamate, L-[^{3}H]proline, and D-[^{14}C]glucose were measured at 20°C using a Millipore filtration technique (Aronson & Sacktor, 1975; Chesney *et al.*, 1973). L-Glutamate transport had a broad pH-optimum, being essentially constant at pH 5.5 to 8.5. Unless noted, the pH of the incubations were at 7.5. The glutamate taken up by the brush border membrane vesicles was accumulated intravesicularly and not metabolized.

RESULTS AND DISCUSSION

Figure 1 compares the microvillus vesicle uptake of L-glutamate with those of L-proline and D-glucose, as a function of time either in a 300 mM buffered mannitol medium or in a medium in which mannitol was

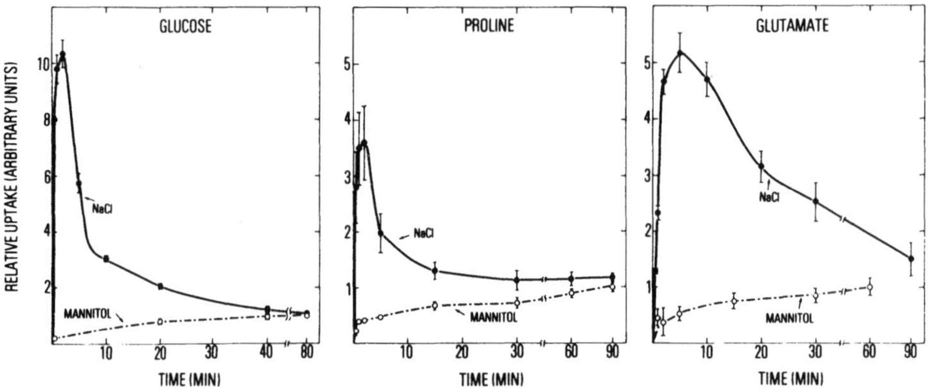

Fig. 1. The effect of a Na^+ gradient (extravesicular > intravesicular) on the initial rates of L-glutamate, L-proline, and D-glucose uptake and in driving the uphill transports of the solutes into renal brush border membrane vesicles. The intravesicular medium was 300 mM buffered mannitol and the extravesicular medium was either the same mannitol solution (○) or 100 mM NaCl in 100 mM mannitol (●), as indicated.

replaced isosmotically by 100 mM NaCl at the initiation of incubation. The presence of the Na^+ electrochemical gradient between the extravesicular and intravesicular media effected marked stimulations of both amino acid and the sugar transport systems. The initial (30 sec) rates of uptake of the amino acids and sugar were approx 10 and 25-times the initial rates in the absence of the gradient, respectively. Accumulation in the membrane vesicles was maximal at 5 min for L-glutamate and about 2 min for L-proline and D-glucose. At the peak of the overshoots, the uptakes of the amino acids were about 5-fold and the uptake of D-glucose was 10-fold the final equilibrium (80–90 min) value. These findings demonstrated that an extravesicular to intravesicular Na^+ electrochemical gradient can drive the movements of L-glutamate, L-proline and D-glucose into renal brush border membrane vesicles against their respective concentration gradients (uphill or concentrative transports), as reported previously (Hammerman & Sacktor, 1977; Aronson & Sacktor, 1975; Schneider *et al.*, 1978; Sacktor, 1980).

The Na^+ gradient-dependent L-glutamate transport system was next examined to determine how alterations in the membrane potential affected its uptake. Modulation of the membrane potential was accomplished by sodium salts comprised of anions of different modes of membrane permeability or was developed by K^+ diffusion potentials in the presence of valinomycin. Fig. 2 (top) compares the effects of a Na_2SO_4 gradient relative to a NaCl gradient on the uptakes of L-glutamate and D-glucose. The Na^+ gradient-dependent uptake of the sugar was strongly inhibited when the relatively impermeant SO_4^{2-} was the anion, in agreement with previous findings (Beck & Sacktor, 1975). In contrast, uptake of L-glutamate was not significantly affected when the less permeable anion was substituted for Cl^- in the salt gradient. In other experiments, reported elsewhere (Beck & Sacktor, 1975; Sacktor, 1980), when the transport of D-glucose was determined in the presence of a salt gradient comprised of 100 mM $NaNO_3$ or NaSCN, the initial rates of uptake with these highly permeable anions were greater than that with a NaCl gradient. The initial rate of L-glutamate uptake, however, was not appreciably altered (Schneider *et al.*, 1978, Sacktor, 1980). These findings show that modification of the membrane potential with anions of different modes of permeability did not alter the Na^+ gradient energized uphill uptake of L-glutamate but did alter that of D-glucose, and suggest that the transport of L-glutamate is electroneutral, in contrast to the electrogenic transport of the sugar.

The role of the membrane potential in the Na^+ gradient-dependent uptake of L-glutamate was examined additionally by comparing L-glutamate and D-glucose uptakes by membrane vesicles using conditions in which K^+ diffusion potentials were induced experimentally and predictably by valinomycin. Brush border membrane vesicles were preloaded with K^+ and then assayed for the Na^+ gradient-dependent transports of L-glutamate and D-glucose, in the presence and absence of valinomycin (Fig. 2, bottom). In the presence of the ionophore, greatly enhanced overshoots were found when D-glucose was the transported solute. In these experiments valinomycin induced the efflux of K^+ down its electrochemical gradient with concomitant generation of a membrane potential, interior negative. The development of this potential accelerated the influx into the vesicle of Na^+ cotransported with the sugar. In contrast, the valinomycin induced K^+ diffusion potential (interior negative) had no effect on the cotransport of Na^+ and L-glutamate. Similar results were obtained when membrane potentials (interior negative) were generated by H^+ diffusion potentials in the presence of the uncoupler FCCP (Schneider & Sacktor, 1980). In additional experiments, reported elsewhere (Schneider & Sacktor, 1980), when K^+ diffusion potentials (interior positive) was generated, Na^+ gradient-dependent D-glucose uptake was markedly inhibited, whereas Na^+ gradient-dependent L-glutamate transport was unaffected. Thus, these findings firmly establish that the concentrative uptake of L-glutamate into membrane vesicles, when energized by a Na^+ gradient, is an electroneutral transport process.

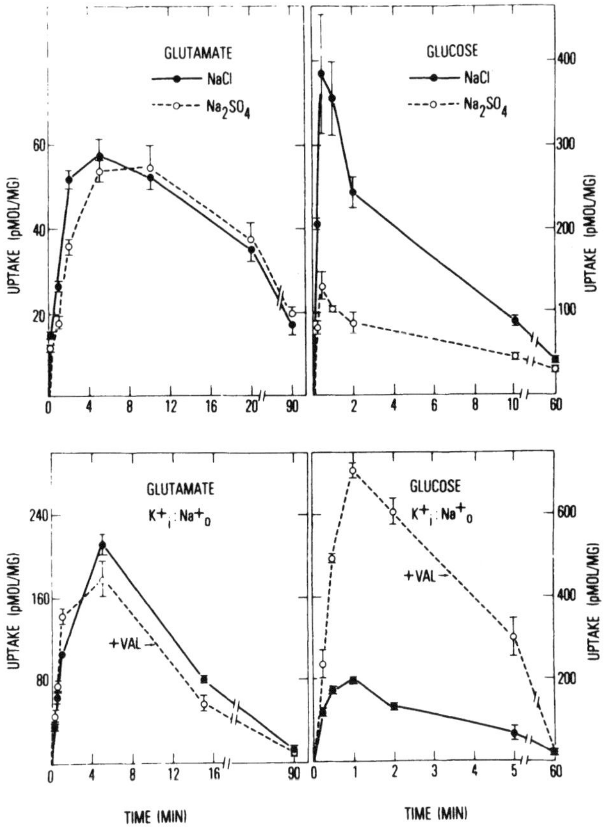

Fig. 2. The effect of the membrane potential on the Na^+ gradient-dependent uptake of L-glutamate and D-glucose. In the experiments illustrated on the top, membrane potentials were altered by sodium salts comprised of a relatively permeant anion, Cl^-, or of an impermeant anion, SO_4^{2-}. In the experiments illustrated on the bottom, K^+ diffusion potentials (inside negative) were developed in KCl preloaded vesicles in the presence of valinomycin.

We previously reported that a K^+ gradient (intravesicular > extravesicular) specifically enhanced the Na^+ gradient-dependent uptake of L-glutamate (Schneider, 1979; Schneider & Sacktor, 1980). Figure 3 illustrates this effect by comparing the Na^+ gradient-dependent transport of L-glutamate with those of L-proline and D-glucose when the membrane vesicles were preloaded with either KCl or mannitol. It was found that L-glutamate transport was increased several-fold when the vesicles were preloaded with K^+. In contrast, the uptakes of L-proline and D-glucose were relatively decreased in the KCl preloaded

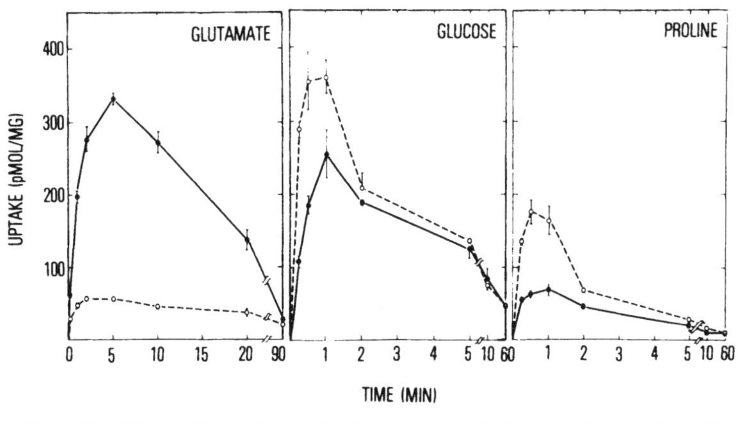

Fig. 3. The effect of a K^+ gradient (intravesicular > extravesicular) on the uptakes of L-glutamate, L-proline, and D-glucose. Membrane vesicles were preloaded with 300 mM buffered mannitol (○) or 100 mM KCl, 100 mM buffered mannitol (●) and incubated in a medium containing 100 mM NaCl and 100 mM mannitol.

vesicles, presumably because a Cl^- electrochemical gradient, which would contribute to the driving force in the electrogenic Na^+-D-glucose or Na^+-L-proline cotransports, is lacking.

A detailed description of the K^+ gradient-dependent transport of L-glutamate was given elsewhere (Schneider, 1979; Schneider & Sacktor, 1980). Important features of the system include the findings that the effect of the intravesicular cation was specific for K^+; only Rb^+ could substitute. The K^+-dependent enhanced L-glutamate uptake required the presence of a K^+ gradient, intravesicular > extravesicular. The larger the K_i^+/K_o^+ ratio the greater was the uptake of the amino acid. At a constant ratio, L-glutamate transport increased with higher concentrations of intravesicular K^+. Moreover, the system showed marked sensitivity to K^+, in that an intravesicular concentration of 10 mM K^+ saturated the transport system and a concentration as low as 1 mM gave half-maximal stimulation. The intravesicular > extravesicular K^+ gradient did not alter the specificity nor the affinity of the uptake process for L-glutamate. Only the V_{max} of the transport was increased. Most importantly, the effect of the K^+ gradient in stimulating the uptake of L-glutamate had an absolute requirement for Na^+. In addition, when Na^+ was present in both the extravesicular and intravesicular media, i.e. in the absence of a Na^+ gradient, a K^+ gradient (intravesicular > extravesicular) energized the uphill uptake of L-glutamate.

This K^+ gradient-energized L-glutamate transport process, like the Na^+ gradient-dependent system, appears to be electroneutral. This view is supported by the experiments illustrated in Fig. 4. In one series of experiments, in which a K^+ gradient but no Na^+ gradient was present (Fig. 4, top), inside negative membrane potentials were established by an extravesicular > intravesicular SCN^- gradient. The permeant anion gradient was sufficient to drive uphill the electrogenic transport of D-glucose. In contrast, the

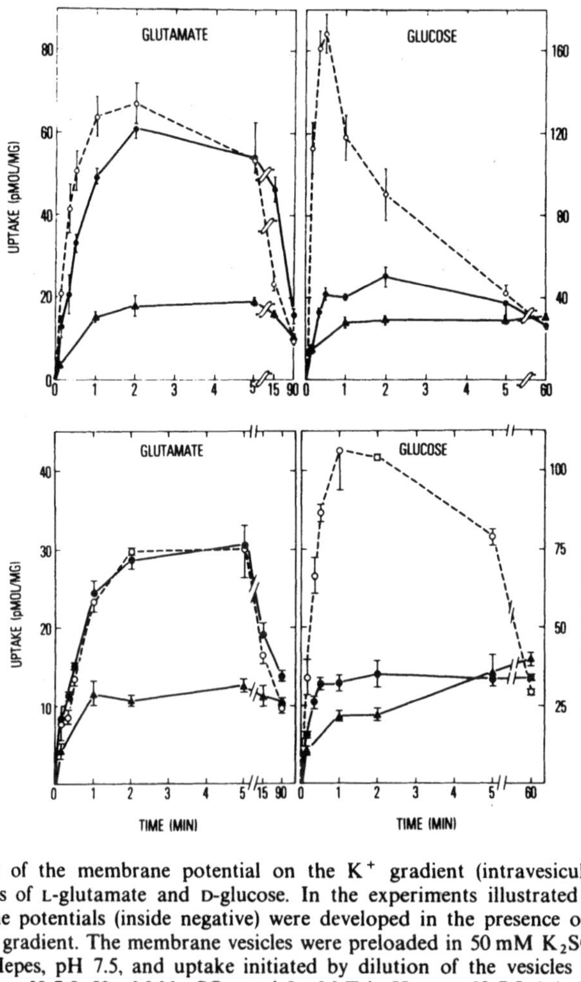

Fig. 4. The effect of the membrane potential on the K^+ gradient (intravesicular > extravesicular)-dependent uptakes of L-glutamate and D-glucose. In the experiments illustrated on the top, SCN^--induced membrane potentials (inside negative) were developed in the presence of a K^+ gradient but absence of a Na^+ gradient. The membrane vesicles were preloaded in 50 mM K_2SO_4, 50 mM Na_2SO_4, and 5 mM Tris–Hepes, pH 7.5, and uptake initiated by dilution of the vesicles in media containing 50 mM Tris sulfate, pH 7.5, 50 mM Na_2SO_4, and 5 mM Tris–Hepes, pH 7.5, (●); 33.3 mM Tris sulfate, pH 7.5, 100 mM NaSCN, and 5 mM Tris–Hepes, pH 7.5 (○); or 50 mM K_2SO_4, 50 mM Na_2SO_4 and 5 mM Tris–Hepes, pH 7.5 (▲). In the experiments illustrated on the bottom, valinomycin-induced K^+ diffusion potentials (inside negative) were developed. Membrane vesicles were preloaded with 50 mM K_2SO_4, 50 mM Na_2SO_4, and 5 mM Tris–Hepes, pH 7.5, and incubated in media containing 50 mM Tris sulfate, pH 7.5, 50 mM Na_2SO_4, and 5 mM Tris–Hepes, pH 7.5, and either valinomycin in ethanol (○) or ethanol alone (●). The ethanol treated vesicles were also incubated in a control medium containing 50 mM K_2SO_4, 50 mM Na_2SO_4, and Tris–Hepes, pH 7.5, (▲).

SCN$^-$ gradient had little affect on the uptake of L-glutamate. In another series of experiments (Fig. 4, bottom) inside negative membrane potentials were developed by a K$^+$ diffusion potential concomitant with the addition of valinomycin. It was found that in the absence of a Na$^+$ gradient, the inside negative membrane potential could drive the concentrative uptake of D-glucose. However, in the parallel experiment, L-glutamate uptake energized by the K$^+$ gradient was not affected. These findings provide strong evidence favoring the hypothesis that the L-glutamate uptake system energized by a K$^+$ gradient as well as the uptake system that is mediated by a Na$^+$ gradient are electroneutral transport processes.

CONCLUSIONS

Using renal brush border membrane vesicles we have shown that both a Na$^+$ gradient (extravesicular > intravesicular), in the absence of K$^+$, and a K$^+$ gradient (intravesicular > extravesicular), in the absence of a Na$^+$ gradient, can energize the concentrative (uphill) transport of L-glutamate. No evidence was obtained that different L-glutamate carriers are involved in the two systems. Since the K$^+$ gradient-dependent and Na$^+$ gradient-dependent uptakes appear to be electroneutral, a direct interaction of K$^+$ with the Na$^+$-L-glutamate carrier is indicated. Furthermore, these observations suggest hypotheses for the stoichiometric relationships between L-glutamate, Na$^+$, and K$^+$ uptakes in the microvillar vesicle system. In the absence of K$^+$, an electroneutral Na$^+$ gradient-dependent L-glutamate uptake indicates a stoichiometry of 1 Na$^+$ to 1 L-glutamate. In the K$^+$ gradient-energized system, which requires the presence of Na$^+$ but does not require a Na$^+$ gradient, an electroneutral process suggests either of two possible stoichiometric relationships: (1) influx of 2 Na$^+$ and 1 L-glutamate per efflux of 1 K$^+$; or (2) influx of 1 Na$^+$, 1 L-glutamate, and 1 H$^+$ per efflux of 1 K$^+$. Preliminary experiments provide some evidence consistent with the latter alternative.

REFERENCES

ARONSON P. S. & SACKTOR B. (1975) The Na$^+$ gradient-dependent transport of D-glucose in renal brush border membranes. *J. biol. Chem.* **250**, 6032–6039.

BECK J. C. & SACKTOR B. (1975) Energetics of the Na$^+$-dependent transport of D-glucose in renal brush border membrane vesicles. *J. biol. Chem.* **250**, 8674–8680.

BECK J. C. & SACKTOR B. (1978a) The sodium electrochemical potential-mediated uphill transport of D-glucose in renal brush border membrane vesicles *J. biol. Chem.* **253**, 5531–5535.

BECK J. C. & SACKTOR B. (1978b) Membrane potential-sensitive fluorescence changes during Na$^+$-dependent D-glucose transport in renal brush border membrane vesicles. *J. biol. Chem.* **253**, 7158–7162.

CHESNEY R. W., SACKTOR B. & ROWEN R. (1973) The binding of D-glucose to the isolated luminal membrane of the renal proximal tubule. *J. biol. Chem.* **248**, 2182–2191.

EVERS J., MURER H. & KINNE R. (1976) Phenylalanine uptake in isolated renal brush border vesicles. *Biochim. biophys. Acta* **426**, 598–615.

FASS S. J., HAMMERMAN M. R. & SACKTOR B. (1977) Transport of amino acids in renal brush border membrane vesicles. Uptake of the neutral amino acid L-alanine. *J. biol. Chem.* **252**, 583–590.

HAMMERMAN M. R. & SACKTOR B. (1977) Transport of amino acids in renal brush border membrane vesicles. Uptake of L-proline. *J. biol. Chem.* **252**, 591–595.

HAMMERMAN M. R. & SACKTOR B. (1978) Transport of β-alanine in renal brush border membrane vesicles. *Biochim. biophys. Acta* **509**, 338–347.

HILDEN S. A. & SACKTOR B. (1979) D-Glucose-dependent sodium transport in renal brush border membrane vesicles. *J. biol. Chem.* **254**, 7090–7096.

KINNE R., MURER H., KINNE-SAFFRAN E., THEES M. & SACHS G. (1975) Sugar transport by renal plasma membrane vesicles. *J. Membr. Biol.* **21**, 375–395.

MCNAMARA P. D., OZOGOVIC B., PEPE L. M. & SEGAL S. (1976) Proline and glycine uptake by renal brush border membrane vesicles. *Proc. natn. Acad. Sci. U.S.A.* **73**, 4521–4525.

ROZEN R., TENENHOUSE H. S. & SCRIVER C. R. (1979) Taurine transport in renal brush–border–membrane vesicles. *Biochem. J.* **180**, 245–248.

SACKTOR B. (1977) Transport in membrane vesicles isolated from the mammalian kidney and intestine. *Current Topics in Bioenergetics*, (Edited by SANADI R.) Vol. 6, pp. 39–81. Academic Press, New York.

SACKTOR B. (1980) Electrogenic and electroneutral Na$^+$ gradient-dependent transport systems in the renal brush border membrane vesicles. *Current Topics in Membranes and Transport*, Vol. 13, (Edited by BRENNER F. & KLEINZELLER A.) Academic Press, New York in press.

SCHNEIDER E. G. (1979) The effect of internal K$^+$ gradient ($K_i^+ > K_o^+$) on the Na$^+$-dependent transport of L-glutamate by rabbit renal brush border membrane vesicles. *Fedn Proc. Fedn Am. Socs exp. Biol.* **38**, 244.

SCHNEIDER E. G. & SACKTOR B. (1980) The effect of internal potassium on the sodium-dependent transport of L-glutamate by renal brush border membrane vesicles. *J. biol. Chem.* Submitted for publication.

SCHNEIDER E. G., HAMMERMAN M. R. & SACKTOR B. (1978) The Na$^+$-dependent transport of L-glutamic acid by renal brush border membranes: evidence for an electroneutral mechanism. *Fedn Proc. Fedn Am Socs exp. Biol.* **37**, 1295.

SEGAL S., MCNAMARA P. D. & PEPE L. M. (1977) Transport interaction of cystine and dibasic amino acids in renal brush border vesicles. *Science* **197**, 169–171.

WEISS S. D., MCNAMARA P. D., PEPE L. M. & SEGAL S. (1978) Glutamine and glutamic acid uptake by rat renal brushborder membrane vesicles. *J. Membr. Biol.* **43**, 91–105.

SYMPOSIUM DISCUSSION

Anner: Is glutamate transport reversible, and if so, how is influx and efflux affected by potassium gradients?

Sacktor: It is reversible. Glutamate efflux is stimulated by a potassium gradient, extravesicular > intravesicular.

Anner: What is the difference between the rate of active transport and passive efflux?

Murer: Passive flux, in the absence of sodium and potassium is less than 10–15% of the total transport.

Lemieux: What about amino acids with an electrical charge different from glutamate?

Sacktor: There are many studies from Murer and from ourselves (*J. Biol. Chem.* **252**, 583 and 591, 1977; *Biochem. biophys. Acta* **426**, 338 1978, and they indicate that most are electrogenic.

Murer: Only sodium-dependent glutamate and aspartate transport are affected by the presence of potassium.

Jorgensen: Do I understand you correctly, that a ternary complex is formed by the amino-acid and two sodium ions and is there no net charge?

Murer: Our conclusion, on the contrary, is that there is a net positive charge, and the reason we looked for this and for the potassium effect was the experiments of Dr Fromter, showing a change in potential. We also differ in terms of the absolute stoichiometry, but that is only theoretical at present; just that there is an excess positive charge!

Sacktor: Our findings suggest that, in the absence of K the cotransport of Na-L-glutamate is electroneutral i.e. there is no net charge. When the cotransport is energised by the K gradient, we have no evidence that the transport system becomes electrogenic.

Silbernagl: Do you have any information on the relative affinity for glutamate and aspartate; in our micro-perfusion experiments the K_m for aspartate was clearly smaller than that for glutamate (Silbernagl, *Klin. Wschr.* **57**, 1009, 1979), while Samarzija & Frömter (*Pflügers Arch. ges. Physiol.* **365**, 58, 1976) in electrophysiological experiments found it the other way round.

Murer: No information; but there is a paper from Segals' laboratory in which two different systems of high and low affinity are described.

Int. J. Biochem., Vol. 12, pp. 235 to 236
© Pergamon Press Ltd 1980. Printed in Great Britain

0020-711X/80/0701-0235$02.00/0

BRUSH BORDER MEMBRANE INJURY AND REGENERATION FOLLOWING RENAL ISCHAEMIA

LEAH M. LOWENSTEIN and JEAN K. PADDOCK
Departments of Medicine and Biochemistry, Boston University School of Medicine, Boston, MA 02118, U.S.A.

In renal ischaemia, one of the first signs of cellular damage is the disappearance of the brush border membrane. If the ischaemia lasts over 60 min in rats, cellular necrosis ensues. When a moderate ischaemic period of 25 min is produced in rats by clamping the renal artery, the brush border disappears in many cells within 15 min of reflow of blood to the kidney. However, within 2 hr, the membrane is partially regenerated, and by 8 hr the cells appear normal histologically (Donohoe *et al.*, 1978). The integrity of the cell is thus preserved, and cellular necrosis does not occur.

The cell membrane plays a crucial role in cellular growth and regeneration. As the laboratories of others and of ourselves have reported, increased phospholipid synthesis is one of the earliest signs of cellular growth (Siegel *et al.*, 1979). For example, when one rat kidney is made ischaemic, followed by little or no reflow of blood, the incorporation of [^{14}C]-choline into phospholipid is increased. (Fig. 1) (Toback *et al.*, 1979).

Today, I wish to discuss studies we have performed on metabolic events during the disappearance and reformation of the brush border membrane following renal ischaemia. This report represents no more than an Abstract of our finding. We studied two major components of the membrane during regeneration: the protein and the phospholipid fractions. We focused on both the regeneration of membrane-bound enzyme activity and the rate of incorporation of radioactive substrates into the regenerating brush borders.

Renal ischaemia was produced in male rats by occluding the left renal artery with a snare for 25 min. The right kidney served as control as did kidneys from sham-operated animals. After the ischaemic period, the blood was allowed to reflow for various time periods up to 24 hr. Kidneys were removed and brush border membranes were prepared by a modification of the method of Booth & Kenny (1974). This consists of gentle homogenization of minced kidney cortex and differential centrifugation of subcellular components in mannitol–Tris buffer until a pellet of brush border membrane is obtained. The pellet from the ischaemic kidney contained correspondingly less brush border protein. Mitochondrial contamination was less than 3% as measured by succinic dehydrogenase activity.

Three membrane-bound enzymes were studied: alkaline phosphatase, gamma glutamyl transpepti-

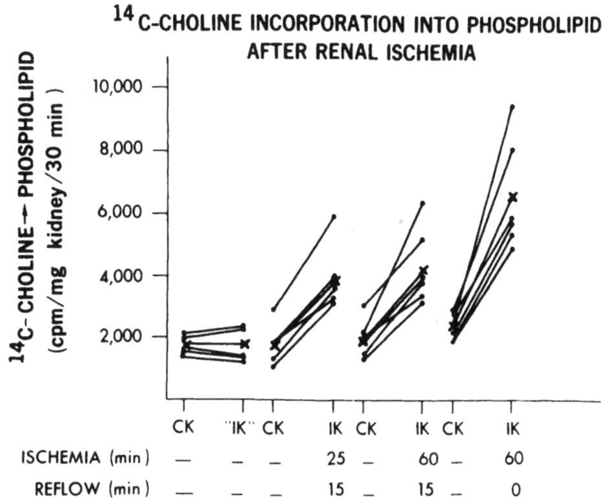

Fig. 1. [^{14}C]-Choline incorporation into renal phospholipid during *in vitro* incubation after various periods of renal artery occlusion and reflow. IK = ischeamic kidney, CK = control kidney, "IK" = sham ischaemic kidney. Ischaemia = minutes of occlusion of renal artery; reflow = minutes of reflow of blood before kidney removed from rat.

dase, and maltase. The enzymatic activities were determined in the homogenate and membrane fraction.

Eight sets of experiments were studied per time point. The values for the activities of all three enzymes were approx 50% of the control values at 15 min of reflow. This was significantly lower than normal. Within 60 min the values returned towards control levels; they were normal by 120 min and remained normal at 24 hr. The curves for all three enzymes—alkaline phosphatase, gamma glutamyl transpeptidase and maltase—were similar, suggesting a non-specific loss of enzyme molecules from the membrane. Values for the sham-operated kidneys did not vary significantly from control values.

In order to determine the rate of the regeneration following renal ischaemia, [^{14}C]-choline and tritiated leucine were injected simultaneously into the animals 25–30 min before killing. The incorporation of the two compounds into phospholipid or protein respectively were measured in the brush border fraction and calculated per mg of brush border protein. Six sets of experiments were measured per time point. The incorporation of tritiated leucine was 4.3 pmols$\cdot$mg^{-1} brush border protein and the incorporation of [^{14}C]-choline into phospholipid was 4.1 pmols$\cdot$mg protein^{-1}. The incorporation of tritiated leucine into protein fell to 30% of control by 30 min of reflow. Within 2 hr, the rate of incorporation returned towards control levels.

In contradistinction, the rate of incorporation of [^{14}C]choline into phospholipid was significantly greater than control values within the first 30 min after reflow. This rate rose to 2.5 times normal by 60 min. Normal values occurred at 24 hr.

Our results suggest that the brush border membrane is rapidly regenerated after a moderate period of renal ischaemia. Since brush borders contain a basic structure of phospholipids and of protein in the form of membrane-bound enzymes, the initial loss of the brush border essentially represents a loss of both cellular enzymes and phospholipids. The cell responds to this loss by rapidly creating new membranes. Increased incorporation of choline into phospholipid or phosphorylcholine is also seen in other forms of rapid growth of the kidney, for instance, during potassium depletion, compensatory growth, recovery from nephrotoxins and the neonatal period.

These studies do not suggest that membranes are formed as a unit with both protein and phospholipid molecules already in place. Rather, our results suggest that the phospholipid and the protein moieties of the membrane may be formed at separate rates during regeneration. One attractive speculation is that the phospholipid scaffolding of the membrane is laid down before the complete insertion of all the protein molecules.

In summary, after 25 min of renal ischaemia, brush border membranes are damaged and largely disappear. This is accompanied by a loss in the membrane-bound enzyme activity. Subsequently, the enzymatic activities of alkaline phosphatase, gamma glutamyl transpeptidase and maltase rapidly return towards normal. Within 2 hr of reflow the activities are normal again. After ischaemia, the rate of incorporation of radioactive leucine into protein is only 30% of normal. However, the rate of incorporation of radioactive choline into phospholipid occurs at a faster rate than normal. This suggests that phospholipid biogenesis or turnover occurs at a faster rate than does protein biogenesis or turnover in the brush border during renal regeneration.

Acknowledgements—We are grateful for the U.S. Public Health Service Grants AM-21596 and HL-18313 for the financial support for this work, and also for funds from the National Science Foundation and Hartford Foundation.

REFERENCES

BOOTH A. G. & KENNY A. J. (1974) A rapid method for the preparation of microvilli from rabbit kidney. *Biochem. J.* **142,** 575–581.

DONOHOE J. F., VENKATACHALAM M. A., BERNARD D. B. & LEVINSKY N. G. (1978) Tubular leakage and obstruction after renal ischaemia: structural–functional correlations. *Kidney Int.* **13,** 208–222.

SIEGEL M. B., LOWENSTEIN L. M. & LEVINSKY N. G. (1979) Choline uptake into renal phospholipids following renal ischaemia in rats. *Circ. Res.* **44,** 62–67.

TOBACK F. G., SMITH P. D. & LOWENSTEIN L. M. (1979) Phospholipid metabolism in the initiation of renal compensatory growth after acute reduction in renal mass. *J. clin. Invest.* **54,** 91–97.

SYMPOSIUM DISCUSSION

Curthoys: Do you know what the turnover rate of brush-border is in the absence of ischaemia?

Lowenstein: McNamara *et al.* (*FEBS Lett.* **41,** 139–142, 1974) found about 68 hr for turnover of microvillous protein.

De Pont: What does the change in enzyme protein mean when the total brush-border protein is altered in response to ischaemia?

Lowenstein: It is difficult to find a suitable denominator for these studies. However, the enzyme activity that we measure decreases more rapidly than the change in total membrane protein.

Brosnan: Is there a marked amino aciduria during the recovery phase?

Lowenstein: During the acute phase there is no urine flow.

Ross: It is possible to measure renal function during the recovery from ischaemia if the kidney is then taken out and perfused. If you do this after 30 min ischaemia, total sodium transport falls by 50% or so, and this is on a line, which is linear with time of ischaemia (Marshall *et al.*, 1979) resulting in zero function after 90 min ischaemia.

Int. J. Biochem., Vol. 12, pp. 237 to 242
0020-711X/80/0701-0237$02.00/0

RENAL HANDLING OF POLYPEPTIDE HORMONES (INSULIN, C-PEPTIDE, h-PTH) AS STUDIED IN THE ISOLATED PERFUSED RAT KIDNEY*

H. J. SCHUREK[1], E. SCHLATTER[1], W. MEIER[1], R. ZICK[1], G. DORN[2], R. HEHRMANN[1] and H. STOLTE[1]

[1]Department Innere Medizin, Medizinische Hochschule, Hannover, and
[2]Nuklearmedizinische Abteilung der Radiologischen Klinik des Universitätskrankenhauses Hamburg-Eppendorf

Abstract—1. Degradation of polypeptide hormones was studied in the isolated perfused rat kidney.

2. Insulin and h-PTH exhibited initially high metabolic clearance rates which levelled off not far above GFR in the steady state phase.

3. In experiments which exhibited a low GFR the renal metabolic clearance rate for insulin was in the same absolute range, i.e. twice that of GFR. C-peptide exhibited a renal metabolic clearance rate twice that of GFR, when the latter was in the normal *in vivo* range.

4. Urinary clearances for insulin and C-peptide were greatly elevated above *in vivo* levels, which is associated with the high albumin filtration in this experimental model and is thought to be due to an overloading of protein reabsorbing mechanisms, hindering peptide hormone reabsorption.

INTRODUCTION

The accumulation of polypeptide hormones in uremic plasma demonstrates the kidney's role in peptide hormone catabolism (Feldman & Singer, 1974; Katz & Emmanouel, 1978). Renal catabolism was shown to be responsible for an important fraction of the total metabolic clearance of polypeptide hormones (Ardaillou & Paillard, 1979; Katz & Rubenstein, 1973; Katz & Emmanouel, 1978). The need to quantitatively distinguish between the extrarenal and renal catabolism has prompted the study of renal catabolism alone by means of the isolated perfused kidney (Hruska *et al.*, 1977; Johnson & Maack, 1977; Kau & Maack, 1977; Martin *et al.*, 1977; Rabkin & Kitabchi, 1978). Using this experimental model, Johnson & Maack (1977) demonstrated that the kidneys account for the major fraction of the total plasma turnover of growth hormone (GH) in the rat. Using a filtering and a nonfiltering kidney they were able to establish the main processes associated with renal catabolism of GH, which were shown to occur in the following sequence: glomerular filtration, tubular reabsorption and degradation. Hruska *et al.* (1977) and Martin *et al.* (1977) using an isolated dog kidney and Kau & Maack (1977) with the isolated rat kidney showed that binding of the intact hormone takes place at the peritubular cell side where fragmentation of the hormone also occurs. C-terminal fragments and intact hormone, which are filtered, are taken up at the luminal cell side. Only a small fraction escapes tubular degradation and can be measured in the end urine; this small fraction accounts for the "urinary clearance". Although C-terminal PTH fragments are biologically inactive, radioimmunoassays of PTH mistakenly identify these fragments as PTH, though the relative specificity differs due to the assay antibodies used (Hehrmann *et al.*, 1979; Katz & Emmanouel, 1978).

* Supported by the Deutsche Forschungsgemeinschaft (Schu 343/2, 4).

Recently published work of Rabkin & Kitabchi (1978) demonstrated a reciprocal relationship between luminal and contraluminal uptake of insulin in an isolated perfused rat kidney. As GFRs in these experiments were less than half of the *in vivo* GFR and *in vivo* experiments at normal GFRs show a renal metabolic clearance rate in the range of GFR (Katz & Emmanouel, 1978; Rabkin & Kitabchi, 1978), the aim of this study was to analyze renal catabolism of peptide hormones in an isolated rat kidney preparation at normal GFR. Glomerular filtration rate in an isolated perfused rat kidney depends critically on the oncotic pressure of perfusate. At a normal oncotic pressure of 20–22 mm Hg, a normal GFR can be obtained in this experimental preparation. This was the rationale behind the selection of a 5.5 g/100 ml albumin perfusate in this study (Schurek *et al.*, 1978, 1980; Stolte *et al.*, 1979).

MATERIALS AND METHODS

Experimental animals were male specified pathogen-free Wistar rats (W cryptorchic, Ztm strain) weighing 190–350 g. All animals had free access to food (Atromin® standard pellets) and tap water immediately prior to the experiment. The animals were anesthetized with 100 mg·kg body weight^{-1} Inactin® (Promonta, Hamburg, FRG). All results are normalized to 1 g kidney weight, using the left, decapsulated kidney as weight basis for calculation. To reach a standardized weight basis the left renal artery was ligated before starting perfusion of the right kidney.

Kidney perfusion technique

The operative technique used has been previously described in detail (Schurek *et al.*, 1975, 1976). The surgical approach was a modification of that reported by Weiss *et al.* (1959), and Nishiitsutsuji-Uwo *et al.* (1967). The right kidney was isolated *in situ* and embedded into a temperature-controlled copper chamber on cotton wool. To simplify the surgical procedure, we inserted a double-barrelled perfusion cannula (o.d. 1.45 mm, i.d. 1.0 mm, inner pressure cannula: o.d. 0.5 mm, i.d. 0.3 mm) into the proximally-clamped aorta. Perfusion was initiated by

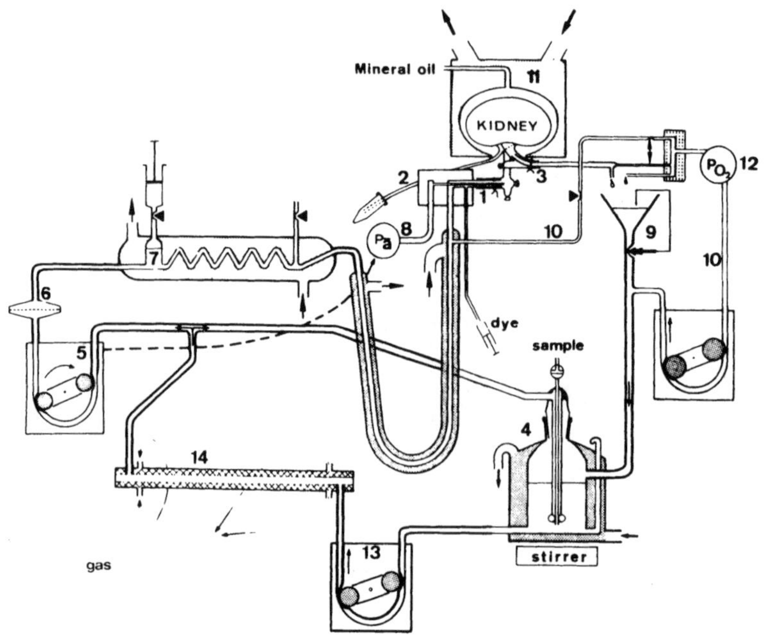

Fig. 1. Schematic diagram of the recirculation perfusion system. 1 = aorta, 2 = ureter, 3 = v. cava, 4 = reservoir, 5 = perfusion pump, 6 = in-line filter, 7 = depulsation chamber, 8 = Statham transducer P23Db, 9 = effluent backflow valve, 10, 12 = bypass for P_{O_2} measurements, 11 = kidney chamber, 13 = pump for driving the oxygenation circuit, 14 = membrane oxygenator. Stippled areas are at 38 C. For dimensions of the cannula see text.

opening the clamp and tying an aortic ligature proximal to the renal artery. The effective perfusion pressure was monitored through the inner cannula and maintained at 100 mm Hg by a servo pump system (Fig. 1). Recirculation was performed through a low-volume membrane oxygenator. The oxygenator was simply constructed from two endplates and the inner frame part of a conventional RP 6 dialyzer. As a membrane we used glassfiber-strengthened silicon 100 μm thick (Detakta, Hamburg, FRG), which was folded around the frame part. To minimize resistance to perfusate flow one side was fitted to the endplate by a 0.3 mm rubber membrane in a frame cut. The end plates were clamped together via two 6 mm thick hard brass plates by 12 U-shaped screw clamps. Filling volume was 6 ml, effective exchange area 775 cm^2. Other parts of the perfusion system are outlined in Fig. 1 and have been previously described in detail (Schurek *et al.*, 1975, 1976; Schurek, 1979; Stolte *et al.*, 1979).

Perfusion medium

As perfusate we used a 5.5 g per 100 ml solution of Cohn fraction V bovine albumin (De Mello & Maack, 1976; Nishiitsutsuji-Uwo, 1967). The perfusate was prepared from a 10 g per 100 ml stock solution of 5 l., predialyzed by an Asahi hollow-fiber dialyzer AM 10 (1.1 m^2) for 8 hr each 2 hr changing dialysate (10 l.). The stock albumin solution was frozen in aliquots of 100 ml after sterile filtration. Buffer composition for dialysis was (mmols$\cdot l^{-1}$): Na^+ 140, K^+ 5, Ca^{2+} 1.25, Mg^{2+} 0.6, Cl^- 106, HCO_3^- 25, HPO_4^{2-} 0.72 and neomycin sulfate 10 mg$\cdot l^{-1}$. An aliquot of the albumin stock was combined with organic compounds to give perfusate (200 ml) with a final composition (mmols$\cdot l^{-1}$): Na^+ 140, K^+ 5, Ca^{2+} 2.5, Mg^{2+} 1.2, Cl^- 100, HCO_3^- 25, HPO_4^{2-} 0.72, urea 6, glucose 8.3, polyfructosan 1 g$\cdot l^{-1}$. Additional substrates used (Schurek *et al.*, 1972, 1975) were (mmols$\cdot l^{-1}$): oxaloacetate 1, pyruvate 2, L-lactate 2, glutamate 2 and the following L-amino acids (De Mello & Maack, 1976) (mmols$\cdot l^{-1}$): methionine 0.5, alanine 2, serine 2, glycine 2, arginine 1, proline 2, isoleucine 1, and aspartic acid 3. As an antidiuretic hormone, pitressin® was added (10 mU$\cdot l^{-1}$). The perfusate was filtered immediately prior to the experiment through a 0.2 μm filter.

Analytical methods and material

Sodium and potassium were analyzed by flame photometry (Il 543 digital flame photometer, Instr. Lab. Inc., Lexington, MA, U.S.A.). Glucose was measured enzymatically by the hexokinase/glucose-6-phosphate dehydrogenase method while polyfructosan was determined by including a hexose–isomerase reaction in the assay (Zwiebel *et al.*, 1969). Methods for the estimation of pO_2 and pH have been previously described (Schurek *et al.*, 1975). h-PTH was extracted and purified from tissue culture of a human parathyroid adenoma (Dorn & Montz, 1977; Dorn *et al.*, 1979). The radioimmunoassay (RIA) for h-PTH was based on the sheep antibody AS 469, which recognizes intact 1–84 hormone and C-terminal fragments (Hehrmann *et al.*, 1976, 1979). C-Peptide was used as the synthetic compound (Novo, Copenhagen, Denmark). For the RIA of C-peptide we used tracer and antibody from Novo. Insulin used was chromatographically pure pig insulin (Novo). For the RIA of insulin (Morgan & Lazarow, 1963) we used tracer and antibody from Hoechst, Frankfurt FRG.

Experimental protocol

After a control perfusion period of 25 min, the peptide hormone was added to a perfusate volume of 100 ml, to reach a concentration range tenfold the *in vivo* value. Five min after hormone administration, 3 clearance periods of 20 min each were performed. Hormone concentration in the perfusate was followed in 5 min intervals for 20 min, thereafter in 10 min intervals. In the insulin experiments, 4 clearance periods, each of 15 min duration were performed.

Calculations

The renal metabolic clearance rate was calculated from the decrease in perfusate immunoreactivity. Calculation

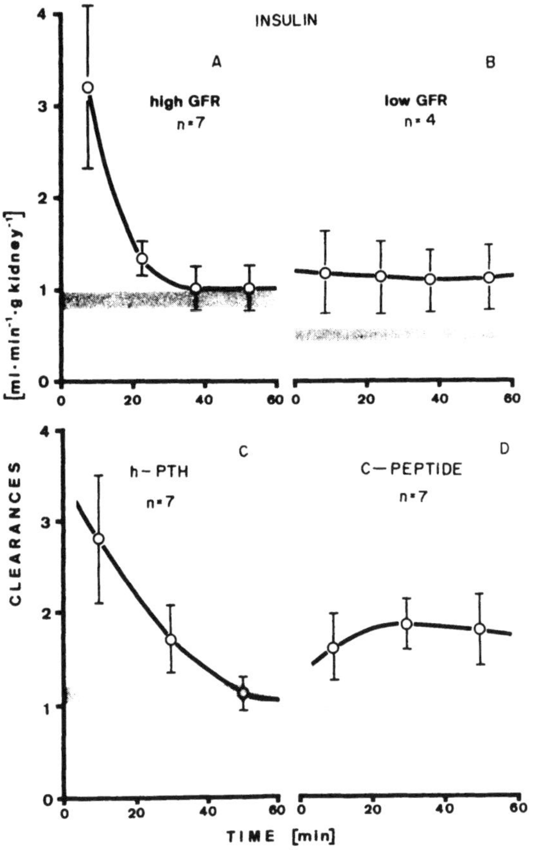

Fig. 2. Renal metabolic clearances of insulin, h-PTH and C-peptide compared to GFR (stippled areas), vs time after the hormone bolus. Hormone application: 25 min after perfusion onset, clearance periods were obtained after 5 more min. Mean values ± SEM.

was corrected for 1 g kidney weight and changes in pool volume:

$$C_{\text{metabolic}} = \frac{V_0 - V}{t}\left[1 - \frac{\ln(C/C_0)}{\ln(V_0/V)}\right]$$

where:

t = duration of clearance period (min)
V_0 = pool volume, initial.
V = pool volume, end of the period.
C_0 = pool concentration, initial.
C = pool concentration, end of the period.

RESULTS

Renal insulin degradation

At normal GFR, renal metabolic clearance for insulin was high initially and levelled off in the subsequent clearance periods as shown in Fig. 2A. The possibility of artifactual results was eliminated since in control experiments without kidney a constant level of immunoreactivity was maintained, confirming the results of Rabkin & Kitabchi (1978). The clearance quotient $C_{\text{Insulin}}/C_{\text{Inulin}}$ was calculated to be 1.23 in the last clearance period, which indicates the major processes in renal catabolism of insulin occur in the following sequence: glomerular filtration—tubular reabsorption—degradation (Bourdeau *et al.*, 1973), when a steady state phase was reached. When GFR was low, as demonstrated in Fig. 2B, the renal metabolic clearance was as high as in the foregoing series, which in this series was twice the inulin clearance rate and indicates a significant fraction of peritubular uptake of insulin. In the study by Rabkin & Kitabchi (1978), comparable results were obtained at a mean GFR below 0.5 ml·g kidney^{-1}·min^{-1}. At normal GFR, the urinary clearance exhibited an increasing fraction of the filtered hormone (Rabkin & Kitabchi, 1978; Schlatter *et al.*, 1979) and reached a rate of larger than 10% of GFR (Table 1). At low GFR, the urinary clearance reached a comparable fraction, which was more than ten times the *in vivo* urinary clearance as reported from humans and in rats (Katz & Emmanouel 1978; Rabkin & Kitabchi, 1978).

Renal PTH degradation

At normal GFR renal metabolic clearance was calculated to be high initially (Fig. 2C), and levelled off to within the range of GFR at a slower rate than observed for insulin. In the initial phase, a significant proportion of h-PTH was taken up from the peritubular cell side. For comparative purposes basic functional data are given in Table 2.

Renal C-peptide degradation

C-Peptide was shown to be significantly degraded from the luminal and peritubular cell side (Katz & Rubenstein, 1973; Katz & Emmanouel, 1978; Rabkin & Kitabchi, 1978). At a normal GFR, comparable results are obtained to those reported by Rabkin & Kitabchi (1978) at low GFR. Renal metabolic clearance rates increased from 1.58 to 1.8 ml·g kidney^{-1}·min^{-1} (Fig. 2D). Increases in urinary clearances were comparable to those of insulin and reached a fraction of 20% of GFR in the last clearance period (Table 2).

DISCUSSION

Renal catabolism of peptide hormones depends mainly on molecular size. Large peptide hormones as erythropoietin are not filtered to a major extent at the glomerular capillary tuft and no arterio–venous extraction has been observed (Ardaillou & Paillard, 1979; Katz & Emmanouel, 1978). Small and medium sized peptide hormones are filtered freely or restricted at the glomerulus in dependence on size and polarity (Ardaillou & Paillard, 1979; Katz & Emmanouel, 1978; Maack, 1975). If arterio-venous extraction exceeds the filtration fraction, it is clear that the hormone is taken up from the peritubular cell side (Ardaillou & Paillard, 1979; Katz & Rubenstein, 1973; Katz & Emmanouel, 1978). The uptake of insulin exceeds the amount of filtered hormone *in vivo*, which seems to be indicative of peritubular uptake. In the isolated perfused rat kidney, uptake was demonstrated to exceed twice the GFR (Rabkin & Kitabchi, 1978). However, when GFR in this model reaches normal *in vivo* levels, the reciprocal relationship between luminal and contraluminal uptake of insulin, as shown by Rabkin & Kitabchi (1978) could be expanded to the normal *in vivo* range if the clearance quotients of the steady state phase are used as a comparison ($C_{\text{Insulin}}/C_{\text{Inulin}}$ = 1.23). It may be speculated that differences from the *in vivo* state may be due to

Table 1. Renal metabolic clearance rate and urinary clearance for insulin at normal and low GFR; vs time. For comparison, relevant functional parameters are added. Mean values ± SEM

Insulin Time (min)	Normal GFR 30–45	45–60	60–75	75–90	Low GFR 30–45	45–60	60–75	75–90
Perfusion flow rate ($ml \cdot g^{-1} \cdot min^{-1}$)	30.3 ± 2.9	37.8 ± 2.7	34.2 ± 2.6	34.3 ± 2.3	28.0 ± 2.7	29.1 ± 3.4	29.2 ± 4.6	29.5 ± 5.4
T_{Na} ($\mu mols \cdot g^{-1} \cdot min^{-1}$)	104 ± 7.9	125 ± 9.2	132 ± 19	117 ± 18	67 ± 7.4	74.5 ± 12.5	75.1 ± 17.4	45.8 ± 20
% Na-reabsorption	92.9 ± 1.6	90.6 ± 1.6	89.4 ± 1.9	89.3 ± 1.9	97.2 ± 0.9	96.5 ± 1.1	91.9 ± 5.7	89.5 ± 8.6
$\dot{Q}_{O_2}$ ($\mu mols \cdot g^{-1} \cdot min^{-1}$)	9.58 ± 0.49	9.78 ± 0.49	9.92 ± 0.47	9.54 ± 0.47	7.55 ± 0.95	7.54 ± 1.33	7.70 ± 2.21	7.39 ± 2.73
C_{Inulin} (GFR) ($ml \cdot g^{-1} \cdot min^{-1}$)	0.76 ± 0.07	0.93 ± 0.08	0.98 ± 0.15	0.86 ± 0.13	0.47 ± 0.05	0.49 ± 0.07	0.46 ± 0.07	0.44 ± 0.15
$C_{Insulin}$ ($ml \cdot g^{-1} \cdot min^{-1}$)	3.22 ± 0.88	1.34 ± 0.19	1.00 ± 0.25	1.02 ± 0.24	1.17 ± 0.39	1.12 ± 0.42	1.07 ± 0.36	1.10 ± 0.36
$C_{Insulin}/C_{Inulin}$	3.97 ± 0.86	1.45 ± 0.18	1.29 ± 0.38	1.23 ± 0.24	2.35 ± 0.58	2.18 ± 0.64	2.22 ± 0.51	2.25 ± 0.39
Urinary clearance ($\mu l \cdot g^{-1} \cdot min^{-1}$)	35 ± 11	58 ± 10	110 ± 21	174 ± 78	39 ± 12	32 ± 13	45 ± 25	56 ± 37
n	7	7	7	7	4	3/4	3/4	3/4

two factors. (1) The high oxygen pressure used in this model may reduce the amount of free SH-groups. (2) The *in vivo* kidney has been shown to extract large amounts of glutathione, a SH-protective agent (Buddecke, 1970; Curthoys *et al.*, 1980; Duckworth, 1976). Therefore, a reduction in glutathione and the increased oxygen pressure may both influence a glutathione–insulin transhydrogenase system in the kidney (Buddecke, 1970), which is thought to be rate limiting for proteolytic hormone degradation. Thus, further studies with manipulation in these systems may show how *in vivo* degradation occurs (Duckworth, 1976).

C-Peptide, which could be shown to be degraded even at normal GFRs with a clearance rate twice that of the GFR is thought to be taken up avidly from both cell sides due to its low molecular weight. Whether there are antiluminal receptor sides facilitating the uptake of this hormone fragment has not been established to date.

The catabolism of PTH is also of increased interest, as this hormone is known to affect the various structures along a normal nephron in different ways (Charbardes *et al.*, 1975). As peritubular fragmentation seems to occur, the fragments produced at this cell side are thought to be filtered and taken up from the luminal cell side in addition to the intact hormone. Therefore, it is difficult to conclude that a major peritubular uptake and degradation of peptides occur when the renal catabolic clearance is found to exceed GFR because measurements of perfusate immunoreactivity include both intact and fragmented hormones. In this experimental series too, a high GFR, comparable to the *in vivo* state may be a prerequisite for the analysis of hormone degradation. Further analysis of hormonal fragments at the end of perfusion may give us more information on the mechanisms involved.

In clinical studies involving kidney transplantation it can be demonstrated that the failure of a transplanted organ is indicated by increasing PTH levels preceding the increase of a freely filtered molecule such as creatinine. This indicates the action of the antiluminal mechanisms in the fragmentation and degrading process (Hehrmann *et al.*, 1979). The increasing urinary clearance of peptide hormones in this experimental model depending upon time, is thought to be due to the high albumin filtration. Albumin clearance was shown to be enhanced (Nishiitsutsuji-Uwo *et al.*, 1967; Schurek *et al.*, 1978; Stolte *et al.*, 1979) and direct analysis by micropuncture methods demonstrated a tenfold increase of the glomerular sieving coefficient for albumin (Schurek *et al.*, 1978, Stolte *et al.*, 1979). A similar phenomenon is known from patients suffering from nephrotic syndrome; namely an enhanced urinary clearance of polypeptide hormones (Maack, 1975) due to an overloading of the tubular reabsorbing capacity.

Table 2. Renal metabolic clearance rate and urinary clearance for h-PTH and C-peptide at normal GFR, vs time. For comparison, relevant functional parameters of the perfused rat kidney are added. Mean values ± SEM

Time (min)	h-PTH 30–50	50–70	70–90	C-peptide 30–50	50–70	70–90
Perfusion flow rate ($ml \cdot g^{-1} \cdot min^{-1}$)	28.8 ± 1.7	30.4 ± 1.8	29.8 ± 2.0	28.5 ± 2.3	28.9 ± 2.3	28.4 ± 2.3
T_{Na} ($\mu mols \cdot g^{-1} \cdot min^{-1}$)	142 ± 9.7	138 ± 13	122 ± 21	118 ± 10	118 ± 8	103 ± 10
% Na-reabsorption	85.2 ± 1.8	84.4 ± 1.8	84.5 ± 3.0	86.0 ± 1.5	85.5 ± 1.4	84.2 ± 2.2
$\dot{Q}_{O_2}$ ($\mu mols \cdot g^{-1} \cdot min^{-1}$)	10.8 ± 0.5	10.8 ± 0.5	10.5 ± 0.5	9.21 ± 0.41	8.66 ± 0.44	7.90 ± 0.46
C_{Inulin} (GFR) ($ml \cdot g^{-1} \cdot min^{-1}$)	1.15 ± 0.09	1.14 ± 0.10	1.00 ± 0.16	0.94 ± 0.08	0.95 ± 0.07	0.84 ± 0.09
$C_{h\ PTH}$ $C_{C\ peptide}$ ($ml \cdot g^{-1} \cdot min^{-1}$)	2.82 ± 0.67	1.84 ± 0.50	0.98 ± 0.17	1.58 ± 0.31	1.85 ± 0.25	1.78 ± 0.34
$C_{h\ PTH}/C_{Inulin}$ $C_{C\ peptide}/C_{Inulin}$	2.71 ± 0.76	1.84 ± 0.62	1.12 ± 0.24	1.65 ± 0.23	1.85 ± 0.19	1.78 ± 0.43
Urinary clearance ($\mu l \cdot g^{-1} \cdot min^{-1}$)	N.M.	N.M.	N.M.	24 ± 9	87 ± 23	200 ± 23
n =	7	7	7	7	7	7

Acknowledgements—We gratefully acknowledge the expert technical assistance of Iris Kilian and the secretarial assistance of Mrs Bahrendt. Dr K. Schindhelm gave valuable advice in the preparation of this manuscript.

REFERENCES

ARDAILLOU R. & PAILLARD F. (1979) Métabolisme rénal des hormones polypeptidiques. *Actualités Nephrologiques de l'Hopital Necker*, pp. 187–205. Flammarion, Paris.

BOURDEAU J. E., CHEN E. R. Y. & CARONE F. A. (1973) Insulin uptake in the renal proximal tubule. *Am. J. Physiol.* **225**, 1399–1404.

BUDDECKE E. (1970) *Grundriss der Biochemie*, 1st edn, p. 315. De Gruyter, Berlin.

CHARBARDÈS D., IMBERT M., CHIQUE A., MONTÉGUT M. & MOREL F. (1975) PTH sensitive adenylate cyclase activity in different segments of the rabbit nephron. *Pflügers Arch. ges. Physiol.* **354**, 229–239.

CURTHOYS N. P., RANKIN B. B. & TSAO B. (1980) Membrane association and orientation of rat renal activities capable of degrading glutathion. *Int. J. Biochem.* **12**, 219–222 (this volume).

DE MELLO G. & MAACK T. (1976) Nephron function of the isolated perfused rat kidney. *Am. J. Physiol.* **231**, 1699–1707.

DORN G. & MONTZ R. (1977) The preparation of human PTH standard from ^{75}Se labelled medium of tissue culture. *Acta endocr., Copenh.* Suppl. **208**, abstract 95.

DORN G., MONTZ R., MOHR H. & DIETEL M. (1979) Further characterization of the h-PTH material P_2 "Hamburg". *Acta endocr.* Suppl. **225**, abstract 403.

DUCKWORTH W. C. (1976) Insulin and glucagon degradation by the kidney—I. subcellular distribution under different assay conditions. *Biochem. biophys. Acta* **437**, 518–530.

FELDMAN H. A. & SINGER I. (1974) Endocrinology and metabolism in uremia and dialysis. A clinical review. *Medicine, Baltimore* **54**, 345–376.

HEHRMANN R., WILKE R., NORDMEYER J. P. & HESCH R. D. (1976) Hochsensitiver, C-terminal-spezifischer Radioimmunoassay für menschliches PTH als Routinemethode. *Dtsch. Med. Wschr.* **101**, 1726–1729.

HEHRMANN R., NORDMEYER J. P., WILKE R. & HESCH R. D. (1979) Radioimmunoassay of human parathyroid hormone. A: Production and characterization of two antisera from sheep. B: Quality control and clinical applicability. *Acta endocr.* (Kbh), submitted for publication.

HRUSKA K. A., MARTIN K., MENNER P., GREENWALT A., ANDERSON C., KLAHR S. & SLATOPOLSKY E. (1977) Degradation of parathyroid hormone and fragment production by the isolated perfused dog kidney. *J. clin. Invest.* **60**, 501–510.

JOHNSON V. & MAACK T. (1977) Renal extraction, filtration, absorption and catabolism of growth hormone. *Am. J. Physiol.* **233**, F185–F196.

KATZ A. J. & RUBENSTEIN A. H. (1973) Metabolism of proinsulin, insulin and C-peptide in the rat. *J. clin. Invest.* **52**, 1113–1121.

KATZ A. J. & EMMANOUEL D. S. (1978) Metabolism of polypeptide hormones by the normal kidney and in uremia. *Nephron* **22**, 69–80.

KAU S. T. & MAACK T. (1977) Transport and catabolism of parathyroid hormone in isolated rat kidney. *Am. J. Physiol.* **233**, F445–451.

MAACK T. (1975) Renal handling of low molecular weight proteins. *Am. J. Med.* **58**, 57–64.

MARTIN K. J., HRUSKA K. A., LEWIS J., ANDERSON C. & SLATOPOLSKY E. (1977) The renal handling of parathyroid hormone. Role of peritubular uptake and glomerular filtration. *J. clin. Invest.* **60**, 808–814.

MORGAN C. R. & LAZAROW A. (1963) Immunoassay of insulin: two antibody system. Plasma insulin levels of normal, subdiabetic and diabetic rats. *Diabetes* **12**, 115–126.

NISHIITSUTSUJI-UWO J. M., ROSS B. D. & KREBS H. A. (1967) Metabolic activities of the isolated perfused rat kidney. *Biochem. J.* **103**, 852–862.

RABKIN R. & KITABCHI A. E. (1978) Factors influencing the renal handling of insulin by the isolated rat kidney. *J. clin. Invest.* **62**, 169–175.

SCHLATTER E., SCHUREK H. J., SCHINDHELM K., ZICK R. & STOLTE H. (1979) Peptide hormones: a comparison of renal handling and dialysis therapy. *Proceedings. EDTA.* Amsterdam 1979.

SCHUREK H. J., BRECHT J. P., BRANDT P., LANGE K., KOLBE H. & KELLER K. (1972) Substrate action on transport and metabolism of the isolated perfused rat kidney. Action of pyruvate, oxaloacetate, butyrate and succinate. *Biochemical Aspects of Renal Function*, (Edited by HOHENEGGER M.) pp. 110–126, Goldmann, München.

SCHUREK H. J., BRECHT J. P., LOHFERT H. & HIERHOLZER K. (1975) The basic requirements for the function of the isolated cell free perfused rat kidney. *Pflügers Arch. ges Physiol.* **354**, 349–365.

SCHUREK H. J., AULBERT E. & EBEL H. (1976) The effect of Ca ion antagonist verapamil on ouabain inhibition of renal sodium reabsorption. Studies in the isolated perfused rat kidney. In *Current Problems in Clinical Biochemistry*, (Edited by SCHMIDT & DUBACH) Vol. 6, pp. 281–288. Huber, Bern.

SCHUREK H. J., SCHWIETZER G., ALT J. & STOLTE H. (1978) Albumin filtration and effective filtration pressure in cortical nephrons in the isolated perfused rat kidney. In *Proceedings of the 7th International Congress of Nephrology*, Montreal, abstract No. 4.

SCHUREK H. J. (1980) Application of the isolated rat kidney in nephrology. *Contributions in Nephrology* Vol. 19, (Edited by STOLTE H. & ALT J. M.) pp. 176–190.

SCHUREK H. J., SCHWIETZER G. & ALT J. M. (1980) Effect of albumin on the hydrodynamics of nephron in perfused rat kidney. *Am. J. Physiol.* Submitted for publication.

STOLTE H., SCHUREK H. J. & ALT J. M. (1979) Glomerular albumin filtration. A comparison of micropuncture studies in the isolated perfused rat kidney with *in vivo* experimental conditions. *Kidney Int.* **16**, 377–384.

WEISS C., PASSOW H. & ROTHSTEIN A. (1959) Autoregulation of flow in isolated rat kidney in the absence of red cells. *Am. J. Physiol.* **196**, 1115–1118.

ZWIEBEL R., HÖHMANN B., FROHNERT P. & BAUMANN K. (1969) Fluorometrisch-enzymatische Mikro- und Ultramikrobestimmung von Inulin und Glucose. *Pflügers Arch. ges. Physiol.* **307**, 127–132.

SYMPOSIUM DISCUSSION

Katz: The perfused kidney should be the ideal system in which to resolve the problem of the excess of whole organ clearance of hormones over the filtered load. However, there is a criticism of this model, i.e. that the blood flow is vastly increased over that *in vivo* so that conclusions about the contribution of the two cell poles may be erroneous. What is your view of this?

Ross: The problem of filtration fraction is to some extent solved by the use of the non-filtering kidney model. In this case, by increasing albumin content and reducing filtration pressure there is no urine production. Under these conditions, you observe what Dr Schurek shows in the early phase of his experiment, a very considerable contraluminal uptake of a number of peptide hormones (Rabkin & Kitabachi, 1978).

Lowenstein: You passed rather rapidly over Dr Rabkin's work, in which he showed considerable uptake of insulin in the perfused kidney which he interpreted to be across the basolateral membrane.

Schurek: The main difference concerns the GFR. At low GFR there may be saturation of receptor sites at an early stage, with subsequent release into the medium.

Ebel: An alternative way to answer the question of the site of entry is to simply measure the binding of PTH to basolateral and brush border membranes. We have collaborated with the group of Dr Hesch and have shown that PTH specifically binds to both types of membranes. Antibody produced to either membrane blocks the PTH binding to the receptor. Thus PTH or its split products may enter the tubular cell from both the contraluminal and luminal side (Hesch R. D. *et al. Contributions in Nephrology* Vol. 13, pp. 104–114. Karger, Basel, 1978).

Schurek: That fits with what is known of PTH degradation in kidney.

Kurokawa: How did you measure PTH degradation?

Schurek: We measured the time course of PTH concentration in the recirculating perfusate. For measurements we used the sheep antibody AS 469 (RIA), as described elsewhere (Hehrmann *et al.*, *Dtsch. Med. Wschr.* **101,** 1736–1729, 1976 and Hehrmann *et al.* Radioimmunoassay of human parathyroid hormone. A: Production and characterization of two antisera from sheep. B: Quality control and clinical applicability. *Acta endocr.*, submitted for publication, 1979). The sheep antibody AS 469 recognizes intact 1–84 hormone and C-terminal fragments.

Chapter 4

Renal work and ATP

Int. J. Biochem., Vol. 12, pp. 243 to 244
© Pergamon Press Ltd 1980. Printed in Great Britain

0020-711X/80/0701-0243$02.00/0

INTRODUCTION

MEASUREMENT OF METABOLISM DURING RENAL WORK

P. DEETJEN
Institut fur Physiologie und Balneologie der Universitat Innsbruck, Fritz-Pregl Strasse 3, Innsbruck, Austria

The topic "measurement of metabolism during renal work" deals with exactly the same question as one of my first papers of almost 20 years ago (Deetjen & Kramer, 1960), when I began to work in renal physiology.

At that time renal physiologists were just beginning to realize that events like "active transport" may take place in the kidney. Thinking along these lines it was not a far step to the assumption that the energy demand for such transport processes may determine renal O_2-consumption.

A hint in this direction was provided by the observation (Fig. 1) that even though O_2-consumption per unit of renal tissue is very high, the arteriovenous O_2-content-difference ($AVDO_2$) is very low. However, it remains constant and independent of renal blood flow as long as the kidney is producing a glomerular filtration rate. When filtration stops, $AVDO_2$ increases inversely to the drop in renal blood flow. Thus, a connection between filtration and O_2-utilization apparently does exist.

More than 90% of the solutes in the glomerular filtrate are sodium salts and most of these salts are reabsorbed together with the solvent when tubular fluid passes through the different sections of the nephron.

It was almost inescapable that our attention became focussed on renal Na-transport and its relation to O_2-consumption. And indeed, there was a clearcut correlation which holds in a great change of experimental variations of Na-load or O_2-delivery (Fig. 2).

When we presented these results it soon became apparent that two other research groups had arrived at the same conclusion. I am very happy that Dr Kiil, who directed one of these groups (Kiil *et al.*, 1961), is with us today and will present the following paper. The other research team was that of Lassen *et al.* (1961) in Copenhagen.

However, when research in subsequent years enlarged our knowledge in many details, the general idea of a close dependence of renal O_2-consumption on active solute transport was confirmed, but it became obvious that the picture is complicated by many influencing and interfering factors.

We now know that not all Na reabsorbed in the kidney undergoes active transport and that the active transport of substances like H^+, Cl^- or glucose contributes significantly to the renal energy requirement. On the other hand, the different parts of the nephron not only metabolize in quite different ways, use different fuels and transport substances in different

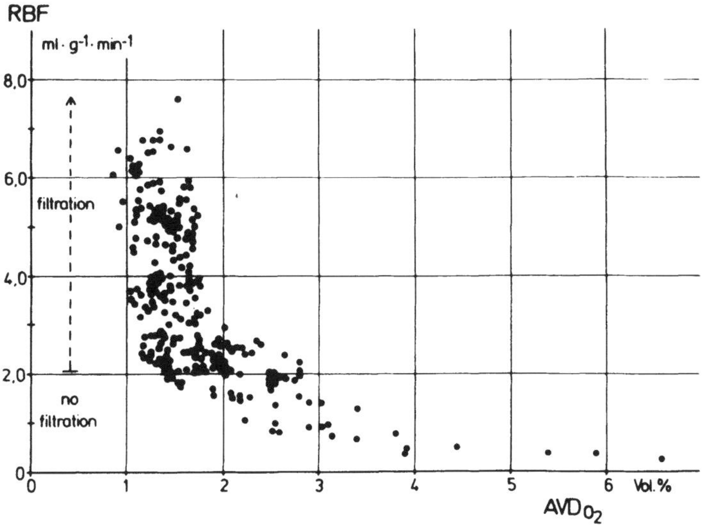

Fig. 1. Relation between renal blood flow (RBF) and arteriovenous oxygen difference ($AVDO_2$) in the dog kidney. The reduction in RBF was experimentally performed by partial occlusion of the renal artery.

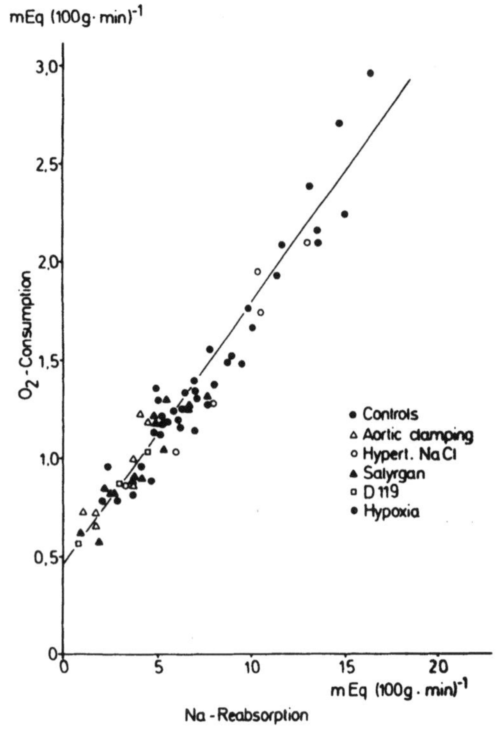

Fig. 2. Relation between renal oxygen consumption and sodium reabsorption under various conditions.

amounts, but also exhibit distinct characteristics and conditions of transport. In the proximal tubule for example, no considerable chemical or electrical gradient influences the transcellular solute flux. Electrolyte transport in this part of the nephron, therefore, can be expected to run rather economically. In more distal parts of the nephron however, chemical as well as electrical gradients require a greater input of energy for the active transport of an equivalent amount of salt.

Thus, the linear correlation between O_2-consumption and sodium transport, which on the basis of equivalents, gives a figure of about 1:30, cannot readily be applied in a calculation of the number of Na ions transported by the energy that is provided by the hydrolization of one molecule of ATP.

To complicate the matter further we have to keep in mind that there exists not only a heterogeneity of metabolic potency in the different parts of one nephron, but that there is also a heterogeneity of metabolism and transport capacity between surface and deeper nephrons. Thus, any overall correlation between total renal energy requirement, metabolism, substance transport, ATP utilization and many other parameters has to be discussed with this reservation in mind.

REFERENCES

DEETJEN P. & KRAMER K. (1960) Na-Rückresorption und O_2-Verbrauch der Niere. *Klin. Wschr.* **14,** 680.

KIIL F., AUKLAND K. & REFSUM H. (1961) Renal sodium transport and oxygen consumption. *Am. J. Physiol.* **201,** 511.

LASSEN N., MUNCK O. & THAYSSEN J. H. (1961) Oxygen consumption and sodium reabsorption in the kidney. *Acta Physiol. scand.* **51,** 371.

Int. J. Biochem., Vol. 12, pp. 245 to 250
© Pergamon Press Ltd 1980. Printed in Great Britain

0020-711X/80/0701-0245$02.00/0

ENERGETICS AND SPECIFICITY OF TRANSCELLULAR NaCl TRANSPORT IN THE DOG KIDNEY

FREDRIK KIIL, OLE M. SEJERSTED and PETTER A. STEEN
University of Oslo, Institute for Experimental Medical Research, Ullevaal Hospital, Oslo 1, Norway

Abstract—1. Ouabain inhibits NaCl reabsorption and oxygen consumption in the dog kidney as expected if transport of sodium by Na-K-ATPase across the peritubular cell membrane was the only energy-requiring transport.

2. The facilitated transport across the luminal cell membrane of NaCl is not specific for chloride, since ouabain and ethacrynic acid inhibit bromide and thiocyanate reabsorption as much as chloride reabsorption.

INTRODUCTION

Na-K-ATPase bound to the cell membrane, pumps sodium out of cells, and *in vivo* and *in vitro* studies on many tissues indicate that three sodium ions are extruded for each ATP split (Bonting & Caravaggio, 1963; Sen & Post, 1964). The basolateral cell membrane of both proximal and distal tubules has a high content of Na-K-ATPase. The simplest conceivable model for transtubular reabsorption is a facilitated, non-energy requiring transport of sodium across the luminal cell membrane, which probably lacks Na-K-ATPase, and an energy requiring transport by Na-K-ATPase across the basolateral membranes. In this model sodium reabsorption varies with changes in the sodium concentration in the cytoplasm close to the basolateral membrane. On the assumption that 6 ATP are generated for each O_2 consumed, the ratios between changes in sodium reabsorption and oxygen consumption would be $\Delta Na/\Delta O_2 = 18$. However, the energetic efficiency of tubular reabsorption of sodium in the kidney as a whole is higher, even if it is assumed that the energy requirements of other transport or metabolic processes do not rise when the tubular reabsorption is raised (Kjekshus *et al.*, 1969).

Studies on the whole kidney indicate that with regard to sodium reabsorption two major tubular cell populations with different characteristics exist. In one system, mainly localized in the proximal tubules, hydrogen ions are exchanged with sodium ions across the luminal cell membrane and the transcellular transport by Na-K-ATPase is restricted to $NaHCO_3$. There is no transcellular NaCl transport in this system. However $NaHCO_3$ extruded into the intracellular space exerts an osmotic force which reabsorbs water and NaCl through the tight junction. This bicarbonate dependent reabsorption of water and NaCl in the proximal tubules does not require energy and accounts for the high $\Delta Na/\Delta O_2$ ratio for the whole kidney (Kiil *et al.*, 1979).

In the diluting segment, osmotic reabsorption can be excluded because the segment is watertight. In this segment NaCl is reabsorbed by the transcellular route. This segment does not reabsorb $NaHCO_3$ whereas NaCl reabsorption can be stimulated by raising sodium concentration in the tubular fluid. Ouabain, a specific inhibitor of Na-K-ATPase, inhibits transcellular sodium reabsorption. In doses compatible with life, ouabain inhibits less than 40% of the total tubular sodium reabsorption during sodium loading.

Sejersted *et al.* (1977) showed in experiments performed during mannitol diuresis in dogs, that NaCl reabsorption and oxygen consumption were reduced by ouabain corresponding to a $\Delta Na/\Delta O_2$ ratio of 14.5 ± 1.3. Because of its vasoconstrictive effect, ouabain reduces glomerular filtration rate (GFR), and hence tubular reabsorption. Measurements were obtained at identical GFR by manipulating the renal perfusion pressure, but an unproven assumption is that the proximal bicarbonate dependent reabsorption of water and NaCl are equal before and after ouabain administration.

These technical shortcomings can now be avoided. After administration of acetazolamide, bicarbonate dependent water and NaCl reabsorption stay constant over a wide range of GFR (Mathisen *et al.*, 1979a). Thus, a reduction in GFR would have no effect on bicarbonate dependent reabsorption. Reductions in sodium reabsorption and oxygen consumption can be completely attributed to the inhibition of Na-K-ATPase activity. The results of such examinations on anaesthetized dogs are reported in the first part of the present study.

A second important question concerning transcellular NaCl reabsorption is, whether the facilitated transport across the luminal cell membrane is specific for chloride (Kiil, 1978). To examine this question we have compared the inhibitory effect of ouabain and ethacrynic acid on chloride, bromide, thiocyanate and iodide reabsorption. Ethacrynic acid was chosen because it may specifically inhibit NaCl transport across the luminal cell membrane (Sejersted *et al.*, 1978).

MATERIALS AND METHODS

Experiments were carried out on mongrel dogs of either sex, weighing from 15 to 23 kg. They were exsanguinated for 300 ml, 2 days before the experiment. The plasma was separated from the red cells and reinfused to increase the renal arteriovenous difference in oxygen saturation (Kiil *et al.*, 1961). Anaesthesia was induced with sodium pentobarbital 25 mg·kg^{-1} intravenously and maintained with additional doses as indicated. Muscle relaxation was obtained with pancuronium bromide 0.2 mg·kg^{-1} and maintained with additional doses of 0.05 mg·kg^{-1}. The dogs were intubated and ventilated with a volume ventilator (modified Cyclator Mark II) to keep a constant P_{CO_2} close to 5 kP during the experiment. Polyethylene catheters were inserted in a femoral vein and artery for infusions, blood sampling and pressure recordings. The tip of the arterial catheter was located just below the origin of the renal arteries and the pressure was recorded by means of a Statham pressure transducer (P23Gb) and a Sanborn amplifier and recorder.

The right kidney was exposed through a retroperitoneal flank incision. The renal vein was cannulated with a soft polyethylene catheter introduced through the contralateral femoral vein. A thin, polyvinyl catheter in the renal artery, the tip pointing upstream, served for infusion of acetylcholine and ouabain. An electromagnetic flowmeter probe (Nycotron, Oslo), fitting the renal artery snugly, permitted continuous recording of renal blood flow (RBF) on the Sanborn recorder. A nylon snare placed on the artery distal to the probe was used for complete occlusion of the artery 3–4 times during the experiment for zero adjustment of the flowmeter reading. The gain of the flowmeter was calibrated according to the RBF values obtained from haematocrit, para-aminohippurate (PAH) clearance and arteriovenous extractions of PAH during three control periods. The ureter was cannulated with a soft polyvinyl catheter. Body temperature was kept constant with the use of heating pads. A priming solution containing inulin (50 mg·kg b.w.$^{-1}$), creatinine (0.04 mg·kg b.w.$^{-1}$) and PAH (120 mg) in 0.9% NaCl solution was injected intravenously, followed by sustained infusion at 2 ml·min^{-1} to obtain arterial plasma concentrations of 20–30 mg per 100 ml, 10–20 mg per 100 ml and 1.0–2.5 mg per 100 ml respectively. $NaBr^{82}$ and NaI^{125} were added to the injectate and infusate to give a stable plasma activity in the individual experiment with a range between experiments of 5000–20,000 counts/min·ml^{-1} and 10,000–30,000 counts/min·ml^{-1} respectively. In the dogs given ethacrynic acid SCN 24 mg·kg^{-1} was added to the injectate and 0.14 mg·kg^{-1}·min^{-1} added to the infusate.

Before control clearance periods 1.5–2 l of 0.9% NaCl was infused intravenously in the course of one hour. The infusate was kept at body temperature, and after this initial volume loading it was infused slightly faster than urine losses. KCl 8–10 mmol·l^{-1}, $CaCl_2$ 3 mmol·l^{-1}, $MgSO_4$ 2 mmol·l^{-1} and KH_2PO_4 1 mmol·l^{-1} were added to all solutions, and additional KCl infused to keep plasma potassium concentration above 4 mmol·l^{-1}. Plasma concentration of bicarbonate was kept constant by infusing $NaHCO_3$ if needed.

Acetazolamide (100 mg·kg b.w.$^{-1}$) was infused intravenously in the course of 3–4 min. After three control clearance periods at steady urine flow, ouabain (90 μg·kg b.w.$^{-1}$) was injected intrarenally in the course of a few minutes in six dogs. To counteract the renal vasoconstrictive effect of ouabain, acetylcholine was infused into the renal artery at a rate of 4 μg·min^{-1} starting before and continuing for at least 10 min after completion of ouabain infusion. These clearance periods were obtained when the haemodynamic changes induced by acetylcholine had subsided.

In the middle of each clearance period before and after ouabain infusion, blood for oxygen determination was collected anaerobically from the artery and renal vein in silicone-treated glass syringes, and oxygen saturation was measured spectrophotometrically using microcuvettes (Refsum & Sveinsson, 1956). Haemoglobin concentration was measured in triplicate with the cyanmethemoglobin method (Hainline, 1958). Oxygen consumption was calculated as previously described (Kiil *et al.*, 1961), but no corrections were made for the oxygen dissolved in urine and renal lymph.

The six dogs not given ouabain received after control clearance periods, ethacrynic acid 3 mg·kg^{-1} intravenously followed by a continuous infusion of 1.5 mg·kg^{-1}·hr^{-1}.

Plasma and urine were analysed for inulin (Rolf *et al.*, 1949) and PAH (Smith *et al.*, 1945) Sodium and potassium were determined on a direct flame photometer using lithium as internal standard (Instrumentation Laboratories I.L. 343). Chloride was measured on a chloride titrator (Radiometer CTN 10). Br^{82} and I^{25} activities were determined in a well-scintillation counter (Selektronik). Blood gases were determined with I.L. electrodes. SCN was determined colourimetrically by an automated modification of Pettigrew and Fell's method (Pettigrew & Fell, 1972).

RESULTS

Energy requirement for transcellular NaCl reabsorption

Table 1 summarizes the effects of acetazolamide and ouabain on renal haemodynamics, electrolyte reabsorption and oxygen consumption. The changes in RBF and GFR induced by ouabain administration were not significant, whereas sodium and chloride reabsorption and renal oxygen consumption were approximately halved. Bicarbonate reabsorption was slightly but significantly reduced. On the assumption that both the inhibition of NaCl reabsorption and $NaHCO_3$ reabsorption were due to reductions in transcellular energy requiring reabsorption, the rates between reductions in sodium and oxygen consumption averaged $\Delta Na/\Delta O_2 = 17.8 \pm 1.5$.

However, if ouabain inhibited the proximal tubular $NaHCO_3$ reabsorption and the bicarbonate dependent water and NaCl reabsorption, two molecules NaCl should be subtracted for each molecule $NaHCO_3$ inhibited (Mathisen *et al.*, 1979b). If this assumption is correct, the average $\Delta Na/\Delta O_2 = 16.6 \pm 1.5$. None of these ratios are significantly different from 18.

Specificity of transcellular NaCl reabsorption

Table 2 summarizes fractional reabsorption of

Table 1. Effect of ouabain on sodium reabsorption and oxygen consumption during acetazolamide infusion

	MABP (mm Hg)	RBF ($ml \cdot min^{-1}$)	GFR ($ml \cdot min^{-1}$)	Na^+ EXCR ($\mu mol \cdot min^{-1}$)	Na^+ REAB ($\mu mol \cdot min^{-1}$)	Cl^- EXCR ($\mu mol \cdot min^{-1}$)	Cl^- REAB ($\mu mol \cdot min^{-1}$)	HCO_3^- EXCR ($\mu mol \cdot min^{-1}$)	HCO_3^- REAB ($\mu mol \cdot min^{-1}$)	O_2 Renal $\dot{V}O_2$ ($\mu mol \cdot min^2$)
Acetazolamide (100 mg·kg b.w.$^{-1}$)	135 ± 7	283 ± 47	41 ± 6	1139 ± 179	4770 ± 733	776 ± 173	4599 ± 715	381 ± 48	474 ± 81	292 ± 48
Ouabain (90 μg·kg b.w.$^{-1}$)	154 ± 9	294 ± 80	37 ± 6	3419 ± 581	1928 ± 357	3154 ± 534	2219 ± 635	474 ± 86	379 ± 74	132 ± 24
Difference	19 ± 10	12 ± 57	−4 ± 2	2281 ± 516	−2842 ± 382	2378 ± 510	−2880 ± 402	93 ± 52	−96 ± 23	−160 ± 30
P	NS	NS	NS	0.025	0.025	0.025	0.025	NS	0.025	0.025

Mean ± SE of experiments in six dogs. Abbreviations: MABP = mean aortic blood pressure; RBF = renal blood flow; GFR = glomerular filtration rate; EXCR = excretion; REAB = reabsorption; Renal $\dot{V}O_2$ = renal oxygen consumption; *P* = probability.

Table 2. Fractional reabsorption of anions

	Thiocyanate	Bromide	Chloride	Iodide
Group I				
Control (C)		0.92 ± 0.04	0.88 ± 0.05	0.69 ± 0.12
Ouabain (O) (90 μg·kg b.w.$^{-1}$)		0.38 ± 0.10	0.35 ± 0.10	0.31 ± 0.07
C − O		0.54 ± 0.09	0.53 ± 0.9	0.38 ± 0.08
O/C		0.41 ± 0.10	0.40 ± 0.10	0.46 ± 0.08
Group II				
Control (C)	0.91 ± 0.04	0.87 ± 0.05	0.82 ± 0.06	0.63 ± 0.07
Ethacrynic acid (E) (3 mg·kg b.w.$^{-1}$)	0.40 ± 0.08	0.36 ± 0.08	0.33 ± 0.06	0.30 ± 0.07
C − E	0.51 ± 0.05	0.51 ± 0.05	0.49 ± 0.04	0.33 ± 0.02
E/C	0.44 ± 0.08	0.41 ± 0.08	0.40 ± 0.06	0.46 ± 0.08

Values are mean ± SE of experiments in six dogs in each of the two groups.

anions. As shown in the upper part of the table, ouabain reduced fractional reabsorption of bromide and chloride to the same extent, whereas the fractional reabsorption of iodine was less reduced. The lower part of Table 2 shows that ethacrynic acid inhibited bromide and thiocyanate reabsorption as much as chloride reabsorption, whereas the inhibitory effect on iodine reabsorption was small.

DISCUSSION

By reducing sodium reabsorption and renal oxygen consumption with ouabain a $\Delta Na/\Delta O_2$ ratio of 17.8 ± 1.5 was obtained. This ratio suggests that the transport across the peritubular cell membrane by Na-K-ATPase of three moles sodium ions for each mol ATP hydrolyzed, is the only energy-requiring step in the transcellular reabsorption of NaCl and that accordingly the transport of NaCl across the luminal cell membrane does not require additional energy.

In our study, bicarbonate reabsorption was also slightly reduced. Transcellular reabsorption of sodium requires the same energy whether chloride or bicarbonate are the accompanying anions (Kiil *et al.*, 1979). However, if $NaHCO_3$ reabsorption in the proximal tubules is inhibited by ouabain, the bicarbonate dependent osmotic reabsorption of water and NaCl would also be inhibited. If this were true, the $\Delta Na/\Delta O_2$ ratio would be slightly higher, and an energy-requiring transport across the luminal cell membrane more probable. However, whereas 1/18 mol of oxygen is consumed for the transport of 1 mol sodium by Na-K-ATPase, our data suggest that the transport across the luminal cell membrane would require less than 1/200 mol oxygen per mol sodium transported. This negligible quantity includes all other energy requiring processes which may be reduced by ouabain administration. Before concluding that transport of NaCl across the luminal cell membrane does not require energy, factors influencing $\Delta Na/\Delta O_2$ are discussed.

The $\Delta Na/\Delta O_2$ ratio is independent of the degree of inhibition. In fact ouabain may stimulate sodium reabsorption by some Na-K-ATPase molecules. By incomplete inhibition, the sodium concentration on the inside of the basolateral membrane would rise and stimulate the activity of the remaining intact molecules. *In vitro* studies suggest that first at concentrations above 50–60 $mmol \cdot l^{-1}$ no further stimulation would be obtained by increasing intracellular sodium concentration. Inhibition of sodium reabsorption by ouabain implies therefore, that intracellular sodium concentration is greatly raised.

In our study the transcellular $NaHCO_3$ reabsorption in the proximal tubules probably was not inhibited at all. The main reason is that the cellular uptake of sodium by the Na^+/H^+ exchange system in the luminal cell membrane may be stimulated by increased supply of $NaHCO_3$, but not by increasing the supply of NaCl (Kiil, 1978). More than 60% of the total amount of Na-K-ATPase is localized in the proximal tubules of dogs (Sejersted *et al.*, 1979). The fractional sodium reabsorption by the bicarbonate dependent system may also be about 60%, but no more than one of three sodium ions are reabsorbed through the cells (Mathisen *et al.*, 1979b). Hence, there is a great surplus of Na-K-ATPase for sodium transport by the bicarbonate dependent system.

Moreover, administration of acetazolamide inhibits $NaHCO_3$ reabsorption and would therefore further reduce the intracellular sodium concentration at the basolateral cell membrane. Inhibition of the bicarbonate dependent sodium transport by ouabain is therefore unlikely, whereas increased delivery of bicarbonate may raise $NaHCO_3$ reabsorption in the distal nephron, and intracellular sodium concentration approaches the saturation level for Na-K-ATPase activity.

Another complication which may influence $\Delta Na/\Delta O_2$ determinations, is the vasoconstrictive effect of ouabain; although it rapidly diminishes, it does not completely disappear. In many studies the inhibitory effect of ouabain on sodium reabsorption has been small because of severe initial vasoconstriction. We solved this problem by infusing ouabain during intrarenal acetylcholine infusion so that the renal vessels are dilated (Lie *et al.*, 1974). Any effect of acetylcholine disappears when the infusion is stopped, whereas the effect of ouabain lasts for hours in dogs. Although RBF recovers, GFR may be more permanently reduced, suggesting persisting intrarenal vasoconstriction. The vasoconstrictive effect may not be evenly divided between all nephrons. Nephron heterogeneity may accordingly be evoked by ouabain.

Increased nephron heterogeneity would, however, have no consequence for the interpretation of the $\Delta Na/\Delta O_2$ ratio. In nephrons with reduced GFR, delivery of NaCl to the diluting segment would be small, whereas it would be high in super-perfused nephrons. Because of the direct proportionality between sodium transport and energy requirement, nephron heterogeneity would not alter the $\Delta Na/\Delta O_2$ ratio. For the same reason, the $\Delta Na/\Delta O_2$ ratio is not dependent on whether ouabain inhibits transcellular NaCl reabsorption completely or incompletely.

The assumption that the oxygen consumption can be taken as an index of ATP generation requires some qualifications. Many naturally occuring substances, such as glycine, glucagon and dopamine, may stimulate renal energy metabolism unrelated to sodium reabsorption (Johannesen *et al.*, 1976, 1977). Elevation of plasma concentration of fatty acids increases oxygen consumption of the heart without increasing its mechanical performance but we have, in an unpublished study, found no evidence of similar effects on renal metabolism.

A more important problem is whether anaerobic metabolism is stimulated. A translation from $\Delta Na/\Delta O_2$ to $\Delta Na/\Delta ATP$ would be impossible if the diluting segment had significant anaerobic metabolism. In our study haematocrit was reduced by bleeding two days prior to the experiment to ensure reliable measurements of renal oxygen consumption. By this procedure GFR and RBF are not reduced because RBF is much larger than necessary for nutritional purposes. There is no release of lactate, as may be encountered when RBF is greatly reduced by constricting the renal artery. Ouabain infusion reduces lactate consumption to insignificant levels. Net release of lactate may increase, although anaerobic metabolism is unlikely. Even if lactate release was the consequence of anaerobic metabolism, the maximal error due to lactate production would be 3–4% in the determination of the $\Delta Na/\Delta O_2$ ratio.

Under conditions of inadequate oxygen supply, as in isolated preparations perfused with oxygenated Ringer solutions, competition between sodium transport and other energy-requiring processes might well exist. Under such conditions the limited supply of oxygen would become available for other purposes after reduction of sodium reabsorption. Consequently, a spuriously high $\Delta Na/\Delta O_2$ ratio would be obtained by ouabain inhibition.

Our study showed that the facilitated transport of NaCl across the luminal cell membrane is not specific for chloride, since ouabain or ethacrynic acid inhibited reabsorption of bromide and thiocyanate as much as chloride reabsorption. Facilitated co-transport across the luminal cell membrane may be energized by the electrochemical potential created by the Na-K-ATPase activity in the basolateral cell membrane. Such a mechanism was postulated by Frizzell *et al.* (1975) for transport of NaCl into the cells of rabbit gallbladders. One condition for such a postulate is that the ratio between extra and intracellular concentrations is higher for chloride than for sodium. In their preparation, intracellular concentrations averaged $66 \pm 3\,mmol \cdot l^{-1}$ for sodium and $84 \pm 3\,mmol \cdot l^{-1}$ for chloride. The ratio between intracellular chloride and sodium concentrations is probably even higher in the diluting segment, but intracellular measurements during high rates of NaCl reabsorption are not available.

A second condition for co-transport of sodium and chloride ions is, that no additional energy is required. Martin & Diamond (1966) examined the energy metabolism of the rabbit gallbladder and found that only 9% of the oxygen uptake of the isolated gallbladder seems to be used for NaCl transport, and that the $\Delta Na/\Delta O_2$ ratio is 25. As already pointed out, a spuriously high $\Delta Na/\Delta O_2$ ratio would be obtained if there is a lack of substrate or oxygen. No conclusions can therefore confidently be drawn from these data concerning the energetics of coupled NaCl transport.

These objections do not apply to the present study. We conclude that NaCl transport across the luminal cell membrane is energized by the Na-K-ATPase mediated transport of sodium across the peritubular cell membrane; the coupled NaCl transport across the luminal cell membrane is not specific for chloride.

Thus, during saline loading the Na-K-ATPase mediated transport across the peritubular cell membrane is the rate limiting step for transcellular NaCl reabsorption, whereas the bicarbonate dependent osmotic NaCl reabsorption in the proximal tubules is not affected. Measurements of heat production in the cortex and outer medulla support this conclusion. The maximal capacity for transcellular NaCl reabsorption is reached when 15–20% of the filtered load is excreted (Monclair *et al.*, 1978). The capacity is greatly reduced at plasma potassium concentrations below $2\,mmol \cdot l^{-1}$ whereas hypokalemia as well as ouabain are without effect on the bicarbonate dependent water and NaCl reabsorption (Monclair *et al.*, 1980).

SUMMARY

During acetazolamide infusion proximal bicarbonate dependent reabsorption of water and NaCl does not vary during variations in GFR over a wide range. To examine the energy requirement of transcellular NaCl reabsorption, ouabain ($90\,\mu g \cdot kg$ b.w.$^{-1}$) was injected into the renal artery of anaesthetized dogs after acetazolamide administration. Ouabain injection halved sodium reabsorption and oxygen consumption. The ratio between the changes, 17.8 ± 1.5, is not different from the ratio expected for Na-K-ATPase mediated sodium transport. Bromide and thiocyanate reabsorption was inhibited as extensively as chloride reabsorption by ouabain or ethacrynic acid. Thus, Na-K-ATPase transport across the basolateral membrane facilitates transport across the luminal cell membrane of sodium together with chloride and other permeable ions without additional energy requirement.

Acknowledgements—The skilled technical assistance of Miss Ann Kristin Andresen, Mrs Åshild Salvesen, Mrs Grethe Laerum, Mrs Anna Croucher and Ove Moen is gratefully acknowledged.

This study was supported by the Norwegian Research Council for Science and the Humanities, the Norwegian Council on Cardiovascular Diseases, Anders Jahre's Fund for the Promotion of Science, and Professor Carl Semb's Medical Research Fund.

REFERENCES

Bonting S. L. & Caravaggio L. L. (1963) Studies on sodium-potassium-activated adenosinetriphosphatase—V. Correlation of enzyme activity with cation flux in six tissues. *Archs Biochem. Biophys.* **101**, 37–46.

Frizzell R. A., Dugas M. C. & Schultz S. G. (1975) Sodium chloride transport by rabbit gallbladder. *J. gen. Physiol.* **65**, 769–795.

Hainline A. (1958) Hemoglobin In *Standard Methods of Clinical Chemistry*, 1st edn, Vol. 2, pp. 49–68. Academic Press, New York.

Johannesen J., Lie M. & Kiil F. (1977) Effect of glycine and glucagon on glomerular filtration and renal metabolic rates. *Am. J. Physiol.* **233**, F61–F66.

Johannesen J., Lie M., Mathisen Ø. and Kiil F. (1976) Dopamine-induced dissociation between renal metabolic rate and sodium reabsorption. *Am. J. Physiol.* **230**, 1126–1131.

Kiil F., Monclair T. & Mathisen Ø. (1979) Energy requirement for sodium reabsorption in the proximal tubules. *Upsala J. med. Sci.* Supplement **26**, 38.

Kiil F., Aukland K. & Refsum H. E. (1961) Renal sodium transport and oxygen consumption. *Am. J. Physiol.* **201**, 511–516.

Kiil F. (1978) Principles of active sodium reabsorption in the kidney. *Scand. J. clin. Lab. Invest.* **38**, 597–602.

Kjekshus J., Aukland K. & Kiil F. (1969) Oxygen cost of sodium reabsorption in proximal and distal parts of the nephron. *Scand. J. clin. Lab. Invest.* **23**, 307–316.

Lie M., Sejersted O. M., Raeder M. & Kiil F. (1974) Comparisons of renal responses to ouabain and ethacrynic acid. *Am. J. Physiol.* **226**, 1221–1226.

Martin D. W. & Diamond J. M. (1966) Energetics of coupled active transport of sodium and chloride. *J. gen. Physiol.* **50**, 295–315.

Mathisen Ø., Holdaas H. & Kiil F. (1979a) *Scand. J. clin. Lab. Invest.* **39**, 297–301.

Mathisen Ø., Monclair T., Raeder M. & Kiil F. (1979b) Coupling of $NaHCO_3$ and NaCl reabsorption in dog kidneys during changes in plasma P_{CO_2}. *Am. J. Physiol.* **236** (3), F232–F239.

MONCLAIR T., MATHISEN Ø. & KIIL F. (1978) Characteristics of transcellular NaCl reabsorption in the kidney. *Scand. J. clin. Lab. Invest.* **38**, 615–626.

MONCLAIR T., SEJERSTED O. M. & KIIL F. (1980) Influence of plasma potassium concentration on the capacity for sodium reabsorption in the diluting segment of the kidney. *Scand. J. clin. Lab. Invest.* **40**, 27–36.

PETTIGREW A. R. & FELL G. S. (1972) Simplified colorimetric determination of thiocyanate in biological fluids, and its application to investigation of the toxic amblyopias. *Clin. Chem.* **18**, 996–1000.

REFSUM H. E. & SVEINSSON S. L. (1956) Spectrophotometric determination of hemoglobin oxygen saturation in hemolyzed whole blood. *Scand. J. clin. Lab. Invest.* **8**, 67–70.

ROLF D., SURTSHIN A. & WHITE H. L. (1949) A modified diphenylamine procedure for fructose or inulin determination. *Proc. Soc. exp. Biol. Med.* **72**, 351–354.

SEJERSTED O. M., MATHISEN Ø. & KIIL F. (1977) Oxygen requirement of renal Na-K-ATPase-dependent sodium reabsorption. *Am. J. Physiol.* **232**, (2), F152–F158.

SEJERSTED O. M., HOLDAAS H. & MONCLAIR T. (1978) Functional differences of ouabain and ethacrynic acid on renal potassium metabolism in dogs. *Scand. J. clin. Lab. Invest.* **38**, 603–614.

SEJERSTED O. M., NICOLAYSEN A., MONCLAIR T. & NICOLAYSEN G. (1979) Distribution of ouabain binding sites along the dog nephron. *Acta physiol. scand.* In press.

SEN A. K. & POST R. L. (1964) Stoichiometry and localization of adenosine triphosphate dependent sodium and potassium transport in the erythrocyte. *J. biol. Chem.* **239**, 345–353.

SMITH H. W., FINKELSTEIN N., ALIMINOSA A. L., CRAWFORD B. & GRABER M. (1945) The renal clearances of substituted hippuric acid derivatives and other aromatic acids in dog and man *J. clin. Invest.* **24**, 388–404.

Int. J. Biochem.. Vol. 12. pp. 251 to 255
0020-711X/80/0701-0251$02.00/0

COMPETITION BETWEEN DIFFERENT METABOLIC DEMANDS FOR OXYGEN CONSUMPTION IN THE KIDNEY

P. SILVA, R. HALLAC, R. SWARTZ and F. H. EPSTEIN
Department of Medicine and Thorndike Laboratory, Harvard Medical School and Beth Israel Hospital, Boston, MA, U.S.A.

Abstract—1. Experiments were done in isolated perfused rat kidneys. When sodium reabsorption (TNa) was increased 42% by raising the pressure of perfusion and thereby increasing glomerular filtration rate 39% oxygen consumption (QO_2) remained unchanged (3.7 vs 3.4 mmol. $min^{-1}.g^{-1}$).

2. In kidneys where gluconeogenesis was stimulated by pretreatment with methylprednisolone (3 mg per 100 g i.m. for 3 days) gluconeogenesis fell 77% when TNa was increased 58% while QO_2 remained constant.

3. Inhibition of gluconeogenesis with 3-mercaptopicolinate (0.15 mM) resulted in an 18% in QO_2 when TNa was increased by 56%.

4. These experiments indicate that TNa and gluconeogenesis can compete for energy requirements in the kidney. The renal tubular cells appear to be able to borrow from non-transport energy requiring processes to pay for the cost of transport.

INTRODUCTION

During the last two decades many investigators have studied the relation between renal energy consumption and function by measuring the relation between oxygen consumption and sodium reabsorption (Deetjen & Kramer, 1961; Kjekshus *et al.*, 1969; Knox *et al.*, 1966; Kramer & Deetjen, 1960; Lassen *et al.*, 1961; Thurau, 1961; Torelli *et al.*, 1966). The chief way in which the relation between sodium reabsorption and energy utilization has been explored has been by measuring the reduction in oxygen consumption after sodium reabsorption has been reduced, either by reducing its filtered load or by inhibiting reabsorption with diuretics. In all of these reports a linear relation between energy consumption and sodium reabsorption has been observed. Implicit in these studies has been the concept that sodium reabsorption is the major energy requiring function of the kidney and therefore, that changes in oxygen consumption associated with changes in sodium reabsorption can be taken to represent the energy cost of sodium reabsorption (Kjekshus *et al.*, 1969).

It seems possible that the linear relation between oxygen consumption and sodium reabsorption observed in such studies might reflect a combination of processes. As the energy required for sodium reabsorption decreases, other energy-requiring processes might also vary in a proportionate manner, thus leading to incorrect conclusions about the energy cost of transport. In the present experiments, oxygen consumption by the isolated perfused rat kidney has been studied during marked changes in glomerular filtration and sodium reabsorption produced by altering perfusion pressure. The effects of these changes in transport on a major non-transport function, gluconeogenesis, has also been measured. The results indicate that changes in sodium reabsorption are not always accompanied by parallel changes in oxygen consumption, since "basal", non-transport energy requirements may be altered by changes in transport.

MATERIALS AND METHODS

Experimental animals

Male rate weighing 300–400 g were used in all experiments. The animals were allowed free access to food (Purina Rat Chow®) and water until the day of the experiment. Animals treated with methylprednisolone were given a dose of 3 mg per 100 g of body weight i.m. for 3 consecutive days prior to the day of the experiment.

Experimental design

The basic experimental protocol consisted of perfusion of an isolated kidney at a constant pressure of either 110 or 150 mm of Hg from the beginning of the experiment. The kidney was obtained from either a control rat or one that had been pre-treated with methylprednisolone for 3 days. Since during the initial minutes of perfusion (usually under 5) the kidney undergoes vasodilatation the pressure was constantly manually adjusted to the desired value. After a control period of 30 min, the pressure was either increased to 150 mm of Hg from 110 or reduced to 110 from 150, and observations continued for an additional thirty minutes. Oxygen consumption, gluconeogenesis, glomerular filtration rate and sodium reabsorption were measured at 10 min intervals. In experiments with control kidneys the pressure was raised to 140 mm of Hg after the first 30 min at 110 and lowered back to the initial pressure after the experimental period.

Isolated rat kidney perfusions

Perfusion of the right kidney was performed according to the technique described by Nishiitsutsuji-Uwo *et al.* (1967) as modified by Ross *et al.* (9). The animals were anesthetized with pentobarbital i.p. (60 mg·kg^{-1}). Heparin, 1000 units, was injected into the femoral vein. The peritoneal cavity was opened and a PE 10 catheter placed in the right ureter. A glass arterial cannula was inserted into the superior mesenteric artery and threaded across the aorta into the right renal artery. Perfusion was started while the cannula was still in the mesenteric artery avoiding thereby any ischemia to the kidney. The kidney was then removed and placed in a constant temperature cabinet where temperature was kept at 37°C. Perfusion medium was recirculated continuously with pulsatile flow at the pressures already stated. Rate of flow of the perfusate was measured using an in-line Brooks® flowmeter installed in series in the arterial line. Perfusion medium consisted of a Krebs–Ringer–Henseleit solution containing ($mM \cdot l^{-1}$) Na 143; Cl 103; K 4.5; Bicarbonate 25; Ca 2.5; Mg 1.2; Phosphate 1.2, at a pH of 7.4 when gassed with 5% CO_2 95% O_2, and bovine serum albumin at a concentration of 6.7 g%. The albumin solution was initially prepared at a 13 g% concentration and dialyzed for 48 hr against a volume 10 times larger of Krebs–Ringer–Henseleit in a Gambro® dialyzer. This procedure allows ultrafiltration and therefore the concentration of the albumin can be kept constant. Two different substrates were used. In the experiments with kidneys obtained from control rats glucose 5 mM was added as the sole exogenous substrate. In the experiments with kidneys obtained from methylprednisolone treated rats pyruvate 5 mM was used as the only substrate.

Oxygen consumption

Oxygen tension was measured using a polarographic (Radiometer®) oxygen electrode maintained at the same temperature as the perfused kidney. Samples for oxygen tension of arterial perfusate were obtained anaerobically with a glass syringe from a self-sealing catheter installed in the arterial line just proximal to the glass arterial cannula. Samples for oxygen tension of venous perfusate were taken anaerobically inside the inferior vena cava with a plastic tipped glass syringe. Care was taken to avoid sampling the perfusate close to the external opening of the vena cava. Renal oxygen consumption was calculated using the arteriovenous oxygen tension difference and the rate of perfusate flow through the kidney.

Gluconeogenesis

Glucose was measured in both plasma and urine using hexokinase (Slien, 1965). The results are expressed in mmols of glucose generated per g of wet kidney weight. The rate of production of glucose was calculated from the rate of change in the total amount of glucose in the recirculating medium. The total amount of glucose in the recirculating medium at the end of each clearance period was calculated from the volume of perfusate and the concentration of glucose at every collection period. Volume of perfusate for every period was calculated back from the final measured volume, the sampling volume, the urine volume and the evaporative loss of water. Due allowances were made for the amount of glucose lost when sampling the recirculating medium and for losses in the urine (the latter was negligible).

Glomerular filtration rate and sodium excretion

Glomerular filtration rate was determined by the clearance of radioactive inulin. Sodium was measured in the perfusate and in the urine by flame photometry and sodium excretion and reabsorption calculated using standard formulas.

Substrates, inhibitors and expression of the results

Glucose and pyruvate were obtained from Sigma Chemical Company and stored as 1 M stock solution in a −20°C freezer. 3-mercaptopicolinate (a gift from Smith, Kline and French Laboratories) was dissolved in Krebs–Ringer–Henseleit immediately before its use and added to the recirculating perfusate at an approximate concentration of 0.15 mM.

Experiments in which for technical reasons no urine flow was established or no stable baseline was obtained in the first 30 min of perfusion were discarded.

RESULTS

Effect of increasing sodium reabsorption on oxygen consumption

(a) *Normal kidneys.* Altering the pressure of perfusion in the isolated perfused rat kidney is followed by parallel changes in glomerular filtration rate and, by consequence, in the filtered load of sodium and the amount of sodium reabsorbed by the tubules. When the pressure of perfusion is raised from 110 to 140 mm of Hg the glomerular filtration rate rises an average of 39% and the rate of sodium reabsorption increases 42%. Oxygen consumption, however, remains relatively constant (Table 1). Reducing the pressure of perfusion to 110 mm of Hg results in a decrease in glomerular filtration rate to the initial values and a similar drop in the rate of sodium reabsorption. Oxygen consumption again remains constant. Lactate formation was not changed by either the increase or the decrease in pressure. These experiments show that a substantial increase in reabsorptive work has occurred in the kidney at apparently no additional cost. Either transport has become suddenly more efficient or the energy derived from oxygen utilization has been diverted to reabsorptive transport from other energy-requiring cellular functions.

(b) *Kidneys in which gluconeogenesis has been stimulated.* There are other energy requiring functions of the kidney among which gluconeogenesis is not only one of the most important but also easy to measure. We have shown previously that when gluconeogenesis is stimulated it can compete with sodium reabsorption for the energy available to the cell (Silva *et al.*, 1975). Accordingly, the effect of increasing sodium reabsorption on oxygen consumption was studied in kidneys in which gluconeogenesis had been stimu-

Table 1. Effect of increasing pressure on perfusion on glomerular filtration rate, sodium reabsorption and oxygen consumption in isolated perfused rat kidneys. Glucose 5 mM was used as the sole exogenous substrate. Values are mean ± SE (6).

	GFR ($ml \cdot min^{-1} \cdot g^{-1}$)	T_{Na} ($\mu Eq \cdot min^{-1} \cdot g^{-1}$)	QO_2 ($\mu mol \cdot min^{-1} \cdot g^{-1}$)
Control (110 mm Hg)	0.36 ± 0.07	48 ± 6	3.7 ± 0.2
Pressure increased (140 mm Hg)	0.50 ± 0.06	68 ± 8	3.4 ± 0.3
Δ	0.14 ± 0.05*	19 ± 6*	−0.3 ± 0.3
Pressure decreased (110 mm Hg)	0.33 ± 0.03	45 ± 4	3.4 ± 0.2
Δ	−0.18 ± 0.05*	−22 ± 7*	−0.1 ± 0.2

* $P < 0.01$

Table 2. Sodium reabsorption, oxygen consumption, glucose and lactate production in isolated perfused kidneys obtained from methylprednisolone treated rats. Five representative experiments

Experiment No.	Pressure of perfusion (mm Hg)	T_{Na} (μEq·min^{-1}·g^{-1})	QO_2 (μmol·min^{-1}·g^{-1})	Glucose production (μmol·min^{-1}·g^{-1})	Lactate production (μmol·min^{-1}·g^{-1})
1	110	17	2.5	0.83	0.65
	150	40	2.7	0.19	0.56
2	150	68	3.4	0.48	0.40
	110	21	3.4	0.85	0.38
3*	110	41	4.3	0.76	0.70
	110	40	3.6	0.18	0.65
4†	110	20	1.9	0.18	0.46
	150	44	2.3	0.12	0.42
5	110	14	3.2	0.90	0.87
	110	13	3.1	0.80	0.80

* 3-mercaptopicolinate was added after the initial control period.
† 3-mercaptopicolinate was added at the beginning of the perfusion.

lated by pre-treatment with methylprednisolone. As shown in representative experiments in Table 2, increasing the pressure of perfusion from 110 to 150 mm of Hg in these kidneys also results in a rise in sodium reabsorption. Oxygen consumption does not change substantially while glucose production decreased. Lactate production remained constant.

Reducing the pressure of perfusion in kidneys of similarly treated rats results in the reverse effects (Table 2). Sodium reabsorption decreases and glucose production increases while oxygen consumption does not change. As in the experiments with normal kidneys, lactate production remained constant.

Effect of inhibiting gluconeogenesis

(a) *On oxygen consumption.* If the energy requirements of gluconeogenesis are reflected in the net oxygen consumption of the isolated perfused rat kidney, inhibiting gluconeogenesis while other factors remain constant should decrease renal oxygen consumption. In Et. 3 of Table 2, after 30 min of perfusion, gluconeogenesis was inhibited with 3-mercaptopicolinate, an inhibitor of phosphoenolpyruvatecarboxykinase (DiTullio *et al.*, 1974). Glucose production decreased to very low levels accompanied by a parallel decrease in oxygen consumption confirming that glucose synthesis in the kidney requires oxidative metabolism. In this experiment neither sodium reabsorption nor lactate production changed.

(b) *On the relationship between sodium reabsorption and oxygen consumption.* When gluconeogenesis was blocked with 3-mercaptopicolinate from the beginning of the experiment, increasing the pressure of perfusion resulted in a rise in sodium reabsorption that was now accompanied by a sharp rise in oxygen consumption. Glucose production, considerably lower than in previous experiments, did not change and neither did lactate production (Table 2, Expt. 4).

DISCUSSION

In marked contrast with the published experiments in which sodium reabsorption was progressively decreased (Deetjen & Kramer, 1961; Kjekshus *et al.*, 1969; Knox *et al.*, 1966; Kramer & Deetjen, 1960; Lassen *et al.*, 1961; Thurau, 1961; Torelli *et al.*, 1966), the experiments reported here show that there is no linear relation between the absolute amount of sodium reabsorption and oxygen consumed. Both in kidneys obtained from normal rats and also in those of methylprednisolone treated rats a large increase in the absolute amount of sdoium reabsorbed is not accompanied by a parallel rise in oxygen consumption. That oxygen consumption remains constant when sodium reabsorption is increased suggests that the increment is reabsorbed without additional cost or that sodium reabsorption now proceeds through a process that demands less energy. Alternatively, it is possible that when the amount of sodium that requires transport is suddenly increased, the renal tubular cells reallocate their available pool of energy to sodium reabsorption from other energy requiring processes. The experiment in kidneys obtained from methylprednisolone treated rats appear to support this. When the amount of sodium reabsorbed was increased, glucose production decreased in parallel while oxygen consumption remained unchanged. Only when gluconeogenesis was blocked was it possible to observe a parallel rise in oxygen consumption accompanying the increment in sodium reabsorption.

This observation is consistent with previous observations of regulation of cellular metabolic processes by energy availability. For example, when the availability of ATP in the renal cortex was reduced by ischemia the uptake of glucose was increased (Hems & Brosnan, 1970). Similarly, in kidney cortex slices, gluconeogenesis from glycerol or dehydroxyacetonephosphate was inhibited by the addition of respiratory chain poisons (Newsholme & Underwood, 1966). In both these examples, the underlying phenomenon is the rapid decline in cellular ATP levels, decreasing ATP available for gluconeogenesis and increasing the demands on the glycolytic pathway. The mechanism of changes in the direction of flow of energy over intracellular metabolic pathways may be complex, involving allosteric regulation of enzyme activities.

Since the ATP cost of gluconeogenesis is known, it is of interest to calculate the balance of ATP spared by the decrease in gluconeogenesis when sodium reabsorption was increased in experiment 1 in Table 2.

The decrease in glucose production would have spared 3.8 ATP which correlates reasonably well with the 3.9 ATP needed for the extra reabsorption of sodium. The assumptions made in this calculation are that 6 mols of ATP are generated per mol of oxygen consumed and that 35 mols of sodium are reabsorbed per mol of oxygen consumed. Appreciating that these assumptions are not rigorously proven, the figures are nevertheless consistent enough to lend support to the contention that under the conditions of these experiments the renal tubular cells show the ability to allocate available energy to different energy requiring processes upon demand.

In summary, these experiments indicate that, at least in the isolated perfused rat kidney, in which non-transport energy requirements utilize a substantial fraction of total oxygen consumption, "basal" oxygen consumption cannot be considered to remain constant as transport is varied. Rather, energy required for transport can be "borrowed" from that used for non-transport functions.

Acknowledgements—The excellent technical assistance of Miss Katherine Spokes and Mrs Pravina Patel is gratefully acknowledged.

This study was supported by grants AM 17199 and AM 18078 of the U.S.P.H.S. Dr Patricio Silva is an Established Investigator of the American Heart Association.

REFERENCES

DEETJEN P. & KRAMER K. (1961) Die Abhangigkeit des O_2-Verbrauchs der Niere von der Na Ruckresorption. *Archs Ges. Physiol.* **273**, 636–650.

DITULLIO N. W., BERKOFF C. E., BLANK B., KOSTOS V., STACK E. J. & SAUNDERS H. L. (1974) 3-mercaptopicolinic acid: an inhibitor of gluconeogenesis. *Biochem. J.* **138**, 387–394.

HEMS D. A. & BROSNAN J. T. (1970) Effect of ischaemia on content of metabolites in rat liver and kidney in vivo. *Biochem. J.* **120**, 105–111.

KJEKSHUS J., AUKLAND K. & KIIL F. (1969) Oxygen cost of sodium reabsorption in proximal and distal parts of the nephron. *Scand. J. clin. Lab. Invest.* **23**, 307–316.

KNOX F. G., FLEMING J. S. & RENNIE D. W. (1966) Effect of osmotic diuresis on sodium reabsorption and oxygen consumption of kidney. *Am. J. Physiol.* **210**, 751–759.

KRAMER K. & DEETJEN P. (1960) Beziehungen des O_2-Verbrauchs der Niere zur Durchblutung und Glomerulusfiltrat. *Archs Ges. Physiol.* **271**, 782–796.

KREBS H. A., SPEAKE R. N. & HEMS R. (1965) Acceleration of renal gluconeogenesis by ketone bodies and fatty acids. *Biochem. J.* **94**, 712–720.

LASSEN N. A., MUNCK O. & THAYSEN J. H. (1961) Oxygen consumption and sodium reabsorption in the kidney. *Acta Physiol. scand.* **51**, 371–384.

NEWSHOLME E. A. & UNDERWOOD A. H. (1966) The control of glycolysis and glyconeogenesis in kidney cortex. *Biochem. J.* **99**, 24c–26c.

NISHIITSUTSUJI-UWO J. M., ROSS B. D. & KREBS H. A. (1967) Metabolic activities of the isolated perfused rat kidney. *Biochem. J.* **103**, 852–862.

ROSS B. D., EPSTEIN F. H. & LEAF A. (1973) Sodium reabsorption in the perfused rat kidney. *Am. J. Physiol.* **225**, 1165–1171.

SILVA P., STOFF J., ROSS B. D. & EPSTEIN F. H. (1975) Relation between sodium transport and gluconeogenesis in the isolated perfused rat kidney. *Kidney Int.* **8**, 490.

SLIEN M. W. (1965) D-Glucose determination with hexokinase and glucose-6-phosphate dehydrogenase. In *Methods of Enzymatic Analysis.* (Edited by BERGMEYER H. U.) pp. 117–123. Academic Press, New York.

THURAU K. (1961) Renal Na-reabsorption and O_2 uptake in dogs during hypoxia and hydrochlorothiazide infusion. *Proc. Soc. expt. Biol. Med.* **106**, 714–717.

TORELLI G., MELLA E., FAELLI A. & COSTANTINI S. (1966) Energy requirements for sodium reabsorption in the *in vivo* rabbit kidney. *Am. J. Physiol.* **211**, 576–580.

UNDERWOOD A. H. & NEWSHOLME E. A. (1967) Control of glycolysis and gluconeogenesis in rat kidney cortex slices. *Biochem. J.* **104**, 300–305.

WILLIAMSON J. R., BROWNING E. T., SCHOLZ R. A., KREISBERG R. A. & FRITZ I. B. (1968) Inhibition of fatty acid stimulation of gluconeogenesis by (+)-decanoylcarnitine in perfused rat liver. *Diabetes* **17**, 194–208.

SYMPOSIUM DISCUSSION

Trimble: Are there any concommitant changes in perfusate flow rate associated with the drugs you use or the pressure changes you induced in these experiments?

Silva: There is a change in flow with changing pressure; the kidney doesn't autoregulate.

Katz: How do the changes in oxygen consumption correspond to the changes in metabolic rate or sodium reabsorption which you describe?

Silva: I was a little too embarrased to show that slide, because they correspond exactly!

Guder: I think there are observations in the literature which are in complete agreement with your suggestion that gluconeogenesis and sodium reabsorption in the proximal tubule use the same ATP. Thus, if you stimulate gluconeogenesis *in vitro* with some hormones, such as PTH, cyclic AMP, catecholamines, or as we have recently shown, with angiotensin II, you observe a 50% increase in glucose synthesis from lactate and pyruvate, without any increase in oxygen consumption. All these substances have been shown in microperfusion experiments to inhibit sodium reabsorption in proximal tubules. On the other hand your observation should not be taken to be generally true for gluconeogenesis as an energy consuming process. While this is the case for lactate and pyruvate, gluconeogenesis from either glutamine or proline actually yields energy (by the oxidation of the extra carbon, beyond the 3 carbons from each molecule converted to glucose, Eds.), so that I would predict that you would not see these effects when you use glutamine as the substrate.

Silva: I agree, that is why we have used pyruvate as carbon source. However, the rate of glutamine oxidation in perfused kidneys is rather low, and insufficient to support adequate sodium reabsorption.

Kiil: Do you think that this competition is only present when the supply of substrates is limited, as in your preparation? It may not apply to the kidney *in vivo* where a great variety of substrates is available.

Silva: It is difficult for me to answer that question from our own studies with individual substrates, but Dr Guder's comment that the phenomenon may occur in other tissue preparations is relevant. It may not apply in vivo when cells are loaded with a variety of substrates.

Ross: If I may make an alternative suggestion for the interpretation of the data which you have shown us: You observe a decrease in the rate at which glucose accumulates in the perfusion medium. This may either be a decrease in the rate of gluconeogenesis or could represent an increase in the rate of glucose consumption. By increasing perfusion pressure, and increasing total sodium reabsorption, you may be increasing the rate of medullary glycolysis.

Silva: That is possible but there are still other alternatives, such as transferring sodium load to other regions of the kidney.

Alleyne: In the experiments in which glucose was the only substrate, did glucose consumption increase in proportion to the increased oxygen consumption?

Silva: We did not measure glucose consumption.

Weiner: My question relates to both Dr Silva's and Professor Kiil's work. Your data suggests that basal metabolism is not a constant, because "basal" metabolism is competing with transport metabolism for available energy sources. If this is so, then the use of the Δ Na/Δ O_2 ratio as an index of the efficiency of sodium transport may not be strictly valid. In fact, it may give a very false idea of the efficiency of sodium transport because conditions which would raise the basal metabolism rate would flatten the curve and actually raise the Δ Na/Δ O_2 ratio, making sodium transport look more efficient than it really is. I wonder if you have a comment on that, or whether Prof Kiil has a comment, since he uses the Δ Na/Δ O_2 ratio in his analysis of the efficiency of bicarbonate and sodium reabsorption.

Silva: My only comment would be to be entirely in agreement with you. This point has concerned us for some time. Indeed our paper at Reisensburg 2 years ato (Swartz *et al.* In *Biochemical Nephrology*, p. 123, Huber, Bern, 1978) showed that basal oxygen consumption was not a fixed entity.

Kiil: We never tried to distinguish between basal metabolism and the other part of metabolism in the kidney. The concept of basal metabolism was introduced by Barcroft (Feature in the *Architecture of Physiological Function*, Cambridge University Press, 1934). There is no evidence that basal metabolism is altered when Na-K-ATPase activity is increased in the intact kidney. Probably all intermediary metabolic steps required to provide the energy for extra sodium transport may be activated, but we are unable to distinguish between these two types of metabolism.

Weiner: My point is that for a long time you have been saying that the Δ Na/Δ O_2 is greater than 20, and that suggests that there is a more efficient type of sodium transport in kidney than say in toad bladder or other tissues in which the ratio is less than 18. What Dr Silva and Epstein's work suggests is that the ratio may be high because the curve is flattened by an increase in the rate of basal metabolism as sodium transport is inhibited. Thus, as you give ouabain, or decrease the glomerular filtration rate and decrease sodium transport there would be a concurrent increase in the rate of other metabolic processes which require ATP. That would raise the intercept and make the curve look flatter, and make one think that sodium transport is a more efficient process in the kidney than it is in other tissues. In this way you could obtain a Δ Na/Δ O_2 ratio of 40 or 50. In the perfused kidney, I have obtained ratios close to infinity because of this flattening of the curve. Now this doesn't mean that the process of sodium transport is becoming less efficient, it just reflects the increasing basal metabolism. The question is, does the ratio Δ Na/Δ O_2 really mean anything at all in the kidney?

Schurek: This may be true. If you compare kidney perfusions conducted with a single substrate with those with several substrates, the oxygen consumption may be doubled, with constant sodium transport. If you increase sodium transport, the rate of oxygen consumption will not be parallel, and the curve flattens. This may be Dr Silva's observation. It may mean that there are processes such as gluconeogenesis, which are highly efficient at low perfusion pressures, and less efficient at higher sodium loads.

Kinne: Well, I should like to stress that we are still faced with the problem of heterogeneity of the kidney in trying to work out the energetics of sodium transport. These discussions may, therefore, not be getting at the true point. What we really would like to do is to measure in one segment of the kidney the active component of transport. Here I should like to remind you that Professor Ullrich always makes the point that in the proximal tubule about 70% of the sodium transport is passive and 30% is active; after correcting for that, the Δ Na/Δ O_2 ratio that you find comes down to the ratio you find in other tissues. I was glad to see that Dr Kiil, by his methods, now gets down to the same point for the proximal tubule. I have a question for Dr Kiil concerning the diluting segment. You mentioned that thiocyanate, bromide and iodide are transported in this segment. Is this thiocyanate transport also inhibited by furosemide? The high permeability of thiocyanate might give a high rate of NaCNS entry by electrical coupling but not by molecular coupling like Na-chloride or Na-iodide.

Kiil: We did not check furosemide, but tested ethacrynic acid and ouabain. The anion order was the same for both inhibitors. I should like to come back to the question raised by Dr Weiner whether sodium transport becomes more efficient because it reduces other types of metabolism. We find that the transcellular transport of sodium requires the same energy, whether it occurs in the diluting segment or in the proximal tubules (Mathisen *et al.*, *Am. J. Physiol.*, In press). $NaHCO_3$ transport requires the same energy as transport of NaCl in the distal tubule, whereas NaCl transport is free in the proximal tubule, because it is an intercellular transport in this segment (Mathisen *et al. Am. J. Physiol.* **236**, F232, 1979). Now let us say that your idea of the energetics may be as good as mine. But you have to explain a number of other phenomena, such as glomerulotubular balance, osmotic diuresis and isosmotic transport. It is the hypothesis which covers most facts which should be examined first.

Epstein: I have a question which concerns your model of the proximal tubule in which the rate of sodium reabsorption was limited by Na:H^+ exchange, but sodium was then pumped out of the cell as sodium bicarbonate, by Na-K-ATPase. Now in the perfused rat kidney, it appears that ouabain does not interfere with Na-bicarbonate reabsorption, but your model would predict that ouabain, by paralysing Na-K-ATPase would limit Na-bicarbonate reabsorption in the dog. I want to ask you whether in the dog, it does?

Kiil: There are as many Na-K-ATPase sites per mm. length of the proximal tubule as there are in the diluting segment. But only one third of the sodium is going through the cells in the proximal tubules (Kiil, *Kidney Int.* **11**, 153, 1977). Therefore there is a surplus of Na-K-ATPase. If we block say 70% of the enzyme, the remaining 30% may do the job. It is very difficult *in vivo* to give ouabain in sufficiently high doses. But under special conditions with high bicarbonate reabsorption caused by high P_{CO_2} we can block 10–20% of Na-bicarbonate reabsorption with ouabain. Under ordinary experimental conditions we are unable to block bicarbonate reabsorption by ouabain at all.

Epstein: You think the reason is that you are not blocking all of the Na-K-ATPase?

Kiil: That's right.

Schwartz: In brain or heart slices there may be a contribution of an electroneutral Ca^{2+}:Na exchange, so that if one inhibits the sodium pump with ouabain, building up sodium there is often an increase in oxygen consumption, both basal and active, due perhaps to an influx of calcium or an increase of ADP. Is this the case in kidney?

Kinne: Well we have a Na^+:Ca^{2+} exchange system in the basolateral membranes, known from membrane work, but I don't know if that has been followed very carefully in the slice.

Schwartz: Oxygen consumption may increase. I am just thinking of that in terms of the question of the peculiar Na/Oxygen ratio....

Epstein: You are postulating that oxygen consumption may increase in response to calcium accumulation; that is an interesting idea.

Int. J. Biochem., Vol. 12, pp. 257 to 261
0020-711X/80/0701-0257$02.00/0

THE USE OF AN UNCOUPLING AGENT TO INVESTIGATE THE REGULATION OF ACTIVE SODIUM TRANSPORT*

MICHAEL W. WEINER
Stanford University Medical Services, Veterans Administration Medical Center, Department of Medicine, 3801 Miranda Avenue (111X), Palo Alto, CA 94304, U.S.A.

Abstract—1. In studies with toad bladders, the uncoupling agent 2,4-dinitrophenol (DNP) reversed the inhibition of CO_2 production produced by direct inhibition of transport.

2. In contrast, DNP did not reverse the inhibition of CO_2 production brought about by metabolic inhibitors.

3. Therefore, the response to DNP distinguished between inhibition of transport and metabolism; this approach may be useful for the investigation of factors that regulate active transport.

INTRODUCTION

The transport of solutes across biological membranes against electrochemical gradients requires energy provided by the metabolic oxidation of substrates. It is generally accepted that ATP is the link between transport and metabolism (Lipmann, 1941; Weiner & Maffly, 1978). According to this view (Fig. 1), ATP is generated by oxidative metabolism and glycolysis; the ATP is utilized by the Na-K-ATPase for ion transport (Hokin & Dahl, 1971), producing ADP. The balance of adenine nucleotides, represented by the phosphorylation state ($ATP/ADP \cdot P_i$) regulates the rate of electron transport (Chance & Williams, 1956; Wilson *et al.*, 1974). It has also been observed that the processes of metabolism and transport are tightly coupled (Weiner & Maffly, 1978; Zerahn, 1956; Cohen & Barac-Nieto, 1973). Direct inhibition of metabolism by respiratory inhibitors such as cyanide (Huf *et al.*, 1975; Strickler & Kessler, 1963) or antimycin A (Strickler & Kessler, 1963) indirectly inhibits sodium transport. Conversely, direct inhibition of sodium transport with ouabain also decreases the rate of metabolism (Coplon & Maffly, 1972). The close relationship between metabolism and transport is thought to be due to the phenomenon of "respiratory control", a term used to indicate that the rate of metabolism is regulated by the phosphorylation state (Chance & Williams, 1956).

COUPLING OF OXIDATIVE METABOLISM AND TRANSPORT
MECHANISM OF 2,4 DINITROPHENOL

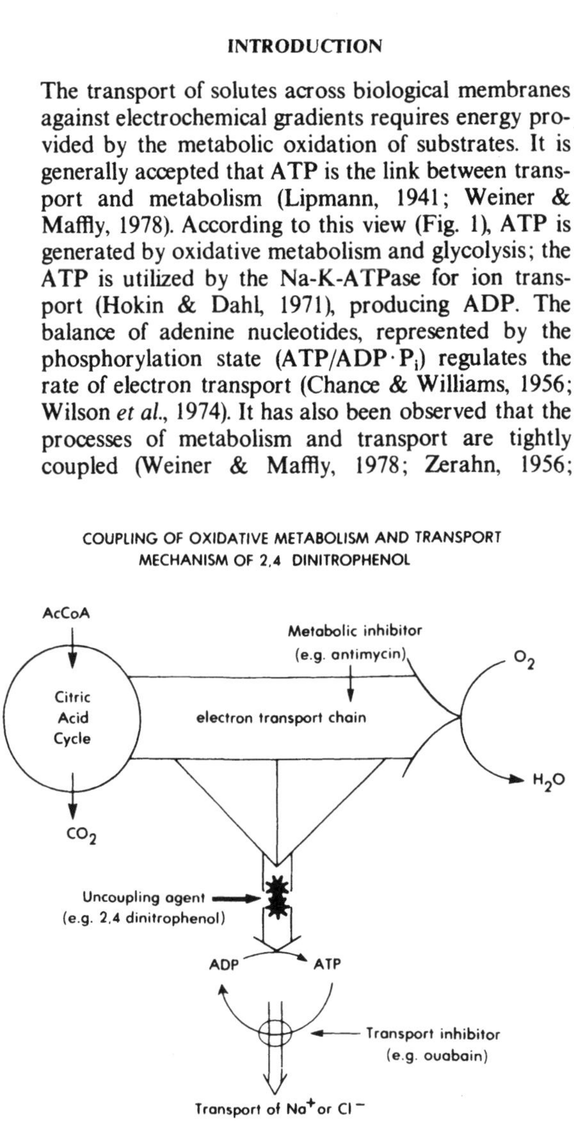

Fig. 1.

A wide variety of physiological factors and pharmacological agents affect active transport and metabolism, but the tight coupling between transport and metabolism has made it difficult to determine their primary site of action. For example, aldosterone stimulates active sodium transport and metabolism (Leaf, 1965). Whether the primary action of this hormone is to stimulate transport directly (Leaf, 1965; Schmidt *et al.*, 1975) or to increase the energy available for transport (Fanestil *et al.*, 1968) continues to be controversial. Similarly, diuretics have been shown to inhibit Na-K-ATPase (Duggan & Noll, 1965; Hook & Williamson, 1965) as well as metabolic pathways which produce energy (Manuel & Weiner, 1976, 1977; Cunarro & Weiner, 1978), but the tight coupling between transport and metabolism has obscured the primary mechanism of these drugs.

The rationale of the present investigation is depicted in Fig. 1. The oxidation reduction reactions of the citric acid cycle generate reducing equivalents which are carried down the electron transport chain to oxygen. The energy produced by electron transport is utilized for ATP synthesis. Metabolic inhibitors inhibit the oxidation-reduction reactions of the citric acid cycle or the respiratory chain (Hochster *et al.*, 1972). In contrast, ouabain directly inhibits Na-K-ATPase (Hokin & Dahl, 1971). The present experiments are based on the well-characterized respiratory-stimulating properties of uncoupling agents to distinguish between direct inhibition of metabolism and direct inhibition of transport. As shown in Fig. 1, inhibition of transport would reduce respiration through the presence of respiratory control, by dimin-

* Portions of this work have been reported elsewhere (Weiner 1979, 1980; Weiner & Winder 1980).

ishing the utilization of ATP. The subsequent addition of an uncoupling agent would be expected to stimulate respiration under these conditions. In contrast, direct inhibition of the reactions of the citric acid cycle or the respiratory chain would reduce respiration and secondarily diminish transport because of diminished ATP production. The subsequent addition of an uncoupling agent would not be expected to stimulate respiration because in this circumstance, respiration is directly limited by the inhibitor, rather than indirectly through the process of respiratory control.

The present experiments were designed to test this rationale with agents known to specifically inhibit active transport or energy metabolism. Experiments using this rationale were then performed to study the mechanism of action of diuretics, and the effects of potassium removal.

MATERIALS AND METHODS

Dominican toad bladders were mounted as a diaphragm between two halves of a glass chamber especially designed for the simultaneous determination of short circuit current (SCC) and CO_2 production (QCO_2). Electrical measurements were made with matched calomel half cells connected to the bathing solutions by 0.11 M KCl–agar bridges. The SCC was applied across the bladder with Ag–AgCl half cells and KCl–agar bridges. The PD was continuously maintained at zero with Mecrolab voltage clamps. The SCC and QCO_2 were recorded continuously on an 8-channel strip-chart recorder. Hemibladders with an initial SCC of less than 50 μA were discarded. The rate CO_2 production by the hemibladders was continuously measured using a modification of the technique described by Coplon *et al.* (1977). This apparatus simultaneously measured the SCC and QCO_2 of four hemibladders. Experiments were performed on paired experimental and control hemibladders obtained from the same toad.

Unless otherwise noted, all experiments were performed using a phosphate-buffered (bicarbonate-free) amphibian Krebs Ringer solution with 10 mM glucose used as the substrate. To prevent growth of bacteria which generate CO_2, the solutions were filtered with 0.20 μm pore size filter and penicillin (0.1 $mg \cdot ml^{-1}$), streptomycin (0.1 $mg \cdot ml^{-1}$) and polymixin B (0.01 $mg \cdot ml^{-}$) were added. All inhibitors were added to both the serosal and mucosal bathing solutions with a syringe and needle through a rubber serum cap.

Experimental design

Initial readings were made after a 30–60 min equilibration period. Then the appropriate compound was added to both mucosal and serosal bathing solutions of the experimental bladders, or the solutions were changed as indicated. To insure that the response to the inhibitor was complete, 30–60 min were allowed to elapse before DNP was added to achieve a final concentration of 10^{-5} M. Measurements were continued for another 30–60 min. Inhibitors were not added to control bladders. However, when DNP was added to the experimental hemibladders, DNP was also added to the control bladders. This allowed a comparison of the response to DNP between the control and experimental hemibladders.

During each experiment, the SCC was continuously monitored in μA, and the QCO_2 was continuously measured in μl per hr per hemibladder. In order to compare the experimental hemibladders with their respective controls, the following formulae were used:

$$\frac{\frac{SCC_t}{SCC_0}\ \text{Experimental}}{\frac{SCC_t}{SCC_0}\ \text{Control}} \times 100 = \%\ \text{control SCC}$$

$$\frac{\frac{QCO_{2_t}}{QCO_{2_0}}\ \text{Experimental}}{\frac{QCO_{2_t}}{QCO_{2_0}}\ \text{Control}} \times 100\%\ \text{control}\ QCO_2$$

Where:

SCC_t = SCC determined at time t

SCC_0 = Initial SCC

QCO_{2_t} = CO_2 production determined at time

QCO_{2_0} = Initial CO_2 production.

Table 1. Effects of inhibitors followed by DNP on respiration

Type of inhibition	Sodium transport after inhibition (SCC % Control)	Respiration after inhibition (QCO_2 % Control)	Respiration after inhibition and DNP (QCO_2 % Control)
Transport inhibition			
Ouabain (10^{-3} M) (n = 12)	40 ± 8***	78 ± 9***	115 ± 12***
Sodium removal† (n = 8)	10 ± 5***	87 ± 3**	93 ± 5
Open circuiting‡ (n = 8)	0	84 ± 2***	114 ± 8
Metabolic inhibition			
Rotenone (10^{-5} M) (n = 9)	54 ± 9***	58 ± 5***	35 ± 7***
Antimycin (10^{-5} M) (n = 9)	45 ± 8***	53 ± 7***	28 ± 6***
Glucose-removal§ (n = 8)	71 ± 4***	76 ± 3***	90 ± 4*

All data is expressed as the mean ± SE. The calculation of % control is given in methods. The inhibitors were applied to the experimental hemibladders, whereas DNP was applied to both experimental and control hemibladders. Asterisks indicate that experimental values are significantly different from control values. (*$P < 0.05$, **$P < 0.01$, ***$P < 0.001$).

† Sodium removal indicates that the mucosal Ringer solution was replaced with a sodium-free (choline) Ringer solution.

‡ Open circuiting indicates that the short circuit current was abolished.

§ Glucose removal indicates that the mucosal and serosal Ringer solutions were replaced with a glucose-free incubation solution.

Table 2. Effects of diuretics and potassium removal, followed by DNP on respiration

Type of inhibition	Sodium transport after inhibition (SCC % Control)	Respiration after inhibition (QCO_2 % Control)	Respiration after inhibition and DNP (QCO_2 % Control)
Amiloride (10^{-4} M) ($n = 4$)	0	85 ± 3**	102 ± 4
Furosemide (5×10^{-4} M) ($n = 9$)	62 ± 19***	86 ± 4***	93 ± 11
Ethacrynic acid (5×10^{-5} M) ($n = 9$)	81 ± 7**	94 ± 23	89 ± 13
Ethacrynic acid (5×10^{-4} M) ($n = 11$)	27 ± 2***	79 ± 6**	55 ± 20***
Potassium-removal† ($n = 8$)	16 ± 5***	59 ± 6**	107 ± 8

All data is expressed as the mean ± SE. Experimental maneuvers were performed on experimental hemibladders, whereas DNP was applied to both experimental and control hemibladders. Asterisks indicate that experimental values are significantly different from control (*$P < 0.05$, **$P < 0.01$, ***$P < 0.001$).

† Potassium removal indicates that the serosal Ringer solution was replaced with potassium-free Ringer solution.

All data are expressed as mean ± SEM. Student's t-test and the paired t-test were used to determine significance. When the term significant is used in the text, it refers to statistical significance ($P < 0.05$).

RESULTS AND DISCUSSION

The first six sets of experiments were designed to test the rationale presented in the Introduction. Table 1 shows that when active sodium transport was directly inhibited with ouabain, by removal of sodium from the serosal solution, or by turning off the short circuit current, sodium transport and respiration were significantly inhibited. However, after the addition of DNP to both experimental and control hemibladders, the rate of respiration was the same, or even greater (in the case of ouabain and open circuiting) in the experimental than in the control hemibladders. Thus, direct inhibition of transport did not inhibit DNP-stimulated respiration.

The lower three sets of experiments in Table 1 show that direct inhibition of metabolism also inhibits sodium transport and respiration. However, after addition of DNP, the respiratory rate was significantly reduced below control. These results contrast with the transport inhibition experiments, and demonstrate that direct inhibition of metabolism significantly inhibits DNP-stimulated respiration.

It is therefore proposed that these findings provide support for the rationale that the respiratory response to DNP can distinguish between direct inhibition of transport and direct inhibition of metabolism.

The experiments presented in Table 2 were designed to utilize this rationale to investigate the mechanism by which diuretics and potassium removal inhibits active transport and metabolism.

Amiloride (10^{-4} M) inhibited sodium transport and reduced respiration, but had no effect on DNP-stimulated respiration. This is consistently with its generally accepted property to inhibit passive sodium diffusion across the mucosal membrane. Furosemide (5×10^{-4} M) also inhibited sodium transport and respiration, but had no significant effect on DNP-stimulated respiration; this suggests a direct pharmacological effect on active transport. A relatively low concentration (5×10^{-5} M) of ethacrynic acid did not significantly inhibit DNP-stimulated respiration, whereas a higher concentration (5×10^{-4} M) did prevent maximal stimulation of QCO_2. This is consistent with the idea that an SH-reactive compound may have a multiplicity of effects, depending upon its concentration.

The relevance of the present findings to the pharmacological action of ethacrynic acid and furosemide on the kidney is uncertain. There are several important differences between the effects of diuretics on toad bladders and on the kidney. Firstly, ethacrynic acid and furosemide primarily inhibit active chloride transport by the thick ascending limb of Henle (Burg *et al.*, 1973; Burg & Green, 1973) while in the present work the diuretics inhibited sodium transport by the toad bladder. Chloride transport by Columbian toad bladders has been reported (Soboslai *et al.*, 1977), but this process appears to be qualitatively different from chloride transport by the loop of Henle. Secondly, higher concentrations of the diuretics are necessary to inhibit sodium transport by toad bladders than those concentrations which inhibit chloride transport in the thick ascending limb. Nevertheless, the present experiments demonstrate that ethacrynic acid and furosemide are capable of directly inhibiting an active transport process in an intact epithelial tissue.

Removal of potassium from the serosal medium inhibits transport and metabolism. The finding that DNP-stimulated respiration was not inhibited (Table 2), supports the idea that serosal potassium availability is necessary for the transport of sodium out of the cell (Essig & Leaf, 1963; Robinson & Knight, 1976).

Experiments with agents which directly stimulate metabolism (i.e. addition of pyruvate) or directly stimulate transport (i.e. a serosal-negative potential difference) indicate that the respiratory response to uncoupling agents can also distinguish between direct stimulation of metabolism and direct stimulation of transport. These results suggest that the use of uncoupling agents may prove to be useful in the investigation of a wide variety of phenomena which regulate biological work functions.

SUMMARY

Agents that directly inhibit sodium transport secondarily reduce the rate of metabolism. Conversely, agents that directly inhibit energy metabolism cause a secondary inhibition of active transport. The aim of the present investigation was to distinguish between these two effects with an uncoupling agent, 2,4-dinitrophenol (DNP). The rates of sodium transport (TNa) and CO_2 production (QCO_2) by paired urinary hemibladders from Dominican toads were simultaneously measured. Ouabain, which directly inhibits sodium transport, inhibited TNa and QCO_2 of toad hemibladders; the subsequent addition of DNP stimulated QCO_2 to a rate similar to that of the control hemibladders. The metabolic inhibitors antimycin A and rotenone also inhibited TNa and QCO_2; in contrast to the results with ouabain, the subsequent addition of DNP did not stimulate QCO_2 in the presence of antimycin A or rotenone. Therefore, the respiratory response to DNP clearly distinguishes between direct inhibition of metabolism and direct inhibition of active transport. The diuretics amiloride (10^{-4} M), furosemide (5×10^{-4} M), and ethacrynic acid (5×10^{-5} M) did not affect DNP-stimulated respiration, consistent with a direct inhibition of active transport. Higher concentrations of ethacrynic acid (5×10^{-4} M) did reduce DNP-stimulated respiration. Removal of potassium from the serosal bathing solution also did not affect DNP-stimulated respiration, suggesting a direct inhibition of transport. These experiments suggest that the present approach may be useful for the investigation of the mechanism of action of drugs, hormones and other biological phenomena.

REFERENCES

BURG M., STONER L., CARDINAL J. & GREEN N. (1973) Furosemide effect on isolated perfused tubules. *Am. J. Physiol.* **225,** 119–124.

BURG M. & GREEN N. (1973) Effects of ethacrynic acid on the thick ascending limb of Henle's loop. *Kidney Int.* **4,** 301–309.

CHANCE B. & WILLIAMS G. R. (1956) The respiratory chain in oxidative phosphorylation. *Adv. Enzymol.* **17,** 65–134.

COHEN J. J. & BARAC-NIETO M. (1973) Renal metabolism of substrate, in relation to renal function. In *Handbook of Physiology,* Section 8, (Edited by ORLOFF J. & BERLINER R. W.) pp. 912–916. American Physiological Society, Washington, DC.

COPLÒN N. S. & MAFFLY R. H. (1972) The effect of ouabain on sodium transport and metabolism of the toad bladder. *Biochim. biophys. Acta* **282,** 250–254.

COPLON N. S., STEELE R. E. & MAFFLY R. H. (1977) Interrelationships of sodium transport and carbon dioxide production by the toad bladder: response to changes in mucosal sodium concentration, to vasopressin and to availability of metabolic substrate. *J. Membr. Biol.* **34,** 289–312.

CUNARRO J. A. & WEINER M. W. (1978) Effects of ethacrynic acid and furosemide on respiration of isolated kidney tubules: the role of ion transport and the source of metabolic energy. *J. Pharmac. exp. Ther.* **206,** 198–206.

DUGGAN D. E. & NOLL R. M. (1965) Effects of ethacrynic acid and cardiac glycosides upon a membrane adenosinetriphosphatase of renal cortex. *Archs Biochem. Biophys.* **109,** 388–396.

ESSIG A. & LEAF A. (1963) The role of potassium in active transport of sodium by the toad bladder. *J. gen. Physiol.* **46,** 505–515.

FANESTIL D. D., HERMAN T. S., FIMOGNARI G. M. & EDELMAN A. (1968) Oxidative metabolism in aldosterone regulation of sodium transport. In *Regulatory Functions of Biological Membranes.* (Edited by JARNEFELT J.) Elsevier, Amsterdam.

HOCHSTER R. M., KATES M. & QUASTEL J. H. (1972) *Metabolic Inhibitors,* Vol. 3. Academic Press, New York.

HOKIN L. E. & DAHL J. L. (1971) The sodium-potassium adenosine-triphosphatase. In *Metabolic Pathways,* 3rd edn, Vol. 6, pp. 270–315. Academic Press, New York.

HOOK J. B. & WILLIAMSON H. E. (1965) Lack of correlation between natriuretic activity and inhibition of renal Na-K-activated ATPase. *Proc. Soc. exp. Biol. Med.* **120,** 358–360.

HUF E. G., DOSS N. S. & WILLS J. P. (1975) Effects of metabolic inhibitors and drugs on ion transport and oxygen consumption in isolated frog skin. *J. gen. Physiol.* **41,** 397–417.

LEAF A. (1965) Transepithelial transport and its hormonal control in toad bladder. *Ergeb. Physiol.* **56,** 216–262.

LIPMANN F. (1941) Metabolic generation and utilization of phosphate bond energy. *Adv. Enzymol.* **1,** 99–162.

MANUEL M. A. & WEINER M. W. (1976) Effects of ethacrynic acid and furosemide on isolated rat kidney mitochondria: Inhibition of electron transport in the region of phosphorylation site II. *J. Pharmac. exp. Ther.* **198,** 209–221.

MANUEL M. A. & WEINER M. W. (1977) Effects of ethacrynic acid and furosemide on phosphorylation reactions of kidney mitochondria: Inhibition of the adenine nucleotide translocase. *Biochim. biophys. Acta.* **460,** 445–454.

ROBINSON B. A. & MACKNIGHT A. D. C. (1976) Relationships between serosal medium potassium concentration and sodium transport in toad urinary bladders. *J. Membr. Biol.* **26,** 269–286.

SCHMIDT U. C., SCHMID J., SCHMID H. & DUBACH H. S. (1975) Sodium and potassium-activated ATPase. A possible target of aldosterone. *J. clin. Invest.* **55,** 655–660.

SOBOSLAI G., MCTIGUE M. & WEINER M. W. (1977) Mechanism of active chloride transport by the urinary bladder of the Columbian toad. *Am. J. Physiol.* **233,** F421–F427.

STRICKLER J. C. & KESSLER R. H. (1963) Effects of certain inhibitors on renal excretion of salt and water. *Am. J. Physiol.* **205,** 117–122.

WEINER M. W. (1979) Uncoupling agents distinguished between the effects of metabolic inhibitors and transport inhibitors. *Science* **204,** 187–188.

WEINER M. W. (1980) Effects of furosemide and ethacrynic acid on sodium transport and CO_2 production of toad bladders: Evidence for direct inhibition of active transport. *J. Pharmac. exp. Ther.* In press.

WEINER M. W. & MAFFLY R. H. (1978) Energy metabolism and active ion transport. In *The Physiological Basis for Disorders of Biomembranes.* Chapter 16, pp. 287–308. (Edited by ANDREOLI T., HOFFMAN J. & FANESTIL D.), Plenum, New York.

WILSON D. F., STUBBS M., OSHINO N. *et al.* (1974) Thermodynamic relationships between the mitochondrial oxidation-reduction reactions and cellular ATP levels in ascites tumor cells and perfused rat liver. *Biochemistry* **13,** 5305–5311.

WINDER C. L. & WEINER M. W. (1980) Effects of metabolic and transport inhibitors on sodium transport and CO_2 production of toad bladders: Use of an uncoupling agent

to distinguish between effects on transport and metabolism. *J. Pharmac. exp. Ther.* In press.
ZERAHN K. (1956) Oxygen consumption and active sodium transport in the isolated and short-circuited frog skin. *Acta Physiol. scand.* **36,** 300–218.

SYMPOSIUM DISCUSSION

Vinay: Is the concentration of DNP critical? If inhibition is incomplete, presumably there could be stimulation or respiration by the effectors?

Weiner: We found 10^{-5} M/2:4 DNP optimal for toad bladder.

Guder: There was some sodium flux even in the presence of DNP. Does that mean that there is respiration-independent transport? Is glucose present in the incubation medium?

Weiner: There is glucose, and I cannot explain the delay in totally inhibiting transport. There are obviously many possibilities, including the generation of ATP by glycolysis.

Kinne: The method is of interest, but you really cannot distinguish in the case of aldosterone whether it has an additional effect. The problem is that DNP itself may have effects on the plasma membrane.

De Pont: Your conclusion that furosemide has a direct effect on transport is not proven by your experiments. It may also have an effect on phosphorylation.

Weiner: At higher concentrations of furosemide, we have observed inhibition of respiration in mitochondria, but at low concentrations, which inhibited short-circuit current of toad bladder there was no effect on respiration.

Radda: Your conclusion concerning the distance of mitochondria from the Na-K-ATPase may be too pessimistic. A number of alternatives are possible; local concentration differences are rather over emphasised. First, in molecular terms the "closeness" of mitochondria to the enzyme is really rather large. There could be a "privileged channel" for ATP to the enzyme which is amenable to study, and finally, the concentration of ATP, as of any charged substance close to a charged polymeric surface, like the inner membrane, is different from the bulk concentration. This too can be studied.

Weiner: It has already been suggested that the ATP concentration in the cell is so far above the K_m of Na-K-ATPase that it cannot be regulatory, but, by analogy with the red cell (Parker & Hoffman, *J. gen. Physiol.* **50,** 893–916, 1969) ATP may be formed in close association to the enzyme site, so that the values for whole cell ATP have little meaning.

Saggerson: With regard to the apparent uncoupling effect of sodium, if there were a Na–Ca exchange, this would discharge calcium from the mitochondria.

Angielski: Not in kidney mitochondria. Here, sodium inhibits calcium efflux. In heart there is a calcium discharge of the type you describe (Crompton *et al. Eur. J. Biochem.* **69,** 453, 1976)

Kirsten: I think that the coupling effect of Na is due to the high ATPase activity of lysosomes. This would be overcome by using digitonin during the preparation.

Int. J. Biochem., Vol. 12, pp. 263 to 267
Pergamon Press Ltd 1980. Printed in Great Britain

ADENOSINE AS A POSSIBLE MEDIATOR OF METABOLIC CONTROL OF GLOMERULAR FILTRATION RATE*

H. OSSWALD, G. NABAKOWSKI and H. HERMES
Abteilung Pharmakologie der Medizinischen Fakultät der Rheinisch-Westfälischen Technischen Hochschule Aachen, Schneebergweg, D-5100 Aachen, Federal Republic of Germany

INTRODUCTION

The possibility of a metabolic control of glomerular filtration rate (GFR) has been considered unlikely to exist as stated by Renkin & Gilmore (1973). This conclusion is based on the assumption that increased metabolism would lead to vasodilatation as in other organs like heart and skeletal muscle. In the kidney renal blood flow (RBF) determines metabolism in as much as increase of RBF leads to an increase of GFR which in turn increases tubular load with sodium chloride and subsequent tubular sodium reabsorption. If increased sodium reabsorption lead to vasodilatation, we would have a case of a positive feedback with no way of regulating constancy of RBF and GFR. Therefore, it was postulated that a vasoconstrictive signal operates in the kidney to limit renal metabolism i.e. mainly tubular sodium chloride reabsorption (Thurau, 1964).

Since adenosine is a vasoconstrictor in the kidney (Osswald, 1975; Osswald *et al.*, 1975, 1978a, 1978b; Thurau, 1964) and since adenosine is present in the normal kidney (Osswald *et al.*, 1977). The question arises whether adenosine plays a role in regulation renal blood flow under physiological conditions (Osswald *et al.*, 1977, 1978; Schnermann *et al.*, 1977).

The present studies were undertaken to measure adenosine tissue content during periods of increased tubular load with sodium chloride and to interfere with the vascular response following high perfusion rates of the loop of Henle using drugs which antagonize and potentiate renal vascular response to adenosine.

MATERIALS AND METHODS

Experiments with hypertonic saline infusion

In Sprague–Dawley rats (mean body weight 212 g) hypertonic sodium chloride (HS) was infused into the thoracic aorta (Osswald *et al.*, 1975) to elevate the femoral arterial plasma sodium concentration to the range of 160–180 mmol·l^{-1}. This manoeuvre increased the tubular sodium load and thus reabsorptive work of the kidney. Left kidney glomerular filtration rate (GFR) was measured by [^{3}H]inulin clearance before and between the 5th and the 9th min after onset of HS infusion. Kidneys were clamped 10 min after start of HS infusion with a Wollenberger clamp precooled to the temperature of liquid nitrogen. The time-lag between removal of the kidney from the rat and complete freeze stop was 1–2 sec. From the $HClO_4$ tissue extracts adenine nucleotides were measured by high pressure liquid chromatography (Jungling & Kammermeier, 1979) and adenosine was measured enzymatically as previously described. (Osswald *et al.*, 1977).

Micropuncture experiments

Sprague–Dawley rats (180–230 g) were prepared for micropuncture. The rectal temperature and the temperature of the paraffin oil bathing the kidney were servo-controlled and kept at 37°C. A pipette, 7–9 μm o.d., connected with a nanoliter perfusion pump (Hampel, Frankfurt), was used to identify the last accessible loop of the proximal tubule using lissamine green stained modified Ringer solution. Two wax blocks were injected into the proximal tubule, one upstream of the perfusion pipette and the other into the first loop of the proximal tubule. A pipette 3–5 μm o.d., connected with a servo-nulling device (Wiederhielm *et al.*, 1964), was inserted upstream of the wax block positioned in the first loop of the proximal tubule to monitor stop flow pressure (SFP) as an equivalent of the hydrostatic pressure in the glomerular capillaries (Osswald *et al.*, 1978a). Tubular load of the loop of Henle with NaCl was varied by setting the infusion pump to values from 0 to 50 nl·min^{-1}.

RESULTS

Experiments with hypertonic saline

The results of this experimental series are summarized in Fig. 1. Under control conditions (group I,

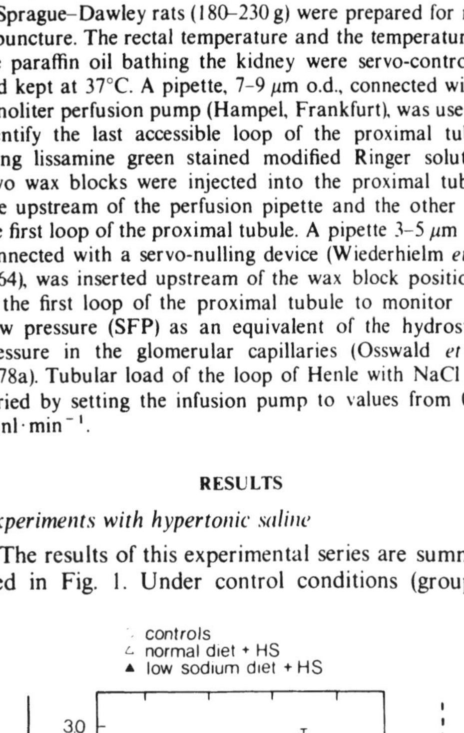

Fig. 1. Tissue levels of ATP (left ordinate, connected with the solid line) and of adenosine (right ordinate, broken line) in relation to the corresponding tubular sodium reabsorption rate (abscissa) of the left kidney in control rats (n = 6), open circles; in rats infused with hypertonic sodium chloride into the thoracic aorta (n = 8), open triangles; and in rats on a low sodium diet infused with hypertonic sodium chloride (n = 7), solid triangles, respectively.

* Supported by the Deutsche Forschungsgemeinschaft

$n = 6$) tubular sodium reabsorption was 64.5 ± 5 μmol·min^{-1}·100 g body weight^{-1}. The corresponding adenine nucleotide tissue content in μmols·g wet weight^{-1} was ATP 2.55 ± 0.05, ADP 0.60 ± 0.09 and for AMP 0.25 ± 0.06, respectively. The adenosine tissue content was 5.69 ± 1.2 nmols·g wet weight^{-1}. Following hypertonic sodium chloride infusion (group II, $n = 8$) tubular sodium reabsorption increased to 82.8 ± 5.9 μmols·min^{-1}·100 g^{-1} whereas ATP tissue levels were lowered to 1.64 ± 0.1 mols·g wet weight^{-1}, those of ADP were 0.47 ± 0.04 and of AMP 0.22 ± 0.05 μmols·g wet weight^{-1} respectively. Adenosine tissue content was slightly elevated to 7.69 ± 1 nmols·g wet weight^{-1}. To further increase the ability of the kidney to reabsorb and high tubular load of sodium chloride we repeated the experiments in rats which were initially sodium depleted by 50 mg·kg^{-1} furosemide and then kept on a low sodium diet for 10–15 days (daily sodium intake was approximately 0.7 mol), a condition associated with hyperaldosteronism. In this group III ($n = 7$) tubular sodium transport rose up to 109 ± 9 μmols·min^{-1}·100 g^{-1}, ATP tissue content was further lowered to 1.05 ± 0.26 μmols·g wet weight^{-1} (ADP, 0.43 ± 0.05; AMP, 0.25 ± 0.05). Adenosine tissue levels were elevated 3-fold above control values to 16.2 ± 1.3 nmols·g wet weight^{-1}. As a result of infusion of hypertonic saline hematocrit (%) decreased from 44.7 ± 2.4 to 34.7 ± 1.4 in group II and from 52.4 ± 1.3 to 38.6 ± 1.1 in group III.

Micropuncture experiments

In these experiments tubular sodium load of functionally isolated loops of Henle was increased to levels above normal range. The vascular response of the afferent arterioles of the glomerulus of the perfused nephron was measured by monitoring the stop flow pressure (SFP) in the early proximal tubules. The original trace in Fig. 2a shows the SFP decrease following the steep increase in endproximal perfusion rate. This vascular response was shown to be the result of afferent arteriolar constriction (Briggs & Wright, 1979). When the adenosine antagonist theophylline was administered intravenously in a dose of 5 μmols·100 g body weight^{-1} the vascular response to high loop perfusion rates was abolished completely. Figure 2b summarizes the results of these experiments.

Another substance was used to interfere with adenosine metabolism. Dipyridamole is known for its inhibition of adenosine uptake from the extracellular

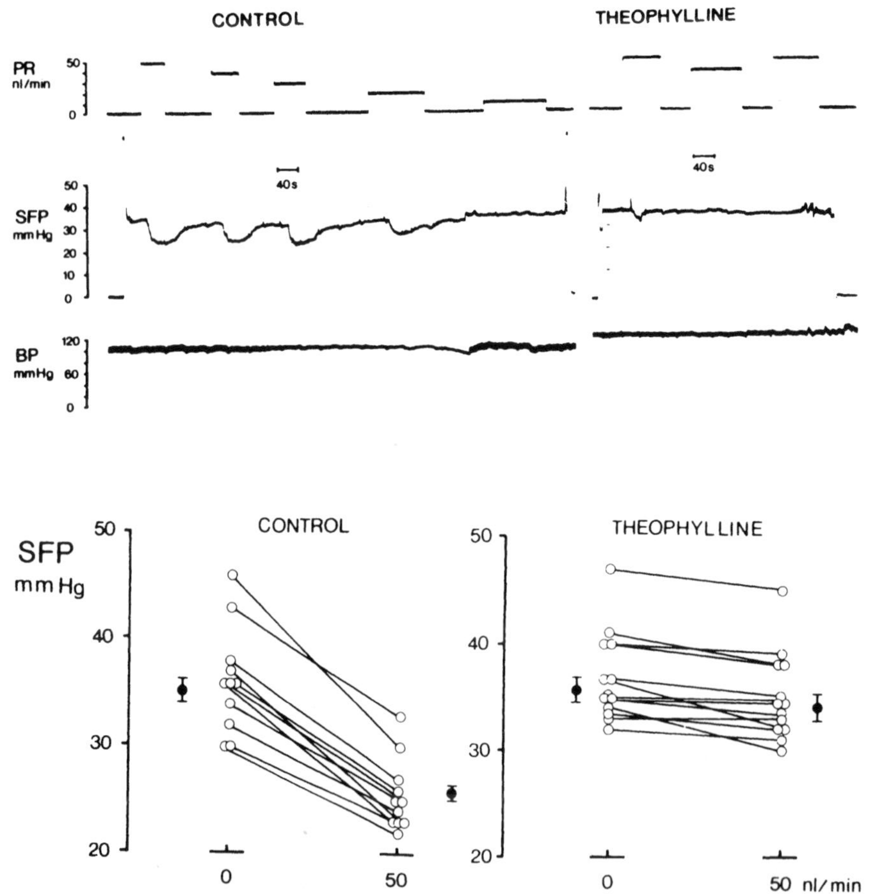

Fig. 2. Upper panel (a). Original trace of endproximal perfusion rate (PR), stop flow pressure (SFP) in the early proximal tubule and arterial blood pressure (BP). Theophylline was administered i.v. at a dose of 5 μmols·100 g body weight^{-1}. Lower panel (b). Stop flow pressures (SFP) before and 15–50 min after theophylline administration in 4 rats. Each line connects the SFP measured at 0 and at 50 ml·min end-proximal perfusion rate in the same nephron.

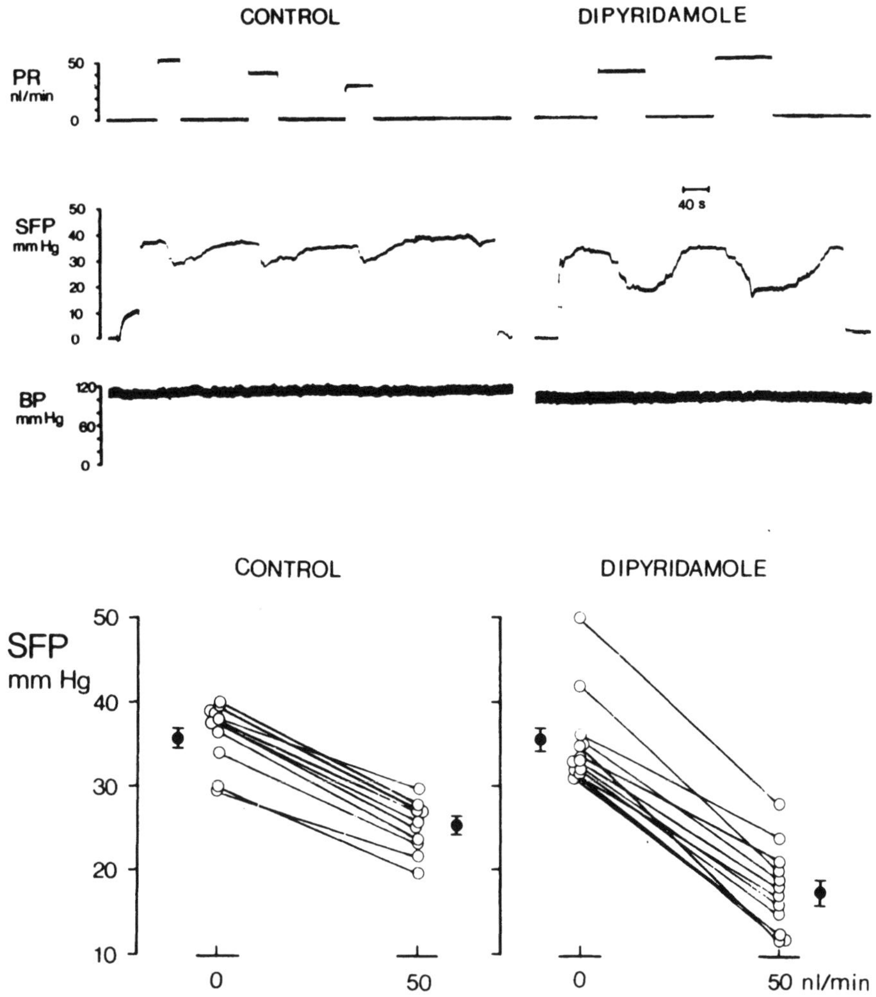

Fig. 3. Upper panel (a). Original trace of endproximal perfusion rate (PR), stop flow pressure (SFP) in the early proximal tubule and arterial blood pressure (BP). Dipyridamole was administered i.v. at a dose of 0.5 mg · 100 g body weight^{-1}. Lower panel (b). Stop flow pressures (SFP) before and 15–50 min after dipyridamole administration in 4 rats. Each line connects the SFP measured at 0 and 50 nl · min^{-1} end-proximal perfusion rate in the same nephron.

space into the cells and thereby potentiating the adenosine effects by elevation of extracellular adenosine concentration (Bunger *et al.*, 1975; Ross & Pfleger, 1972; Schrader *et al.*, 1972). As shown in Fig. 3a i.v. administration of 0.5 mg/100 g body weight dipyridamole potentiates the SFP response to elevation of endproximal perfusion rate from 0 to 50 nl · min^{-1}. This experimental series is summarized in Fig. 3b. Systemic blood pressure was not changed by theophylline or dipyridamole.

DISCUSSION

It is generally assumed that in the kidney metabolic vasodilatation would be disadvantageous because increased renal blood flow would further increase the work load of the kidney via an increase in the filtered load of sodium (Thurau, 1964). In this study the idea of a metabolic vasoconstriction was tested by two different types of experiments. The infusion of hypertonic sodium chloride increased acutely the amount of tubular reabsorbed sodium. The tissue levels of ATP were lowered and those of adenosine elevated (Fig. 1). These results provide a basis to suggest a metabolic control of renal blood flow and glomerular filtration rate via increased intrarenal generation of adenosine which is a vasoconstrictor in the kidney (Osswald, 1975; Osswald *et al.*, 1975, 1978a, 1978b; Thurau, 1964). However, in the experiments with hypertonic saline we did not see a significant decrease in GFR. This can be explained by the two vasodilatatory stimuli applied to the kidney: hyperosmotic vasodilation (Young & Rostorfer, 1973) and extracellular volume expansion due to hypertonic saline infusion into the aorta.

For this reason, in the micropuncture experiments an increase of the tubular load with sodium was achieved without changes in blood osmolality and hematocrit. The high perfusion rate of the loop of Henle is associated with an increase of sodium chloride reabsorption of the ascending limb (Schnermann *et al.*, 1977). The vasoconstriction seen during high loop perfusion rates was originally described by Schnermann and is known as tubulo-glomerular feedback (see Schnermann & Briggs, 1979). It is not possible at present to measure *in vivo* ATP levels or adenosine generation in the perfused Henle's loops. However, it is possible to interfere with the vascular response of the glomerulus to high loop perfusion rates using substances of known mechanism of action. In an earlier study we demonstrated that theophylline can abolish the reduction of stop flow pressure following high loop perfusion rates (Schnermann *et al.*, 1977). The concentration of intratubular infused theophylline was 5 mmols$\cdot l^{-1}$. Such a high concentration of theophylline may inhibit the cyclic adenosine monophosphate phosphodiesterase. To avoid this possible action of theophylline a much lower dose of theophylline (5 μmols$\cdot 100\,g^{-1}$) was injected intravenously. The half maximal inhibition of adenosine actions by theophylline is seen at concentrations of $2\text{–}5 \times 10^{-6}$ mols$\cdot l^{-1}$ (Alfonso, 1970; Ally & Nakatsu, 1976; Bunger *et al.*, 1975; Ebert & Schwabe, 1973; Hedqvist *et al.*, 1978; Osswald, 1975; Osswald *et al.*, 1977; Sattin & Rall, 1970; Schaumann *et al.*, 1970). It can be assumed that no phosphodiesterase inhibition in the kidney occurred at the theophylline dose used in the present experiments (Fredholm *et al.*, 1978). Therefore, the effect of theophylline to inhibit the tubulo-glomerular feedback response (Fig. 2) is likely to be the result of an adenosine antagonism. This conclusion is further supported by our finding that dipyridamole potentiates the vasoconstriction induced by elevation of endproximal perfusion rates from zero to 50 nl$\cdot$min^{-1} (see Fig. 3). Dipyridamol is known to inhibit the uptake of adenosine into the cells (Ross & Pfleger, 1972; Schrader *et al.*, 1972). It can be used as a tool to elevate extracellular adenosine concentration. Since theophylline and dipyridamole have opposite effects on the tubulo-glomerular feedback and since both substances inhibit at high concentrations the cAMP phosphodiesterase (Fredholm *et al.*, 1978) is is highly unlikely that the observed effects on the tubulo-glomerular feedback are mediated by phosphodiesterase inhibition. The observed effects are rather mediated by their known adenosine antagonistic and synergistic action.

The tubulo-glomerular feedback can be abolished by inhibition of the sodium chloride reabsorption of the ascending limb of Henle's loop with high ceiling diuretics like furosemide (Wright & Schnermann, 1974). Thus, the sodium chloride transport of the ascending limb has to be intact in order to transmit a constrictive signal to the afferent arteriols when the sodium chloride load is acutely increased. We suggest that adenosine can function as the mediator of such a signal transmission from the ascending limb of Henle's loop to the afferent arteriole of the glomerulus in response to an increased sodium chloride transport rate. It is possible that this concept may not hold for the deep cortical region since continuous infusion of adenosine into the renal artery leads to constriction of the afferent arteriols mainly in the outer cortex and induces vasodilatation in the deep cortex (Osswald *et al.*, 1978*a*).

REFERENCES

AFONSO S. (1970) Inhibition of coronary vasodilating action of dipyridamole and adenosine by aminophylline in the dog. *Circ. Res.* **26,** 743–752.

ALLY A. J. & NAKATSU K. (1976) Adenosine inhibition of isolated rabbit ileum and antagonism by theophylline. *J. Pharmac. exp. Ther.* **199,** 208–215.

BRIGGS J. P. & WRIGHT F. S. (1979) Feedback control of glomerular filtration rate: site of the effector mechanism. *Am. J. Physiol.* **236,** F40–F47.

BÜNGER R., HADDY F. J. & GERLACH E. (1975) Coronary responses to dilating substances and competitive inhibition by theophylline in the isolated perfused guinea pig heart. *Pflügers Arch. ges Physiol.* **358,** 213–224.

EBERT R. & SCHWABE U. (1973) Studies on the antilipolytic effect of adenosine and related compounds in isolated fat cells. *Naunyn-Schmiedeberg's Arch. exp. Path. Pharmak.* **278,** 247.

FREDHOLM B. B., HEDQUIST P. & VERNET L. (1978) Effect of methylxanthines and related compounds on rabbit renal cyclic nucleotide phosphodiesterase, 5′-nucleotidase and adenosine deaminase. *Biochem. Pharmac.* **27,** 2845–2850.

HEDQVIST P., FREDHOLM B. B. & ÖLUNDH S. (1978) Antagonistic effects of theophylline and adenosine on adrenergic neuroeffector transmission in the rabbit kidney. *Circ. Res.* **43,** 592–598.

JÜNGLING E. & KAMMERMEIER H. (1979) Rapid assay of adenine nucleotides or creatine compounds respectively in extract of cardiac tissue by paired reverse phase high performance liquid chromatography. *Analyt. Biochem.* In press.

OSSWALD H. (1975) Renal effects of adenosine and their inhibition by theophylline. *Naunyn-Schmiedeberg's Arch. exp. Path. Pharmak.* **288,** 79–86.

OSSWALD H., SCHMITZ H.-J. & HEIDENREICH O. (1975) Adenosine response of the rat kidney after saline loading, sodium restriction and hemorrhagia. *Pflugers Arch. ges. Physiol.* **357,** 323–333.

OSSWALD H., SCHMITZ H.-J. & KEMPER R. (1977) Tissue content of adenosine, inosine and hypoxanthine in the rat kidney after ischemia and postischemic recirculation. *Pflügers Arch. ges. Physiol.* **371,** 45–49.

OSSWALD H., SPIELMAN W. S. & KNOX F. G. (1978a) Mechanism of adenosine mediated decrease in glomerular filtration rate. *Circ. Res.* **43,** 465–469.

OSSWALD H., SCHMITZ H.-J. & KEMPER R. (1978b) Renal action of adenosine: effect on renin secretion in the rat. *Naunyn-Schmiedeberg's Arch. exp. Path. Pharmak.* **303,** 95–99.

RENKIN E. M. & GILMORE J. P. (1973) Glomerular filtration. In *Handbook of Physiology,* Section 8: Renal Physiology, Chap. 9, p. 220. (Edited by ORLOFF J. & BERLINER R. W.) American Physiological Society, Washington, DC.

ROSS H. & PFLEGER K. (1972) Kinetics of adenosine uptake by erythrocytes, and the influence of dipyridamole. *Mol. Pharmac.* **8,** 417–425.

SATTIN A. & RALL T. W. (1970) The effect of adenosine and adenine nucleotides on the cyclic adenosine 3′:5′ phosphate content of guinea pig cerebral cortex slices. *Mol. Pharmac.* **6,** 13.

SCHAUMANN W., JUHRAU W. & DIETMANN K. (1970) Antagonismus der Kreislaufwirkungen von Adenosin durch Theophyllin. *Arzneim.-Forsch.* **20,** 372–377.

SCHNERMANN J., OSSWALD H. & HERMLE M. (1977) Inhibitory effect of methylxanthines on feedback control of glomerular filtration rate in the rat kidney. *Pflügers Arch. ges. Physiol.* **369,** 39–48.

SCHNERMANN J. & BRIGGS J. P. (1979) Reduktion des Glomerulumfiltrates (GFR) bei akuter Hypernatriämie (Hyper-Na) durch tubulo-glomeruläre Rückkopplung. *XIII Symposion der Gesellschaft für Nephrologie,* 7–10 Oktober, Berlin.

SCHRADER J., BERNE R. M. & RUBIO R. (1972) Uptake and metabolism of adenosine by human erythrocyte ghosts. *Am. J. Physiol.* **223,** 159–166.

THURAU K. (1964) Renal hemodynamics. *Am. J. Med.* **36,** 698–719.

WIEDERHIELM C. A., WOODBURG J. W., KIRK S. & RUSHMER R. F. (1964) Pulsatile pressures in the microcirculation of frog's mesentery. *Am. J. Physiol.* **207,** 173–176.

WRIGHT F. S. & SCHNERMANN J. (1974) Interference with feedback control of glomerular filtration rate by furosemide, trifloxin, and cyanide. *J. clin. Invest.* **53,** 169–170.

YOUNG D. B. & ROSTORFER H. H. (1973) Blood flow and filtration rate responses to alterations in renal arterial osmolarity. *Am. J. Physiol.* **225,** 1003–1008.

SYMPOSIUM DISCUSSION

Silva: Have you done similar experiments with inosine? I ask the question because you may be looking at the conversion of adenosine to ATP and to cyclic AMP.

Osswald: No, cAMP content is much lower in the kidney than is ATP. Inosine is not vasoactive in the kidney. The cyclic AMP system is difficult to check because you have to look at the juxtaglomerular apparatus, in order to explain afferent vasoconstriction, and I am not aware of any measurements of cAMP in these cells, following administration of adenosine.

Bogusky: Were you able to measure appreciable differences in inosine content of the urine or tissues after adenosine vasoconstriction?

Osswald: No, but if adenosine is given in sodium-depleted rats, the kidneys become ischaemic, and then there is an increase in inosine and hypoxanthine tissue content (Osswald *et al. Pflügers Arch. ges. Physiol.* **371,** 45–49, 1977). Under normal conditions, there was no hypoxia after giving adenosine, and adenosine in these amounts is not a substrate sufficient to change tissue levels of inosine or hypoxanthine.

Deetjen: In which way do you think that adenosine formed in the renal tissue reaches the afferent arteriole?

Osswald: Adenosine is formed from ATP hydrolysis associated with active sodium transport. I don't know the precise site of formation of adenosine in relationship to the macula densa. It may be that adenosine is formed by the epithelium of the ascending thick limb of Henle's loop in a little distance away from the macula densa; adenosine formation in the medulla or in the proximal tubule would not make sense, because here are no resistance vessels. We see adenosine as the link between the sodium transport signal and the vascular response.

Jorgenson: What you suggest is that the release of adenosine depends on the function of 5′ nucleotidase and passage across a membrane.

Osswald: Yes, but 5′-nucleotidase is not the only enzyme necessarily involved in adenosine formation. There is another pathway of adenosine formation which involves S-adenosylhomocysteine hydrolase. The understanding of intracellular adenosine metabolism is incomplete at present.

Kirsten: Did you notice any effect of adenosine on total renal blood flow?

Osswald: Yes, but the response depends upon the Na-dietary status of the animals. Infusion of adenosine results in a temporary fall in blood flow, which recovers within 3–5 min to preinfusion levels. Rats on a low sodium diet show a slightly decrease of RBF during adenosine infusion, whereas rats on a high sodium diet respond to adenosine infusion with an increase of RBF during steady state (Osswald *et al. Naunyn-Schmiedeberg's Arch. exp. Path. Pharmak.* **303,** 95–99, 1978). GFR remains depressed and micropuncture showed that the outer cortex is constricted during adenosine infusion, while the deep cortex is dilated. The sum of total renal vascular resistance is not changed (Osswald *et al. Circ. Res.* **43,** 465–469, 1978).

Int. J. Biochem., Vol. 12, pp. 269 to 275
0020-711X/80/0701-0269$02.00/0

FLUORESCENCE OF PYRIDINE NUCLEOTIDE AND FLAVOPROTEINS AS AN INDICATOR OF SUBSTRATE OXIDATION AND OXYGEN DEMAND OF THE ISOLATED PERFUSED RAT KIDNEY

HOLGER FRANKE[1], CLYDE H. BARLOW[2] and BRITTON CHANCE[2]
[1]Department of Nephrology, University of Kiel, 23 Kiel, Federal Republic of Germany and
[2]Johnson Research Foundation, School of Medicine, University, of Pennsylvania, Philadelphia, PA 19174, U.S.A.

Abstract—To evaluate the relationship between renal function and mitochondrial redox state the following photometric techniques were applied to the isolated perfused rat kidney and correlated to changes of experimental conditions:

1. Surface fluorescence of reduced pyridine nucleotides (PN) and oxidized flavoproteins (FP) was recorded simultaneously with a double beam fluorometer.
2. PN-fluorescence was monitored continuously with a DC-fluorometer.
3. Photographs of PN-fluorescence were taken with a large format camera.

The results led to the following conclusions:

1. Since a close relationship exists between FP- and PN-fluorescence during normoxic-anoxic transitions, PN-fluorescence of renal cortex reflects mainly the mitochondrial redox state, while the cytoplasmic signal seems of minor importance.
2. In spite of the high flow rate and the high O_2-saturation of the perfusate, renal function during isolated perfusion with dextran is limited by O_2-delivery to tissue, as demonstrated by the more oxidized mitochondrial redox state at low perfusion temperatures (28, 20, 14°C) compared to 38°C.
3. Calculated on the base of PN-reduction L-lactate seems to be more utilized for oxidative phosphorylation of kidney cortex than L-glutamine. D-glucose had no effect on PN-fluorescence indicating that D-glucose is not oxidized in renal cortex in large amounts. This finding is supported by the fact that during perfusion with D-glucose in the absence of other substrates renal function was not different from substrate-free perfusion.
4. The PN-fluorescence photographs show the repetitive pattern characteristic for tubular organisation at the kidney surface demonstrating morphological and metabolic heterogeneity.

INTRODUCTION

Information about the metabolic state of intact tissues so far are obtained mostly by analyses of tissue contents as well as by analyses of the extracellular fluid components. However, these methods do not provide a continuous control of tissue respiration and in addition determination of intracellular components is connected to tissue disruption. Optical methods on the other hand have the distinct advantage that they allow continuous monitoring without complicated analytical work and without disruption of the tissue.

It was shown in the past that surface fluorescence of reduced pyridine nucleotides (PN) is responsive to the redox state of the mitochondria (Chance, 1964, 1976; Chance *et al.*, 1972; Mayevsky & Chance, 1974). The chief drawback of the PN-fluorescence as an indicator of the mitochondrial redox state, the distribution of PN in both the mitochondrial and the cytoplasmic space, seems to be of minor importance since it was demonstrated that more than 80% of the fluorescence signal is due to the mitochondrial space (Chance, 1976). In addition, the relationship between the PN- and flavoprotein signals was tested in this study during normoxic–anoxic transitions.

To evaluate in the isolated rat kidney perfused with plasma substitutes the effectiveness of O_2-delivery to the capillary space, from where the O_2 diffuses to the mitochondria and to study the validity of several substrates for the oxidative phosphorylation of the renal cortex, PN-fluorescence changes were correlated to changes of perfusion temperature, substrate-free perfusion and reintroduction of several substrates. In addition the corresponding Na-reabsorption rates were determined. Finally to obtain information about the total surface area and about a possible heterogeneity of the PN-fluorescence signal, fluorescence photographs were taken of the kidney surface.

Since the PN-redox state is controlled first by the utilizable substrates present at the mitochondria, secondly by the energy requirement, and thirdly by the intracellular O_2-concentrations, differences from the results obtained from experiments on isolated mitochondria, observed in the perfused rat kidney may be due to marginal O_2-delivery to the mitochondrial space.

MATERIALS AND METHODS

Perfusion technique

Male adult albino rats of the Wistar strain, weighing 180–220 g, were used for all experiments. Operation and perfusion procedure was carried out as described elsewhere in detail (Franke *et al.*, 1971, 1976). The experiments were started with no reference to the feeding cycle. For studies of the influence of substrates on the PN-redox state the animals were starved for 24 hr before the experiments.

The kidneys were perfused in a single-pass system, i.e. the perfusion fluid was not recycled. The perfusion pressure was adjusted to 112 mm Hg, the O_2-consumption was calculated on the base of the PO_2 av-difference—determined with two Clark-type electrodes—and the flow rate.

For the perfusion a modified Krebs–Henseleit buffer was used. As a plasma substitute either dextran (mol. wt. 40,000, ischemia experiments) or hydroxyethyl starch was added.

Fluorometric techniques

During normoxic–anoxic transitions flavoprotein and PN-fluorescence were determined simultaneously with a time-sharing fluorometer (Chance *et al.*, 1972). As a light source either a Hg-arc lamp or a xenon lamp was used. FP-excitation wavelength was 436 nm, FP-fluorescence was measured at 570 nm. The excitation wave length for PN was 366 nm, the fluorescence response was recorded at 460 nm.

However, since it seemed necessary to correct for changes in tissue opacity, PN-oxidation–reduction changes were continuously monitored by measuring the surface fluorescence of reduced pyridine nucleotide with a DC-fluorometer (Chance *et al.*, 1974). The fluorometer was attached to the surface of the perfused rat kidney utilizing a trifurcated fibre optics light pipe with 45 ± 4% of the fibres two branches (excitation and fluorescence) and 10 ± 1% of the fibres in the third branch (reflectance at 366 nm). All fibres were randomly mixed at the 4 mm common end. PN-fluorescence emission was corrected for changes in tissue opacity by a 1:1 subtraction of reflectance changes at the excitation wavelength of 366 nm from the PN-fluorescence (Jobsis, 1963; Mayevsky & Chance, 1974).

The photographs of PN-fluorescence emission from the kidney surface were obtained with a custom built camera using a high-speed plain film (Kodak Royal X-pan). As a light source for excitation a strong xenon flash with a 34–375 nm filter in front was used. The camera lens was covered by a 450–510 nm filter. For these experiments total darkness at the moment of the flash was necessary. All negatives and prints were developed under identical conditions to recognize changes of mitochondrial redox state.

RESULTS

Simultaneous recording of FP- and PN-fluorescence

In Fig. 1 the oxidation–reduction changes of FP and PN during a normoxic-anoxic transition is shown. To alternate aerobic and anaerobic perfusates 95% O_2 + 5% CO_2 and 95% N_2 + 5% CO_2 was equilibrated with the perfusates in duplicate vessels each at the same perfusion pressure.

It can be seen that after introduction of anaerobic medium into the kidney a first slow reduction occurs followed by a rapid phase of both, FP and PN of about 30%. After reintroduction of O_2-saturated fluid both systems show a fast recovery to control conditions.

PN-fluorescence response to ischemia and Na-reabsorption at different temperatures

In Table 1 the influence of different perfusion temperatures on the response of PN-fluorescence to a normoxic-ischemic transition and the Na-reabsorption at 38, 28, 20 and 14°C is given. Original records of PN-fluorescence changes during normoxic-ischemic cycles were published prevously (Franke *et al.*, 1976).

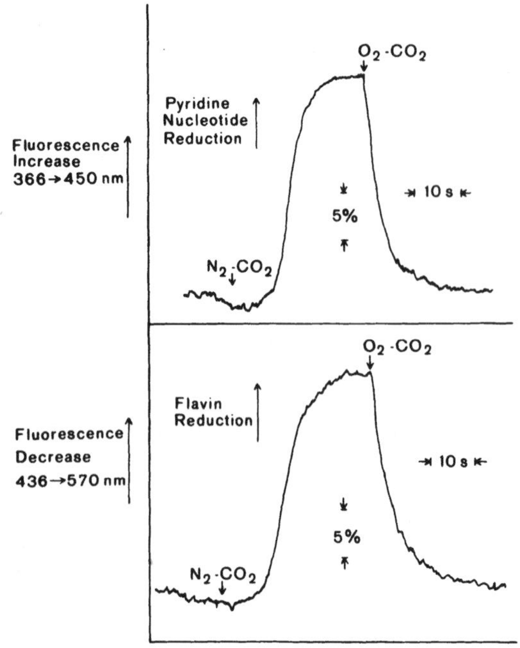

Fig. 1. Simultaneously monitored fluorescence of flavoproteins (lower chart) and pyridine nucleotide (upper chart) during a normoxic-anoxic cycle. FP-excitation wave length was 436 nm, the fluorescence response was determined at 570 nm. PN-excitation wave length was 366 nm, PN-fluorescence was measured at 460 nm. In both systems after introduction of anoxic perfusate a fast reduction of about 30% occurred. After reintroduction of O_2-saturated fluid a fast recovery was observed.

The PN-fluorescence increase during the rapid phase of PN-reduction became, in contrast to our expectations, larger at lower temperatures indicating that the system was more oxidized than at 38°C. Only when the perfusion temperature was lowered from 20 to 14°C, was an increase of PN-fluorescence obtained.

Substrate-linked PN-reduction

Figure 2 shows the influence of a perfusion with no substrates present in the medium on PN-fluorescence. The fact that endogenous substrates were still present in the tissue is demonstrated by a decrease of respiration from 0.142 to 0.074 $ml \cdot g^{-1} \cdot min$ and by a simultaneous decrease of PN-fluorescence by 13%. It can be postulated that after this pretreatment most of the endogenous substrates were consumed or washed out

Table 1. Influence of different perfusion temperatures on Na-reabsorption, the induction time between the beginning of ischemia and PN-reduction, and the fractional PN-redox change during a normoxic-ischemic transition

Perfusion temperature (°C)	Na-reabsorption (control = 100%)	Induction time (sec)	F_{NADH} (%)
38	100 ± 3.43	12.0 ± 1.2	100 ± 4.3
28	68.7 ± 1.19	19.0 ± 1.8	143 ± 5.1
20	48.4 ± 1.79	30.5 ± 2.8	171 ± 4.6
14	30.8 ± 2.15	64.3 ± 5.4	157 ± 4.1

ΔF_{NADH}: control condition at 38 C = 100%

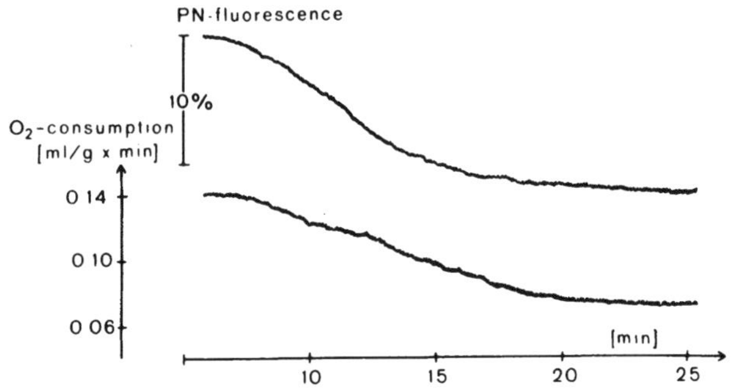

Fig. 2. PN-fluorescence (upper trace) and O_2-consumption (lower trace) of the kidney during perfusion with substrate-free medium. O_2-consumption and PN-fluorescence decreased indicating exhaustion of endogenous substrates.

and that the PN-redox level reached represents almost state 2 (Chance & Hollunger, 1963). Starting from this state a substrate-linked PN-reduction should be observed, if the introduced substrate (PN-dependent) is utilized for oxidative phosphorylation. This is demonstrated in Fig. 3: in the upper trace the influence of L-lactate followed by a normoxic-ischemic cycle is shown. L-lactate at a concentration of 1.8 mM (i.e. the highest concentration which still affected PN-redox state) induced a PN-reduction of 13%. Ischemia was followed by an additional PN-reduction of 29%. The middle trace shows a titration curve of L-glutamine. The highest effective L-glutamine concentration induced a PN-reduction of only 6%. The corresponding Na-reabsorption rates fit well the PN-redox changes. Introducing L-lactate at a concentration of 1.8 mM into the kidney maintained 65% of the Na-net-transport of control organs. L-glutamine on the other hand maintained only 40% of control values.

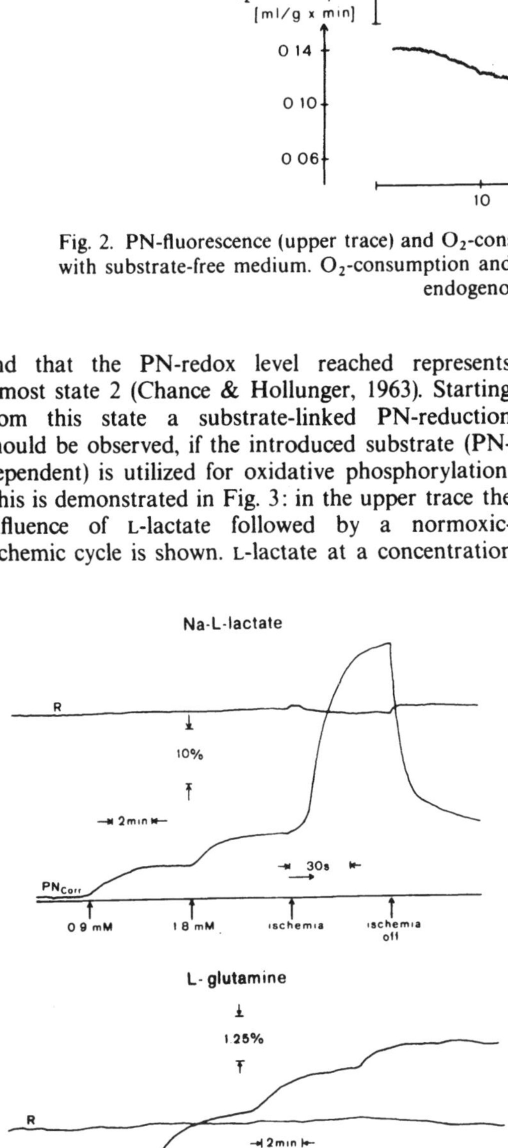

Fig. 3. Titration of PN-fluorescence with L-lactate (upper chart), L-glutamine (middle chart), and D-glucose (lower chart). (R: reflectance; PN_{corr}: corrected PN-fluorescence). It is evident that the most distinct influence on the PN-redox state was with L-lactate. The effect of L-glutamine was much smaller, while the PN-redox state in the presence of D-glucose remained unchanged.

In the lower chart D-glucose in concentrations of 5 and 10 mM was tested. No significant influence of D-glucose on the PN-fluorescence of kidney cortex was found. The next figure (Fig. 4) demonstrates the

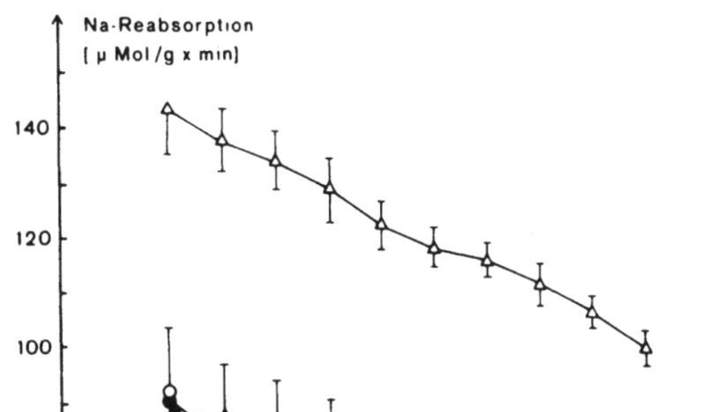

Fig. 4. Na-reabsorption of the rat kidney during 60 min of perfusion with different substrates. While Na-reabsorption was not significantly different in the groups perfused either substrate-free or with D-glucose as the sole substrate, a sufficient Na-reabsorption was obtained with the mixture of substrates. However, in the presence of other substrates D-glucose raised $\dot{T}_{Na}$ by more than 50% compared to the control conditions.

effect of D-glucose in detail: the first group was perfused without any substrate present in the medium; the next group was perfused with D-glucose (5 mM) in the absence of other substrates. The third group was perfused with a mixture of substrates (L-lactate, pyruvate, octanoate, L-glutamine) but without D-glucose and the last group with the above mentioned substrate mixture + 5 mM D-glucose. It can be seen that both the substrate-free and the D-glucose perfused kidneys show a continuous decrease of Na-reabsorption from more than 90 to less than 20 μmols$\cdot$g$^{-1}\cdot$min after 60 min of perfusion. The mixture of substrates was able to support a Na-reabsorption rate between 89 and 63 μmols$\cdot$g$^{-1}\cdot$min, while additional infusion of 5 mM D-glucose was followed by a marked increase of the Na-net-transport of more than 50% compared to the substrate mixture without D-glucose.

PN-fluorescence photography

The results presented so far are obtained by continuous monitoring of PN-fluorescence emission via a light tube from a circumscribed point of tissue surface. Evidently no information can be obtained with this method from areas not positioned directly under the fibre optics. This may be observed by fluorescence photography as demonstrated by Fig. 5. On the left side PN-fluorescence at a perfusion pressure of 125 mm Hg is shown, on the right side the PN-redox state at a perfusion pressure of only 80 mm Hg. Since negatives and prints were developed under identical conditions, intensity and dimension of the fluorescing areas are comparable. It is evident that at lower perfusion pressures PN-fluorescence intensity increases, while at the same time the fluorescing areas expand.

DISCUSSION

As demonstrated by Fig. 1 a close relationship between the FP- and PN-fluorescence signal exists in the cortex of the rat kidney, similar to that shown previously for other tissues. (Chance *et al.*, 1972; Chance, 1976). Moreover, the mitochondrial volume ratio of the renal cortex was determined to be as high as 35% (Pfaller & Rittinger, 1980), which is comparable to heart muscle (Page *et al.*, 1971). It can be assumed for this reason that in the rat kidney also the PN-fluorescence reflects mainly the mitochondrial space.

Since the absolute amount of PN cannot be determined by surface fluorometry, it is necessary to calculate the PN-redox state from transitions from the condition of interest to another defined state. It can be postulated that PN-fluorescence during anoxia or ischemia (state 5 (Chance & Hollunger, 1963)) is almost identical under all experimental conditions. Thus a normoxic-anoxic (ischemic) transition provides information regarding the initial state.

This leads to the conclusion that during perfusion at different temperatures PN is more oxidized at lower temperatures than at 38°C (Table 1). However, it is to be expected that with decreasing metabolic activity, as indicated by the increasing induction time between the start of ischemia and the beginning of the rapid phase of PN-reduction, the PN-redox state becomes more reduced (Chance, 1964) rather than more oxidized. The fact that PN is more oxidized at 28 and 20°C proves that O_2-delivery to tissue must be marginal during isolated perfusion at 38°C and approaches a balance at lower temperatures. This balance may be reached at 14°C where for the first time an increase of PN-fluorescence was observed suggesting that at 14°C the O_2-delivery to the tissue is sufficient to cover the demand.

However, it must be kept in mind that these experiments were carried out on kidneys perfused with dextran. Since distinctly better function can be obtained with hydroxyethyl starch or bovine albumine (Little & Cohen, 1974), O_2-delivery may be better in these preparations.

Starting from state 2 conditions (Chance & Hollunger, 1963) which were approached by substrate-free perfusion, introduction of a PN-dependent substrate into the kidney led to a reduction of PN (Fig. 3): a PN-fluorescence increase of 13% was obtained by L-lactate, while 65% of the control values of Na-reabsorption could be maintained. Both, the PN-reduction and the Na-net-transport were much less enhanced under the influence of L-glutamine, and no effect was measured, when D-glucose was infused.

These results indicate that the amount of PN-reduction correlates well to the obtained functional state and the respiration. In the case of D-glucose the unchanged PN-fluorescence gave evidence that this substrate is not oxidized in large amounts in the renal cortex. Moreover, the functional data show that D-glucose in the absence of other substrates is not able to effectively support renal function. On the other hand D-glucose had a distinct influence in the presence of other substrates, where Na-reabsorption was raised by more than 50% compared to control values (Fig. 4).

The results demonstrate that continuous monitoring of PN-fluorescence is a helpful tool for further evaluation of the relationship between substrate and O_2-delivery, the energy requirement for active transport and the mitochondrial redox state of the renal cortex.

SUMMARY

The relationship between renal function and mitochondrial redox state was studied in the isolated perfused rat kidney by continuous monitoring of PN- and FP-fluorescence. PN-oxidation-reduction changes during ischemic cycles at different temperatures indicate that in the applied preparation O_2-delivery to tissue is marginal. Perfusion without substrates reduced PN-fluorescence by 13%. Reintroduction of substrates induced reduction of PN. The most pronounced effect on PN-redox state was found for L-lactate, while under the action of D-glucose PN-fluorescence remained unchanged. Correspondingly D-glucose in the absence of other substrates did not maintain sufficient Na reabsorption rates. Fluorescence photography demonstrates heterogeneity of the fluorescence signal obtained utilizing a fibre optics light pipe.

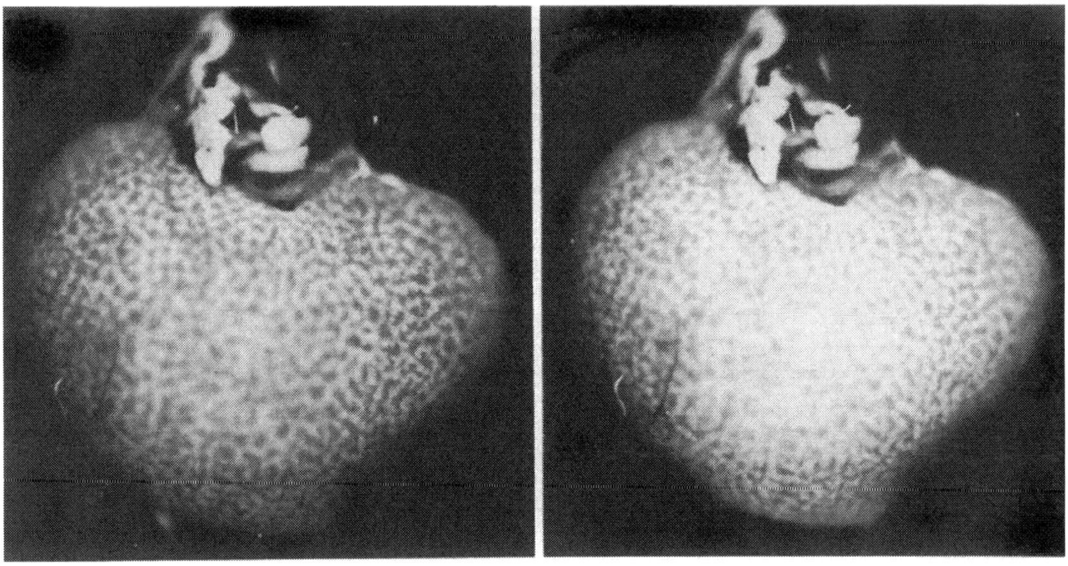

Fig. 5. Fluorescence photography of perfused rat kidney at two different states. (Left picture: perfusion pressure 125 mm Hg, right picture perfusion pressure 85 mm Hg). Reducing O_2-delivery to tissue by lowering the perfusion pressure was followed by an increase in fluorescence intensity, while at the same time the fluorescing areas expand.

REFERENCES

CHANCE B. & HOLLUNGER G. (1963) Inhibition of electron and energy transfer in mitochondria. I. Effects of amytal, thiopental, rotenone, progesterone, and methylene glycol. *J. biol. Chem.* **278,** 418–431.

CHANCE B. (1964) Continuous recording of intracellular reduced pyridine nucleotide changes in skeletal muscle *in vivo*. *Tex. Rep. Biol. Med.* **22,** 836–841.

CHANCE B., GRAHAM N. & MAYER D. (1972) A time-sharing fluorometer for the readout of intracellular oxidation–reduction states of NADH and flavoprotein. *Rev. Sci. Intr.* **42,** 951–957.

CHANCE B., SALKOVITZ I. A. & KOVACH A. G. B. (1972) Kinetics of mitochondrial flavoprotein and pyridine nucleotide in perfused rat heart. *Am. J. Physiol.* **223,** 207–218.

CHANCE B., MAYEVSKY A., GOODWIN C. & MELA L. (1974) Factors in oxygen delivery to tissue. *Microvasc. Res.* **8,** 276–282.

CHANCE B. (1976) Pyridine nucleotide as an indicator of the oxygen requirements for energy-linked functions of mitochondria. *Circ. Res.* **38,** 31–38.

FRANKE H., HULAND H., WEISS CH. & UNSICKER K. (1971) Improved net sodium transport of the isolated rat kidney. *Res. exp. Med.* **156,** 268–282.

FRANKE H., BARLOW C. H., & CHANCE B. (1976) Oxygen delivery in perfused rat kidney: NADH fluorescence and renal functional state. *Am. J. Physiol.* **231,** 1082–89.

JÖBSIS F. (1963) Spectrophotometry of intact muscle. I. Components of the respiratory chain. *J. gen. Physiol.* **46,** 905–928.

LITTLE J. R. & COHEN J. J. (1974) Effect of albumin concentration on function of isolated perfused rat kidney. *Am. J. Physiol.* **226,** 512–517.

MAYEVSKY A., & CHANCE B. (1974) A long-term method for the measurement of NADH fluorescence in intact rat brain with chronically implanted cannula. In *Oxygen Transport to Tissue*, (Edited by BICHER & BRULEY) pp. 276–288. Plenum, New York.

PAGE E., MCCALLISTER L. P. & FOWER B. (1971) Stereological measurements of cardiac ultrastructures implicated in excitation–contraction coupling. *Proc. natn. Acad. Sci. U.S.A.* **68,** 1465–66.

PFALLER W. & RITTINGER M. (1980) Quantitative morphology of the rat. *Int. J. Biochem.* **12,** 17–22 (this volume).

SYMPOSIUM DISCUSSION

Kinne: My question concerns whether respiration is substrate controlled or oxygen controlled.

Franke: I think respiration is controlled from three sites: the first, the energy requirement (that means the ADP + P_i levels in the tissue), the second is oxygen, and the third is substrate supply. The case which I have shown here is the kidney from 24 hr starved animals, perfused for 20–30 min, substrate-free. In this instance the system becomes more oxygenated, and I think that this was due to a lack of substrate. Even if you have an oxygen deficiency, you may be able to get substrate deficiency when you perfuse substrate-free. I don't think this is a contradiction.

Weiner: Dr Franke, on your last slide you indicated that the fluorescence of the surface would be dependent on two things. First is the redox state of the pyridine nucleotides. Second is dilation or constriction of the vessels of the tubular surface. Is it possible then that when you change oxygen tension, substrates, flow, or other variables, you would change the actual surface area which is fluorescing. Therefore is the total pyridine nucleotide fluorescence which you measure is not specific for the pyridine nucleotide content of the tissue or is it affected by the changing surface area of fluorescent tissue?

Franke: Well, I think this is partly compensated for. When you carry out manoeuvres like this, you also see changes in tissue opacity, and the advantage of this method is that it is possible to make corrections for these changes. Under the conditions that I have shown of normoxic–anoxic cycles, it is unlikely that there are such changes. Possibly the vessels collapse completely when there is complete ischemia and there is a fluorescent change which is not correctable. Nevertheless, the fluorescence is identical under these conditions, and we use it to calculate the ratio of reduced to oxidised pyridine nucleotide.

Vinay: In many systems, fluorescence tends to increase when temperature falls.

Franke: That is true for this system too, at lower temperatures than 10°C. Then we observe a marked increase. As you know, deep frozen tissues have a much greater pyridine nucleotide fluorescence. However, it is not a matter for concern in these experiments.

Int. J. Biochem., Vol. 12, pp. 277 to 281
© Pergamon Press Ltd 1980. Printed in Great Britain

0020-711X/80/0701-0277$02.00/0

^{31}P NMR STUDIES ON KIDNEY INTRACELLULAR pH IN ACUTE RENAL ACIDOSIS

G. K. RADDA, J. J. H. ACKERMAN*, P. BORE†, P. SEHR and G. G. WONG
Department of Biochemistry, University of Oxford

and

B. D. ROSS, Y. GREEN, S. BARTLETT and M. LOWRY
Department of Clinical Biochemistry, Radcliffe Infirmary, Oxford

Abstract—1. Phosphorus nuclear magnetic resonance (^{31}P NMR) provides a non-destructive method for the quantitative observation of the most abundant phosphate-containing metabolites in isolated perfused kidney and in kidneys inside an anaesthetised animal.

2. In this paper, the NMR method is introduced and the intracellular pH changes following acute renal acidosis are measured (from the resonance position of P_i) for the isolated perfused rat kidney.

3. The results are discussed in relation to the biochemical data obtained by freeze extraction.

INTRODUCTION

In this paper we shall describe a study of acute renal acidosis using the technique of nuclear magnetic resonance, NMR. Since this is probably the first time that NMR studies on the perfused kidney have been presented at these meetings (or in the literature), it is appropriate to provide a brief introduction to the method (for a more detailed discussion see Radda & Seeley, 1979).

WHAT IS NMR?

It is a way of observing the magnetic properties of atomic nuclei within molecules when these molecules are placed in a highly homogeneous magnetic field. One essentially measures the absorption of radiofrequency radiation which is selective for particular nuclei. In biology the most useful nuclei are ^{13}C, hydrogen and ^{31}P, although practically every nucleus in the periodic table has an isotope that is observable by NMR. In 1974 we demonstrated that when the spectrometer is tuned to observe the phosphorus nucleus, good signals can be obtained from metabolites that are contained in intact skeletal muscle preparations (Hoult *et al.*, 1974). Since then the interfacing of physiological techniques with the NMR measurements on a whole variety of organs including kidney, have been perfected by us (Garlick *et al.*, 1977; Sehr *et al.*, 1977) and others (Jacobus *et al.*, 1977). We shall first illustrate the kind of measurements one can make by NMR in intact systems.

WHAT DO WE MEASURE BY NMR?

Figure 1 shows a typical phosphorus NMR spectrum of a rat heart perfused in the Langendorff mode, beating in the spectrometer. In the spectra we plot frequency against the intensity of the absorption. From the position of the signal, the resonance frequency, we can identify the chemistry of the molecule that we are looking at. In Fig. 1 we can clearly assign, in comparison with proper standards, the peaks to the β, α, γ phosphates of ATP, phosphocreatine and to inorganic phosphate inside the cell and in the perfusion medium outside the cell. The reasons why we see two inorganic phosphate signals will be described below because this is the key to some of the results we wish to discuss in relation to our renal work. So the position tells us about chemistry and therefore provides identification. The intensity or the area under the signal is proportional to the number of nuclei we are observing. You do not have to assume an extinction coefficient and since the radiofrequency penetrates the tissue right through one is measuring directly the total amount of the metabolite that gives rise to a particular signal. The third piece of information is related to the width of the lines, and some other NMR properties that one can measure independently, that tell us something about molecular motion. Very crudely, when the signal is narrow one is dealing with a highly mobile small molecule, while for macromolecules the signal will be broad. This is the reason why we do not see phospholipids and DNA within the tissue. Thus, from the sharpness of the resonance, we can find out something about the conditions that the particular metabolite finds itself in.

In addition, there is a special method that allows one to look at rates of reactions catalysed by enzymes in tissues even though the reaction is at equilibrium or in the steady state (Brown *et al.*, 1978). For a perfused heart it is possible to measure the rate at which the phosphate group—from the γ-phosphate of ATP is transferred to phosphocreatine and that for the reverse reaction.

The P_i resonance and pH

Why do we see two inorganic phosphate (P_i) signals? The position of the resonance is very sensitive to the chemical environment of the nucleus so much so

* Present address: Department of Chemistry, University of Washington, St Louis, MO, U.S.A.

† Present address: Department of Surgery, University of Brisbane, Brisbane, Australia.

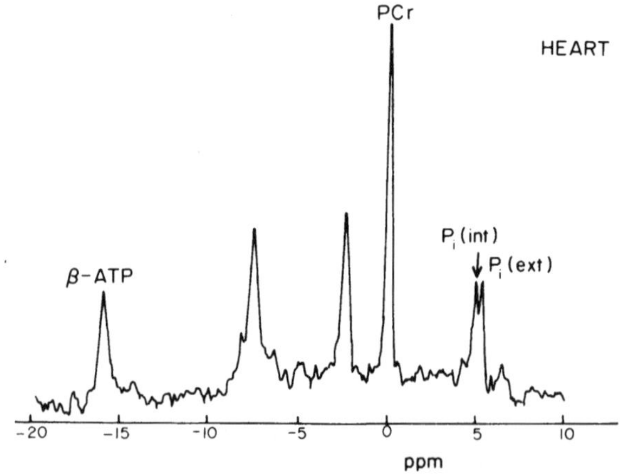

Fig. 1. High resolution ^{31}P NMR spectrum of Langendorff-perfused rat heart. The spectrum represents the Fourier transform average of 480 sampling pulses of 45° and with a 1 sec repetition interval. The spectrum is expanded to display 2.2 kHz. Peak assignments are: β-ATP = β-phosphate of adenosine 5′-triphosphate; PCr = phosphocreatine; P_i (int.) = intracellular inorganic phosphate; and P_i (ext.) = Krebs–Henseleit buffer inorganic phosphate.

that when a phosphate group is protonated, i.e. in the mono-ionic form, or unprotonated, in the di-ionic form, the signals occur at different positions. It is well known (Hoult *et al.*, 1974) that if you take a solution of inorganic phosphate and phosphocreatine and change the pH (in the range of 5.5–7.5) the P_i signal shifts compared to that of phosphocreatine that has no ionisable phosphate in this pH range. From appropriate calibration procedures (Gadian *et al.*, 1979) the position of the inorganic phosphate line gives a direct readout of intracellular pH vs extracellular pH depending on where the phosphate is located. Thus we have a sensitive way of measuring tissue pH.

If NMR is so simple why has it not been used before to study tissue? The reason is that the method is inherently insensitive and two major technical developments were required. One was the introduction of superconducting magnets at high fields and the other the introduction of the so-called Fourier Transform method (Farrar & Becker, 1971).

In the conventional or "continuous wave" NMR spectrometers the frequency range was slowly "scanned" to obtain the spectrum. As a single scan took 10–15 min, signal accumulation by repeated scanning was a very time-consuming process. In Fourier Transform NMR an intense pulse of radiofrequency that lasts for about 1–100 μsec is applied. Pulsing greatly increases the spread of radiation frequency and in this way allows all nuclei of a particular type to be excited simultaneously. The receiver is switched on immediately after the pulse and collects (as a voltage change) the decay in the "magnetization" of the nuclei. The process is repeated at relatively rapid intervals (1–20 sec) and the successive signals are added coherently in a computer memory. Accumulation of data is terminated when adequate signal-to-noise has been obtained. The conventional absorption vs frequency spectrum is obtained from the signal by the mathematical operation of Fourier transformation. So when we talk about the number of scans in presenting the spectra, it is the number of times we repeat the pulses before we get the signal that we regard as acceptable in terms of signal-to-noise.

NMR STUDIES ON PERFUSED KIDNEY

We shall only discuss one problem here, that of acute renal acidosis. The metabolic adaptation of the kidney in acute acidosis involves enzyme induction, increased gluconeogenesis, enhanced ammonia production and ammonia excretion into an acid urine (see Pitts, 1973; Tannen, 1978). This complex of events, which occurs as an homeostatic response to a change in blood pH, can be reproduced in the isolated kidney. Tannen & Ross (1979) found that the isolated perfused rat kidney responds to acute metabolic acidosis by (1) decrease in urine pH, (2) diuresis, (3) natriuresis, (4) an increased rate of ammonia production and (5) decreased kidney 2-oxoglutarate concentration. Studies with an inhibitor of gluconeogenesis demonstrated that the fall in 2-oxoglutarate concentration is not due to its increased consumption along that pathway (Ross & Tannen 1979). However, this metabolite is a reactant on the pathway of ammonia production by glutamate dehydrogenase activity from glutamate.

$$\text{Glutamate} + \text{NAD} \rightleftharpoons \text{2-oxoglutarate} + \text{NADH} + NH_3 + H^+$$

This is a near-equilibrium reaction (Krebs & Vinay, 1975) and can be written as

$$K = \left(\frac{[\text{NADH}]}{[\text{NAD}]}\right) \times \left(\frac{[\text{2-oxoglutarate}] \times [NH_3]}{[\text{glutamate}]}\right) \times [H^+]$$

In this mass action-ratio two constituents are unknown: (a) the ratio reduced:oxidized coenzyme, NADH/NAD and (b) the $[H^+]$. The rapid fall in

Table 1. Function of the isolated kidney perfused in the magnet in the absence of inorganic phosphate

	Mean ± SEM
Perfusate pH	7.38 ± 0.10 (3)
GFR (ml·min^{-1})	0.48 ± 0.06 (4)
U/P inulin	7.5 ± 0.8 (6)
% Na reabsorption	96.6 ± 0.9 (3)
Total Na^+ reabsorbed μmol·min^{-1}	67.7 ± 15.9 (3)

Kidneys perfused in the absence of inorganic phosphate give functions that do not differ significantly from results obtained by Ross & Tannen (1979) in the presence of inorganic phosphate.

oxoglutarate concentration may be a reflection of a change in either of these components of the equilibrium reaction. There is no satisfactory method of assessing the ratio NADH:NAD *in vivo*, but the pH of an intact kidney can be determined by NMR.

In order to do that we have to perfuse the kidney inside the spectrometer. The kidney is placed in the "probe" surrounded by a radio-frequency coil. The conventional perfusion system has to be modified to interface it with the NMR measurement. The modifications include changes in the length of the perfusion circuit, therefore in the perfusion volume and consequently in the perfusion pressure required. In addition, because we were trying to use the position of the intracellular phosphate to measure intracellular pH we had to leave out the phosphate from the perfusion medium. It is essential to establish first that under these conditions the biochemistry and function of the kidney remain the same as in the conventional perfusion system. The comparison shown in Table 1 demonstrates that this is indeed the case.

It turns out, rather remarkably, that in the absence of phosphate in the perfusion medium all the functions in the kidney that we have measured are retained, although the intracellular to extracellular phosphate ratio is of the order of 29:1 compared to the normal 3:1.

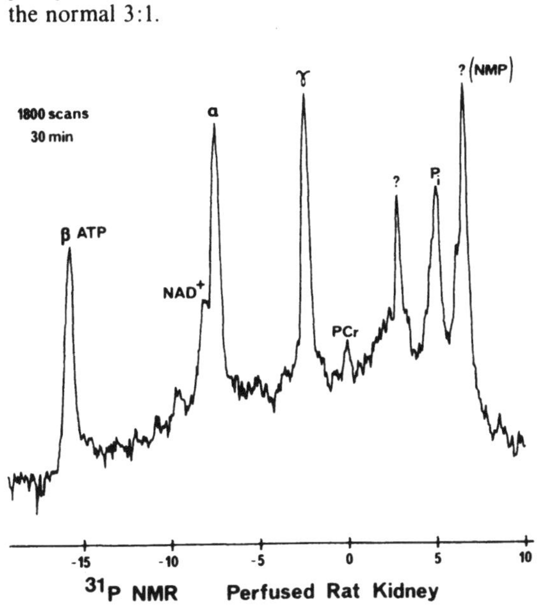

Fig. 2. ^{31}P NMR spectrum of perfused rat kidney. Perfusion conditions as in Table 2 using phosphate-free buffer.

Figure 2 shows the kinds of ^{31}P NMR spectra we can collect from perfused kidneys. This spectrum was collected in 30 min though the time resolution of our spectrometer for obtaining acceptable spectra is currently of the order of 1–2 min. The different peaks one can see correspond to ATP (β, α and γ phosphate). The β phosphate peak contains contributions from ADP and therefore the difference between the β and γ phosphate signals tells us how much ADP is present. We see a very small amount of phosphocreatine, a large peak of inorganic phosphate and an intense signal, which in position corresponds to nucleotide monophosphate AMP and IMP. This peak appears to be much larger than expected from conventional analytical methods and indicate the need for further analysis. Finally, in many kidneys we find an unexpected signal from a metabolite present in very high concentrations. It corresponds to a phosphodiester and we have not yet sorted out its role. We shall now focus on the inorganic phosphate signal. Two of its features are relevant: (i) from its position we can read out the average pH in the kidney as 7.2, (ii) compared to heart and other tissues we have studied, the inorganic phosphate signal in the kidney is considerably broader, implying that there is heterogeneity in pH of about 0.5 pH units within the kidney tissue.

By measuring the P_i peak positions we can follow the intrarenal pH changes during acute acidosis. This is induced by adding HCl to the perfusion medium, the medium pH starting at 7.4. As the pH of the perfusion medium is decreased, shown on the dotted line in Fig. 3 the intracellular pH of the kidney follows this change. The final average pH drop is 0.3 pH units. In the outside medium the pH drop is 0.5 in this experiment.

At the same time, we can observe the acidification of the urine and ammonia production. In addition, at the end of an experiment, we can take the kidney out, freeze–clamp it and do the usual biochemical analysis.

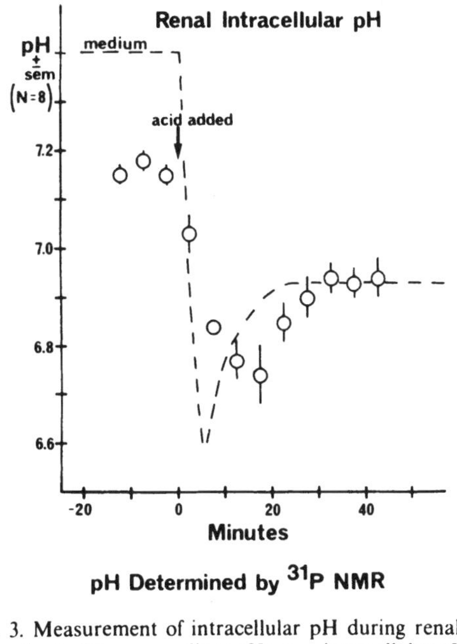

Fig. 3. Measurement of intracellular pH during renal acidosis. Dotted line = medium pH; O = intracellular pH determined from the position of the P_i resonance.

Table 2. Metabolites of the kidney perfused in the absence of inorganic phosphate

Metabolite	Metabolite concentration (μmols·g dry wt^{-1}) No phosphate	Control with phosphate
ATP	5.62 ± 0.21 (7)	7.1 ± 0.53 (7)
ADP	3.03 ± 0.49 (7)	2.14 ± 0.33 (5)
AMP	1.11 ± 0.36 (7)	1.37 ± 0.57 (5)
P_i	8.64 ± 0.82 (12)	12.86 ± 0.90 (16)
Total adenine nucleotide	9.80 ± 0.88 (7)	10.98 ± 0.64 (4)
$\frac{ATP}{ADP \times P_i}$	0.22 ± 10^{-3} M	0.26×10^{-3} M

Kidneys of fed rats were perfused for 90 min before freeze–clamping. The perfusion medium of 7.5 g% bovine serum albumin, containing 0.5 mM glutamine and 5 mM D-glucose, was prepared by dialysis against Krebs–Henseleit saline from which K_2HPO_4 was omitted. This perfusion medium contained 0.09 mM phosphate, compared with 1 mM in the control. Control figures are taken from Ross & Tannen (1979).

Table 3. Effect of acute acidosis on metabolites of kidney perfused in the absence of inorganic phosphate

	No phosphate		*P* (7.4 vs 6.9)	Control	
Mean pH	7.38 ± 0.10 (6)	6.85 ± 0.04 (10)		7.4	6.9
2-oxoglutarate	1.99 ± 0.24 (6)	0.32 ± 0.08 (7)	<0.01	2.63 ± 0.19 (8)	0.67 ± 0.05 (7)
NH_3	20.00 ± 1.07 (9)	11.54 ± 1.46 (15)	<0.001	20.7 ± 0.92 (7)	11.83 ± 0.84 (5)
Glutamate	9.97 ± 0.68 (9)	6.56 ± 0.31 (13)	<0.01	14.34 ± 0.39 (8)	9.56 ± 1.05 (7)
$\left[\frac{[\text{2-oxoglutarate}]\ NH_3}{[\text{glutamate}]}\right]$ (for wet weight)	0.69 ± 0.09 (5) $\times 10^{-3}$ M	0.11 ± 0.03 (6) $\times 10^{-3}$ M	<0.01	0.71 ± 0.01 (8)	0.14 ± 0.03 (6)

Experimental conditions as in Table 2: after 40 min, the pH of the perfusate was lowered by addition of N HCl. Results obtained under similar conditions, but in the presence of inorganic phosphate, are taken from Ross & Tannen (1979).

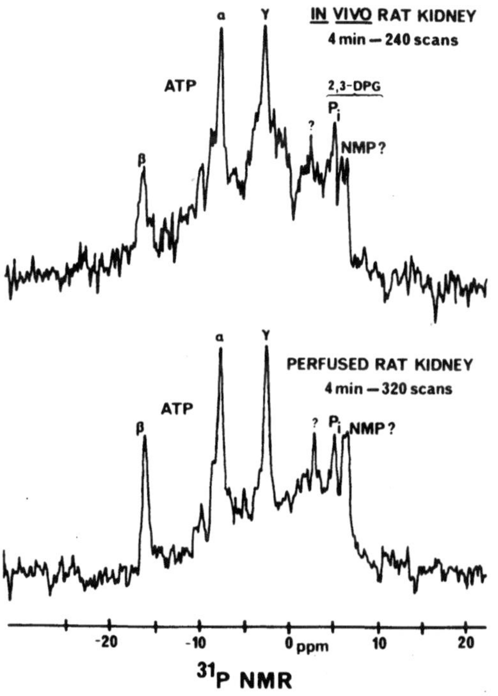

Fig. 4. ^{31}P NMR spectra of *in vivo* and perfused rat kidneys.

Measurements of adenine nucleotides and other metabolites are summarized in Table 2. Even in the absence of inorganic phosphate in the perfusion medium the oxoglutarate concentration in acidosis decreases considerably, as does tissue ammonia while glutamate only changes by a small amount (Table 3). The mass action ratio considerably decreases, to 15% of its original value. We can therefore conclude on the basis of the NMR experiments that the intracellular pH change of 0.2–0.3 is not sufficient to account for the change in the mass action ratio. The expected pH change should be of the order of 0.7 if this alone were responsible for the fall in tissue concentration of 2-oxoglutarate.

EXTENSION OF THE NMR METHOD TO OTHER PROBLEMS

Finally, we should mention that the kinds of measurements we described can be applied to the study of many other problems particularly when one considers that they can also be extended to measurements of kidneys inside an animal. We have perfected the operative techniques that allow us to expose the kidney so that the radio-frequency coil can be put around the organ in the animal. The whole animal is then placed in the spectrometer. In Fig. 4 we show the phosphorus NMR spectra we see from a perfused rat kidney compared to that of an *in vivo* rat kidney. It is rewarding to see that the two are very similar. Clearly one can study kidneys both in the isolated form and within the whole animal by the non-destructive NMR method.

REFERENCES

Brown T. R., Gadian D. G., Garlick P. B., Radda G. K., Seeley P. J. & Styles P. (1978) Creatine kinase activities in skeletal and cardiac muscle measured by saturation transfer NMR. In *Frontiers of Biological Energetics: Electrons to Tissues* (Edited by Dutton L., Leigh J. & Scarpa A.) pp. 1341–1351. Academic Press, New York.

Farrar T. C. & Becker E. D. (1971) *Pulse and Fourier Transform NMR—Introduction to Theory and Methods.* Academic Press, New York.

Gadian D. G., Radda G. K., Richards R. E. & Seeley P. J. (1979) ^{31}P NMR in living tissue: the road from a promising to an important tool in biology. In *Biological Applications of Magnetic Resonance* (Edited by Shulman R. G.) pp. 463–537. Academic Press, New York.

Garlick P. B., Radda G. K., Seeley P. J. & Chance B. (1977) Phosphorus NMR studies on perfused heart. *Biophem. biophys. Res. Commun.* **77,** 195–202.

Hoult D. I., Busby S. J. W., Gadian D. G., Radda G. K., Richards R. E. & Seeley P. J. (1974). Observations of tissue metabolites using ^{31}P nuclear magnetic resonance. *Nature* **252,** 285–287.

Jacobus W. E., Taylor G. J., Hollis D. P. & Nunnally R. L. (1977) Phosphorus nuclear magnetic resonance of perfused working hearts. *Nature* **265,** 756–758.

Krebs H. A. & Vinay P. (1975) Regulation of renal ammonia production. *Med. Clin. N. Am.* **59,** 591–603.

Pitts R. F. (1973) In *Handbook of Physiology,* Section 8: Renal Physiology. (Edited by Orloff J. & Berliner R. W.) pp. 455–496.

Radda G. K. & Seeley P. J. (1979) Recent studies on cellular metabolism by nuclear magnetic resonance. *A. Rev. Physiol.* **41,** 744–769.

Ross B. D. & Tannen R. L. (1979) Effects of decrease in bicarbonate concentration in metabolism of the isolated perfused rat kidney. *Clin. Sci.* **57,** 103–111.

Sehr P. A., Radda G. K., Bore P. J. & Sells R. A. (1977) A model kidney transplant studied by phosphorus nuclear magnetic resonance. *Biochem. biophys. Res. Commun.* **77,** 1256–1262.

Tannen R. L. (1978). Ammonia metabolism. *Am. J. Physiol.* **235,** F265–F277.

Tannen R. L. & Ross B. D. (1979) Ammoniagenesis by isolated perfused kidney: the critical role of urinary acidification. *Clin. Sci.* **56,** 353–364.

SYMPOSIUM DISCUSSION

Osswald: How do the values for tissue content of adenine nucleotides obtained with NMR methods compare in μmols·g wet weight^{-1} with other methods?

Radda: The adenine nucleotide concentrations given in this paper were obtained by conventional enzymatic assay because the conditions required to get quantitive data and pH measurements are somewhat different. We have done careful measurements in the heart, comparing NMR values with those from freeze–clamped extracts, and the conclusion is that we see 100% of the ATP and phosphocreatine by NMR. I think the result will be the same for the kidney ATP.

Osswald: What is the total adenine nucleotide content?

Ross: Total adenine nucleotides of perfused kidney are about 3.5 μmols·g wet weight^{-1}, and ATP about 1.3 μmols, both of which compare closely with the figures obtained for non-perfused kidneys (Nishiitsutsuji-Uwo *et al., Biochem. J.,* **103,** 352, 1967).

Halperin: Despite the fact that you don't add phosphate to your perfusion medium is there phosphate in the urine? Urine pH is very much lower than tissue pH. Would that influence the mean pH that you are recording?

Ross: The phosphate content of the urine in the phosphate-free perfused kidneys was 0.15–0.2 mM, when the medium contained less than 0.09 mM and the tissue P_i was 3 mM, so we consider that the urine contributes very little to the signal that we observed.

Koepsel: Did you try to distinguish bound from free ATP, is this possible with this technique?

Radda: From the width of the lines, we can say that we only see mobile ATP, and ADP and we should not see the bound ATP which would give rise to a broad signal. It is interesting that in kidney, in contrast to heart and other muscles, that we see free ADP. In muscle ADP is much more completely bound whereas in kidney it is free, as you might expect.

Vinay: When kidney tubules are incubated in phosphate-free medium they can maintain a phosphate gradient of more than 10, and have a completely normal intracellular phosphate concentration.

Weiner: Why is it necessary to perfuse with phosphate-free medium when you can also study the kidney *in vivo*, with phosphate present in the blood?

Radda: We wanted the defined conditions of perfused kidney to induce the metabolic changes of acidosis. The reason phosphate must be omitted from the medium is concerned with the presence of albumin in the perfusion medium. This so alters the NMR characteristics of the phosphate that we cannot separate internal from external phosphate, as is possible with the perfused heart.

Kinne: Where do the pH changes take place, in the cytoplasm or the mitochondrion?

Radda: That is one of the key issues here. Most of the signal is from the cytosol, so that we are measuring cytoplasmic pH. The evidence for this comes from another tissue, the barnacle muscle, in which micro-pH electrode (most probably in the cytosol, and not in the mitochondria!) give the same value as NMR. It also depends upon the total phosphate distribution and the majority of the phosphate in total volume that we see is in the cytoplasm, so that the majority of the signal we see arises in the cytoplasm.

Kinne: There is thought to be a large pH gradient across the mitochondrial membrane. In what way does the gradient influence the signal?

Radda: The signal is directly proportional to the number of molecules, so that if the phosphate concentration in mitochondria was substantially higher than the cytoplasm (so that the majority of tissue phosphate was mitochondrial) then you would observe mitochondrial pH: but that is not the case.

Vinay: Estimation of cytosolic pH from the LDH equilibrium might answer Dr Kinne's question. Have you done that, and does it agree with the NMR findings?

Radda: We measure a pH drop of 0.3 units on acidification, and I don't therefore have to explain why this doesn't agree with the other method of calculation.

Int. J. Biochem., Vol. 12, pp. 283 to 286

0020-711X/80/0701-0283$02.00/0

INTRODUCTION

ENERGETICS OF ACTIVE TRANSTUBULAR TRANSPORT; FUNCTION OF THE Na-K-ION PUMP

PETER LETH JØRGENSEN
Institute of Physiology, University of Arhus, 8000 Arhus C, Denmark

INTRODUCTION

The kidney is the only mammalian tissue from which the Na-K-pump can be prepared in pure, undenatured form. Pure renal Na-K-ATPase has been available for 5–6 yr (Jørgensen, 1975). Its protein structure and reaction mechanism have been studied intensively. In contrast to this detailed information about the pure Na-K-ATPase many basic questions concerning the functions of the Na-K-pump in kidney tubules cannot be answered at present. The kidney cell membranes are equipped with numerous transport molecules but only the Na-K-pump and perhaps one or two other proteins are capable of coupling ATP splitting to active cation transport. However, few transport functions in kidney tubules can unambiguously be attributed to the Na-K-pump. In this introduction I shall try to discern some of the unsolved questions concerning the renal Na-K-pump and to identify physiological problems which may be solved through studies on the renal Na-K-pump.

STRUCTURE OF THE RENAL NA-K-PUMP

Ligand binding experiments show that the proteins of renal Na-K-ATPase that have been purified in membrane-bound form are organized in dimeric units ($\alpha_2\beta_2$) of mol wt 270,000–286,000 consisting of two α-subunits with mol wt 104,000 and two sialoglycoproteins (β-subunits) with mol wt close to 40,000 (Jørgensen 1974, 1977). A proteolipid with mol wt close to 10,000 may constitute a γ-subunit of Na-K-ATPase as it is covalently labelled by a photoaffinity derivative of ouabain (Forbush *et al.*, 1978). Electron microscopy after negative staining show surface particles (30–50 Å diameter, $13{,}000 \cdot \mu m^{-2}$) corresponding to protein units containing one α-subunit. Dimeric intramembraneous particles (80–90 Å diameter, $6600 \cdot \mu m^{-2}$) observed after freeze fracture and rotatory replication are proposed to represent the unit with mol wt 280,000 ($\alpha_2\beta_2$) (Deguchi *et al.*, 1977; Maunsbach *et al.*, 1979).

Purification of Na-K-ATPase always involves the use of detergents and may therefore be achieved at the expense of structural and functional alterations. It is therefore not known whether the Na-K-pump in the native renal cell membrane has the same structure as that observed for the purified Na-K-ATPase. One way to examine the structure of the Na-K-pump is to look at the molecule after reconstitution into phospholipid vesicles. In the process of reconstitution excess lipid is added and the density of protein particles in the vesicle membrane can be varied at will. We observed active cation transport in vesicle preparations containing on an average less than one particle per vesicle. A linear relationship was observed between the rate of active sodium transport and the number of particles per vesicle in the range from 0 to about 16 intramembraneous particles (90 Å diameter) per vesicle with diameter 900 Å (Skriver *et al.*, 1979). The intramembraneous particle in the vesicle membrane has the same size as the protein particle in the pure membrane-bound Na-K-ATPase (80–90 Å diameter) (Maunsbach *et al.*, 1979). This provides evidence that the $\alpha_2\beta_2$-unit with mol wt 280,000 can catalyze active coupled Na-K-transport. These observations should only be extrapolated to the native renal Na-K-pump with caution, since the turnover number of the reconstituted Na-K-pump molecules is only about $\frac{1}{4}$ of the turnover number of the Na-K-pump in the cell membrane. This discrepancy may be due to inactivation by the detergent used in the reconstitution procedure. Recent studies of ligand binding led to the proposal that Na-K-ATPase in the cell membranes of the outer medulla of mammalian kidney are organized in tetramers ($\alpha_4\beta_4$) or even in octamers ($\alpha_8\beta_8$) (Hansen *et al.*, 1979). It therefore remains a possibility that larger oligomers than the dimer ($\alpha_2\beta_2$) are required to catalyze Na-K-ion transport at the rates which are observed in intact cells (for references see Jørgensen, 1975).

THE AMOUNT OF NA-K-ATPASE IN KIDNEY TUBULES

Identification of a unit of renal Na-K-ATPase ($\alpha_2\beta_2$) with a maximum turnover rate close to $10{,}000\,\text{ATP} \cdot \text{min}^{-1}$ (Jørgensen, 1975) forms a basis for quantitative analysis of the amount of Na-K-pump sites in isolated tubules. Techniques have been developed for quantitative analysis of Na-K-ATPase in isolated tubules from rabbit kidney (Schmidt & Horster, 1978). The data in Table 1 are recalculated to units of enzyme activity per cm tubule length to facilitate comparison with the transport data which are obtained in isolated perfused rabbit kidney tubules. In terms of enzyme units per gram tubule the Na-K-ATPase activities in proximal convoluted segments are 2–4-fold lower than in the medullary thick ascending limb of Henle. However, this difference in activity becomes much smaller when expressed in units per

Table 1. Na-K-ATPase activities and solute transport capacities in isolated rabbit kidney tubule segments

	Na-K-ATPase activity in isolated segments	Net transport across isolated segments Na$^+$	J_{max} glucose	J_{max} aminoacids
	pmol ATP/sec·cm	pmol/sec·cm		
PCT	2.8–6.4	35	13	5
MTAL	8.5	4–40		
$CTAL_{neonatal}$	0.6	2.1		
$CTAL_{mature}$	3.5	9–13		
CCD	3.2	3.5–12		
MCD	2.5	—		

Na-K-ATPase activities were determined by Schmidt & Horster (1978). The transport capacities were determined in isolated prefused segments by Kokko *et al.* (1971), Tune & Burg (1979, 1976), Barfuss & Schafer (1979), Horster (1978) and Schwartz & Burg (1978). Abbreviations: PCT: proximal convoluted tubule. MTAL and CTAL: medullary and cortical thick ascending limbs of Henle. CCD and MCD: cortical and medullary collecting ducts.

cm tubule length, because the brush border membrane which is devoid of Na-K-ATPase forms a substantial fraction of the mass of proximal tubule cells.

The main problem in relating the Na-K-ATPase activities to the transport capacities in isolated tubules is that the turnover rate per pump molecule in the intact cells and the stoichiometry of the active cation transport are unknown. Using a Na:ATP ratio of 3, there is a surprisingly good agreement between the Na-K-ATPase activities and the transport capacities of the isolated tubules in Table 1. However, this agreement may turn out to be coincidental since the degree of exposure of latent Na-K-ATPase sites is uncertain and some inactivation of pump sites may occur during freeze drying.

Techniques for determining the concentration of Na-K-pump sites by measuring the ouabain binding capacity in isolated tubules have not yet been developed.

IDENTIFICATION OF NA-K-PUMP FUNCTIONS IN KIDNEY TUBULES

The main problem in defining the role of the Na-K-pump in transtubular transport is that methods for controlling and monitoring cytoplasmic cation activities and ATP concentrations are not available. Operationally the Na-K-pump in kidney tubules can therefore only be studied by varying Na$^+$ and K$^+$ concentrations in luminal and peritubular fluids and by specific inhibition with ouabain. Inhibition by ouabain and manipulation with luminal Na$^+$ and peritubular K$^+$ are therefore the important tools for identifying Na-K-pump functions in kidney tubules.

The transport processes in Table 1 and in Figs 1 and 2 have been shown to depend on luminal Na$^+$ and peritubular K$^+$ and to be inhibited by ouabain. In rabbit kidney tubules, inhibition by 10^{-5} M ouabain a few minutes after application is direct evidence for participation of the Na-K-pump in the transport process. The Na-K-pump is extremely sensitive to extracellular K$^+$. Removal of K$^+$ may therefore not always totally abolish Na-K-exchange. Studies of the concentration dependence may be more profitable since the dependence of the rate of Na-K-transport on extracellular K$^+$ is a characteristic feature of the Na-K-pump. Recently, it was observed that peritubular K$^+$ stimulates transtubular transport in isolated proximal tubules along a sigmoid curve with a $K_{\frac{1}{2}}$ for K$^+$ close to 1 mM at 149 mM Na$^+$ (Cardinal & Duchesneau, 1978). This is similar to the dependence of Na-K-transport in red cell on extracellular K$^+$ (Glynn & Karlish, 1975). Although direct evidence for recycling of K$^+$ across the basolateral membrane has not been obtained, the effects of ouabain and peritubular K$^+$ on the transtubular transport suggest that coupled Na-K-transport prevails at the basolateral membrane like in the vesicles reconstituted with pure renal Na-K-ATPase.

The failure to establish a direct relation between the rate of transtubular Na$^+$ transport and influx of

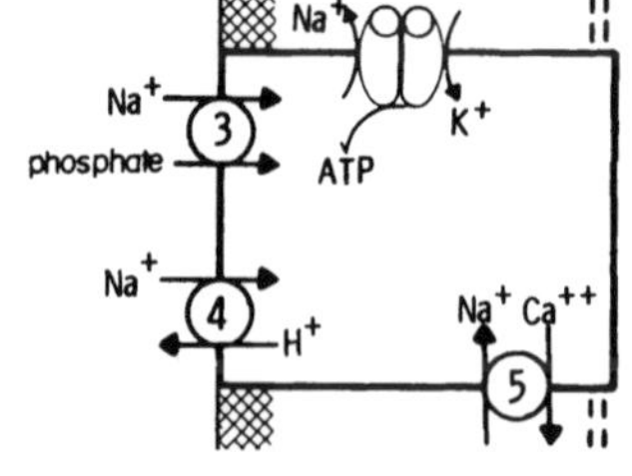

Fig. 1. The modes of transtubular Na$^+$ transport in proximal convoluted tubules. The Na-K-pump couples ATP hydrolysis to active Na$^+$ transport from cytoplasm to extracellular fluid and creates electrochemical Na$^+$ gradients from extracellular fluid to cytoplasm. The carriers mediating Na$^+$ coupled active transport of solutes are placed in numerical order.

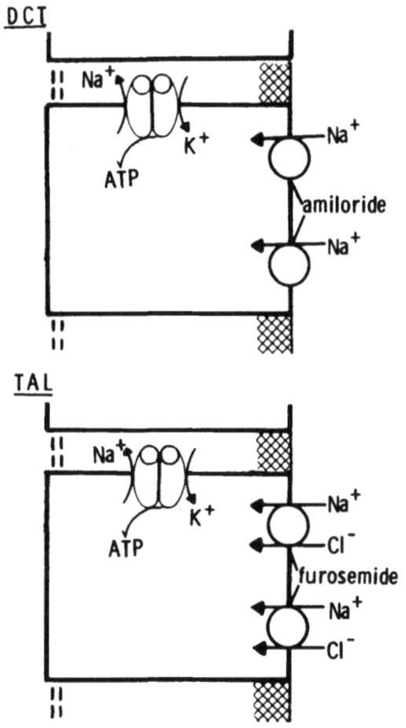

Fig. 2. Model for primary active Na^+ transport and secondary active Cl^- transport in medullary and cortical thick ascending limbs of Henle. Coupled electroneutral entry of Na^+ and Cl^- is mediated by a cotransport system for NaCl which is sensitive to furosemide like in other epithelia (Nellans *et al.*, 1973; Eveloff *et al.*, 1978). In distal tubules and collecting ducts the entry of Na^+ is mediated by an amiloride sensitive carrier mechanism (Burg, 1976).

K^+ across the basolateral membrane or the K^+ activity in the cytoplasm has been used as an argument against involvement of the Na-K-pump in transtubular transport (Schultz, 1978). This may not be justified in kidney since the problems involved in analysis of the cytoplasmic pool of K^+ remain unsolved. The mitochondrial pool of K^+ is not immediately available for exchange with the cytoplasm. This, together with the high rates of transport and the high permeability of the basolateral membrane for K^+, may explain that the small cytoplasmic pool of K^+ in the space between the mitochondria and the cell membrane cannot be identified in the intact kidney tissue.

FUNCTION OF THE NA-K-PUMP IN DISCRETE NEPHRON SEGMENTS

The fraction of filtered Na^+ which is reabsorbed by the Na-K-pump is subject to species variation and internal regulatory control. Studies on intact dog and rat kidney show that 30–50% of filtered Na^+ is reabsorbed by the Na-K-pump (Besarab *et al.*, 1976; Sejersted *et al.*, 1977). This estimate agrees with the analysis on isolated tubules which suggest that the Na-K-pump is responsible for 1/3 of net Na^+ reabsorption in proximal tubules and that all Na^+ reabsorption in thick ascending limbs of Henle, distal convoluted tubules and collecting ducts is driven by the Na-K-pump.

A model based on a unifying concept of the function of the Na-K-pump in active transtubular transport is proposed in Figs 1 and 2. It is obvious that the Na-K-pump drives transport processes of widely different characteristics in the discrete nephron segments, but this diversity of the transport processes does not reside within the Na-K-pump *per se*. The nature and direction of the transport processes depend on the sodium coupled transport elements in the cell membranes in conjunction with the conductances of the tight junctions and basement membranes. The Na-K-pump couples ATP hydrolysis to active Na^+ transport from cytoplasm to the extracellular fluid. Maintenance of the resulting electrochemical gradient for Na^+ across the cell membrane is the prime function of the Na-K-pump. The Na^+ conductance of the cell membrane *per se* is low and the entry of Na^+ along the gradient created by the Na-K-pump is governed by specific carrier mechanisms. The control of the Na-K-pump turnover rate by the cytoplasmic Na^+ activity links the carriers and the Na-K-pump into intgrated transport systems which provide the characteristic features of the active solute reabsorption in the discrete nephron segments.

The carriers mediating Na^+ coupled active transport of solute are placed in numerical order in Figs 1 and 2. Consult the recent article by Kinne & Schwartz (1978) for a resumé of their properties. In proximal tubule cells, the Na-K-pump drives active reabsorption of Na^+ in tight coupling with secondary active transport of other solutes (Fig. 1). The sodium cotransport systems can be demonstrated in vesicles of brush border and basolateral membranes, but these carriers have not been isolated and their structure is unknown. The observation that the maximum capacity (J_{max}) for glucose reabsorption is in the same range as the capacity for Na^+ transport estimated from the content of Na-K-ATPase in proximal tubules (Table 1) suggests that the capacity for Na^+ transport may be rate limiting in certain conditions and thus determine the magnitude of the T_{max} for glucose.

The hypothesis for primary active Na^+ transport and secondary active Cl^- transport in the TAL (Fig. 2) has been discussed in detail before (Jørgensen, 1976).

In distal convoluted tubules and collecting ducts Na^+ reabsorption against steep electrochemical gradients is ouabain sensitive (for ref. see Burg, 1976). The role of the Na-K-pump in these segments is therefore less controversial than in proximal tubules and in Henle's loop. The main questions are whether the Na-K-pump participates in acute and chronic adaptation of the transport capacity and whether the pump is a target for hormonal control. Chronic adaptation of the Na^+ transport capacity in collecting ducts have been shown to be accompanied by a marked change in area of basolateral membrane infoldings (Wade *et al.*, 1979), but the amount of Na-K-ATPase has not been measured in these conditions.

Acknowledgement—Supported by the Danish Medical Research Council.

REFERENCES

Barfuss D. W. & Schafer J. A. (1979) Active aminoacid absorption by proximal convoluted and proximal straight tubules. *Am. J. Physiol.* **236**, F149–F162.

BESARB A., SILVA P. & EPSTEIN F. H. (1976) Multiple pumps for sodium reabsorption by the perfused kidney. *Kidney Int.* **10,** 147–153.

BURG M. B. (1976) Mechanisms of action of diuretic drugs. In *The Kidney.* (Edited by BRENNER B. M. & RECTOR F. C.) Vol. 1, pp. 737–762. Saunders, Philadelphia.

CARDINAL I. & DUCHESNEAU D. (1978) Effect of potassium on proximal tubular function. *Am. J. Physiol.* **234,** F381–F385.

DEGUCHI N., JØRGENSEN P. L. & MAUNSBACH A. B. Ultrastructure of the sodium pump. Comparison of thin sectioning, negative staining and freeze fracture of purified, membrane-bound Na, K-ATPase. *J. Cell Biol.* **75,** 619–634.

EVELOFF J., KINNE R., KINNE-SAFFRAN E., MURER H., SILVA P., EPSTEIN F. H., STOFF J., & KINTER W. B. (1978) Coupled sodium and chloride transport into plasma membrane vesicles prepared from dogfish rectal gland. *Pflügers Arch. ges. Physiol.* **378,** 87–92.

FORBUSH B., KAPLAN J. H. & HOFFMAN J. F. (1978) Characterization of a new photoaffinity derivative of ouabain: Labelling of the large polypeptide and of a proteolipid component of the Na-K-ATPase. *Biochemistry* **17,** 3667–3676.

FRÖMTER E. (1979) Solute transport across epithelia: What can we learn from micropuncture studies on kidney tubules. *J. Physiol.* **288,** 1–31.

GLYNN I. M. & KARLISH S. J. D. (1975) The sodium pump. *A. Rev. Physiol.* **37,** 13–53.

HANSEN O., JENSEN J., NØRBY J. G. & OTTOLENGHI P. (1979) A new proposal regarding the subunit composition of Na,K-ATPase. *Nature* **280,** 410–412.

HORSTER M. Loop of Henle functional differentiation *in vitro* perfusion of the isolated thick ascending segment. *Pflügers Arch. ges Physiol.* **378,** 15–24.

JØRGENSEN P. L. (1974) Purification and characterization of Na,K-ATPase. IV. Estimation of the purity and of the molecular weight and polypeptide content per enzyme unit in preparations from the outer medulla of rabbit kidney. *Biochim. biophys. Acta* **356,** 53–67.

JØRGENSEN P. L. (1975) Isolation and characterization of the components of the sodium pump. *Q. Rev. Biophys.* **7,** 239–274.

JØRGENSEN P. L. (1976) The function of Na,K-ATPase in the thick ascending limb of Henles loop. *Curr. Prob. clin. Biochem.* **6,** 190–199.

JØRGENSEN P. L. (1977) Purification and characterization of Na,K-ATPase. VI. Differential tryptic modification of catalytic functions of the purified enzyme in presence of NaCl and KCl. *Biochim. biophys. Acta* **466,** 97–108.

KINNE R. & SCHWARTZ J. L. (1978) Isolated membrane vesicles in the evaluation of the nature, localization, and regulation of renal transport processes. *Kidney Int.* **14,** 547–556.

KOKKO J. P., BURG M. B. & ORLOFF J. Characteristics of NaCl and water transport in the renal proximal tubule. *J. clin. Invest.* **50,** 69–76.

MAUNSBACH, A. B. SKRIVER E. & JØRGENSEN P. L. (1979) Ultrastructure of purified Na,K-ATPase membranes. In *Sodium, Potassium-ATPase: Structure and Kinetics.* (Edited by SKOU J. C. & NØRBY J. G.) pp. 3–13. Academic Press, New York.

NELLANS H. N., FRIZZELL R. A. & SCHULTZ S. G. (1973) Coupled sodium-chloride influx across the brush border of rabbit ileum. *Am. J. Physiol.* **225,** 467–475.

SCHMIDT U. & HORSTER M. (1977) Na,K-activated ATPase: activity maturation in rabbit nephron segments dissected *in vitro. Am. J. Physiol.* **233**(1), F55–F60.

SCHULTZ S. G. (1978) Is a coupled Na,K-exchange "pump" involved in active transepithelial Na transport? A status report. In *Membrane Transport Processes.* (Edited by HOFFMAN J. F.) Vol. 1. pp. 213–227. Raven Press, New York.

SCHWARTZ G. J. & BURG M. B. (1978) Mineralcorticoid effects of cation transport by cortical collecting tubulus *in vitro. Am. J. Physiol.* **235,** F576–585.

SEJERSTED O., MATHISEN Ø. & KIIL F. Oxygen requirement of renal Na,K-ATPase dependent sodium reabsorption. *Am. J. Physiol.* **232,** F152–F158.

SKRIVER E., MAUNSBACH A. B. & JØRGENSEN P. L. (1980) Ultrastructure of Na,K-transport vesicles reconstituted with purified renal Na,K-ATPase. *J. Cell Biol.* in press.

TUNE B. M. & BURG M. B. (1971) Glucose transport by proximal renal tubules. *Am. J. Physiol.* **221,** 580–585.

WADE I. B., O'NEILL R. G., PRYOR J. L. & BOULPAEP E. Modulation of cell membrane area in renal collecting tubules by corticosteroid hormones. *J. Cell Biol.* **81,** 439–445.

Int. J. Biochem., Vol. 12, pp. 287 to 293
© Pergamon Press Ltd 1980. Printed in Great Britain

0020-711X/80/0701-0287$02.00/0

STRUCTURE, FUNCTION AND REGULATION OF Na–K-ATPase*

ARNOLD SCHWARTZ†, ROBERT J. ADAMS, WILLIAM J. BALL JR, JOHN H. COLLINS, SHARMILA S. GUPTE, LOIS K. LANE, ANITA S. REEVES and EARL T. WALLICK
Department of Pharmacology and Cell Biophysics, University of Cincinnati College of Medicine, 231 Bethesda Avenue, Cincinnati, OH 45267, U.S.A.

Abstract—1. The Na–K-ATPase consists of a large chain (α) and a small chain (β) and possibly a proteolipid chain (γ), of molecular weights 100,000, 45,000 and about 13,000 respectively.

2. Various fluorescent-labelled probes when incorporated into purified lamb kidney Na–K-ATPase, reveal important conformational changes that appear to be modified by cations, including calcium.

3. The regulation of ouabain binding to the Na–K-ATPase involves interaction of both Na^+ and K^+ at an "external" site.

4. Vanadate may be involved in regulation of the sodium pump, by interaction with an "internal" site. This produces modification of an "external" K^+ site. Both ATPase activity and ouabain binding are affected by this trace metal.

5. A search is ongoing for endogenous factor(s) that specifically interact with the digitalis receptor and the Na–K-ATPase.

INTRODUCTION

There is now little doubt that the Na–K-ATPase is the *in vivo* sodium pump. Thus far, kidney medulla is the only mammalian tissue from which it has been possible to purify the Na–K-ATPase. The kidney enzyme is similar to those isolated from non-mammalian sources, in that it consists primarily of a $M_r = 95{,}000$ catalytic (α) subunit and a $M_r \simeq 40{,}000$ glycoprotein (β) subunit in a 1:1 molar ratio ($\alpha_2\beta_2$; $M_r \simeq 275{,}000$). The purified kidney Na–K-ATPase also appears to be quite similar to preparations which have been partially purified from mammalian brain, cardiac and skeletal muscle (e.g. phosphorylated α subunit, affinities for ATP, cations and ouabain). In spite of extensive studies over the last few years, the minimum molecular constituents of the enzyme complex are not known, and we still do not understand the mechanism by which the enzyme regulates ion transport *in vivo*. In our efforts to better understand the structure-function relationship of the Na-K-ATPase and to identify *in vivo* regulators of the sodium pump, we are currently (a) using fluorescent probes and antibodies to study lipid–protein interactions and conformational changes in the enzyme complex; (b) determining the amino acid sequence of the lamb kidney Na–K-ATPase proteins and (c) investigating factors which may be responsible for the *in vivo* regulation of the sodium pump.

PROBES OF Na–K-ATPase STRUCTURE AND FUNCTION

It is generally accepted that the coupling of ATP hydrolysis with the transport of Na^+ and K^+ across the cell membrane is mediated via conformational changes in the Na–K-ATPase. Our early experiments with circular dichroism and fluorescence spectroscopy using a crude Na–K-ATPase preparation also suggested that conformational changes in the Na–K-ATPase occurred with the binding of cardiac glycosides to the enzyme (Lindenmayer & Schwartz, 1970; Nagai *et al.*, 1970). These studies were hampered, however, by the lack of a purified enzyme. More recently, we have utilized the purified Na–K-ATPase from lamb kidney (Lane *et al.*, 1973, 1979) to study conformational changes. A fluorescent phospholipid, dansyl phosphatidyl ethanolamine (DPE), was incorporated into the purified Na–K-ATPase fraction (DPE-NKA) and into lipids extracted from the enzyme (Gupte *et al.*, 1979). The addition of Mg^{2+}, or lower concentrations of Ca^{2+}, resulted in a concentration-dependent enhancement in the fluorescence of both DPE-NKA (20%) and DPE-lipids (50%). Monovalent cations reversed the divalent cation-induced fluorescence enhancement. The binding of divalent cations to phospholipid head groups is known to increase membrane rigidity, and the binding of monovalent cations reverses this effect. Presumably, the changes in DPE fluorescence are reporting these alterations in membrane fluidity. The apparent binding constants for Mg^{2+} and Ca^{2+} which were derived from the fluorescence enhancement experiments agree with those obtained previously from direct ^{45}Ca binding (Table 1).

It is clear that the divalent cation site that regulates ouabain binding to the Na–K-ATPase (K_D = 0.20 mM) is *not* the same as that which causes an increase in the fluorescence of DPE (Table 1, 0.95 mM). The site which regulates ouabain binding is probably on the enzyme protein, while the site affecting DPE is associated with lipids.

Fluorescence intensity of DPE incorporated into the bulk lipids (as above) and fluorescence energy transfer from tryptophans or tyrosines to DPE incorporated into the Na–K-ATPase boundary lipids was

* This work was supported by grants from the National Institutes of Health (HL 22619, T32 HL 07382, AM 20875, HL 00555 and F32 HL 05802).

† Dr Schwartz is a Senior Visiting Fellow of the Josiah Macy Foundation, at the University of Oxford, Departments of Biochemistry and Physiology.

Table 1. Comparison of divalent cation binding to Na–K-ATPase

Apparent dissociation constants (mM)		
Na–K-ATPase	Lipids	Methods
Ca^{2+}:		
0.115	0.185	DPE fluorescence*
0.131	0.147	^{45}Ca binding†
Mg^{2+}:		
0.95	0.83	DPE fluorescence*
0.83	—	Microcalorimetry‡
1.10	—	Phosphorylation from [$^{32}P_i$]‡
0.20	—	[^3H]ouabain binding in presence of Mg^{2+} alone§

* Gupte *et al.* (1979)
† Gervais *et al.* (1977)
‡ Kuriki *et al* (1976)
§ Mandel *et al.* (1979)

measured to determine if the conformational changes which are thought to occur in the Na–K-ATPase protein during ligand binding and ATP hydrolysis cause structural changes in the associated lipids. Thus far, no changes in DPE fluorescence or fluorescence energy transfer as a result of ouabain binding, phosphorylation or other "states" of the enzyme have been detected (Gupte *et al.*, unpublished observations).

The fluorescent sulfhydryl probe 2-(4′-maleimidylanilino)naphthalene 6-sulfonic acid (MalANS), which reacts covalently with sulfhydryl groups on the α subunit of the Na–K-ATPase has also been used in an attempt to detect conformational changes in the enzyme protein (Gupte & Lane, 1979). We found that the rate and the magnitude of the reaction of MalANS with Na–K-ATPase sulfhydryl groups was increased by the presence of divalent cations (1–5 mM) and higher concentrations (100 mM) of monovalent cations. The effect of the divalent cations appeared to be due to their interaction with the lipids (K_D Mg^{2+} = 0.70 mM). The site of action of the monovalent cations is not known, but it did not appear to be due to a specific effect of the cations on the enzyme protein. Pre-treatment of the Na–K-ATPase with ouabain had no effect on the rate or the magnitude of the MalANS reaction, but ATP did reduce both the rate and the magnitude of MalANS labeling and partially protected against the loss of enzyme activity.

The alkylation of enzyme sulfhydryl groups by MalANS caused a parallel loss of Na–K-ATPase activity and Na^+-dependent phosphoenzyme formation that was proportional to the amount of MalANS bound to the enzyme and to the increase in fluorescence intensity. The ouabain binding capacity of the enzyme was not significantly reduced by sulfhydryl alkylation. This suggests (a) that phosphorylation may not be required for ouabain binding and (b) that the ouabain binding site probably does not contain a reactive sulfhydryl group.

Antibodies to the Na–K-ATPase have also been used to study conformational changes in the enzyme. This technique has great potential due to the high degree of specificity in the enzyme-antibody interaction (e.g. our earlier study indicated that Na–K-ATPase antibody fractions could detect structural differences between native enzyme and the enzyme–ouabain complex (McCans *et al.*, 1974)).

Antibodies to the purified lamb kidney Na–K-ATPase have been raised in rabbit, and the γ-globulin fractions prepared from the antisera have been shown to inhibit 50–70% of the Na–K-ATPase and 30% of the K^+-dependent *p*-nitrophenyl phosphatase activities. In contrast, Askari & Rao (1972) and Koepsell (1979) have reported that antibodies prepared against the rat brain and kidney enzymes inhibit ATP hydrolysis more than 90%. When measured under enzyme turnover conditions (MgATPNaK), the γ-globulin fraction raised against the lamb kidney enzyme stimulated ouabain binding while under Mg^{2+} only binding conditions, ouabain binding was inhibited. This is consistent with our earlier suggestion (Michael *et al.*, 1977) that the γ-globulin fraction contains different populations of Na–K-ATPase antibodies which bind to different conformational states of the enzyme.

More recently, an ^{125}I-protein A immunoadsorbent binding technique has been utilized to demonstrate that antibodies raised against native Na–K-ATPase bind to the denatured and purified α and β subunits, as well as to the native enzyme. Carboxymethylation and succinylation of the -SH and ε-NH_2 groups of the α subunit reduce the reactivity of the protein with the antibody by approx 50%. These results indicate that only a fraction of the antibody binding to the α subunit is dependent upon the native conformation of the protein.

STRUCTURAL STUDIES

We are currently in the process of determining the complete amino acid sequence of the protein subunits of the lamb kidney Na–K-ATPase. The α and β subunits have been purified by SDS-hydroxyapatite chromatography and delipidated on Sepharose or BIO Gel A-5m (Lane *et al.*, 1979). Following carboxymethylation of -SH groups, succinylation of ε-NH_2 groups, and removal of SDS, the α subunit has been digested with trypsin. Sephadex G-50 chromatography of the trypsin-digested α subunit resolves the peptides into an aggregated, hydrophobic fraction and three well-defined, water-soluble fractions. The hydrophobic fraction accounts for about 24% of the total protein and contains approximately six peptides which have a relatively high content of non-polar amino acids (including all of the tryptophan) and a low content of charged amino acids. These peptides are presumably derived from membrane-bound segments of the molecule, suggesting that the polypeptide chain of the α subunit traverses the cell membrane several times. Thus far, 14 water-soluble peptides, ranging in size from 3 to 17 amino acid residues, and containing a total of 138 amino acid residues have been purified. It has been demonstrated that the hydrophobic fraction and two of the water-soluble fractions of α subunit tryptic peptides from Sephadex G-50 can react with γ-globulin raised against native Na–K-ATPase. Polyacrylamide gel electrophoresis and Protein A binding to peptide–antibody complexes suggest that complete digestion of the α subunit has occurred and that at least some of the peptides are immunologically reactive.

Recently we have isolated a chloroform-methanol soluble, low molecular weight protein from the "purified" lamb kidney Na–K-ATPase (Collins *et al.*, 1979). Based on amino acid analysis, and assuming a molecular weight of 13,500, approx 0.8 mol of this protein (termed the γ protein) per mol of α subunit can be isolated. The amino acid composition of the γ protein is quite different from those of proteolipids associated with the Ca-ATPase of sarcoplasmic reticulum (Maclennan *et al.*, 1972) or the proton-translocating ATPascs of mitochondrial and bacterial membranes (Blondin, 1979; Filligame, 1976). The amino acid composition of the γ protein is, however, quite similar to the composition of a low molecular weight protein isolated from a beef heart membrane fraction, which could be phosphorylated by cAMP-dependent protein kinase (Dowd & Schwartz, 1975).

REGULATION OF Na–K-ATPase

Recently there has been much interest in the identification of endogenous factors which might regulate the activity of the sodium pump *in vivo*. It has been suggested that the sodium pump is regulated by (a) cAMP-dependent protein kinase phosphorylation of the Na–K-ATPase or of a small molecular weight protein associated with the enzyme (b) the concentration of cations (c) trace metals such as vanadate, and (d) as yet unidentified, endogenous substances which act like cardiac glycosides ("Endodigin").

It has been demonstrated that the activity of kidney Na–K-ATPase can be influenced by a variety of substances, such as trace metals, adrenal steroids, and cardiac glycosides (Schwartz *et al.*, 1975). There is also evidence suggesting that cAMP-dependent protein kinase phosphorylation of the Na–K-ATPase or of low molecular weight proteins associated with the enzyme may regulate Na–K-ATPase activity (see Schwartz *et al.*, 1975; Adams, 1978). In view of this, the isolation of a low molecular weight protein (γ protein) from the purified lamb kidney Na-K-ATPase is exciting because this protein may be an integral part of the enzyme complex. As described above, the amino acid composition and molecular weight of the γ protein is similar to that of a protein isolated from cardiac sarcolemma, which was phosphorylated by cAMP-dependent protein kinase (Dowd & Schwartz, 1975). Recently, two other groups reported that photoaffinity derivatives of ouabain covalently labeled a

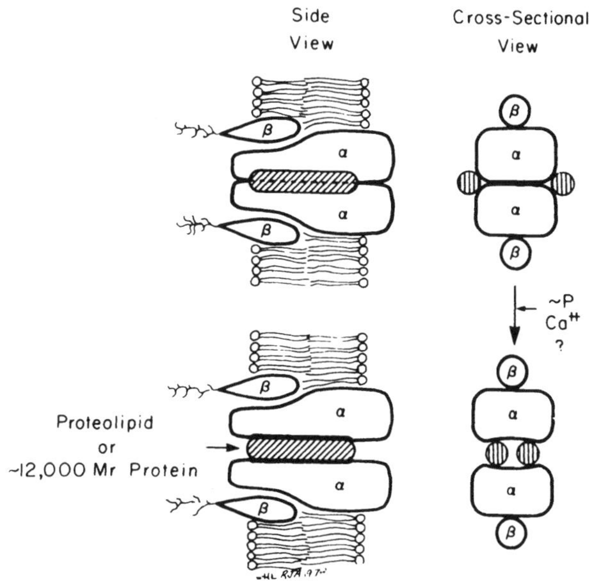

Fig. 1. Schematic representation of possible association of low molecular weight protein with the Na–K-ATPase. A low molecular weight protein, (isolated from kidney and possibly proteolipid in nature, M_r = 13,500) shown as the hatched area, may be structurally and functionally associated with the Na–K-ATPase. The enzyme is represented as dimers of catalytic (α) and glycoprotein (β) subunits embedded in the phospholipid bilayer of the plasma membrane. The low molecular weight component, tentatively designated the γ protein of the Na-K-ATPase, may act as an integral functional subunit involved in cation transport or may function as a regulatory protein which is modulated by phosphorylation, calcium binding or other factors (see text for discussion). We emphasize that the location of this putative subunit (or its derivation) in the membrane is unknown.

small molecular weight protein in both crude and purified Na–K-ATPase fractions (Forbush *et al.*, 1978; Rogers & Lazdunski, 1978). The data suggest that this protein is in close proximity to the ouabain binding site on the α subunit. It is also interesting to speculate that the γ protein may be functionally analogous to the proteolipid of the sarcoplasmic reticulum Ca-ATPase, which is believed to form a Ca^{2+} transport channel (Fig. 1).

Evidence for the regulation of Na–K-ATPase by another membrane protein has been reported by Lelievre *et al.* (1979). These investigators found that Ca^{2+}, in combination with a $M_r = 34{,}000$ protein from the intracellular surface of the plasma membrane, caused a 300-fold change in the ouabain sensitivity of Na–K-ATPase of EDTA-treated plasma membranes isolated from murine plasmocytoma cells. Although it remains to be seen whether such a "ouabain sensitivity conferring factor" exists in other cell types, these results, in view of other recent reports, suggest that membrane proteins may play a role in the regulation of Na–K-ATPase.

It is known from kinetic studies on inhibition of enzymatic activity by ouabagenin (Wallick *et al.*, 1974) and from direct binding studies (Wallick & Schwartz, 1974) that physiological ligands such as Mg^{2+}, Na^+, K^+, ATP and inorganic phosphate (P_i) regulate [^{3}H]ouabain binding as well as modulate enzymatic activity and transport of sodium and potassium in intact systems. We have recently examined the binding of [^{3}H]ouabain in the presence of magnesium plus inorganic phosphate. If the magnesium concentration is held constant at 5 mM, the apparent K_D for phosphate is 0.1 mM. If phosphate is held constant at 5 mM, the apparent K_D for magnesium is 0.1 mM. Other investigators (Kuriki *et al.*, 1976) have reported much larger K_D values for magnesium and inorganic phosphate derived from studies of phosphorylation (Table 1). If phosphorylation of the enzyme is necessary to induce ouabain binding, the affinities for the magnesium and phosphate sites that regulate the two processes should be the same. Although the source of enzyme for these two studies is different, it suggests that ligand sites that regulate phosphorylation are different from the sites that regulate ouabain binding.

We have suggested that in the presence of magnesium and ATP a single monovalent cation site (which can competitively bind sodium or potassium) allosterically modulates ouabain binding (Lindenmayer & Schwartz, 1973). When potassium is bound to this site, ouabain binding is prevented. When sodium is bound to this site, ouabain can bind. Since the affinity for this site is higher for potassium than for sodium, we further suggested that this modulation site is a potassium site for enzyme activity, and by extrapolation, is an extracellular potassium transport site in intact cells. We now have evidence that this monovalent cation site also regulates vanadate binding (Wallick *et al.*, 1979).

We found that sodium orthovanadate inhibited Na–K-ATPase isolated from both rat and lamb kidneys with an I_{50} of 0.6 μM for both enzymes. Vanadate also inhibited *p*-nitrophenyl phosphatase activity. Vanadate did not alter the number of ouabain sites nor did it alter the rate of dissociation of ouabain from the ouabain–enzyme complex. The rate of ouabain association in the presence of magnesium alone was stimulated by vanadate, indicating that vanadate can substitute for inorganic phosphate in the regulation of ouabain binding; vanadate is 1000 times more effective than phosphate. In the presence of magnesium plus ATP plus sodium plus potassium, vanadate decreased the rate of binding by increasing three-fold the apparent affinity of the enzyme for potassium at the site that modulates ouabain binding. The similarity of the affinities for potassium, as estimated from the effect of vanadate on [^{3}H]ouabain binding and from the effect of vanadate on Na–K-ATPase activity (Cantley *et al.*, 1978), suggests that the potassium site which regulates ouabain binding and the potassium site which regulates vanadate binding are identical. These results further suggest that vanadate binding, ouabain binding and ATPase activity are all regulated by a common potassium site.

The possibility that endogenous, "hormone-like" substances can regulate Na–K-ATPase is intriguing. It is now well established that the endogenous substances, endorphins and enkephalins bind to the opiate receptor. It is interesting to speculate that an endogenous substance (which we have named "Endodigin") exists which binds to the cardiac glycoside receptor. At present the evidence to support such a contention is very limited. Flier *et al* (1979) recently reported that the serum of *Bufo marinus* contains a substance (possibly a bufadienolide) that inhibits Na–K-ATPase and [^{3}H]ouabain binding to the enzyme. This work was confirmed in our laboratory and was extended to show that a toad serum extract produces a positive inotropic effect similar to that of ouabain (Schwartz & Adams, 1980). Haddy *et al.* (1979) have reported that the blood of volume-expanded, hypertensive animals contains a "slowly acting ouabain-like humoral agent". Adrenal steroids and, in particular, the progesterone derivatives, progestins, appear to have "digitalis-like" properties. The progestin, chlormadinone acetate, inhibits Na–K-ATPase activity, Na^+ transport in myocardium and inhibits [^{3}H]ouabain binding to Na–K-ATPase (LaBella *et al.*, 1979; Schwartz *et al.* unpublished observations).

These preliminary data encourage us to continue to search for an endogenous substance which might regulate the functions of the sodium pump *in vivo*.

REFERENCES

ADAMS R. J. (1978) Positive inotropic action of sanguinarine. University of Arkansas for Medical Sciences, Little Rock, Arkansas. Doctoral Dissertation.

ASKARI A. & RAO S. N. (1972) Na^+,K^+-ATPase complex: Effects of anticomplex antibody on the partial reactions catalyzed by the complex. *Biochem. biophys. Res. Commun.* **49,** 1323–1328.

BLONDIN G. A. (1979) Resolution of the mitochondrial N,N'-dicylohexylcarbodiimide binding proteolipid fraction into three similar sized proteins. *Biochem. biophys. Res. Commun.* **87,** 1087–1094.

CANTLEY L. C. JR, CANTLEY L. G. & JOSEPHSON L. (1978) A characterization of vanadate interactions with the (Na,K)-ATPase. *J. biol. Chem.* **253,** 7361–7368.

COLLINS J. H., LANE L. K. & REEVES A. A. (1979) Structural studies on lamb kidney Na–K-ATPase. *Abstracts of the XIth International Congress of Biochemistry*. July 8–13, 1979, Toronto, Canada, p. 450.

DOWD F. & SCHWARTZ A. (1975) The presence of cyclic AMP-stimulated protein kinase substrates and evidence for endogenous protein kinase activity in various Na^+, K^+-ATPase preparations from brain, heart and kidney. *J. mol. cell. Cardiol.* **7,** 483–497.

FILLINGAME R. H. (1976) Purification of the carbodiimide-reactive protein component of the ATP energy-transducing system of *Escherichia coli*. *J. biol. Chem.* **251,** 6630–6637.

FLIER J. S., MARATOS-FLIER E., PALLOTTA J. A. & MCISAAC D. (1979) Endogenous digitalis-like activity in the plasma of the toad *Bufo marinus*. *Nature* **279,** 341–343.

FORBUSH B. III, KAPLAN J. H. & HOFFMAN J. F. (1978) Characterization of a new photoaffinity derivative of ouabain: Labeling of the large polypeptide and of a proteolipid component of the Na,K-ATPase. *Biochemistry* **17,** 3667–3676.

GERVAIS A., LANE L. K., ANNER B. M., LINDENMAYER G. E. & SCHWARTZ A. (1977) A possible molecular mechanism of the action of digitalis. Ouabain action on calcium binding to sites associated with a purified sodium-potassium-activated adenosine triphosphatase from kidney. *Circ. Res.* **40,** 8–14.

GUPTE S. S. & LANE L. K. (1979) Reaction of purified (Na,K)-ATPase with the fluorescent sulfhydryl probe 2-(4′-maleimidylanilino)naphthalene 6-sulfonic acid. *J. biol. Chem.* **254,** 10362–10367.

GUPTE S. S., LANE L. K., JOHNSON J. D., WALLICK E. T. & SCHWARTZ A. (1979) The interaction of divalent cations with (Na,K)-ATPase. *J. biol. Chem.* **254,** 5099–5103.

HADDY F. J., PAMNANI M. B. & CLOUGH D. L. (1979) Humoral factors and the sodium-potassium pump in volume expanded hypertension. *Life Sci.* **24,** 2105–2118.

KOEPSELL H. (1979) Characteristics of antibody inhibition of rat kidney (Na^+ + K^+)-ATPase. *J. Membr. Biol.* **44,** 85–102.

KURIKI Y., HALSEY J., BILTONEN R. & RACKER E. (1976) Calorimetric studies of the interaction of magnesium and phosphate with (Na^+,K^+)-ATPase: Evidence for a ligand-induced conformational change in the enzyme. *Biochemistry* **15,** 4956–5961.

LABELLA F. S., Bihler I. & Kim R. S. (1979) Progesterone derivative binds to cardiac ouabain receptor and shows dissociation between sodium pump inhibition and increased contractile force. *Nature* **278,** 571–573.

LANE L. K., COPENHAVER J. H. JR, LINDENMAYER G. E. & SCHWARTZ A. (1973) Purification and characterization of and [^{3}H]ouabain binding to the transport adenosine triphosphatase from outer medulla of canine kidney. *J. biol. Chem.* **248,** 7197–7200.

LANE L. K., POTTER J. D. & COLLINS J. H. (1979) Large-scale purification of lamb kidney Na,K-ATPase and its protein subunits. *Prep. Biochem.* **9,** 157–170.

LELIEVRE L., ZACHOWSKI A., CHARLEMAGNE D., LAGET P. & PARAF A. (1979) Inhibition of Na^+,K^+-ATPase by ouabain: Involvement of calcium and membrane proteins. *Biochim. biophys. Acta.* **557,** 399–408.

LINDENMAYER G. E. & SCHWARTZ A. (1970) Conformational changes induced in Na^+,K^+-ATPase by ouabain through a K^+-sensitive reaction: Kinetic and spectroscopic studies. *Archs Biochem. Biophys.* **140,** 371–378.

LINDENMAYER G. E. & SCHWARTZ A. (1973) Nature of the transport adenosine triphosphatase-digitalis complex. IV. Evidence that sodium and potassium competition for a common site modulates the rate of glycoside interaction. *J. biol. Chem.* **248,** 1291–1300.

MACLENNAN D. H., YIP C. C., ILES G. H. & SEEMAN P. (1972) Isolation of sarcoplasmic reticulum proteins. *Cold Spring Harb. Symp. quant. Biol.* **37,** 469–477.

MANDEL F., WALLICK E. T. & SCHWARTZ A. (1977) Mg-stimulated ouabain binding to purified Na,K-ATPase from kidney. *Fedn Proc. Fedn. Am. Socs exp. Biol.* **36** (3), 274. (Abstract).

MATSUI H. & SCHWARTZ A. (1968) Mechanism of cardiac glycoside inhibition of the (Na^+,K^+)-ATPase from cardiac tissue. *Biochim. biophys. Acta* **151,** 655–663.

MCCANS J. L., LANE L. K., LINDENMAYER G. E., BUTLER V. P. JR & SCHWARTZ A. (1974) Effects of an antibody to a highly purified Na,K-ATPase from canine renal medulla: Separation of the "holoenzyme antibody" into catalytic and cardiac glycoside receptor-specific components. *Proc. natn. Acad. Sci. U.S.A.* **71,** 2449–2452.

MICHAEL L., WALLICK E. T. & SCHWARTZ A. (1977) Modification of (Na^+,K^+)-ATPase function by purified antibodies to the holoenzyme. *J. biol. Chem.* **252,** 8476–8480.

NAGAI K., LINDENMAYER G. E. & SCHWARTZ A. (1970) Direct evidence for the conformational nature of the Na^+,K^+-ATPase system: Fluorescence and circular dichroism studies. *Archs Biochem. Biophys.* **139,** 252–254.

ROGERS T. B. & LAZDUNSKI M. (1978) Photoaffinity labelling of a small protein component of a purified (Na^+-K^+)ATPase. *FEBS Lett.* **98,** 373–376.

SCHWARTZ A. & ADAMS R. J. (1980) Studies on the digitalis receptor. Circ. Res. In press.

SCHWARTZ A., LINDENMAYER G. E. & ALLEN J. C. (1975) The sodium-potassium adenosine triphosphatase: Pharmacological, physiological and biochemical aspects. *Pharmac. Rev.* **27,** 3–134.

SCHWARTZ A., MATSUI H. & LAUGHTER A. H. (1968) Tritiated digoxin binding to (Na^+ + K^+)-activated adenosine triphosphatase: Possible allosteric site. *Science* **159,** 323–325.

WALLICK E. T., DOWD F., ALLEN J. C. & SCHWARTZ A. (1974) The nature of the transport adenosine triphosphatase-digitalis complex. VII. Characteristics of ouabagenin-Na,K-adenosine triphosphatase interaction. *J. Pharmac. exp. Ther.* **189,** 434–444.

WALLICK E. T., LANE L. K. & SCHWARTZ A. (1979) Biochemical mechanism of the sodium pump. *A. Rev. Physiol.* **41,** 397–411.

WALLICK E. T., LANE L. K. & SCHWARTZ A. (1979) Regulation by vanadate of ouabain binding to (Na^+,K^+)-ATPase. *J. biol. Chem.* **254,** 8107–8109.

WALLICK E. T. & SCHWARTZ A. (1974) Thermodynamics of the rate of binding of ouabain to the sodium, potassium-adenosine triphosphatase. *J. biol. Chem.* **249,** 5141–5147.

SYMPOSIUM DISCUSSION

Kinne: Some discussion is required since I have the impression that there are differences of opinion as to how many monomers are together in the membrane, how many ATP binding sites, how many ouabain binding sites and so on.

Osswald: I have a question for Dr Schwartz. You said that vanadate would stimulate adenylate cyclase at concentrations around 10^{-4} *M*. This must be outside the range of any physiological importance.

Schwartz: Actually, it is effective in stimulating cyclase over the range 10^{-6}–10^{-4} M (Schwabe *et al.*, *Nature* **277,** 143–145, 1979). The observed effects of vanadate on purified Na–K-ATPase are well within the concentrations found in vivo, but for the effect on adenylate cyclase it depends very much on which species of vanadate is present within the cell, something which is presently not clear.

Osswald: Which membrane did you use to demonstrate a stimulatory effect of vanadate on adenylate cyclase?

Schwartz: Guinea-pig heart cell membrane preparation (Grupp *et al.*, *Biochem. biophys. Res. Commun.* **88,** 440–447, 1979).

Silva: You suggested that vanadate might be a physiological regulator. What is the K_i and what concentration do you expect within the cell?

Schwartz: The I_{50} depends upon the conditions and varies between 28–600 nM. (Wallick *et al.*, *J. biol. Chem.*

254, 8107–8109, 1979; Cantley *et al.*, *J. biol. Chem.* **253,** 7361–7368, 1978).

Ross: You suggest that there may be a physiological modulator of Na–K-ATPase in cells. As an alternative to your idea of vanadate, McGeogh *et al.* (*Lancet* **ii,** 17–18, 1978) have found that human myeloma light chain, of molecular weight 22000 inhibits the enzyme at a concentration of 10^{-6} M. Whilst this is an unlikely inhibitor, and we do not yet know its mode of action, Dr McGeogh and Dr Falconer Smith have recently shown that smaller molecular weight fragments of the same protein are also inhibitors; light chain is of course present in many cells.

Silva: I should like to comment on vanadium ion as a diuretic. But there has only been one case of work reported to date and that is Grantham's, of a paper showing that vanadium is capable of inducing diuresis. In my hands, vanadium induces intense vasoconstriction of the kidney and you have to raise your concentration to about 10^{-4} M to produce some increase and sometimes it is just a fleeting increase in sodium excretion. Other investigators that I have talked to have not been able to reproduce Grantham's experiment, in terms of diuresis.

Osswald: It is true that you cannot easily produce diuresis in anaethetized animals. You will kill the dog if vanadate is injected too rapidly, but you can infuse it slowly and the manoeuvre Grantham used was to infuse potassium. He used sodium chloride plus potassium and then you can use lower doses and measure the GFR and rejection rate of sodium and show that it is higher. You can see a diuresis but in animals under narcosis the effect is less.

Silva: May I add comment to that? I also use the isolated perfused rat kidney in which, of course, you do not have any problem as with the heart, but you could have a vascular problem. When you infuse it slowly so that you do not have a vascular problem, you get about a 10–15% increase in sodium excretion, which is not a very big effect for a drug which should be inhibiting sodium-potassium ATPase.

Robinson: Could I just comment on the proteolipid? We have found that 2–5% of brush border is proteolipid of about 14,000 molec. weight but yet these membranes have no sodium-potassium ATPase or virtually none. This suggests that it is not a protein which is specifically associated with the ATPase (Kramers M. T. C., D.Phil. Thesis; University of Oxford, 1974).

Schwartz: This is always the problem that you may think the proteolipid is associated with the enzyme during the preparation and later it turns out to be a contaminant.

Epstein: Just a footnote to your mention of "endigin". The Chinese have used dried toad skins for thousands of years to treat heart failure. Dr. Jeffrey Flier at Beth Israel Hospital has recently published the finding of endogenous ouabain-like substances in the serum as well as the tissues in a number of amphibians, (*Nature*, 1979).

Weiner: Can I ask the contributors what is the current thinking about the adaptations in Na – K-ATPase which have been observed in response to diet or changes in GFR. Is this *de novo* protein synthesis, or changes in the assembly of the various sub-units that don't require changes in synthesis;

Ebel: In my view rapid changes of Na – K-ATPase activity might be more due to a change in enzyme specific activity rather than to a change in enzyme concentration. As to the mechanism of enzyme activation many possibilities exist. A simple example is that small local changes of Na and K might immediately cause significant changes of specific Na – K-ATPase activity since the enzyme is characterized by an allosteric kinetic behavior.

Weiner: Yes, but many of the studies are with isolated enzyme, measured with added ATP, under optimal conditions, and none of these other factors are relevant, so that they are measuring the amount of enzyme. There is usually a good correlation between ouabain binding sites and ATPase activity under optimal conditions, yet uninephrectomy, methylprednisolone and high-protein diet, among other things, affect the amount of Na – K-ATPase in the kidney. My question is, is that through increased synthesis, decreased degradation or some other mechanism?

Jorgensen: I think that there is evidence for a true increase in the concentration of sodium pump sites per unit weight of tissue, or as in this case of potassium adaptation, in pump sites per unit of tubule length. In the thick ascending limbs the changes in Na – K-ATPase activity may be due to adaptation to the loads of sodium. After a chronic sodium load you may observe an increase of the amount of enzyme by up to 50%. The concentration of sites is obtained directly, if the activity is measured in conditions in which there is a constant maximum turnover rate per site. To examine the question whether aldosterone affects the amount of Na – K-ATPase, the activity should be measured in the collecting ducts in the conditions described by Schwartz & Burg (*Am. J. Physiol.* **235,** F576–585, 1978). They produced a beautiful curve relating variations in endogenous aldosterone to a four-fold variation in net sodium transport across the collecting duct. Another group (Wade *et al. J. Cell Biol.* **81,** 439–445, 1979) looked at the ultrastructure of the collecting ducts in the same condition and found a drastic change in the area of the basolateral membrane infoldings, suggesting that the adaptation to the different hormone levels may be explained by a change in area of the basolateral infoldings which contain the Na – K-pump sites.

Schwartz: Relevant to the question of ATPase control: In duck nasal salt gland, in response to sodium loading, there is an increase in the number of ouabain binding sites, correlated directly with induction of cyclic AMP, and both the increase in binding sites and the cAMP response were prevented by inhibitors of protein synthesis (C. Hegrary).

Kinne: Perhaps we should ask Dr Epstein to report on a system in which there is very rapid adaptation of sodium pumping.

Epstein: As Dr Kinne suggests, there are really two problems. One relates to a chronic increase in the enzyme activity over a period of time, presumably accomplished by protein synthesis and basolateral membrane synthesis. Another question which is perhaps more difficult to answer, is what about the increase in ATP hydrolysis due to Na – K-ATPase activity which occurs when transport is thrown into gear very abruptly. We have been interested in looking at this in the shark rectal gland, which as we reported 2 years ago, secretes chloride in a way that is turned on by cyclic AMP. Chloride secretion is dependent upon Na – K-ATPase, in an indirect way, since it depends upon the co-transport of sodium with chloride, across the basolateral membrane, into the rectal gland, and down a gradient that is maintained and sustained by the activity of Na – K-ATPase. When you stimulate the perfused rectal gland with cyclic AMP, the oxygen consumption goes up several times. Practically all of the increase is ouabain-inhibitable, so that the ouabain-inhibitable oxygen consumption may increase 6–10 fold, a tremendous increase in what we take to be an indirect measurement of Na – K-ATPase. This occurs in minutes, and raises the question as to what "turns on" the ATPase. I think a natural first hypothesis for a nephrologist was that it was due to an increase in the admission of sodium into the cell, and a stimulation through internal sodium concentration. We realised that if that were the case, the sodium concentration on the inside of the membrane would have to start very low, since if it were already at K_m (half-maximal for Na – K-ATPase stimulation) the most it could do would be to double it. In fact, the internal Na^+ is at or slightly above the K_m for the enzyme in this tissue, that is about 50 60 mM. Moreover, we found, when we measured the intra-cellular sodium concentration (using inulin, subtracting extracellular Na^+) that after stimulation, it did not go up, it went down! So that suggested that the Na – K-ATPase was stimulated by some other event. This might be the regulatory protein that people have speculated about, analogous to "calmodulin". Other possibilities might include a change in the configuration of this transmembrane protein that has to do with the potential across the membrane.

Newsholme: A question to Dr Epstein. In relation to the point he made, this poses a problem of "sensitivity" in control. How could a very small increment in sodium concentration produce a very large increase in the activity of the system? This is a general point which underlies the discussion. If you have a "leak" mechanism, allowing sodium back into the cell, as well as an exit sodium transport system, you produce what we call a translocation cycle which can make the system extremely sensitive to small increments in sodium. It doesn't then matter what the absolute concentration of sodium is: you then have a system which has improved the sensitivity over and above the absolute concentration. So my question to De Epstein is the general one, how important is the sodium leak?

Epstein: It may be very important.

Weiner: Leaf *et al.* have published work in toad bladder which deals with that specific point. Their conclusion is that in toad bladder, which is a tight epithelium there is virtually no back-leak of sodium, except through the transport pathway. In proximal tubule, or leaky epithelia, the situation may be very different.

Jorgenson: Did you look at the time course of potassium adaptation, Dr Doucet? In addition, was it the freezing or the osmotic shock which exposed enzyme activity?

Doucet: To your first question the answer is no; we did not study the time course of this adaptation. The earlliest experiments were performed after 12 days of treatment and at this time the effect was already maximal; no further change in ATPase activity was observed during the next month of K-loading. About your second question, we studied separately the effect of the two permeabilisation steps, and both the hypoosmotic and the thermic shock increased the activity.

Ebel: Perhaps one important factor which might be involved in short term regulation of Na – K-ATPase and other membrane bound enzymes is the lipid microenvironment. It is well known that the specific activity of lipid dependent enzymes such as the Na – K-ATPase is dependent on lipid fluidity or viscosity (Kimelberg & Papahadjopoulos *J. biol. Chem.* **259**, 1071–1080, 1974). Lipid fluidity, however, is influenced by a variety of factors. For example small local changes of surface charge, of pH, of divalent cation concentration might be able to alter very rapidly local microviscosity. This would effect enzyme mobility and the conformational changes involved in allosteric enzyme activation or inhibition.

Int. J. Biochem., Vol. 12, pp. 295 to 299
© Pergamon Press Ltd 1980. Printed in Great Britain

0020-711X/80/0701-0295$02.00/0

OPERATION OF THE RENAL Na^+–K^+-PUMP IN ARTIFICIAL MEMBRANES

BEATRICE M. ANNER
Department of Pharmacology, Ecole de Médecine CH-1211 Geneva 4, Switzerland

Abstract—1. Na^+–K^+-ATPase was purified from the outer medulla of rabbit kidneys and incorporated into artificial vesicular membranes (liposomes). Within 60 min of the addition of ATP to the liposomes, the intravesicular Na^+ concentration rose from 20 to about 65 mM whereas the K^+ concentration dropped from 50 to about 30 mM.

2. Alkylation of SH groups on the reconstituted pump protein with *N*-ethylmaleimide inactivated 30% of the ATP-driven Na^+-transport. K^+-transport appeared unaffected.

3. Occupation of the phosphorylation site by the natriuretic vanadate abolished the total Na^+-transport capacity of the reconstituted Na^+–K^+-pump.

4. From the results described it appears that the *in vitro* system may be a useful model for simulating effects of extrinsic agents on the renal Na^+–K^+-pump.

INTRODUCTION

It is likely that the renal Na^+–K^+-pump (Na^+–K^+-ATPase) is responsible for most, if not all, the Na^+ reabsorption in the thick ascending loop of Henle (Schmidt & Dubach, 1969; Epstein & Silva, 1974; Jørgensen, 1976).

When the Na^+–K^+-ATPase from the renal outer medulla was purified and incorporated into phosphatidylcholine-liposomes, a functional pump was obtained which performed coupled active Na^+ and K^+ transport and was inhibited by ouabain (Anner *et al.*, 1976, 1977; Goldin, 1977).

Examination of the purified Na^+–K^+-transport system in artificial membranes led to the characterization of possible transport pathways which may be cautiously extrapolated to the *in vivo* situation (Anner 1980).

In the present work, the reconstituted Na^+–K^+-pump was chemically modified either by alkylating SH groups with *N*-ethylmaleimide or by blocking the phosphorylation site with vanadate, and the resulting alteration of the Na^+ and K^+ transport capacity was determined. It appeared that only a labile fraction of the active Na^+-transport was suppressed by the *N*-ethylmaleimide treatment. In contrast, the potent natriuretic vanadate (Balfour *et al.*, 1978) totally abolished Na^+-transport.

The results encourage the use of the *in vitro* system as a model for establishing transport patterns of the renal Na^+–K^+-pump.

MATERIALS AND METHODS

Preparation of soluble Na^+–K^+-ATPase

Na^+–K^+-ATPase from the outer medulla of rabbit kidneys was purified to a specific activity of 800–1200 μmol $P_i \cdot mg\ protein^{-1} \cdot hr^{-1}$ according to the angle rotor procedure described by Jørgensen (1974). For solubilization, 1 mg Na^+–K^+-ATPase protein was suspended at 0°C in 500 μl of a 1% sodium cholate solution in buffer A (20 mM NaCl, 50 mM KCl, 50 mM choline choline chloride, 5 mM $MgCl_2$, 30 mM imidazole, 1 mM L-cystein chloride, 1 mM EDTA, pH 7.1). The suspension was stirred for 60 sec at 22°C and then centrifuged 15 min at 100,000 *g*. The clear supernatant contained about 50% of the initial Na^+–K^+-ATPase protein. The method of Lowry *et al.* (1951) was used for determination of protein, except that 0.1% sodium dodecyl sulfate was present.

Incorporation of Na^+–K^+-ATPase into liposomes

Reconstitution was performed by a technique developed from previous procedures (Goldin & Tong, 1974; Hilden *et al.*, 1974; Anner *et al.*, 1977). A hexane solution containing 1 g per 10 ml egg phosphatidylcholine (Sigma type III-E) was dried under a stream of N_2 in a rotavapor. To 20 mg dried phospholipid 2.5 ml of the 1% cholate solution in buffer A were added and the lipid was dissolved by rotating at 22°C. For reconstitution, an aliquot of the 1% cholate–lipid solution was added to an aliquot of the 1% cholate–enzyme solution (in ice) at a 1:1 ratio and the mixture was dialysed for 90 hours at 5°C against a 1000-fold excess of buffer A.

Electron micrographs revealed a homogenous population of 1000 Å vesicles which contained Na^+–K^+-pump particles spanning the lipid bilayer (Skriver *et al.*, in preparation).

Transport measurements

Aliquots of the liposomes suspension were loaded with ^{22}Na and ^{86}Rb and isotope equilibration was followed by passing 10 μl samples over Sephadex-G-50 (medium) columns (1 × 20 cm) and collecting the eluted liposomes for scintillation counting. Active transport was initiated by adding 5 mM Tris–ATP to the liposomes; this induced accumulation of Na^+ in the liposomes and extrusion of K^+ from the liposomes. The ATP had been freed from vanadate by treatment with Dowex WX2 resin (Hudgins & Bond, 1977).

RESULTS

Transport pattern of the renal Na^+–K^+-pump in liposomes

For the experiments shown in Fig. 1, the liposomes had been prepared in 20 mM NaCl and 50 mM KCl, and were then equilibrated with ^{22}Na and ^{86}Rb (not shown). The rate constants for passive equilibration were 0.014 min^{-1} for K^+ and 0.013 min^{-1} for Na^+, indicating that the permeability of the liposomes for Na^+ and K^+ is not much different (Anner, 1980).

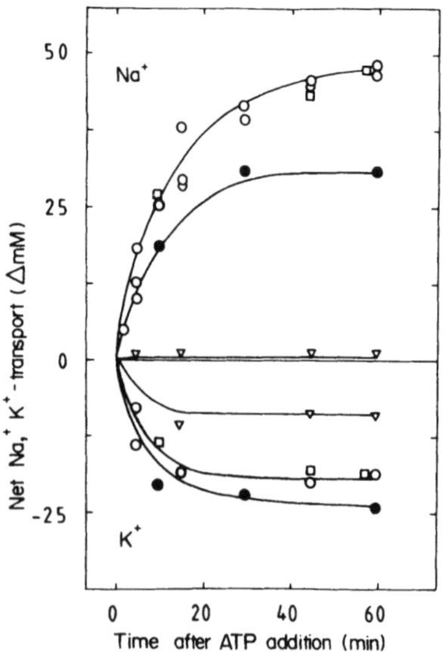

Fig. 1. Net Na^+ and K^+ transport in phosphatidylcholine-liposomes reconstituted with purified renal Na^+–K^+-ATPase in buffer A (20 mM NaCl, 50 mM KCl) as explained in Materials and Methods. After equilibration of separate batches with ^{22}Na or ^{86}Rb (a K^+ congener in this system) at 25°C, active transport was initiated by adding to aliquots of liposomes ATP (○), ATP and 5–10 sec later N-ethylmaleimide (●), ATP plus vanadate (▽) or plus ouabain (□). Final concentrations were: ATP 5 mM, N-ethylmaleimide 1.5 mM, vanadate (Na_3VO_4) 1 mM, ouabain 1 mM. At the times indicated on the abcissa, the isotope content of the liposomes was determined as described in Materials and Methods, and net transport was calculated from the difference between the radioactivity of liposomes incubated in presence or absence of the inhibitor with or without ATP.

At isotopic equilibrium, ATP was added to a final concentration of 5 mM. As a result, the internal Na^+ concentration increased from 20 to 68 mM, while the internal K^+ concentration fell from 50 to 30 mM within 60 min; this yielded stable steady state gradients of 48 mM for Na^+ and of 20 mM for K^+.

As the permeability of the liposomes for Na^+ and K^+ is equal, the size of the Na^+-gradient relative to the size of the K^+-gradient expresses the respective number of Na^+ and K^+ ions that have been transported by the pump within a given time unit. In consequence, determination of the ratio of the Na^+ to the K^+ gradient at steady state brings useful information about the coupling ratio of Na^+:K^+ transport.

Figure 1 also illustrates that no inhibitory effect of ouabain on net Na^+ and K^+ fluxes was observed within 60 min of the addition of 5 mM ATP plus 1 mM ouabain. In previous work the incubation time in presence of ouabain was extended to several hours and inhibition of active transport became apparent as ouabain slowly penetrated the liposomes (Anner *et al.*, 1977).

The confinement of the ATP activation to outer pump sites and of the ouabain inhibition to inner pump sites in liposomes ascertains the structural integrity of the purified and reconstituted Na^+–K^+-pump.

Reduction of the ATP-driven Na^+-transport by N-ethylmaleimide

Alkylation of SH groups of the Na^+–K^+-ATPase protein with N-ethylmaleimide has been extensively used for determining the role of SH groups for partial enzyme reactions (Schwartz *et al.*, 1975). Essentially, the N-ethylmaleimide-treated enzyme still undergoes phosphorylation by ATP, but dephosphorylation by K^+ is inhibited at 0°C (Post *et al.*, 1969) and slowed down at 22°C (Wallick *et al.*, 1978), and ADP:ATP exchange activity is increased; this results in an overall 80% decrease in enzyme turnover.

It was of interest to treat the reconstituted Na^+–K^+-ATPase with N-ethylmaleimide, as the SH groups of the pump protein facing outwards will be the first target of N-ethylmaleimide, while the protein parts inside the liposomes will be protected as long as the alkylating agent has not entered the liposomes.

In Fig. 1 a typical experiment is shown, where in the presence of 1.5 mM N-ethylmaleimide, the Na^+-gradient formed by the reconstituted pump reached only 31 mM within 60 min as compared to the 48 mM gradient formed by the untreated pump within the same time period. In contrast, the K^+-gradient built by the modified pump reached 24 mM, which was about 4 mM above control values. Accordingly, the ratio of the Na^+ to the K^+ gradient attained about 1.2, whereas the Na^+:K^+ gradient ratio of the untreated pump was about 2.4.

The observation that a 30% fraction of the ATP-driven Na^+-transport was rapidly inactivated by N-ethylmaleimide raised the question whether a distinct class of SH groups was responsible for the labile Na^+-transport component. The results shown in Fig. 2 support this contention: although the concentration of N-ethylmaleimide was increased from 0.5 to 4 mM, the reduction of the Na^+-transport capacity recorded at 30 min after the addition of ATP and N-ethylmaleimide plateaued around 20–30%. Beyond 4 mM N-ethylmaleimide, active Na^+-transport fell off suddenly, as depicted in Fig. 2.

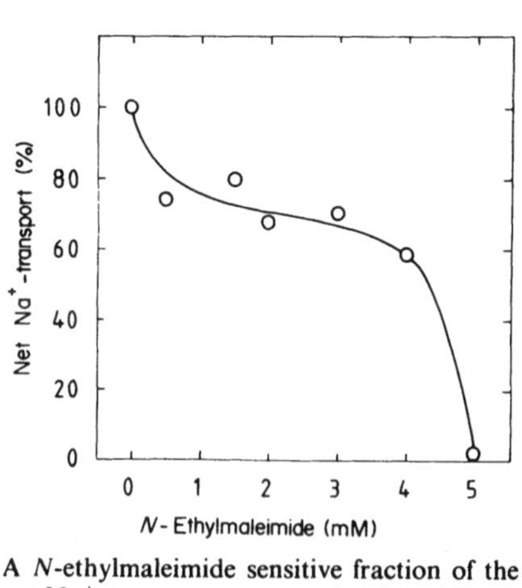

Fig. 2. A N-ethylmaleimide sensitive fraction of the ATP-dependent Na^+-transport was revealed by adding increasing concentrations of N-ethylmaleimide 5–10 sec after the ATP to liposomes which were prepared, incubated and processed as described in Materials and Methods and in Fig. 1. The ATP-dependent Na^+-gradient formed within 30 min in presence of N-ethylmaleimide was compared to the 100% gradient formed in absence of N-ethylmaleimide.

Inactivation of the ATP-driven Na^+-transport by vanadate

Vanadate inactivates the Na^+–K^+-ATPase by binding tightly to the phosphorylation site (Cantley *et al.*, 1978).

In Fig. 1 it is shown that vanadate abolishes the ATP-driven Na^+-transport. Indeed, the Na^+-content of liposomes which were incubated in the presence of 5 mM ATP, 5 mM $MgCl_2$ plus 1 mM vanadate was undistinguishable from the control values obtained in a medium containing the vanadate, the $MgCl_2$ but not the ATP.

A question remains as to the inhibition of the ATP-driven K^+-transport by vanadate: even though the Na^+-transport was completely blocked by vanadate, up to 50% of the net K^+-transport was still apparent (Fig. 1).

DISCUSSION

The present work has examined the question whether the renal Na^+–K^+-pump reconstituted in liposomes presents a model for studying the modulation of the active Na^+–K^+-transport by extrinsic agents.

N-ethylmaleimide, ouabain and vanadate were selected as modifiers because their interaction with isolated Na^+–K^+-ATPase is precisely known (for reviews see Schwartz *et al.*, 1975; Glynn & Karlish, 1975), as summarized in Scheme I. *N*-ethylmaleimide

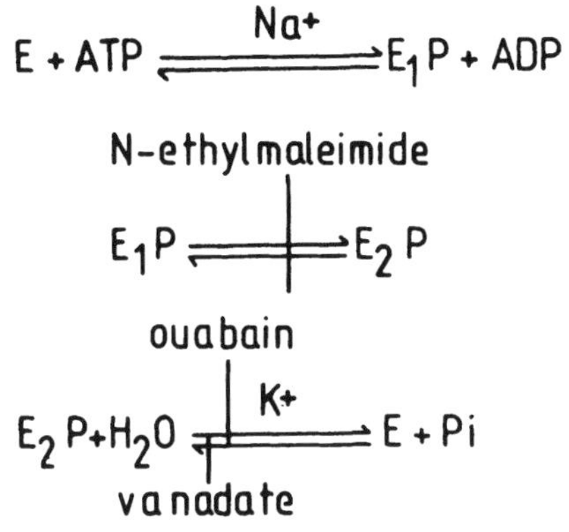

slows down the transition of the enzyme from an ADP sensitive form (E_1P) to a K^+ sensitive form (E_2P). Ouabain binds to a steroid site and abolishes ATP hydrolysis by blocking the K^+-stimulated dephosphorylation of the phosphoenzyme. Finally, vanadate occupies directly the phosphorylation site and so hinders the interaction of Na^+–K^+-ATPase with ATP (Cantley *et al.*, 1978).

N-ethylmaleimide-treatment of the reconstituted Na^+–K^+-pump caused a 20–30% reduction of the Na^+-transport capacity, while the K^+-transport capacity appeared unchanged or slightly increased. These results imply that reactive SH groups which are exposed on the liposome surface are concerned primarily with a 25% fraction of the active Na^+-transport mediated by the renal Na^+–K^+-pump. In other words, a component of the Na^+-transport seems to be labile, and not directly coupled to counter-transport of K^+ ions. In previous work, where Na^+–K^+-ATPase had been modified selectively by trypsinolysis prior to reconstitution, an even more pronounced transport defect, specific for Na^+, had been detected (Anner & Jørgensen, 1979; Jørgensen & Anner, 1979). *N*-ethylmaleimide treatment as well as graded trypsinolysis lower the rate of the E_1P to E_2P transition. Both treatments also remove a fraction of the Na^+-transport capacity of the reconstituted enzyme. In contrast, the K^+-transport capacity of the pump, associated possibly with the ATP binding and the first phosphorylation step, appears to be rather resistant to chemical or enzymatic modification.

The Na^+–K^+-pump is strictly asymmetrical (Glynn & Karlish, 1975). After reconstitution, the probability that the catalytic ATP site finds itself at the inner or at the outer side of the liposomes is equal (Hilden *et al.*, 1974). Therefore the cardiac glycoside ouabain can not be simply used as a pump inhibitor. Indeed, ouabain binds to the protein part which is located at the membrane side opposed to the ATP site. As a matter of fact, only catalytic sites facing outwards are activated by ATP, which itself does not permeate the lipid bilayer within the time interval required to accomplish a transport assay (unpublished results). Because ouabain does not permeate either, the ATP-activated pumps are not affected by external ouabain.

In contrast, vanadate is an ideal inhibitor, as it acts at the ATP site which faces outwards. Indeed, as shown herein and in previous work (Anner & Jørgensen, 1979), the interaction of vanadate with the reconstituted Na^+–K^+-pump abolishes active Na^+-transport. Despite the blocking of the net Na^+-flux, some residual net K^+-flux is still apparent. The origin of the vanadate-resistant K^+-transport has not yet been determined. At the same time, vanadate happens to be the most potent natriuretic presently known (Balfour *et al.*, 1978). It is tempting to relate the natriuretic effect of vanadate to the block of the active Na^+-transport demonstrated in the purified *in vitro* transport system.

In conclusion, the results contained in the present report reveal that fundamental properties of the Na^+–K^+-pump are preserved throughout purification and reconstitution and that in consequence, the *in vitro* system may be used as a model to characterize normal as well as chemically modified transport pathways of the renal Na^+–K^+-pump.

SUMMARY

The renal Na^+-K^+-pump (Na^+-K^+-ATPase) was purified from the outer medulla of rabbit kidneys and incorporated into phosphatidylcholine-liposomes. The *in vitro* system was used to attempt chemical modification of the purified Na^+–K^+-transport system to study the flexibility of the Na:K coupling.

When ATP was added to the liposomes, the reconstituted pump formed stable steady state gradients of about 45 mM for Na^+ and of about 20 mM for K^+ within 60 min at 25°C. The buffered incubation medium contained essentially 20 mM NaCl, 50 mM KCl, 5 mM $MgCl_2$ and 50 mM choline chloride; the pH was 7.10 at 20°C. The liposomes were equally permeable for Na^+ and K^+ in the absence of ATP.

It was examined whether SH groups influenced the transport pattern of the reconstituted Na^+–K^+-

pump. To that end, SH groups on the phosphorylated pump protein were alkylated by adding 0.5 to 4 mM *N*-ethylmaleimide at 5–10 sec after the ATP. As a result, the Na^+-gradient formed by the modified pump reached only 70–80% of the Na^+-gradient built up by the untreated pump within 30 min. Conversely, *N*-ethylmaleimide-treatment increased the K^+-gradient, so the final result was a decrease of the $Na^+:K^+$ transport ratio of the pump from about 2.4 to about 1.2.

When the phosphorylation site of the reconstituted Na^+–K^+-pump was blocked with vanadate, a potent natriuretic, the Na^+-gradient was reduced to zero.

In general, it is concluded that the *in vitro* system will be a useful tool to investigate the transport patterns of the renal Na^+–K^+-pump in various physiological or pathological conditions.

Acknowledgement—I wish to thank Mrs M. Moosmayer for excellent technical assistance.

REFERENCES

ANNER B. M. (1980) Reconstitution of the Na^+,K^+-transport system in artificial membranes. *Acta Physiol. scand.* (Suppl.) In press.

ANNER B. M. & JØRGENSEN P. L. (1979) Defective Na^+ transport by phospholipid vesicles reconstituted with selectively modified Na^+,K^+-ATPase. *Na,K-ATPase: Structure and Kinetics* (Edited by SKOU J. C. & NØRBY J. G.) pp. 87–97. Academic Press, New York.

ANNER B. M., LANE L. K., SCHWARTZ A. & PITTS B. J. R. (1977) A reconstituted Na^+,K^+-pump in liposomes containing purified (Na^+ + K^+)-ATPase from kidney medulla. *Biochim. biophys. Acta* **467**, 340–345.

ANNER B. M., PITTS B. J. R., LANE L. K. & SCHWARTZ A. (1976) Renal medulla Na,K-ATPase reconstituted in vesicles: coupled sodium and potassium transport. *Pharmacologist* **18**, 239.

BALFOUR W. E., GRANTHAM J. J. & GLYNN I. M. (1978) Vanadate-stimulated natriuresis. *Nature* **275**, 768.

CANTLEY L. C., CANTLEY L. G. & JOSEPHSON L. (1978) A characterization of vanadate interactions with the (Na,K)-ATPase. *J. biol. Chem.* **253**, 7361–7368.

EPSTEIN F. H. & SILVA P. (1974) Role of sodium, potassium ATPase in renal function. *Ann. N.Y. Sc. Sci.* **242**, 519–526.

GLYNN I. M. & KARLISH S. J. D. (1975) The sodium pump. *A. Rev. Physiol.* **37**, 13–55.

GOLDIN S. M. (1977) Active transport of sodium and potassium ions by the sodium and potassium ion-activated adenosine triphosphatase from renal medulla. *J. biol. Chem.* **252**, 5630–5642.

GOLDIN S. M. & TONG S. W. (1974) Reconstitution of active transport catalyzed by the purified sodium and potassium ion-stimulated adenosine triphosphatase from canine renal medulla. *J. biol. Chem.* **249**, 5307–5315.

HILDEN S., RHEE H. M. & HOKIN L. E. (1974) Sodium transport by phospholipid vesicles containing purified sodium and potassium ion-activated adenosine triphosphatase. *J. biol. Chem.* **249**, 7432–7440.

HUDGINS P. M. & BOND G. H. (1977) (Mg^{2+} + K^+) dependent inhibition of Na,K-ATPase due to a contaminant in equine muscle ATP. *Biochem. biophys. Res. Commun.* **77**, 1024–1029.

JØRGENSEN P. L. (1974) Isolation of (Na^+ + K^+)-ATPase. *Meth. Enzym.* **32**, 227–290.

JØRGENSEN P. L. (1976) The function of (Na^+,K^+)-ATPase in the thick ascending limb of Henles loop. *Current Problems in Clinical Biochemistry*, Vol. 6, Renal Metabolism in Relation to Renal Function (Edited by SCHMIDT U. & DUBACH U. C.) pp. 190–199. Hans Huber, Berne.

JØRGENSEN P. L. & ANNER B. M. (1979) Purification and characterization of Na^+,K^+-ATPase. VIII Altered Na:K transport ratio in vesicles reconstituted with purified Na^+,K^+-ATPase that has been selectively modified with trypsin in presence of NaCl. *Biochim. biophys. Acta* **555**, 485–492.

LOWRY O. H. ROSEBROUGH N. J., FARR A. L. & RANDALL R. J. (1951) Protein measurement with the folin phenol reagent. *J. biol. Chem.* **193**, 265–276.

POST R. L., KUME S., TOBIN T., ORCUTT B. & SEN A. K. (1969) Flexibility of an active center in sodium-plus-potassium adenosine triphosphatase. *J. gen. Physiol.* **54**, 306–326.

SCHMIDT U. & DUBACH U. C. (1969) Activity of (Na^+ + K^+)-stimulated adenosinetriphosphatase in the rat nephron. *Pflugers Arch. ges. Physiol.* **306**, 219–226.

SCHWARTZ A., LINDENMAYER G. E. & ALLEN J. C. (1975) The sodium-potassium adenosine triphosphatase: pharmacological, physiological and biochemical aspects. *Pharmac. Rev.* **27**, 3–134.

WALLICK E. T., ANNER B. M., RAY M. V. & SCHWARTZ A. (1978) Effect of temperature on phosphorylation and ouabain binding to *N*-ethylmaleimide-treated (Na^+,K^+)-ATPase. *J. biol. Chem.* **253**, 8778–8786.

SYMPOSIUM DISCUSSION

Koepsell: Can you tell me how many SH-groups you labelled with *N*-ethylmaleimide under the conditions you used? As you know, there are about 36 SH-groups in the enzyme and depending upon the conditions and the ligands, we have found that we can titrate a different number of SH-groups.

Anner: That would be very interesting to do in liposomes, as only the SH-groups of the activated part of the enzyme can be attacked by the *N*-ethylmaleimide, and the other groups are protected.

Epstein: I should like to ask Dr Anner, and perhaps anyone else who has worked with reconstituted liposomes, a question which has to do with the proportion of Na^+ and K^+ that is transported. If indeed the passive permeability to sodium and potassium is the same in these membranes, and if 3 sodium ions are transported in, but 2 potassium ions are transported out, does that mean that the liposome swells? If not, how does it work? In addition, can you alter the ratio by substituting anions of varying mobilities, to which the liposome membrane is more or less permeable?

Anner: The answer to that question is not yet clear. It may be that the liposomes swell slightly. On the other hand there may be counter-transport of protons out of the liposome.

Jorgensen: I know that you can demonstrate thiocyanate uptake as an expression of the potential of the liposomes and Hokin would say that it is a proton which takes the ride out in exchange for the sodium.

De Pont: I should like to question Dr Jørgensen about his statement that at physiological ionic concentrations the pump would work at only 1/5th of its maximal capacity. This conclusion is reached by extrapolating data from the test tube, where the ions are in equal concentrations on both sides of the plasma membrane, to the physiological situation, where the ionic concentrations at both sides are different. Is such an extrapolation permissible?

Jørgensen: The assumption is that the apparent affinities of extracellular and cytoplasmic cation sites differ so much that you can look at the two sites separately in titrations *in vitro*. The extracellular potassium sites are fully loaded with potassium at concentrations above 2 mM. At extracellular concentrations (5 mM) the turnover rate of the pump will therefore depend upon the intracellular Na/K ratio. This can be tested by looking at actual turnover rates in cells. This has not been done in kidney, but in sickle cells, Ehrlich cells and red cells you find that the turnover rate is between 1000 and 3000 ATP per minute, i.e. about 10–30% of the maximum turnover, which is 10,000 $ATP \cdot min^{-1}$.

Int. J. Biochem., Vol. 12, pp. 301 to 305
0020-711X/80/0701-0301$02.00/0

INDICATIONS OF SEVERAL NUCLEOTIDE BINDING SITES ON THE Na^+-K^+-ATPase MOLECULE

HERMANN KOEPSELL
Max-Planck-Institut für Biophysik, Kennedyallee 70, 6000 Frankfurt am Main 70, Federal Republic of Germany

Abstract—1. The effect of different ATP concentrations on the inhibition of purified membrane-bound Na^+-K^+-ATPase by different inhibitors was investigated.

2. Trypsin, the SH-group reagent 5,5'dithiobis(2-nitrobenzoic acid) and the covalently binding ATP analogue 6-((3-carboxy-4-nitrophenyl)thiol)-9-β-D-ribofuranosyl-purine 5'triphosphate were employed as inhibitors.

3. The effects of ATP on enzyme inhibition were observed in three concentration ranges different from those previously employed to determine the high affinity ATP binding.

4. The data suggest that four types of nucleotide binding sites are present on the Na^+-K^+-ATPase molecule.

INTRODUCTION

The mechanism of the coupled transport of Na^+ and K^+ as mediated by the Na^+-K^+-ATPase is not understood. The reason for this is that despite intensive investigation the enzyme structure and the number and location of ligand binding sites are not known. It is not unequivocally known whether the functioning Na^+-K^+-ATPase complex in the membrane is a dimer consisting of two catalytic and two glycoprotein subunits (Kyte, 1975; Giotta, 1976) or whether it is composed of more than two monomers (Haase & Koepsell, 1979). The total number of ionic, ouabain and nucleotide binding sites in the functioning Na^+-K^+-ATPase complex has also not been determined.

Binding of ligands to the Na^+-K^+-ATPase can be measured directly with radioactive ligands or indirectly by observing effects of ligand binding to the enzyme structure. Such ligand-induced structural alterations can be either detected by physical methods or by measuring the enzyme response to different inhibitors. For methodological reasons the direct measurement of ligand binding is frequently restricted to the high affinity range. However, observing the alterations in enzyme structure in the presence of ligands is considered a useful tool for the detection of lower affinity binding sites. In the present study, information was obtained on low affinity ATP binding to the Na^+-K^+-ATPase by measuring the effects of a wide range of ATP concentrations (0.001–10 $mmol \cdot l^{-1}$) on the inhibition of Na^+-K^+-ATPase activity by different inhibitors. The results suggest that besides the high affinity binding site(s) which have been observed directly (Nørby & Jensen, 1971; Hegyvary & Post, 1971; Koepsell, 1978), several low affinity ATP binding sites are present on the enzyme.

MATERIALS AND METHODS

Materials

Highly purified membrane-bound Na^+-K^+-ATPase with a specific activity of 30–36 μmol ATP split per mg protein per min was prepared from rat kidney outer medulla and freed from tightly bound nucleotides by gel chromatography in the presence of Mg^{2+} as previously described (Koepsell, 1978, 1979). Nb-S^6ITP was synthesized according to Höckel *et al.* (1978). DTNB was obtained from Sigma (London) and ATP(Na_2) from Boehringer GmbH (Mannheim). The Tris salt of ATP was prepared by ion exchange chromatography. Other chemicals were purchased as described earlier (Koepsell, 1978, 1979).

Methods

Protein determination and Na^+-K^+-ATPase assay—Protein was determined after precipitation with 10% trichloroacetic acid and solution in 1 M NaOH and 10% SDS according to Lowry *et al.* (1951) using bovine serum albumin as a standard. Na^+-K^+-ATPase activity was assayed optokinetically by the pyruvate kinase–lactate dehydrogenase linked system as previously described (Koepsell, 1978). The reaction was started by adding 20 μl of enzyme-containing solution to 1 ml of pre-warmed reaction mixture.

ATP effects on trypsin inactivation—The nucleotide free enzyme was incubated at 37°C with trypsin (6 $\mu g \cdot ml^{-1}$) in a buffer containing 25 $mmol \cdot l^{-1}$ imidazole, pH 7.5, NaCl, KCl and ATP as indicated in Results. The ionic strength was kept constant by the addition of choline chloride. After a 40 min incubation, the digestion was stopped by adding soybean trypsin inhibitor (weight ratio of inhibitor to trypsin, 7.5). The samples were immediately assayed for Na^+-K^+-ATPase activity.

ATP effects on DTNB inactivation—Nucleotide free enzyme (0.1 mg protein per ml) was incubated with 24 $\mu mol \cdot l^{-1}$ DTNB at pH 8.4 in the presence of Tris–HCl, EDTA and ATP as indicated in Results. After a 20 hr incubation at 0°C, samples were diluted 50 times in the assay buffer and analyzed for Na^+-K^+-ATPase activity. The amount of free DTNB which was transferred to the assay medium did not influence the measurement of the Na^+-K^+-ATPase activity. Controls were incubated under the same ligand conditions without addition of DTNB. The inhibition of Na^+-K^+-ATPase activity is expressed as a percentage of the controls.

ATP effects on the inactivation by Nb-S^6ITP—The inactivation of Na^+-K^+-ATPase by covalent labelling with Nb-S^6ITP was measured under the same experimental conditions as the inactivation by DTNB. Incubation time, Nb-S^6ITP concentration and ligand conditions are indicated in Results.

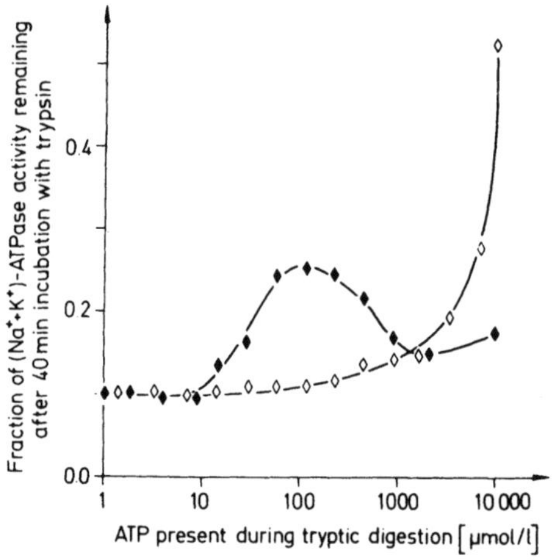

Fig. 1. Effect of ATP on the trypsin inactivation of membrane-bound Na^+-K^+-ATPase in the presence of Na^+ or K^+. Purified Na^+-K^+-ATPase (0.1 mg protein per ml) was incubated at 37°C for 40 min with trypsin (6 μg per ml) in a buffer containing varying concentrations of ATP, 25 mmol·l^{-1} imidazole–HCl, pH 7.5, and in addition 150 mmol·l^{-1} NaCl (◆) or 150 mmol·l^{-1} KCl (◇). The digestion was stopped by adding trypsin inhibitor and the remaining Na^+-K^+-ATPase activity was immediately assayed.

RESULTS

The effect of ATP concentrations varying from 0.001–10 mmol·l^{-1} on the inactivation of the purified membrane-bound Na^+-K^+-ATPase by different inhibitors was investigated. Trypsin, the SH-group reagent DTNB and the ATP analogue Nb-S^6ITP were employed as inhibitors. ATP effects were observed in three different concentration ranges. The half maximal ATP concentrations for these effects were about 3 μmol·l^{-1}, in the range of 20 to 30 μmol·l^{-1} and in the range of 0.6 to 8 mmol·l^{-1}.

The ATP dependence of inactivation of the purified membrane-bound Na^+-K^+-ATPase by trypsin was measured in the presence of NaCl or KCl. The enzyme was incubated for 40 min at 37°C with trypsin in a buffer containing 25 mmol·l^{-1} imidazole–HCl, pH 7.5, varying concentrations of ATP plus 150 mmol·l^{-1} NaCl or 150 mmol·l^{-1} KCl. From Fig. 1 it can be seen that in the presence of NaCl, ATP decreased the trypsin inactivation at low ATP concentrations (half maximal effect about 28 μmol·l^{-1}), whereas it increased the trypsin inactivation at high ATP concentrations (half maximal effect about 0.6 mmol·l^{-1}). In the presence of KCl the trypsin inactivation of the enzyme was only affected by high ATP concentrations. ATP concentrations in the range 0.2–10 mmol·l^{-1} markedly decreased the inactivation of the enzyme (Fig. 1).

To measure the effect of ATP on the inactivation of membrane-bound Na^+-K^+-ATPase by DTNB, the enzyme was incubated at 0°C with 24 μmol·l^{-1} DTNB in the presence of 50 mmol·l^{-1} Tris–HCl, pH 8.4, 2 mmol·l^{-1} EDTA and varying ATP concentrations. After 20 hr the residual Na^+-K^+-ATPase activity was measured and compared to a control. It was found that inactivation by DTNB was increased by ATP in a concentration range of 5 to 200 μmol·l^{-1} (Fig. 2). From experiments in which the time course of DTNB inactivation in the presence of different ATP concentrations was measured, a half-maximal ATP concentration of 23 μmol·l^{-1} was determined and positive cooperativity with a Hill coefficient of 1.6 was obtained.

The effects of varying ATP concentrations on the inactivation of membrane-bound Na^+-K^+-ATPase by 0.4 mmol·l^{-1}Nb-S^6ITP were investigated under the same experimental conditions as the ATP effects on the inactivation by DTNB. Under the given experimental conditions Nb-S^6ITP binds covalently to the enzyme. Kinetic studies (Koepsell & Hulla, in preparation) strongly suggest that the covalent labelling occurs at the catalytic sites of the enzyme. Measuring the effects of high ATP concentrations (0.1–10 mmol·l^{-1}) on the Na^+-K^+-ATPase inactivation induced by covalent labelling with Nb-S^6ITP the expected result was obtained that the Na^+–K^+-ATPase was protected by ATP (Fig. 3a). For this ATP effect a $K_{0.5}$ value of 2.2 mmol·l^{-1} was calculated from experiments in which the time course of inactivation in the presence of different ATP concentrations was measured. Plotting the data according to the Hill equation positive cooperativity with a Hill coefficient of 1.6 was obtained. When the effects of low ATP concentrations (0.1 to 250 μmol·l^{-1}) on the Nb-S^6ITP inactivation were measured the unexpected result was obtained that low ATP concentrations increased the inactivation of the enzyme (Fig. 3b). For this ATP effect a $K_{0.5}$ value of 3 μmol·l^{-1} and negative cooperativity with a Hill coefficient of 0.7 were determined. The finding that μmolar concentrations of ATP increase the inhibition of 0.4 mmol·l^{-1} Nb-S^6ITP indicates that the ATP analogue cannot substitute for ATP at this ATP binding site(s).

DISCUSSION

The present data suggest that beside the high affinity ATP binding site(s), detected by measuring the

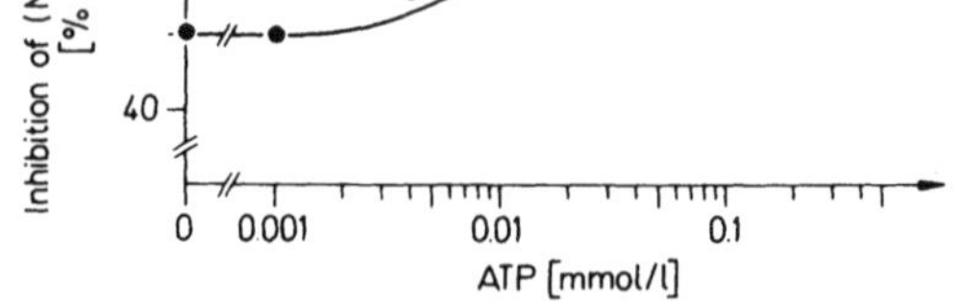

Fig. 2. Effect of ATP on the inactivation of membrane-bound Na^+-K^+-ATPase by DTNB. The enzyme (0.1 mg protein per ml) was incubated at 0°C with 24 μmol·l^{-1} DTNB in the presence of 50 mmol·l^{-1} Tris–HCl, pH 8.4, 2 mmol·l^{-1} EDTA plus the indicated ATP concentrations. After 20 hr the Na^+-K^+-ATPase activity was determined and compared to controls which were incubated without DTNB. The ionic strength was kept constant with choline chloride.

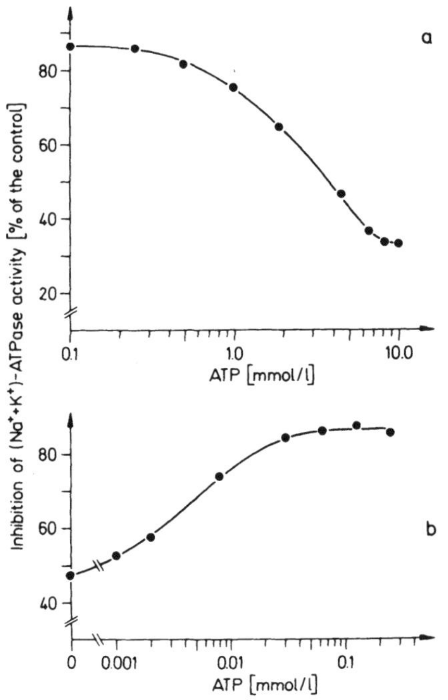

Fig. 3. Effects of (a) high and (b) low ATP concentrations on the inactivation of membrane-bound Na$^+$-K$^+$-ATPase by Nb-S^{6}ITP. The incubation of the enzyme (0.1 mg protein per ml) was performed with and without 0.4 μmol·l^{-1} Nb-S^{6}ITP at 0°C in the presence of 50 mmol·l^{-1} Tris–HCl, pH 8.4, plus varying ATP concentrations. After 20 hr the Na$^+$-K$^+$-ATPase activity was measured and the inhibition by Nb-S^{6}ITP was calculated. The ionic strength was kept constant with choline chloride.

ATP binding directly, nucleotide binding sites with lower affinity are also present in the enzyme. Since nucleotide binding was detected indirectly in the present study, the calculated half maximal ATP concentrations which lead to alterations in inhibitor action can only with reservations be considered as estimates of $K_{0.5}$ values for nucleotide binding. It cannot be excluded that nucleotide binding sites may have been altered by a reaction of the enzyme and inhibitor at non inhibitory sites. Furthermore, the possibility must be considered that the observed ATP-dependent alteration of the enzyme structure is not due to the nucleotide binding but to a successive kinetic step. This applies especially to the trypsin digestion experiments which were performed in the presence of NaCl or KCl. Moreover, it has to be carefully determined in future experiments whether the nucleotide effects seen in the DTNB and Nb-S^{6}ITP inactivation experiments in the presence of 2 mM EDTA, are solely due to the presence of ATP or whether some hydrolysis of ATP may have occurred so that they could be due to the presence of ADP.

Despite these reservations the observed ATP effects seem to indicate that several nucleotide binding sites are present on the Na$^+$-K$^+$-ATPase. In Table 1 the half maximal concentrations which are required for the observed nucleotide effects are taken as estimates of $K_{0.5}$ values for ATP binding. They are listed together with data from studies in which high affinity ATP binding and the ATP dependence of the Na$^+$-K$^+$-ATPase activity was measured (Koepsell, 1978). It can be seen that four different $K_{0.5}$ values can be estimated for the nucleotide binding. Since either negative or positive cooperativity was obtained for each of these $K_{0.5}$ values, it may be assumed that

Table 1. Nucleotide binding sites of the Na$^+$-K$^+$-ATPase complex

Affinity range	Estimated $K_{0.5}$ value for nucleotide binding	Hill coefficient	Method to detect the nucleotide binding	Proposed number of nucleotide binding sites
I	0.55 μmol·l^{-1}	0.6	Measurement of ATP binding (Koepsell, 1978)	2
II	3 μmol·l^{-1}	0.7	ATP effect on the inactivation by Nb-S^{6}ITP	2
III	28 μmol·l^{-1}	ND	ATP effect on the inactivation by trypsin in the presence of Na$^+$	2
	23 μmol·l^{-1}	1.6	ATP effect on the inactivation by DTNB	
IV	1.9 mmol·l^{-1}	0.86	ATP dependence of the Na$^+$-K$^+$-ATPase activity (Koepsell, 1978)	2
	0.6 mmol·l^{-1}	ND	ATP effect on the inactivation by trypsin in the presence of Na$^+$	
	8 mmol·l^{-1}	ND	ATP effect on the inactivation by trypsin in the presence of K$^+$	
	2.2 mmol·l^{-1}	1.6	ATP dependence of the inactivation by Nb-S^{6}ITP	

Summary of data which suggest that on the Na$^+$-K$^+$-ATPase molecule nucleotide binding sites are present in four different affinity ranges (I, II, III, IV). $K_{0.5}$ values for nucleotide binding were estimated (a) from ATP binding measurements (Koepsell, 1978), (b) from measurements of the ATP dependence of the Na$^+$-K$^+$-ATPase activity (Koepsell, 1978) and (c) from the half maximal ATP concentrations which were determined for ATP effects on the inhibition of Na$^+$-K$^+$-ATPase activity by trypsin, DTNB and Nb-S^{6}ITP.

more than one nucleotide binding site is present in each affinity range. Thus the data suggest that at least eight nucleotide binding sites with different affinities are present in the functioning Na^+-K^+-ATPase complex.

The differential effects of low and high ATP concentrations on the inactivation of Na^+-K^+-ATPase activity by covalent labelling of the catalytic sites of the enzyme with Nb-S^{6}ITP (Koepsell & Hulla, in preparation) suggest that at least two structurally different nucleotide binding sites may be present in the enzyme. Whether the nucleotide binding sites with a $K_{0.5}$ of 2.2 mmol·l^{-1} may represent the catalytic sites and those with a $K_{0.5}$ of 3 μmol·l^{-1} regulatory sites has to be elucidated in the future.

Information concerning the number of nucleotide binding sites may help us to understand the subunit composition of the functioning Na^+-K^+-ATPase complex in the membrane. At present the interpretation of such data is difficult since the number of nucleotide binding sites per catalytic subunit, at which all the nucleotide binding sites are supposed to be located, has not been determined. In general it may be stated that the presence of a large number of nucleotide binding sites with different affinities suggests that the Na^+-K^+-ATPase may be an oligomeric enzyme consisting of monomers which exhibit negative cooperativity. This view is supported by the recent finding of Hansen *et al.* (1979) that the number of high affinity nucleotide binding sites in the Na^+-K^+-ATPase can be increased two times by mild detergent treatment which also leads to an increase in the Na^+-K^+-ATPase activity. Thus if the idea is correct that negatively cooperative interactions are the reason for the detected high number of different nucleotide binding sites, the reported data fit with the hypothesis, which we recently raised on the basis of morphological findings (Haase & Koepsell, 1979), that the Na^+–K^+-ATPase complex in the membrane may be a tetramer. According to this concept each monomer of this complex is composed of a catalytic and a glycoprotein subunit and may contain two nucleotide binding sites.

SUMMARY

The effect of different ATP concentrations (0.001–10 mmol·l^{-1}) on the inactivation of purified Na^+-K^+-ATPase by (a) trypsin, (b) 5,5′dithiobis(2-nitrobenzoic acid) (DTNB), and (c) 6-((3-carboxy-4-nitrophenyl)thiol)-9-β-D-ribofuranosylpurine 5′triphosphate (Nb-S^{6}ITP) was measured. Depending on the inhibitor employed, ATP effects were observed in three different concentration ranges (half maximal ATP effects at 3 μmol·l^{-1}, in the range of 20–30 μmol·l^{-1} and in the range of 0.6–8 mmol·l^{-1}). For these effects either negative or positive cooperativity was obtained. In this study it was assumed that the ATP concentrations where the half maximal effects were observed correlated to the $K_{0.5}$ values for ATP binding. The data suggest, therefore, that in addition to the high affinity ATP binding sites, which have been detected by ATP binding measurements, three other types of nucleotide binding sites with lower affinities are present on the enzyme. The presence of four types of nucleotide binding sites would support the hypothesis that the Na^+-K^+-ATPase complex in the membrane is composed of four monomers, each of which consists of a catalytic and a glycoprotein subunit.

Acknowledgement—I want to thank M. Porz for her skilful and conscientious technical assistance.

REFERENCES

GIOTTA G. J. (1976) Quaternary structure of (Na^+ + K^+)-dependent adenosine triphosphatase. *J. biol. Chem.* **251**, 1247–1252.

HAASE W. & KOEPSELL H. (1979) Substructure of membrane-bound Na^+-K^+-ATPase protein. *Pflügers Arch. ges. Physiol.* **381**, 127–135.

HANSEN O., JENSEN J., NORBY J. G. & OTTOLENGHI P. (1979) A new proposal regarding the subunit composition of (Na^+ + K^+) ATPase. *Nature* **280**, 410–412.

HEGYVARY C. & POST R. L. (1971) Binding of adenosine triphosphate to sodium and potassium ion-stimulated adenosine triphosphatase. *J. biol. Chem.* **246**, 5234–5240.

HÖCKEL M., HULLA F. W., RISI S. & DOSE K. (1978) Kinetic studies on bacterial plasma membrane ATPase (F_1). Nucleotide-induced long term inactivation of ATP hydrolyzing activity is linked to the formation of multiple "tight" enzyme nucleotide complexes. *J. biol. Chem.* **253**, 4292–4296.

KOEPSELL H. (1978) Characteristics of antibody inhibition of rat kidney (Na^+-K^+)-ATPase. *J. Membr. Biol.* **44**, 85–102.

KOEPSELL H. (1979) Conformational changes of membrane-bound (Na^+-K^+)-ATPase as revealed by trypsin digestion. *J. Membr. Biol.* **48**, 69–94.

KYTE J. (1975) Structural studies of sodium and potassium ion-activated adenosine triphosphatase. The relationship between molecular structure and the mechanism of active transport. *J. biol. Chem.* **250**, 7443–7449.

LOWRY O. H., ROSEBROUGH N. J., FARR A. L. & RANDALL R. J. (1951) Protein measurement with the folin phenol reagent. *J. biol. Chem.* **193**, 265–275.

NORBY J. G. & JENSEN J. (1971) Binding of ATP to brain microsomal ATPase. Determination of the ATP-binding capacity and the dissociation constant of the enzyme-ATP complex as a function of K^+ concentration. *Biochim. biophys. Acta* **233**, 104–116.

SYMPOSIUM DISCUSSION

Schwartz: While the details of multiple binding sites for ATP are important for understanding the mechanism, Dr Radda has told us that the ATP content is several orders of magnitude higher than the values you are discussing. How do you fit this proposal into a physiological control?

Koepsell: The actual ATP concentration in the microenvironment of the Na^+-K^+-ATPase is not known. Furthermore I cannot be absolutely sure at the moment whether the effects which I have described are specifically due to ATP. There may be some effect of ADP since the possibility of some ATP hydrolysis has not been excluded.

Jørgenson: You would agree that you are measuring apparent affinities here; you should consider that binding constant and constants for the equilibrium between conformations of the proteins may interact in a way to give you "apparent" constants in your measurements that do not reflect binding of ATP.

Koepsell: I would agree that in these studies we do not show direct binding. The justification for such studies is the fact that it is technically difficult to measure ATP binding directly in these different affinity ranges. By such measurements we get a feeling for how ATP interacts with the enzyme. I don't think that I have unequivocally proved the existence of the different ATP binding sites.

Jorgenson: There is one further point. Just by adding a little potassium, you could create, in binding studies, nearly all the values you have been able to show here with the inhibitors. As you know our studies show that there is an equilibrium between the E_1 form and the E_2 form of the enzyme, and that this equilibrium is governed by potassium and ATP. Thus, by adding potassium, you can create whatever binding constants for ATP you want.

Koepsell: Yes, we are aware of that, and have done many studies with sodium and potassium. The studies reported here were performed in the absence of potassium or in the presence of a fixed potassium concentration. The study deals only with ATP, and I think we are observing ATP effects in conditions under which the enzyme does not turn over.

Jorgenson: But this implies that your compounds do not alter the equilibrium between the conformations.

Koepsell: Yes, this is a critical point which must be carefully controlled in the future.

Int. J. Biochem., Vol. 12, pp. 307 to 313
0020-711X/80/0701-0307$02.00/0

USE OF MONO- AND BIFUNCTIONAL GROUP-SPECIFIC REAGENTS IN THE STUDY OF THE RENAL Na^+–K^+-ATPase

J. J. H. H. M. de Pont, B. M. Schoot* and S. L. Bonting
Department of Biochemistry, University of Nijmegen, Nijmegen, The Netherlands

Abstract—1. Mono- and bifunctional reagents are useful tools for studying Na^+–K^+-ATPase. They can provide information on (a) classes of functional groups; (b) effect on partial reactions as compared to overall enzyme activity; (c) protection by ATP; (d) conformational changes induced by ions; (e) importance of free mobility of subunits for enzyme activity.

2. In this paper the effects of a number of these reagents, reacting with arginine, sulfhydryl and amino groups, on purified Na^+–K^+-ATPase from rabbit kidney outer medulla are surveyed.

INTRODUCTION

Na^+–K^+-ATPase is responsible for the active transport of sodium and potassium ions across mammalian membranes (Bonting, 1970; Jørgensen, 1975; Glynn & Karlish 1975; Schuurmans Stekhoven & Bonting, 1981). The enzyme consists of two protein subunits: the α or catalytic subunit with a molecular weight of 100,000 and the β subunit, a glycoprotein, with a molecular weight of 50,000. There are two α subunits per mol of enzyme, but the number of β subunits (1 or 2) has not yet been established with certainty. In addition, the enzyme complex is associated with phospholipids, removal of which leads to inactivation of the enzyme. After de-lipidation with detergents or phospholipases, reconstitution of enzyme activity can be obtained. Acidic phospholipids are particularly suitable in this respect (Wheeler & Whittam, 1970; Kimelberg & Papahadjopoulos, 1972), leading to the conclusion that these phospholipids would be essential for the enzyme activity. However, gentle removal or conversion of phospholipids with various types of phospholipase C and with phosphatidylserine decarboxylase in highly purified (Na^+–K^+)ATPase from rabbit kidney outer medulla has shown that the enzyme has no specific requirement for either phosphatidylserine or phosphatidylinositol (de Pont *et al.*, 1978).

The relation between structure and function of the Na^+–K^+-ATPase system, which due to the complexity of the transport system has not yet been resolved, can be studied by means of group-specific reagents. By studying the effect of treatment with such a reagent on the overall activity of the enzyme and its partial reactions various types of information can be obtained, particularly when ligands which influence the activity of the enzyme are present during the reaction with the group-specific reagent. In this way the existence of different conformational states of the enzyme can be established.

MATERIALS AND METHODS

Na^+–K^+-ATPase is purified from rabbit kidney outer medulla according to Jørgensen (1974). ATP tightly bound to the enzyme is removed as described previously (de Pont *et al.*, 1977). The activity of the enzyme amounts to 1000–2000 μmol ATP split·mg protein^{-1}·hr^{-1} and ouabain-insensitive activity is undetectable.

Modification with the following reagents is carried out as described before: butanedione (de Pont *et al.*, 1977); *N*-ethylmaleimide (Schoot *et al.*, 1977); 5,5′-dithiobis-(2-nitrobenzoic acid) (DTNB) (Schoot *et al.*, 1978), dimethyl 3,3′-dithiobispropionimidate (de Pont, 1979). Modification with trinitro benzene sulfonic acid (TNBS) (BDH Chemicals Ltd, Poole, England) is carried out in 0.2 M triethanolamine pH 8.5 with 0.5 mg·ml^{-1} protein and 100 μM TNBS for 15 min at 20°C, whereupon the reaction is stopped by filtration over Sephadex G 25 coarse (100 × 5 mm) equilibrated with the triethanolamine buffer. Amidination is carried out in 0.2 M triethanolamine (pH 8.5) with 0.5–1 mg·ml^{-1} Na^+–K^+-ATPase and 25 mM ethylacetimidate (Eastman Kodak Co., Rochester, NY, U.S.A.) for 30 min at 25°C, whereupon the reaction is stopped by dilution in the triethanolamine solution or by gel filtration. Acetylation is carried out in half-saturated sodium acetate (pH 8.5) and 10 mM acetic anhydride (Merck, Darmstadt, G.F.R.) with 50 μg·ml^{-1} Na^+–K^+-ATPase for 1 hr at 25°C, whereupon the reaction is stopped by 10-fold dilution, followed by centrifugation for 10 min at 300,000 *g*.

Cross-linking with dithiobis (succinimidyl propionate) (DTSP) (Pierce Chem. Co., Rockford, IL, U.S.A.) is carried out in 5 mM sodium phosphate buffer (pH 7.0) with 100 μg·ml^{-1} Na^+–K^+-ATPase and 1–2 mg·ml^{-1} DTSP for 2 min at 23°C. DTSP is first dissolved in dimethylformamide and diluted so that the final dimethyl formamide concentration is 5%. The reaction is stopped by addition of an equal volume 50 mM lysine. Thereafter the mixture is incubated for 30 min at 37°C with or without dithioerythritol in order to cleave the cross link. In the incubation media, ions, CDTA and ATP are present in the indicated concentrations.

Assays of Na^+–K^+-ATPase and its partial reactions are carried out according to the methods previously described (Schoot *et al.*, 1978) immediately after stopping the modification reaction.

Free amino groups present in the enzyme preparation before and after chemical modification are determined fluorimetrically using the Fluram reagent according to Böhlen *et al.* (1973), except that 1% SDS is added to all samples before adding Fluram.

RESULTS AND DISCUSSION

Classification of functional groups

In a series of investigations we have modified argi-

*Present address: European Molecular Biology Laboratory, Grenoble Outstation, Grenoble, France.

nine (de Pont *et al.*, 1977), sulfhydryl (Schoot *et al.*, 1977, 1978) and amino groups (to be published). By the application of different modifying agents it is in principle possible to subdivide functional groups in classes, as we have done for sulfhydryl groups in rabbit kidney outer medulla Na^+–K^+-ATPase (Schoot *et al.*, 1978). Treatment of the enzyme with 5,5'-dithiobis-(2-nitrobenzoic acid) (DTNB) in the presence of 1% sodium dodecyl sulfate shows that 36 sulfhydryl groups per mol enzyme (mol wt 250,000; Kepner & Macey, 1968) react with DTNB under release of 5-thio-2-nitrobenzoic acid. In the absence of sodium dodecyl sulfate only 12 sulfhydryl groups react, indicating that 24 sulfhydryl groups react with DTNB only under denaturating conditions. When the enzyme is pretreated with *N*-ethylmaleimide, DTNB under native conditions no longer reacts with sulfhydryl groups, whereas in the presence of sodium dodecyl sulfate it reacts with maximally 10 sulfhydryl groups. This means that *N*-ethylmaleimide has reacted under native conditions with 26 sylfhydryl groups, including the 12 which can react with DTNB under these conditions.

It is thus possible to divide the sulfhydryl groups into three classes:

Class A, containing 12 sulfhydryl groups, reacting both with DTNB and *N*-ethylmaleimide.

Class B, containing (at least) 14 sulfhydryl groups, reacting with *N*-ethylmaleimide but not with DTNB.

Class C, containing (at most) 10 sulfhydryl groups, which react with neither DTNB or *N*-ethylmaleimide in the absence of detergent.

By using ATP as a protecting agent we have shown that in class A as well as in class B there is at least one essential sulfhydryl group. The difference in reactivity of the various sulfhydryl groups is probably due to their localization in more or less hydrophobic parts of the enzyme molecule.

By means of labeled *N*-ethylmaleimide and sodium dodecyl sulfate gel electrophoresis it can be shown that 34 of the 36 sulfhydryl groups are located in the catalytic α subunit (Schoot *et al.*, 1979).

Effect on partial reactions

In addition to the overall Na^+–K^+-ATPase activity several so-called partial reactions can be measured in the enzyme preparation. These include ATP binding, phosphorylation by ATP or inorganic phosphate, ATP–ADP exchange, [^{3}H]ouabain binding and the K^+-stimulated phosphatase activity. We have compared the effects of six monofunctional group specific reagents on Na^+–K^+-ATPase and K^+-stimulated *p*-nitrophenylphosphatase activities. Table 1 shows that upon treatment with *N*-ethylmaleimide and acetic anhydride both activities are inhibited to the same extent. The other reagents affect the K^+-stimulated phosphatase activity less than the Na^+–K^+-ATPase activity. This suggests that fewer of the affected functional groups are required for proper functioning of the K^+-stimulated phosphatase activity of the Na^+–K^+-ATPase system than for the operation of the total Na^+–K^+-ATPase system.

The different effects of the two sulfhydryl reagents *N*-ethylmaleimide and DTNB can be explained by the fact that the former reacts with sulfhydryl groups of both class A and B, whereas the latter reacts only with those of class A. There is apparently at least one sulfhydryl group of class B, which is essential for both the ATPase and the phosphatase activity.

The different effects of the various amino groups modifying reagents are more difficult to explain. Half inhibition of the Na^+–K^+-ATPase activity by reaction with ethylacetimidate requires modification of

Table 1. Effects of chemical modifying reagents on the overall activity and the K^+-stimulated *p*-nitrophenylphosphatase activity of Na^+–K^+-ATPase

Modifying reagent	Modified group	Na^+–K^+-ATPase activity	K^+-stimulated *p*-nitrophenyl phosphatase activity
		Inhibition (%)	
N-ethylmaleimide*	–SH	50	50
		80	80
DTNB†	–SH	50	36
		80	66
Butanedione‡	–arg	50	15
		80	30
Acetic anhydride§	$-NH_2$	50	52
		80	83
TNBS§	$-NH_2$	50	40
		80	69
Ethylacetimidate§	$-NH_2$	50	22
		80	42

Na^+–K^+-ATPase is modified as described under Materials and Methods. For each reagent residual K^+-stimulated *p*-nitrophenylphosphatase activity was plotted against residual Na^+–K^+-ATPase activity. Percentage inhibition of the K^+-stimulated *p*-nitrophenylphosphatase activity at 50 and 80% Na^+–K^+-ATPase inhibition, respectively, was read from these plots. Values from * Schoot *et al.* (1977); † Schoot *et al.*, 1978; ‡ de Pont *et al.*, 1977 and § unpublished results.

Table 2. Effects of butanedione on overall activities and partial reactions of Na^+-K^+-ATPase

	Inhibition (%)
Na^+-K^+-ATPase activity	79 ± 1.2
Na^+ dependent phosphorylation by ATP (37°C)	78 ± 1.1
Phosphorylation by P_i	35 ± 2.5
K^+-stimulated *p*-nitrophenylphosphatase activity	30 ± 3.0

Na^+-K^+-ATPase is incubated for 30 min at 25°C in 125 mM sodium borate buffer (pH 7.5), containing 5 mM $MgCl_2$ and 5 mM butanedione. The various activities are determined as described under Materials and Methods and expressed as percent inhibition of the activities of a control preparation treated in the same way without butanedione. Values are means of three experiments with SEM.

25% of the amino groups. In the case of acetic anhydride 20% modification is sufficient to reach this degree of inhibition. With TNBS only a very small number of amino groups needs to be modified (less than 10%) for 50% inhibition of the Na^+-K^+-ATPase activity. The inequality of the inhibition of the K^+-stimulated *p*-nitrophenylphosphatase activity and the Na^+-K^+-ATPase activity suggests that the different amino group reagents affect different classes of amino groups. The class which is specifically modified by acetic anhydride seems to contain amino groups which are important for both enzyme activities.

Modification of arginine residues with butanedione inhibits the K^+-stimulated *p*-nitrophenylphosphatase activity much less than the Na^+-K^+-ATPase activity (Table 1). We have also investigated the effect of butanedione on the phosphorylation by ATP and inorganic phosphate. Table 2 shows that the phosphorylation by ATP is inhibited to the same degree as the Na^+-K^+-ATPase activity, whereas the phosphorylation by inorganic phosphate is inhibited in parallel with the K^+-stimulated *p*-nitrophenylphosphatase activity. The equal sensitivity of the Na^+ dependent phosphorylation and the Na^+-K^+-ATPase activity towards butanedione can be explained by assuming that modification with butanedione primarily prevents binding of ATP to the enzyme and thus all reactions that require this step. The lower sensitivity of the K^+-stimulated *p*-nitrophenylphosphatase activity and the phosphorylation by inorganic phosphate suggest that the arginine group in the binding centre is less essential for the binding of *p*-nitrophenylphosphate and inorganic phosphate than for ATP binding.

Protecting effects of ATP

The enzyme has a very high affinity for ATP (K_D = 0.12–0.22 μM; Hegyvary & Post, 1971; Nørby & Jensen, 1971). The binding of ATP is maximal in the absence of Mg^{2+}, Na^+ and K^+ions. In the presence of Mg^{2+} and Na^+ ions the enzyme is phosphorylated and thus the original ATP-binding site is vacated. When chemical modification is carried out in the presence of ATP and in the absence of Mg^{2+} (endogenous Mg^{2+} complexed by CDTA), the rate of inactivation by several of the reagents is markedly reduced. The apparent K_d for ATP calculated from the protection curves with the method of Scrutton & Utter (1965) varies with the reagent used (Table 3). In the presence of Mg^{2+} (and Na^+) ions the protection by ATP is much less or is completely absent.

The protecting effect of ATP in the absence of Mg^{2+} can be explained in two ways: (a) there is a specific functional group present in the ATP binding centre which is protected when ATP is bound to the enzyme; (b) the interaction of ATP with the enzyme induces a conformation by which an essential group outside the ATP binding centre is shielded. The lower the ATP concentration necessary for 50% protection, the more likely it would seem to be that the functional group under consideration is located in the ATP binding centre. The lowest ATP concentration, which protects against chemical modification, has been found with butanedione (Table 3). An arginine residue has been assumed to be present in the substrate or cofactor binding centre for many enzymes in which negatively charged substrates or cofactors play a role (Riordan *et al.*, 1977), including several ATPases, such as chloroplast ATPase (Andreo & Vallejos, 1977), mitochondrial ATPase (Marcus *et al.*, 1976), Ca^{2+}-Mg^{2+}-ATPase (Murphy, 1976) and K^+-H^+-ATPase (Bonting *et al.*, 1980). Hence, we suggest that an arginine residue is also involved in the

Table 3. Affinity of ATP for Na^+-K^+-ATPase obtained from modification experiments in the presence of ATP

Modifying reagent	K_D (μM)
N-ethylmaleimide*	12
DTNB†	5
butanedione‡	0.8
TNBS	11

Values for the apparent dissociation constant K_D are obtained by means of the method of Scrutton & Utter (1965). Data from *Schoot *et al.* (1977). †Schoot *et al.* (1978) and ‡de Pont *et al.* (1977) are presented. Experiments with TNBS (100 μM) were carried out in 0.2 M triethanolamine (pH 8.5) with 0.5 mg·ml^{-1} Na^+-K^+-ATPase. In all experiments 2–5 mM CDTA was present to complex endogenous Mg^{2+}. With acetic anhydride and *N*-ethylacetimidate the protecting effect of 5 mM ATP was so small that calculation of a K_D value was not possible.

ATP binding centre of Na^+–K^+-ATPase. This suggestion is further supported by the fact that K^+ ions diminish both the rate of inhibition by butanedione (de Pont *et al.*, 1977) and the ATP binding to the enzyme (Hegyvary & Post, 1971), indicating that K^+ ions induce a conformational change in the enzyme, which buries the essential arginine group in such a way that reaction with ATP and butanedione is hindered.

Interpretation of the inhibitory effects of ATP on the modification of sulfhydryl groups by DTNB and *N*-ethylmaleimide is more difficult. High- and low-affinity binding sites and ATP-induced conformational changes may be involved in these protecting effects. The fact that the rate of inhibition by butanedione is decreased after pretreatment with DTNB suggests that an essential sulfhydryl group is located near the ATP binding centre.

A similar situation exists for the modification of amino groups. Here inactivation with the amino group reagent TNBS, under conditions where it reacts with a very small number of these groups, can be antagonized by low ATP concentrations. However, ATP has only a very minor protecting effect on the amino group modification by ethylacetimidate or acetic anhydride. In this case many more amino groups need to be modified in order to obtain comparable inactivation of the Na^+–K^+-ATPase activity. This indicates that ethylacetimidate and acetic anhydride inactivate the Na^+–K^+-ATPase in a rather non-specific way, whereas TNBS inactivates through reaction with a few strategically located, important amino groups.

Effect of ions

Na^+, K^+ and Mg^{2+} ions play an important role in the mechanism of action of Na^+–K^+-ATPase. One possible way by which these ions exert their effects is by inducing changes in the conformation of the enzyme protein. Such conformational changes may result in the exposure or shielding of important functional groups, leading to increase or decrease of the inhibitory effects of the modifying reagents.

Nearly all studies with butanedione have been carried out in a sodium borate buffer (de Pont *et al.*, 1977). Replacement of sodium ions by potassium ions decreases inhibition by butanedione. The effect of K^+ ions is already half-maximal at a K^+:Na^+ ratio of only 0.034, suggesting that a K^+ specific site is involved in this effect. Addition of Mg^{2+} ions does not change the effect of butanedione, at least when the enzyme is free of bound ATP.

Mg^{2+}, Na^+ and K^+ ions have marked effects on the inactivation of Na^+–K^+-ATPase by *N*-ethylmaleimide and DTNB. Mg^{2+} ions cause a large and Na^+ ions a small increase in the inactivation due to treatment by these two reagents (Schoot *et al.*, 1979). With *N*-ethylmaleimide the effect of Na^+ ions is lost at higher (>30 mM) Na^+ concentrations. The effects of both ions are larger with DTNB than with *N*-ethylmaleimide as the inactivating reagent. With 5 mM K^+ present in the inactivation medium, there is a slight protecting effect, while higher K^+ concentrations (>10 mM) do not influence the inactivation by *N*-ethylmaleimide, but increase the inactivation by DTNB. These results indicate that Mg^{2+}, K^+ and Na^+ ions have, depending on their concentrations, effects on the conformational state of Na^+–K^+-ATPase, leading to changes in the exposure of essential sulfhydryl groups. The difference between the effects of these ions on the inactivation caused by *N*-ethylmaleimide and DTNB confirms that different sulfhydryl groups are involved in the inactivation process of these reagents.

Modification of amino groups by TNBS, but not by ethylacetimidate or acetic anhydride, can be influenced by the above cations. Fig. 1 shows that Na^+ ions slightly increase the inactivation of both Na^+–K^+-ATPase and K^+-stimulated *p*-nitrophenylphosphatase activities. Mg^{2+} ions have a similar effect as Na^+ ions (not shown). On the other hand, K^+ ions markedly protect both enzyme activities against inactivation by TNBS. This effect is half-maximal at 0.3 mM K^+ concentration in the absence of Na^+. However, in the presence of 10 mM Na^+ ions, the K^+ concentration necessary for 50% protection is 40 mM (Fig. 2). This indicates that a K^+ sensitive site, with high affinity for Na^+, may be involved in the protecting effect. It may be a site located on the inner side of the membrane, since similar sites have been found at the inner face of the human erythrocyte membrane (Garay & Garrahan, 1973). The similarity of the effects of these cations for the Na^+–K^+-ATPase and K^+-stimulated *p*-nitrophenylphosphatase activities indicates that occupation of the cationic binding sites leads to conforma-

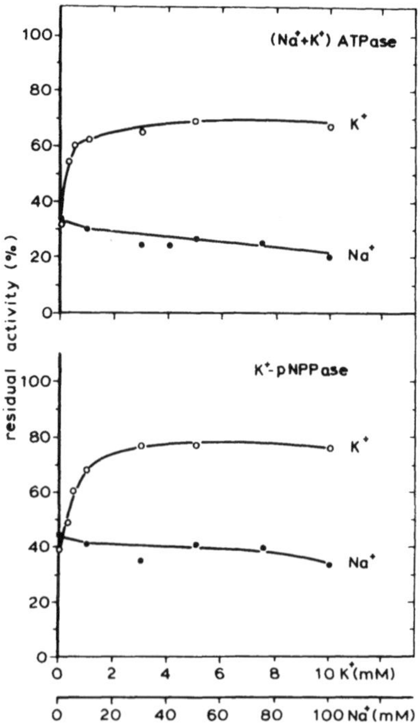

Fig. 1. Effect of Na^+ and K^+ ions on inactivation of Na^+–K^+-ATPase by TNBS. Na^+–K^+-ATPase (0.6 mg·ml^{-1}) was treated with 100 μM trinitrobenzene sulfonate (TNBS) in 0.2 M triethanolamine (pH 8.5) with 0–10 mM K^+ or 0–100 mM Na^+ present. Incubation was for 30 min at 20°C. After gel filtration both enzyme activities were determined as described under Materials and Methods. Activities are expressed as percent of the activity of a sample treated in the same way without TNBS.

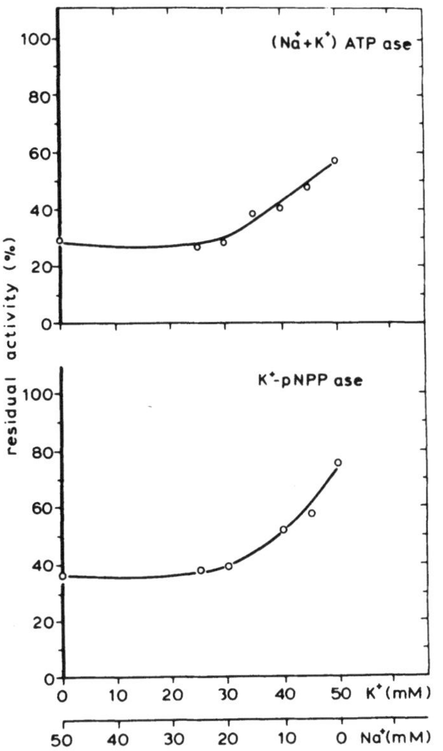

Fig. 2. Effect of replacement of Na^+ by K^+ ions on the inactivation of Na^+–K^+-ATPase by TNBS. Conditions are the same as in Fig. 1, except that the sum of Na^+ and K^+ ions is kept at 50 mM.

tional changes, influencing the exposure of reactive amino groups involved in both these activities.

Subunit interaction

The Na^+–K^+-ATPase complex contains two different subunits, the catalytic or α subunit, and the glycoprotein or β subunit. When the enzyme is treated with bifunctional amino group reagents, such as dimethylsuberimidate (Kyte, 1972), dimethyl 3,3′-dithiobispropionimidate (de Pont, 1979) and dithiobis (succinimidylpropionate), the major product is an αβ dimer. Surprisingly, the same product is found after treatment with the monofunctional reagent ethylacetimidate (Sweadner, 1977; de Pont, unpublished observations). This is due to the fact that an *N*-alkylimidate is formed as an intermediate (Browne & Kent, 1975), which can react with a second amino group nearby. The latter amino group then lies on another subunit, hence the formation of a cross link between an α and β subunit follows.

Bifunctional reagents reacting with sulfhydryl groups, such as Cu^{2+} phenanthroline (Kyte, 1975; Giotta, 1976; Liang & Winter, 1977; Huang & Askari, 1978; Schoot, 1978), bis maleimidomethyl ether (Schoot, 1978) and *p*-azophenyl *N,N′* dimaleimide (Schoot, 1978), form primarily an α_2 dimer, at least in the absence of detergent. In the presence of digitonin or Triton-X-100, Cu^{2+} phenanthroline also leads to the formation of an αβ dimer (Liang & Winter, 1977; Huang & Askari, 1979). The failure of bifunctional sulfhydryl reagents to form αβ dimers under native conditions can be explained by the fact that the β subunit has no reactive sulfhydryl groups under these conditions (Schoot *et al.*, 1979).

These studies indicate that the Na^+–K^+-ATPase system contains at least two α subunits and one β subunit in close proximity. However, the exact number of the two subunits in the native enzyme cannot easily be estimated since small amounts of larger oligomers are formed in addition to the αβ and α_2 dimers. The fluidity of the plasma membrane enables the formation of intermolecular cross links, which complicates the interpretation of the electropherograms.

Reaction of Na^+–K^+-ATPase with bifunctional reagents is accompanied by a loss of Na^+–K^+-ATPase activity. This activity loss can be due both to the modification of functional groups as such, and to restriction of the mobility of one or more subunits which are essential for enzyme activity. The second possibility seems to be indicated by the results obtained with cleavable bifunctional agents, such as dimethyl 3,3′ dithiobispropionimidate (DTP) and dithiobis(succinimidylpropionate) (DTSP). Both reagents have an internal disulfide bridge, which can be split by the addition of sulfhydryl compounds like dithioerythritol without affecting the links with the amino groups. Table 4 shows the effect of addition of dithioerythritol on the activities of Na^+–K^+-ATPase and K^+-stimulated *p*-nitrophenylphosphatase after prior treatment with either DTP or DTSP. Concen-

Table 4. Effect of cleavable bifunctional reagents on the overall activity and the K^+-stimulated *p*-nitrophenylphosphatase activity of Na^+–K^+-ATPase

	−DTE	+DTE	*n*
Na^+–K^+-ATPase activity (% of control)			
DTP	50 ± 4.5	84 ± 2.9	6
DTSP	49 ± 3.8	64 ± 3.9	9
K^+-stimulated *p*-nitrophenylphosphatase activity (% of control)			
DTP	67 ± 4.1	87 ± 2.1	6
DTSP	60 ± 4.4	70 ± 3.1	9

Na^+–K^+-ATPase was treated with either 0.2–0.4 $mg \cdot ml^{-1}$ dimethyl 3,3′dithiobispropionimidate (DTP) or 1–2 $mg \cdot ml^{-1}$ dithiobis(succinimidylpropionate) (DTSP) as described under Materials and Methods. After gel filtration and incubation with or without 10 mM dithioerythritol for 30 min at 25°C the activities of Na^+–K^+-ATPase and K^+-stimulated *p*-nitrophenylphosphatase were determined and expressed as percent of the activities in the absence of DTP and DTSP. Values are given as means with standard error for *n* experiments.

tration of the latter reagents and incubation times have been chosen in such a way that the residual Na^+–K^+-ATPase activity in the absence of dithioerythritol is approximately 50%. The K^+-stimulated *p*-nitrophenylphosphatase activity is inhibited somewhat less. Addition of dithioerythritol leads to reactivation of both enzyme activities. The effect is largest when DTP is used. The (partial) recovery of both enzyme activities indicates that at least the α subunit must be fully mobile in order to achieve full enzyme activity. Recovery of enzyme activity is only partial, since modification of the amino groups as such persists after cleavage of the reagent. The larger recovery by dithioerythritol after treatment with DTP than with DTSP could be due to a minor contribution of the effect of amino group modification by the former reagent.

CONCLUSIONS

Mono- and bifunctional modifying reagents are useful tools in the study of a complex enzyme system like Na^+–K^+-ATPase. The most important findings of our studies up to now are:

(1) An essential arginine residue is involved in the ATP binding centre of the enzyme.

(2) Sulfhydryl groups and some amino groups are important for the enzyme activity.

(3) Mg^{2+}, Na^+, K^+ and possibly ATP induce conformational changes in the enzyme.

(4) The K^+-activated *p*-nitrophenylphosphatase activity is less sensitive to some forms of chemical modification than the Na^+–K^+-ATPase.

(5) Free mobility of at least the α subunit is essential for enzyme activity.

Acknowledgements—The skilled technical assistance of Mrs S. E. van Emst-de Vries and Mrs A. van Prooijen-van Eeden is gratefully acknowledged.

REFERENCES

Andree C. S. & Vallejos R. H. (1977) An essential arginyl residue in the soluble chloroplast ATPase. *FEBS Lett.* **78**, 207–210.

Bohlen P., Stein S., Dairmon W. & Udenfriend S. (1973) Fluorimetric assay of proteins in the nanogram range. *Archs Biochem. Biophys.* **155**, 213–220.

Bonting S. L. (1970) Na-K activated ATPase and cation transport. In *Membrane and Ion Transport* (Edited by Bittar E. E.) pp. 257–363. Wiley Interscience, London.

Bonting S. L., Pont J. J. H. H. M. de, Amelsvoort J. M. M. van & Schrijen J. J. (1980) Transport ATPases in anion and proton transport. *Ann. N.Y. Acad. Aci.* In press.

Browne D. T. & Kent S. B. H. (1975) Formation of non-amidine products in the reaction of primary amines with imido esters. *Biochem. biophys. Res. Commun.* **67**, 126–138.

Garay R. P. & Garrahan P. J. (1973) The interaction of sodium and potassium with the sodium pump in red cells. *J. Physiol., Lond.* **231**, 297–325.

Giotta G. J. (1976) Quarternary structure of (Na^+–K^+)-dependent adenosine triphosphatase. *J. biol. Chem.* **251**, 1247–1252.

Glynn I. M. & Karlish S. J. D. (1975) The sodium pump. *A. Rev. Physiol.* **37**, 13–55.

Hegyvary C. & Post R. L. (1971) Binding of ATP to sodium and potassium ion stimulated ATPase. *J. biol. Chem.* **246**, 5234–5240.

Huang W. & Askari A. (1978) Na^+, K^+-ATPase: On the nature of the "cross-linked" subunits obtained in the presence of *o*-phenanthroline and cupric ion. *Biochem. biophys. Res. Commun.* **82**, 1314–1319.

Huang W. & Askari A. (1979) (Na^+–K^+)-ATPase: Effects of detergents on the crosslinking of subunits in the presence of Cu^{2+} and *o*-phenanthroline. *Biochim. biophys. Acta* **578**, 547–552.

Jørgensen P. L. (1974) Purification and characterization of (Na^+–K^+)-ATPase III. Purification from the outer medulla of mammalian kidney after selective removal of membrane components by sodium dodecyl sulfate. *Biochim. biophys. Acta* **356**, 36–52.

Jørgensen P. L. (1975) Isolation and characterization of the components of the sodium pump. *Q. Rev. Biophys.* **7**, 239–274.

Kepner G. R. & Macey R. I. (1968) Molecular weight estimation of membrane bound ATPase by in vacuo radiation inactivation. *Biochem. biophys. Res. Commun.* **30**, 582–587.

Kimelberg H. K. & Papahadjopoulos D. (1972) Phospholipid requirements for (Na^+–K^+)-ATPase activity: head group specificity and fatty acid fluidity. *Biochim. biophys. Acta* **282**, 277–292.

Kyte J. (1972) Properties of the two polypeptides of sodium and potassium dependent adenosine triphosphatase. *J. biol. Chem.* **247**, 7642–7649.

Liang S.-M. & Winter C. G. (1977) Digitonin-induced changes in subunit arrangement in relation to some *in vitro* activities of the (Na^+,K^+)-ATPase. *J. biol. Chem.* **252**, 8278–8284.

Marcus F., Schuster S. M. & Lardy H. D. (1976) Essential arginyl residues in mitochondrial ATPase. *J. biol. Chem.* **251**, 1775–1780.

Murphy A. J. (1976) Arginyl residue modification of the sarcoplasmic reticulum ATPase protein. *Biochem. biophys. Res. Commun.* **70**, 1048–1054.

Nørby J. G. & Jensen J. (1971) Binding of ATP to microsomal ATPase. Determination of the ATP binding capacity and the dissociation constant of the enzyme–ATPase complex as a function of K^+ concentration. *Biochim. biophys. Acta* **233**, 104–116.

Pont J. J. H. H. M. de (1979) Reversible inactivation of (Na^+–K^+)-ATPase by use of a cleavable bifunctional reagent. *Biochim. biophys. Acta* **567**, 247–256.

Pont J. J. H. H. M. de, Schoot B. M., van Prooijen-van Eeden A. & Bonting S. L. (1977) An essential arginine residue in the ATP-binding centre of (Na^+–K^+)ATPase. *Biochim. biophys. Acta* **482**, 213–227.

Pont J. J. H. H. M. de, van Prooijen-van Eeden A. & Bonting S. L. (1978) Role of negatively charged phospholipids in highly purified (Na^+–K^+)-ATPase from rabbit kidney outer medulla. Studies on (Na^+–K^+)-activated ATPase, XXXIX. *Biochim. biophys. Acta* **508**, 464–477.

Riordan J. F., McElvany K. D. & Borders C. L. Jr (1977) Arginyl residues: anion recognition sites in enzymes. *Science* **195**, 884–886.

Schoot B. M. (1978) Functional groups of Na–K-ATPase. Thesis, University of Nijmegen, Nijmegen, The Netherlands.

Schoot B. M., Schoots A. F. M. Pont J. J. H. H. M. de, Schuurmans Stekhoven F. M. A. H. & Bonting S. L. (1977) Studies on (Na^+–K^+)-activated ATPase. XLI. Effects of *N*-ethylmaleimide on overall and partial reactions. *Biochim. biophys. Acta* **483**, 181–192.

Schoot B. M., Pont J. J. H. H. M. de & Bonting S. L. (1978) Studies on (Na^+–K^+)-activated ATPase XLII. Evidence for two classes of essential sulfhydryl groups. *Biochim. biophys. Acta* **522**, 602–613.

SCHOOT B. M., PONT J. J. H. H. M. DE & BONTING S. L. (1979) Functional groups of Na-K ATPase. In *Sodium, potassium-ATPase: Structure and Kinetics* (Edited by SKOU J. C & NØRBY J. G.) pp. 193–204. Academic Press, New York.

SCHUURMANS STEKHOVEN F. M. A. H. & BONTING S. L. (1981) Transport ATPases. *Physiol. Rev.* In press.

SCRUTTON M. C. & UTTER M. F. (1965) Pyruvate carboxylase V. Interaction of the enzyme with adenosine triphosphate. *J. biol. Chem.* **240,** 3714–3723.

SWEADNER K. J. (1977) Crosslinking and modification of Na,K-ATPase by ethyl acetimidate. *Biochem. biophys. Res. Commun.* **78,** 962–969.

WHEELER K. P. & WHITTAM R. (1970) The involvement of phosphatidylserine in adenosine triphosphatase activity of the sodium pump. *J. Physiol. Lond.* **207,** 303–328.

Int. J. Biochem., Vol. 12, pp. 315 to 318
© Pergamon Press Ltd 1980. Printed in Great Britain

0020-711X/80/0701-0315$02.00/0

PROTEIN METABOLISM OF RENAL BASOLATERAL MEMBRANES IN RAT*

H. EBEL and A. GEBHARDT
Institute of Clinical Physiology, Klinikum Steglitz, Freie Universität Berlin, Federal Republic of Germany

Abstract—1. The incorporation of [^{3}H]phenylalanine into protein of renal basolateral membranes (BLM) and endoplasmic reticulum(ER) has been measured *in vivo*.

2. Maximal incorporation was achieved within 30 min in ER and after 10–12 hr in BLM. Thus BLM protein might be synthetized by the ER.

3. Protein degradation in BLM and ER followed first-order kinetics. The apparent half life times were 60–61 hr for both BLM and ER.

4. The turnover of single Triton X100 soluble proteins was heterogenous. Half life times of the 155,000 and 97,000 dalton proteins, containing Na – K-ATPase subunits were 66 and 86 hr, respectively.

5. It is suggested that rapid hormonal induced changes of ion transport may not be primarily mediated by a change in turnover of specific BLM proteins.

INTRODUCTION

In recent years our knowledge of ion transport and its hormonal regulation has increased considerably. Much progress has been made to identify and analyse transport proteins such as the Na – K-ATPase (for review see Wallick *et al.*, 1979) and others (for review see Korenbrot, 1977). Also hormone receptor proteins have been isolated (Roy *et al.*, 1975; Malbon & Zull, 1977). However, the dynamic turnover of these specific proteins and its relationship to transport processes remains to be elucidated. Therefore we started studying protein metabolism of renal basolateral membranes.

MATERIALS AND METHODS

Animals

For experiments male Sprague–Dawley rats (Zentralinstitut für Versuchstierkunde, Hannover, Germany) with a body weight of 180–200 g were used. The animals were kept under constant light and temperature conditions and had free access to food (Altromin®) and water.

Isotope administration

Protein synthesis or degradation was followed by measuring the *in vivo* incorporation of L-[4-^{3}H]-phenylalanine (Amersham, England, No TRK 204). Usually a dose of 100 μCi · 100 g body weight^{-1} was given in 100 μl of 0.9% NaCl. The isotope was intracardially injected during a short ether narcosis.

Membrane isolation

Various times after isotope administration the animals were killed by bleeding. Kidneys were removed and placed on ice. The cortex was dissected with a razor blade. Homogenization and isolation of basolateral membranes-(BLM) of single rats was performed as outlined in detail previously (Ebel *et al.*, 1976). In principle, a 1350–2500 g pellet was subjected to discontinuous sucrose density gradient centrifugation at 95,000 ***g*** for 120 min. The BLM accumulated at the density interface of $d = 1.14/1.15$. Endoplasmic reticulum(ER) was isolated as described by Rollestone (1972). Briefly, a 10,000–100,000 ***g*** pellet was subjected to discontinuous sucrose gradient centrifugation for at least 18 hr at 130,000 ***g***. ER accumulated at the interface between 1.3 and 2.0 M sucrose.

Protein extraction of membranes

For counting of radioactivity, samples of BLM and ER were precipitated and washed with trichloroacetic acid (final concentration 5% w/v). Then lipid was extracted by washing with ethanol and ether. The remaining protein was dissolved in 0.5 N NaOH at 90°C.

Gel electrophoresis

For gel electrophoresis the BLM were solubilized in 0.05% Triton X 100 as described by Banerjee *et al.* (1970). Gel electrophoresis of the Triton solubilized membranes was conducted according to the method of Davis (1964). Triton X100, 0.05% was included in the gel. The acrylamide concentration was 5%. Cylindrical precision bore glass tubes of 0.5 × 7.5 cm were used.

For the counting of radioactivity single gel slices were solubilized according to Tishler & Epstein (1968) with H_2O_2. Then NCS (Amersham–Searle) and a toluene-based scintillator were added. For protein analysis gels were stained with Coomassie Blue according to Chrambach *et al.* (1967). PAS staining was performed as described by Kapitany & Zebrowski (1973). For densitometry a Hewlett–Packard integrator type 3380A was used connected with a Zeiss spectrophotometer PM Q II equipped with a disc-scanning attachment. For histochemical identification of various phosphatases the split phosphate was localized with the method of Wachstein & Meisel (1957). Aminopeptidase was stained according to Nachlas *et al.* (1960). Alkaline phosphatase was determined by the method of Seligman *et al.* (1951). For identification of Na – K-ATPase phosphorylation from ATP^{32} was used (Post & Sen, 1967).

Counting of radioactivity

For counting of radioactivity a liquid scintillation spectrometer (Tricarb model 3385) was used. Quenching correction was made by means of automatic external standardization. Specific activity was expressed in dis/min per mg protein or in dis/min per gel slice. The scintillator used for trichloroacetic acid extracted proteins contained PPO

* Supported in part by a grant of the Deutsche Forschungsgemeinschaft.

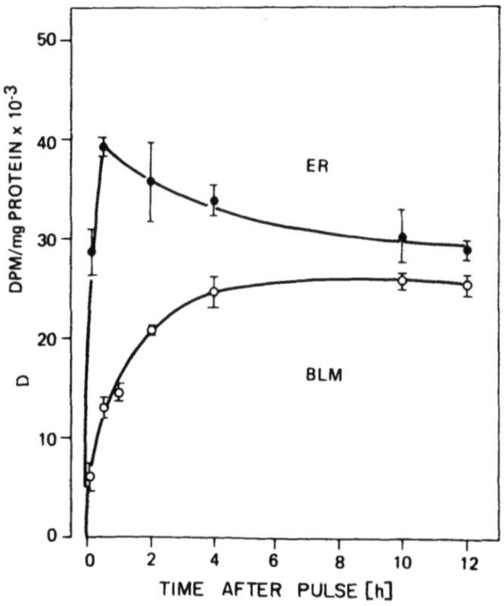

Fig. 1. Incorporation of L-[^{3}H]phenylalanine into basolateral membranes(BLM) and endoplasmic reticulum(ER) protein of rat kidney cortex. A dose of 100 μCi · 100 g body weight^{-1} in a volume of 100 μl 0.9% NaCl was injected intracardially in ether narcosis.

3 g, POPOP 150 mg, naphthalene 100 ml, dioxan 300 ml and ethyleneglycol monoethylether 300 ml. The scintillator used for solubilized gel slices was composed of PPO 7.5 g, POPOP 0.25 g in toluene 2.5 l.

Protein determination

Protein was determined with the method of Lowry *et al.* (1951). Bovine serum albumin was used as standard.

RESULTS AND DISCUSSION

First a dose–response curve was established. Two hours after administration of [^{3}H]phenylalanine (^{3}H-PA) isotope incorporation into BLM protein was linear within the dose range tested at least up to 150 μCi · 100 g body weight^{-1}. For ER a more curvilinear plot was obtained.

Next, the effect of a potent inhibitor of protein synthesis on ^{3}H-PA incorporation was tested. Cycloheximide 300 mg · kg^{-1} solubilized in 0.9% NaCl was injected intraperitoneally. The inhibitor was administered 20 min before pulse labelling. At this time the effect was maximal. It was found that cycloheximide almost completely inhibited ^{3}H-PA incorporation into BLM protein. In a 2 hr pulse the inhibition averaged 92%.

Figure 1 demonstrates the time–course of ^{3}H-PA incorporation into total membrane protein. The endoplasmic reticulum is characterized by a rapid increase of isotope incorporation. Maximal labeling was achieved within 30 min. Quite in contrast the BLM were characterized by a slower incorporation rate with maximal labeling at 10–12 hr. The sequence of maximal labeling of membrane protein observed in this and other studies (for latest review see Morré *et al.*, 1979) is consistent with the assumption that the proteins of plasma membranes as well as that of the BLM subfraction are synthetized by the endoplasmic reticulum and are then transferred and inserted possibly via the Golgi-apparatus.

After maximal labeling the specific activity of BLM and ER declined in a first order process, at least up to 96 hr. From the decay of specific activity the rate constant of degradation has been calculated according to the equation reported by Schimke & Doyle (1970). Despite rather different times for maximal labeling the apparent half life times of BLM and ER were the same and in the range of 60–61 hr. By autoradiography of fucosylglycoproteins in mouse kidney a similar value in the range of 80 hr has been reported for BLM of proximal tubule cells (Haddad *et al.*, 1977). Also for rat liver plasma membranes values ranging from 40 to 73 hr have been reported (Arias *et al.*, 1969, Franke *et al.*, 1971, Narayan and Chandrasekhara, 1971). It should be noted that in contrast to BLM in this study the turnover of renal brush borders appeared to be a second order process (Quirk *et al.*, 1973). As to whether this really indicates different turnover mechanisms of BLM and brush borders remains to be clarified. Perhaps one explanation is that the brush borders were contaminated by other subcellular membranes that may have a different turnover time.

In order to study the turnover of single BLM proteins the membranes were partially solubilized with Triton X100 and subsequently separated by polyacrylamide gel electrophoresis. As can be seen in Table 1 at least 14 protein bands with different mobilities could be detected. Most characteristic was a single large band (number 4) exhibiting a molar weight of 155,000, representing 32% of the Triton-soluble proteins. One or more glycoproteins were present. Histochemical methods showed that several enzymes were assembled in this band. These were 5′-nucleotidase, alkaline phosphatase and aminopeptidase. In experiments with AT^{32}P the main peak of Na stimulated phosphorylation was localized in the band 7 protein, molar weight 97,000 daltons. This is identical with the value reported several times for the catalytic subunit of Na – K-ATPase (for review, see Wallick *et al.*, 1979). Most interestingly, a smaller second peak was localized in the band 4 protein with 155,000 daltons. Previously Clarke (1975) has reported that Triton X-100 solubilized Na – K-ATPase is split into a subunit containing one catalytic and one glycoprotein unit with a molar weight of 141,000 daltons which is in the range of our value for band 4 protein.

After this preliminary characterization of the Triton-soluble BLM proteins ^{3}H-PA incorporation of these proteins was measured. We preferred single isotope administration rather than double isotope labeling since we were interested to evaluate absolute turnover instead of relative turnover of single proteins.

As first, isotope incorporation into Triton-soluble BLM proteins was investigated after a 2 hr pulse. As expected the ^{3}H-PA incorporation followed the protein profile. It is concluded that in the gel isotope incorporation into protein is preferentially measured.

The result of a first approach to determine the turnover of single BLM proteins is shown in Fig. 2. The percentage decay of specific activity is plotted for proteins with different molar weights. Obviously the apparent turnover of single membrane proteins was

Table 1. Analysis of the Triton X100 soluble (0.05%) BLM proteins separated on a 5% polyacrylamide gel. Proteins were stained with Coomassie Blue, sugars with the PAS method. For densitometry a Hewlett–Packard integrator type 3380A was used connected to a Zeiss PMQ II spectrophotometer equipped with a disc-scanning attachment.

Band No.	Apparent molecular weight × 10^{-3}	Coomassie Blue staining (%)	PAS reaction
1	430	3.1	
2	245	3.0	+
3	195	15.6	+
4	155	32.0	+
5	128	17.6	
6	110	6.8	+
7	97	9.2	
8	85	0.9	+
9	64	3.1	
10	52	1.8	
11	44	1.2	
12	32	1.2	+
13	21	1.8	+
14	14	1.6	

not uniform. The same conclusion has been reached by other authors measuring relative degradation rates with the double isotope method in plasma membranes of rat liver (Dehlinger & Schimcke, 1971; Landry & Marceau, 1975) and in intestinal brush borders (Alpers, 1972). No clear cut relationship between molar size and turnover time could be detected by us as was described by most of the authors using the double isotope technique.

For a more accurate determination of the apparent half life times of single proteins, in another experiment a higher dose of ^{3}H-PA was given. 500 μCi · 100 g body weight^{-1} instead of 100 μCi · 100 g body weight^{-1} were injected. ^{3}H-PA incorporation was measured for 10, 48 and 96 hr. For the proteins with a molar weight of 155,000 daltons containing a Na – K-ATPase subunit as well as other enzymes an apparent half life time of 66 hr was calculated. For the proteins with a molar weight of 97,000, also containing a Na – K-ATPase subunit, the apparent half life time was in the range of 86 hr. However, because of the low counts this value may be only semi-quantitative. Proteins with longer turnover times were also detected, for example 181 hr for the proteins with 245,000.

It is clear that there are many difficulties involved in determining true half life times, such as the possible reincorporation of the label, and the unknown specific activity of the phenylalanin precursor pool. Therefore our data must be regarded with some caution. Probably the most accurate value is that for the 155,000 dalton proteins. The arguments are as follows: (1) the peak contained enough activity for accurate counting, (2) the amount of protein included in this peak was rather reproducible from gel to gel, (3) the apparent half life times of the total BLM protein and of the peak proteins that represented 30% of the Triton-soluble proteins were very similar.

If the apparent turnover times for total and single BLM proteins are really close to the real turnover times then it might be asked if rapid hormonal induced changes of ion transport could be primarily mediated by a change in turnover time of specific BLM proteins. It is probable that the rapid, several-fold increase in specific activity of Na – K-ATPase one hour after the administration of aldosterone

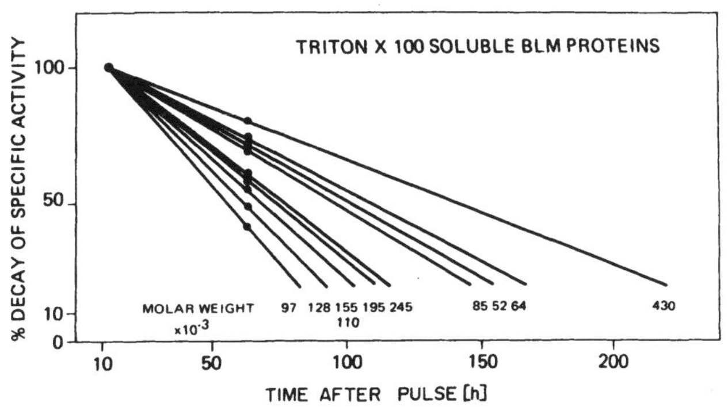

Fig. 2. Percentage decay of specific activity of single Triton X100 soluble (0.05%) membrane proteins of different molar weights. The proteins were separated on a 5% polyacrylamide gel. Maximal labelling was set as 100%.

(Schmidt *et al.*, 1975) can be explained by a change in enzyme activity rather than in enzyme concentration.

Acknowledgement—We want to thank Miss M. Hristova and Miss M. Naegele for their skilfull technical assistance.

REFERENCES

Alpers D. H. (1972) The relation of size to the relative rates of degradation of intestinal brush border proteins. *J. clin. Invest.* **51**, 2621–2630.

Arias J. M., Doyle D. & Schimcke R. T. (1969) Studies on the synthesis and degradation of proteins of endoplasmic reticulum of rat liver. *J. biol. Chem.* **12**, 3303–3315.

Banerjee S. P., Dwosh J. L., Kanna V. K. & Sen A. K. (1970) Solubilization of guinea pig (Na^+ + K^+)-ATPase with Lubrol W and Triton X-100. *Biochim. biophys. Acta* **211**, 345–355.

Chrambach A., Reisfeld, R. A., Wyckoff M. & Zaccari J. (1967) A procedure for rapid and sensitive staining of protein fractionated by polyacrylamide gel electrophoresis. *Analyt. Biochem.* **20**, 150–154.

Clarke S. (1975) The size and detergent binding of membrane proteins. *J. biol. Chem.* **250**, 5459–5469.

Davis B. J. (1964) Disc electrophoresis II. Method and application to human serum proteins. *Ann. N.Y. Acad. Sci.* **121**, 404–427.

Dehlinger P. J. & Schimcke R. T. (1971) Size distribution of membrane proteins of rat liver and their relative rates of degradation. *J. biol. Chem.* **246**, 2574–2583.

Ebel H., Aulbert E. & Merker H. J. (1976) Isolation of the basal and lateral plasma membranes of rat kidney tubule cells. *Biochim. biophys. Acta* **433**, 531–546.

Franke W. W., Morré D. J., Deumling B., Cheetham, R. D., Kartenbeck J., Jarasch E. D. & Zentgraf H. W. (1971) Synthesis and turnover of membrane protein in rat liver: an examination of the membrane flow hypothesis. *Z. Naturforsch.* **26b**, 1031–1039.

Haddad A., Bennett G. & Leblond C. P. (1977) Formation and turnover of plasma membrane glycoproteins in kidney tubules of young and adult mice, as shown by radioautography after an injection of ^{3}H-fucose. *Am. J. Anat.* **148**, 241–273.

Kapitany R. A. & Zebrowski E. J. (1973) A high resolution PAS stain for polyacrylamide gel electrophoresis. *Analyt. Biochem.* **56**, 361–369.

Korenbrot J. J. (1977) Ion transport in membranes. Incorporation of biological ion-translocating proteins in model membrane systems. *A. Rev. Physiol.* **39**, 19–49.

Landry J. & Marceau N. (1975) The relative rates of degradation of the plasma membrane glycoproteins from normal rat liver. *Biochim. biophys. Acta* **389**, 154–161.

Lowry O. H., Rosebrough N. J., Farr A. L. & Randall R. J. (1951) Protein measurement with the Folin phenol reagent. *J. biol. Chem.* **193**, 265–275.

Malbon C. C. & Zull J. E. (1977) Studies of binding of parathyroid hormone to a detergent dispersed preparation from bovine kidney cortex plasma membranes. *J. biol. Chem.* **252**, 1079–1083.

Morré D. J., Kartenbeck J. & Franke W. (1979) Membrane flow and interconversions among endomembranes. *Biochim. biophys. Acta* **559**, 71–152.

Nachlas M. M., Monis B., Rosenblatt D. & Seligman A. M. (1960). Improvement in the histochemical localization of leucine aminopeptidase with a new substrate, l-leucyl-4-methoxy-2-naphylamide. *J. biophys. biochem. Cytol.* **7**, 261–264.

Narayan K. A. & Chandrasekhara N. (1971) Turnover of the plasma membrane and microsomal proteins of rat liver containing primary hepatoma nodules. *Biochem. J.* **124**, 953–955.

Post R. L. & Sen A. K. (1967) ^{32}P-labeling of a (Na^+ + K^+)-ATPase intermediate. In *Methods in Enzymology* Vol. 10, pp. 773–776, Academic Press, New York.

Quirk S. J., Byrne J. & Robinson G. B. (1973) Studies on the turnover of protein and glycoprotein components in rabbit kidney brush borders. *Biochem. J.* **132**, 501–508.

Rollestone F. S. (1972) The binding of ribosomal subunits to endoplasmic reticulum membranes. *Biochem. J.* **129**, 721–731.

Roy C., Rajerison R., Bockaert J. & Jard S. (1975) Solubilization of the (8-lysine) vasopressin receptor and adenylate cyclase from pig kidney plasma membranes. *J. biol. Chem.* **250**, 7885–7893.

Schimke R. T. & Doyle D. (1970) Control of enzyme levels in animal tissues. *A. Rev. Biochem.* **39**, 929–976.

Schmidt U., Schmid J. & Dubach U. C. (1975) Sodium- and potassium-activated ATPase. A possible target of aldosterone. *J. clin. Invest.* **55**, 655–660.

Seligman A. M., Chauncey H. H., Nachlas M. M., Mannheimer L. H. & Ravin H. A. (1951) The colorimetric determination of phosphatases in human serum. *J. biol. Chem.* **190**, 7–15.

Tishler P. V. & Epstein C. J. (1968) A convenient method of preparing polyacrylamide gels for liquid scintillation spectrometry. *Analyt. Biochem.* **22**, 89–98.

Wachstein M. & Meisel E. (1957) Histochemistry of hepatic phosphatases at a physiological pH. With special reference to the demonstration of bile caniculi. *Am. J. clin. Pathol.* **27**, 13–23.

Wallick E. T., Lane L. K. & Schwartz A. (1979) Biochemical mechanisms of the sodium pump. *A Rev. Physiol.* **41**, 397–411.

SYMPOSIUM DISCUSSION

Osswald: Do you think that there may be a difference between the half-life of the labelling and the half-life of function? It appeared that the function disappeared faster than the label of an important side chain.

Ebel: All that I wanted to say is that the biological regulation of Na – K-ATPase might be performed by two mechanisms: immediate adaptation to biological needs by a rapid change of enzyme activity and long term adaptation by a change of enzyme concentration.

Osswald: But protein synthesis may not be affecting all of the membrane proteins at the same rate.

Ebel: We estimate the half life of Na – K-ATPase turnover to be in the range of 60–81 hr. Thus, in 1 hr approximately 1% of the enzyme is renewed. However, in the distal convolution aldosterone has been reported to increase specific activity of Na – K-ATPase by about 400% within 1 hr (Schmidt *et al.*, 1975, see above). Therefore, the rapid increase in enzyme activity may not be explained by a change of enzyme turnover.

Int. J. Biochem., Vol. 12, pp. 319 to 324
© Pergamon Press Ltd 1980. Printed in Great Britain

0020-711X/80/0701-0319$02.00/0

EFFECT OF ALDOSTERONE ON INCORPORATION OF [^{3}H]LEUCINE INTO BRUSH BORDER MEMBRANES OF RAT KIDNEY

R. KIRSTEN, J. ASSMUTAT, K. NELSON and U. RÜSCHENDORF
Department of Clinical Pharmacology, University of Frankfurt, Sandhofstraße Nr. 74, D-6000 Frankfurt am Main 70, Federal Republic of Germany

Abstract—1. To determine whether a correlation between aldosterone activated sodium transport and renal protein synthesis exists, the incorporation of [^{3}H]leucine into proteins from different regions of the rat kidney was compared between adrenalectomized and aldosterone substituted adrenalectomized rats.

2. Aldosterone (5 μg·100 g body weight^{-1}) or diluent was administered s.c. 1, 2 or 3 hr and [^{3}H]leucine (350 μCi per rat) was injected i.v. 0.5, 1 or 2 hr prior to kidney removal. The kidneys from 10 rats (5 diluent and 5 aldosterone treated) were dissected into 3 zones (outer and inner cortex and medulla) and luminal plasma membranes (brush borders) were prepared. From these 1 mg protein of outer and inner cortex and 200 μg of medulla protein were subjected to polyacrylamide gel electrophoresis. The protein bands were identified under u.v.-light, cut into slices and [^{3}H]leucine incorporation measured.

3. The total membrane fractions were solubilized in SDS-mercaptoethanol and electrophoretically separated into 18 consistently reproduceable protein peaks. Molecular weights of the relevant proteins were estimated at 19,000 to 221,000 by comparing them to reference proteins subjected to the same procedure.

4. The amount of label incorporated into proteins was dependent on the exposure time to [^{3}H]leucine and aldosterone. Maximum labelling occurred one hour after injection of [^{3}H]leucine. The maximum effect of aldosterone on label incorporation was found 2 hr after aldosterone substitution. Two hours after aldosterone substitution the isotope ratios of aldosterone/diluent in the total membrane fraction were: outer cortex—1.24 ($P < 0.05$), inner cortex—1.22 ($P < 0.05$), medulla—1.68 ($P < 0.01$). Aldosterone specifically increased ($P < 0.01$) the amount of label incorporated into six proteins of cortex and medulla.

5. These results are the first evidence of in vivo effects of aldosterone on proteins in kidney membranes participating in sodium transport and correlate with the data showing a maximum labelling of lipids matching the minimum Na^{+}:K^{+} ratio in the urine of adrenalectomized rats after aldosterone replacement (Kirsten *et al.*, 1977, 1978).

INTRODUCTION

Numerous findings have led to the proposition that the synthesis of new proteins is included in the aldosterone mediated renal sodium reabsorption process. The most convincing evidence supporting the role of protein synthesis is the occurrence of a latent period between exposure to aldosterone and the onset of the physiological effect. Events occurring during this latent period are:

(1) Binding of aldosterone to specific receptors (Edelman & Fanestil 1970; Fanestil & Edelman, 1966; Marver *et al.*, 1972).

(2) Stimulation of RNA-synthesis (Edelman & Fanestil 1970; Porter, 1975).

(3) DNA-dependent protein synthesis (Chu & Edelman, 1972; Trachewsky & Yang, 1975).

(4) Increases in both activity and induction of mitochondrial key enzymes (Kinne & Kirsten, 1968; Kirsten & Kirsten, 1972; Law & Edelman, 1978).

We recently noted that aldosterone stimulated sodium transport across the renal tubule is accompanied by an increase in turnover of lipid fractions in the apical membranes of cortical and medullary cells. This paper addresses the question of whether the proteins of these membranes are involved as well during the latent period, which precedes the increased handling of sodium.

MATERIALS AND METHODS

Animals, tissue preparation

Male Sprague–Dawley rats weighing 120–175 g were maintained on Altromin pellets (standard diet 1324) and tap water (for intact rats) or 0.9% NaCl (for adrenalectomized rats) *ad libitum*. The rats, 7–12 days after adrenalectomy, were sacrificed by a blow to the head, the kidneys rapidly removed, chilled and dissected into outer and inner cortex and medulla. Brush border membranes were isolated according to Wilfong & Neville (1970).

Injection of aldosterone and [^{3}H]leucine

Aldosterone (Ciba AG, Wehr, West Germany) (5 μg·100 g body weight^{-1}) was injected s.c. 1, 2 or 3 hr before membrane preparation. [^{3}H]leucine (Amersham-Buchler, Braunschweig, West Germany) (350 μCi) was injected in the same rats either 0.5, 1 or 2 hr prior to membrane preparation.

Protein yields and enzyme studies

Protein was determined according to Beisenherz *et al.* (1953). Enzyme studies, as criteria for purity and enrichment of membrane preparations, were performed as cited by Fleischer & Kervina (1974).

Polyacrylamide gel electrophoresis

After treatment with sodiumdodecylsulphate (f.c. 1%) and β-mercaptoethanol (f.c. 1%) as described by Weber & Osborn (1969) 1 mg protein from cortex and 200 μg protein from medulla were subjected to polyacrylamide gel electro-

Table 1. Tissue and protein yields after zonal dissection of kidneys

Kidney zone	Fresh weight (g) (Values in parentheses = % of total) Aldosterone	Diluent	Ratio ALDO:DIL
Outer cortex	5.4 (49)	5.0 (49)	1.08
Inner cortex	4.4 (40)	4.0 (39)	1.10
Medulla	1.2 (11)	1.2 (12)	1.00
Total	11.0 (100)	10.2 (100)	1.08

Kidney zone	Protein yield (mg) (Values in parentheses = % of total) Aldosterone	Diluent	Ratio ALDO:DIL
Outer cortex	3.23 (51)	3.04 (52)	1.12
Inner cortex	2.79 (45)	2.59 (44)	1.08
Medulla	0.26 (4)	0.25 (4)	1.04
Total	6.28 (100)	5.88 (100)	1.07

Kidneys of 5 rats used in each preparation. Each value represents the mean of 4 experiments. All ratios aldo:dil are not significantly different.

phoresis for 7 hr (40 mA, 60–80 V, length 8 cm, thickness 7 mm). The protein bands were quantitated under u.v.-light (280 mm) (Aron, 1975). After staining with Amido Black the bands were scanned at 660 nm (Racusen, 1973). Thereafter, the gel was cut into 36 slices and radioactivity was measured by liquid scintillation. The molecular weights of the relevant proteins were estimated by comparing them to reference proteins subjected to the same procedure (Weber & Osborn, 1969).

RESULTS

Yields

Table 1 shows that no significant differences were apparent either in fresh weight or protein yield between aldosterone and diluent pretreated kidney preparations. The upper part of the table lists the freshweight yields from the starting material. The average yields from outer, inner cortex and medulla were 5, 4 and 1.2 g, respectively. No differences could be established between the diluent and aldosterone group. 49% of the harvested membranes originated from the outer cortex, about 40% from the inner cortex and the medulla accounted for about 11%. The lower part of the table shows that 3 mg membrane protein were harvested from the outer cortex, about 2.7 mg from the inner cortex and 0.25 mg from the medulla. No significant differences between diluent and aldosterone pretreated preparations could be found.

Criteria of purity

Specific activity of the membranes relative to the starting homogenate was evaluated by measuring alkaline phosphatase as reference enzyme. The ratio of activity in the brush border membranes to activity in homogenate was 12 ± 2. The degree of contamination, determined by measuring the activities of the enzymes characteristic for other cell particles. (Na-K-ATPase, glucose-6-phosphatase, citrate synthase, acid phosphatase, lactic dehydrogenase and galactosyltransferase) was comparable to that reported in the literature (Sacktor, 1977; Wilfong & Neville, 1970).

Optimization of [^{3}H]leucine and aldosterone injections

Figure 1 depicts the results of two different experimental designs. The left side of the figure shows that the leucine injection was kept constant at 1 hr exposure time, while the aldosterone or diluent injection was varied—1, 2 or 3 hr. The injection of diluent, regardless of whether it was injected 1, 2 or 3 hr before membrane preparation did not change the incorporation of [^{3}H]leucine. However, varying the injection time of aldosterone (1, 2 or 3 hr before membrane preparation) did have an effect on the incorporation of [^{3}H]leucine. Maximum incorporation occurred 2 hr after aldosterone injection, and 3 hr after injection the effect was no longer apparent. On the right side of the figure the exposure time to aldosterone was kept constant at 2 hr (maximum effect) and the injection time of [^{3}H]leucine (0.5, 1 or 2 hr) was varied. The highest incorporation occurred 1 hr after [^{3}H]leucine injection.

[^{3}H]leucine incorporation into renal zones

Table 2 shows that the outer cortex membranes incorporated more [^{3}H]leucine, 49,200 dis/min per mg protein than the proteins of the inner cortex with 39,700 dis/min and the medulla with 5700 dis/min. In all three zones aldosterone pretreated kidney membranes incorporated significantly more [^{3}H]leucine than control membranes. The average ratio dis/min-aldosterone:dis/min-diluent is 1.25. The medulla proteins show the lowest absolute incorporation per mg protein with 5700 dis/min (for aldosterone) and 3400 dis/min (for diluent), but the highest difference between aldosterone and diluent, with a ratio aldo:dil of 1.68.

Separation of membrane proteins

Figure 2 represents an example of a profile from an absorbance record at 660 nm of gel separated cortical membrane proteins. The solid curve shows 18 distinguishable protein bands with corresponding molecular weights ranging from 19,000 to 221,000. There

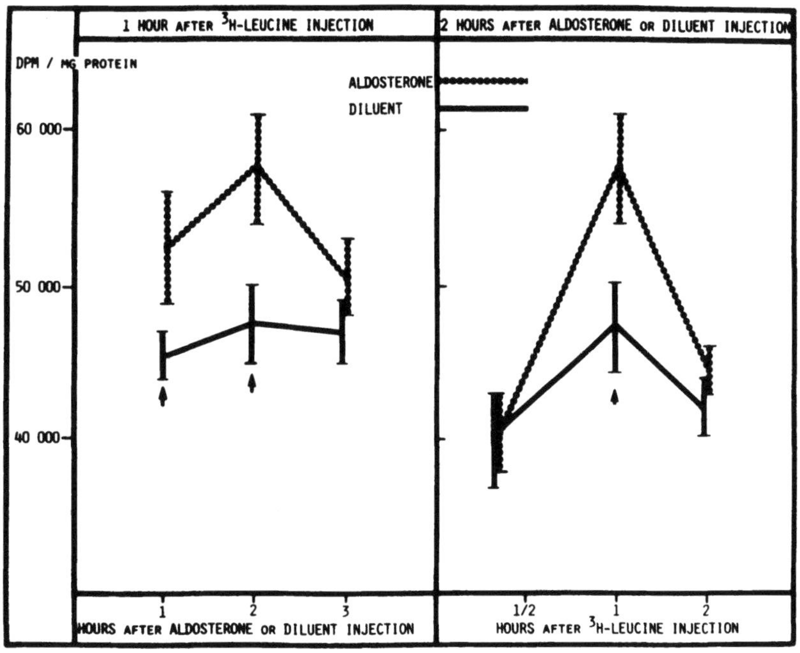

Fig. 1. Time–course of incorporation of [^{3}H]leucine into proteins of renal brush border membranes. Kidneys of 5 rats used in each preparation. Each value represents the mean of 4 experiments ± SEM. Arrows indicate $P < 0.02$.

was no appreciable difference in band profiles from cortex and medulla. The hatched columns indicate dis/min per mg protein and point out that the degree of labelling is not uniform. For example, the protein with the molecular weight of 87,000 is relatively small in amount but high in degree of labelling. Proteins with molecular weights between 47,000 and 147,000, with a maximum at 105,000 incorporated the largest amounts of label, that is about 3000 dis/min per mg protein.

Aldosterone sensitive membrane proteins

Figure 3 shows that aldosterone significantly increased the amount of label incorporated into 6 different proteins. The largest differences in incorporation between aldosterone and diluent pretreated membranes occurred in proteins with molecular weights of 118,000 and 105,000 ($P < 0.01$). Proteins with molecular weights of 147,000, 134,000, 63,000 and 47,000 showed aldosterone caused differences with $P < 0.05$.

Evidence of ^{3}H label incorporated as leucine

To decide whether we were dealing with incorporation of metabolic products of leucine or leucine itself, the renal brush border membranes from aldosterone and diluent pretreated rats were hydrolysed and subjected to ion exchange chromatography. The single amino acids were collected and the radioactivity counted. 73% of the total radioactivity was recovered in the leucine fraction and was characteristic for both aldosterone and diluent pretreated samples. Figure 4 shows a typical chromatogram with the occurrence of ^{3}H label in the leucine fraction.

DISCUSSION

This study was designed to investigate in vivo effects of physiological doses of aldosterone on pro-

Table 2. ^{3}H-label incorporation into proteins of brush border membranes

Kidney zone	[^{3}H]Leucine incorporation (dpm/mg protein × 10^3) (Values in parentheses = % of total) Aldosterone	Diluent	Ratio ALDO:DIL
Outer cortex	49.2 (52)	39.6 (52)	1.24*
Inner cortex	39.7 (42)	32.6 (43)	1.22*
Medulla	5.7 (6)	3.4 (4)	1.68*
Total	94.6 (100)	75.6 (100)	1.25*

* $P < 0.01$.

Values measured 1 hr after injection of [^{3}H]leucine and 2 hr after injection of aldosterone. Each value represents the mean of 4 experiments.

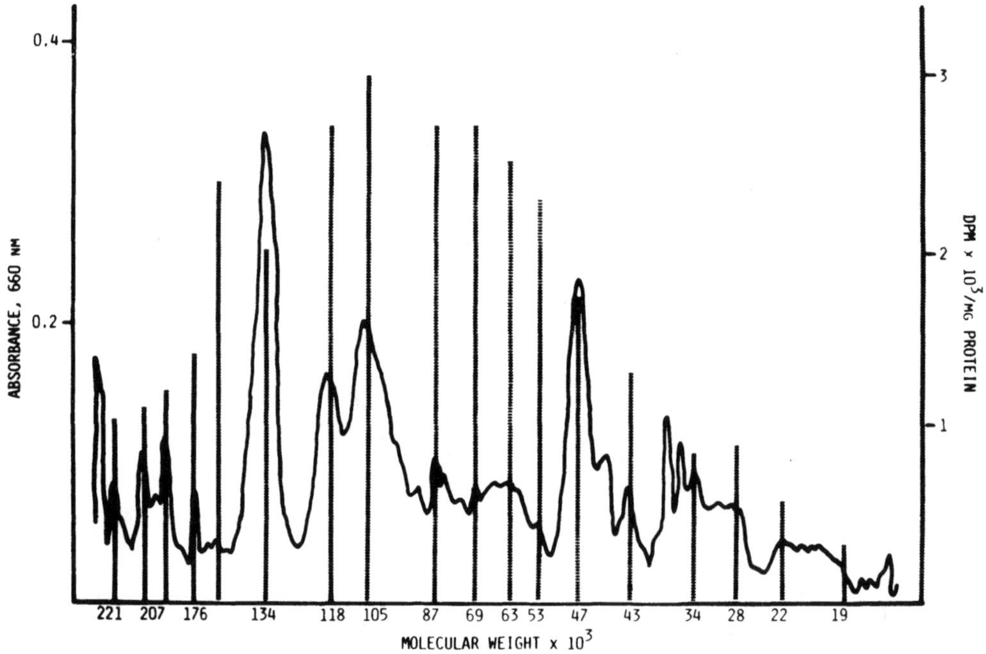

Fig. 2. Renal brush border proteins. Polyacrylamide gel scan (solid curve) and [^{3}H]leucine incorporation into proteins identified by molecular weight (hatched columns). Scan of 1 mg cortical membrane protein.

teins in kidney membranes participating in sodium transport.

The measurement of specific marker enzymes and contaminating enzymes in the brush border membranes are evidence that the observed effects are intrinsic to the membranes and not to contaminating subcellular organelles.

No significant differences in yields between aldosterone and diluent pretreated preparations could be found, implying that the higher degree of incorporation induced by aldosterone is indeed due to higher induction and not to differences in yield.

Although the medulla proteins showed the lowest absolute incorporation of [^{3}H]leucine per mg protein,

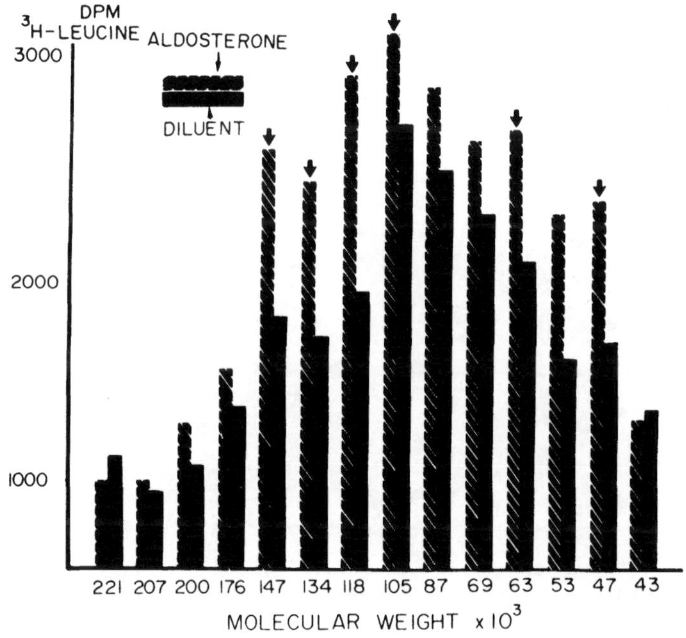

Fig. 3. Aldosterone induced increases of [^{3}H]leucine in proteins of the brush border membrane. (1 hr after [^{3}H]leucine injection and 2 hr after aldosterone injection.) Each value represents the mean of 4 experiments. Arrows indicate $P < 0.02$ (cortical membrane preparation).

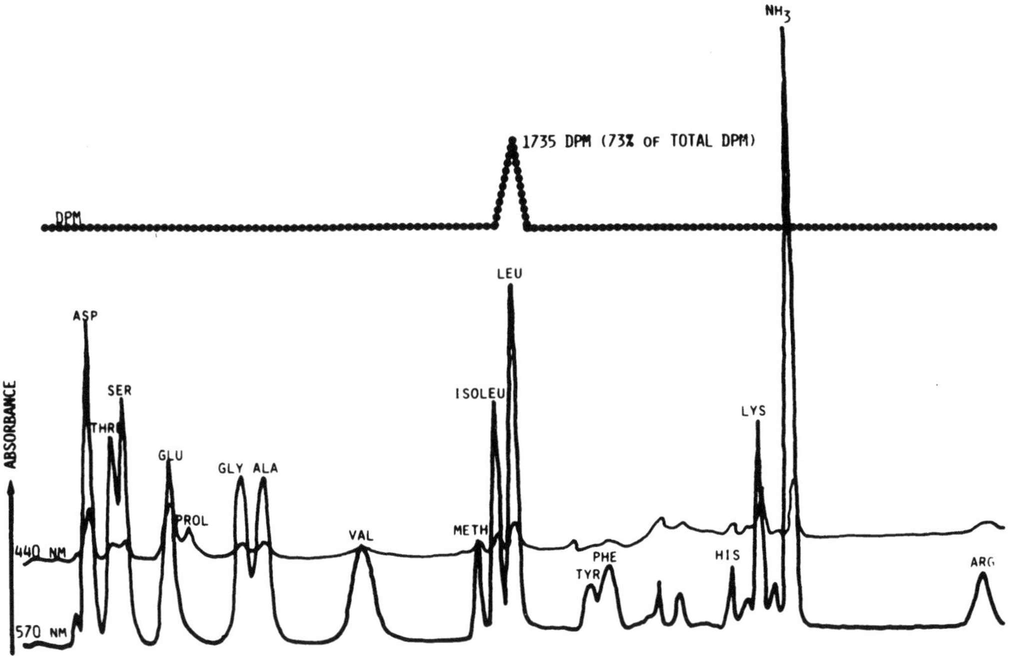

Fig. 4. Amino acid chromatogram of hydrolysed renal brush border membranes. Proteins hydrolysed in 6 N HCl. Total dis/min in hydrolysate was 2380.

the ratio of aldosterone:diluent was the highest, indicating that aldosterone may play an active part in the medulla of the kidney where the loop of Henle is located.

The identification of [^{3}H]leucine in the hydrolysed proteins and insignificantly small amounts in all other amino acids exclude the possibility that breakdown products of leucine which might have entered unknown metabolic pathways were our main concern. The data allow us to conclude that the increase in incorporation of [^{3}H]leucine is stimulated by aldosterone.

The results reported here demonstrate that not only the lipid fractions of the brush border membranes are effected by aldosterone (Kirsten, 1978) but that the protein fraction is influenced as well. These data do not allow conclusions as to whether the effects of aldosterone primarily result in increased permeability or surface area of brush border membranes. However, the point at which maximal incorporation of [^{3}H]leucine occurs (2 hr after aldosterone injection) precedes the minimum sodium:potassium ratio in the urine of aldosterone pretreated adrenalectomized rats, indicating that these protein changes belong to early events in the aldosterone induced process.

Acknowledgement—This work was supported by the Deutsche Forschungsgemeinschaft.

REFERENCES

Aron C. G. (1975) The use of Isco instruments for quantitation of protein by uv absorption in electrophoresed polyacrylamide gels. Isco Applications Research Bulletin No. 8, 3rd edn., Isco, Nebraska.

Beisenherz G., Boltze H. J., Bücher Th. Czok R., Garbade K. H., Meyer-Arendt E., Pfleiderer G. (1953) Diphosphofructose-Aldolase, Milchsäure-Dehydrogenase und Pyruvat-Kinase aus Kaninchenmuskulatur in einem Arbeitsgang. *Z. Naturforsch.* **8b**, 555.

Chu L. L. H. & Edelman I. (1972) Cordycepin and α-Amanitin: inhibitors of transcription as probes of aldosterone action. *J. Membr. Biol.* **10**, 291–310.

Edelman I. & Fanestil D. D. (1970) Mineralocorticoids. In *Biochemical Actions of Hormones* (Edited by Litwack G.), Vol. 1, pp. 321–364. Academic Press, New York.

Fanestil D. D. & Edelman I. (1966) Characteristics of the renal nuclear receptors for aldosterone. *Proc. Natn. Acad. Sci., U.S.A.* **56**, 872–879.

Fleischer S. & Kervina M. (1974) Subcellular fractionation of rat liver. In *Methods of Enzymology* (Edited by Colowick S. & Kaplan N. O.), Vol. 31, pp. 6–41.

Kinne R. & Kirsten R. (1968) Der Einfuß von Aldosteron auf die Aktivität mitochondrialer und cytoplasmatischer Enzyme in der Rattenniere. *Pflugers Arch. ges. Physiol.* **300**, 244–254.

Kirsten R. & Kirsten E. (1972) Redox state of pyridine nucleotides in renal response to aldosterone. *Am. J. Physiol.* **223**, 229–235.

Kirsten R., Nelson K., Rabah E., Rüschendorf U., Scholz Th., Stüve J. & Ulbricht R. (1978) Response of renal lipid metabolism to aldosterone. *Curr. Problems clin. Biochem.* **8**, 389–396.

Kirsten R., Nelson K., Rüschendorf U., Seger W., Scholz Th. & Kirsten E. (1977) Effects of aldosterone on lipid metabolism and renal oxygen consumption in the rat. *Pflügers Arch. ges. Physiol.* **368**, 189–194.

Law P. Y. & Edelman I. (1978) Induction of citrate synthase by aldosterone in the rat kidney. *J. Membr. Biol.* **41**, 41–64.

Marver D., Goodman D. & Edelman I. (1972) Relationships between renal cytoplasmic and nuclear aldosterone-receptors. *Kidney Int.* **1**, 210–223.

Porter G. A. (1975) Action of aldosterone on transepithelial sodium transport. In *Enzyme Induction* (Edited by Parke D. V.), pp. 105–141. Plenum Press, London.

Racusen D. (1973) Stoichiometry of the amido black reaction with proteins. *Analyt. Biochem.* **52,** 96.

Sacktor B. (1977) The brush border of the renal proximal tubule and the intestinal mucosa. In *Mammalian Cell Membranes.* (Edited by Jamieson G. A. & Robinson D. M.), Vol. 4, pp. 221–254. Butterworth, London.

Trachewsky D. & Yang H. Y. (1975) Alteration in the labelling of renal ribosomal protein by aldosterone. *J. Steroid Biochem.* **6,** 1157–1164.

Weber K. & Osborn M. (1969) The reliability of molecular weight determination by dodecylsulfate-polyacrylamide gel electrophoresis. *J. biol. Chem.* **244,** 4406–4412.

Wilfong R. F. & Neville D. U. (1970) The isolation of a brush border membrane fraction from rat kidney. *J. biol. Chem.* **245,** 6106–6112.

SYMPOSIUM DISCUSSION

Ebel: Our data on turnover time of renal basolateral membrane proteins apparently are different from your data in renal brush border membranes. While we found a rate constant of 0.01128 hr^{-1} for degradation of total basolateral membrane protein you report a 26% increase of brush border protein synthesis only one hour after aldosterone administration. Now, since you achieved a maximum of isotope incorporation after such a short time my question is whether this might be due to a contamination with Golgi vesicles?

Kirsten: We have done all the controls for possible contaminating enzymes.

Schoolwerth: I wonder if the specific activity of the leucine remains constant during your experiment?

Kirsten: We found 73% of our radioactivity in the leucine fraction and could find none elsewhere.

INDEX

Printed in Dunstable, United Kingdom

91897634R00205